A Decade of HAART

The Development and
Global Impact of Highly Active
Antiretroviral Therapy

A Decade of HAART
The Development and Global Impact of Highly Active Antiretroviral Therapy

Edited by

José M. Zuniga

Alan Whiteside

Amin Ghaziani

John G. Bartlett

Managing Editor

Lynn-Marie Holland

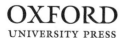

OXFORD
UNIVERSITY PRESS

OXFORD
UNIVERSITY PRESS

Great Clarendon Street, Oxford, OX2 6DP,
United Kingdom

Oxford University Press is a department of the University of Oxford.
It furthers the University's objective of excellence in research, scholarship,
and education by publishing worldwide. Oxford is a registered trade mark of
Oxford University Press in the UK and in certain other countries

Published in the United States of America by Oxford University Press
198 Madison Avenue, New York, NY 10016, United States of America

British Library Cataloguing in Publication Data

Data available

Library of Congress Cataloging in Publication Data

Data available

ISBN 978-0-19-922585-9

Foreword

Luc Montagnier and Robert Gallo

Highly active antiretroviral therapy (HAART) for HIV/AIDS, the tenth anniversary of which this book celebrates, has its roots in basic research on animal retroviruses that began over 40 years ago. At that time, retroviruses causing leukaemia or sarcoma in chickens and mice were the main models upon which our knowledge of retrovirus replication was built. In 1970, the key enzyme that initiates the reverse transcription of viral RNA, reverse transcriptase (RT), was discovered in the Rous sarcoma and murine leukaemia viruses. At about the same time, another key enzyme, a protease specific to the cleavage of the precursor polypeptide of nucleocapsid proteins, was also found in the same avian viruses. The advent of modern molecular biology, together with genetics, then contributed to the unravelling of the complete genome structure of these animal retroviruses. This research was stimulated, at least in part, by the possibility that similar retroviruses would exist in humans and cause some leukaemias and other cancers.

A specific funding initiative, the Virus Cancer Program, was established to foster the search and discovery of human retroviruses in the United States at the National Cancer Institute (NCI) in the 1970s. However, as this search proved unsuccessful, most research groups turned their efforts to the study of the cellular genes carried by retroviruses and involved in cancer, the so-called oncogenes. Likewise, the pharmaceutical industry paid little attention to the design of possible inhibitors of the retroviral key enzymes during this period. The discovery (by one of us, Robert Gallo) in the late 1970s of a real human retrovirus (HTLV) involved in an unusual form of leukaemia did nothing to alter this attitude.

The situation changed dramatically when a new, lethal disease—acquired immune deficiency syndrome (AIDS)—was identified in 1981. In 1983–4, its causative agent was identified. This agent was a new retrovirus that belonged to a less-publicized subfamily, that of retro-lentiviruses, not close to the subfamily of oncogenic retroviruses. Representatives of this group were already known to cause long-lasting wasting diseases in animals (e.g. sheep, goats, horses) but lacked signs of immune suppression. The discovery of the human immunodeficiency virus (HIV) led to the isolation of similar viruses in non-human primates.

The rapid growth of the HIV epidemic in developed and developing countries, together with the pressure brought to bear by groups of people living with the disease, were strong incentives to find medical solutions as quickly as possible. The discovery of HIV thus paved the way to three main avenues of application:

+ *Diagnostics* of HIV infection by detection of specific antibodies in blood reduced the risk of infection by blood transfusion and blood products, allowed accurate epidemiological studies and provided the basis for a rational approach to prevention. It also greatly helped in convincing scientists of the causative role of HIV in AIDS (1984–5).

+ *A preventive vaccine* was the obvious way to ensure prevention of HIV infection. However, all attempts, from the classical inactivated virus to more sophisticated recombinant constructs or purified subunits, have so far proved unsuccessful and have been impeded by the lack of a reliable and preferably small animal model. Additionally, two obstacles have not been fully overcome, namely: the integration of viral DNA into the cellular genome; and the high variability potential of the virus. The road to a therapeutic vaccine may, therefore, be easier.

♦ *Viral inhibitors*: Although screening for RT inhibitors was carried out in the 1970s, there was little interest in their pursuit because of the lack of known human retroviruses at the time. After HIV was shown to be the cause of AIDS, intense screening for RT inhibitors was undertaken in several European and North American laboratories in collaboration with pharmaceutical companies. This began in early 1984. The companies first provided compounds previously synthesized for other purposes, such as nucleoside analogues for cancer chemotherapy. Thus, Samuel Broder and his co-workers at the NCI tested several compounds that had been developed at Burroughs Wellcome and had properties suggesting they might inhibit the RT of HIV, which included azidothymidine, or AZT. This analogue, synthesized as early as 1972, was not developed for cancer therapy, as it was found to be too toxic in animal studies. However, seen as the lesser of two evils, Broder and his co-workers used it in clinical trials for patients with advanced AIDS. Short-term effects were beneficial, while a one-year trial showed no benefits for morbidity and mortality. Besides toxicity, the main problem was the rapid development of mutations in the RT gene, giving rise to highly resistant variants. The problem was found, in fact, for all viral inhibitors used in monotherapy. However, the work with AZT was a major step forward. Indeed, it was the first time in medicine that a compound was proven in the clinic to minimize viral titres.

The initial success of AZT stimulated the synthesis and trial of other nucleoside inhibitors, zalcitabine (ddC), didanosine (ddI) and lamivudine (3TC), all acting by competition with normal nucleotides incorporated in DNA. The pioneering work of the Louvain group in Belgium led to the development of a new class of RT inhibitors that bind to the catalytic site of the enzyme. Here, too, resistant mutants rapidly emerged, but research with this new family steadily led to the improved drugs now utilized in the present triple antiretroviral therapy regimens.

The pharmaceutical industry then turned its efforts to the second virus-specific enzyme, the HIV encoded protease. Owing to its reduced size, its conformational 3D structure became readily available, which in turn opened the door to a rational molecular design of inhibitors. Among many screened components, a few protease inhibitors emerged that were active in clinical trials but not always with good bioavailability.

As the catalogue of viral inhibitors increased, several bold clinicians, among them Jacques Leibovitch in France, and Broder and Martin Hirsch in the United States, thought of using combinations of several inhibitors in AIDS patients. The reasoning was that even though the virus had an extraordinary capacity of mutating, it was unlikely that its changes would be sufficient to avoid three different inhibitors acting at different levels. The risk of emergence of multi-resistant mutants was, therefore, much lower.

Unlike many fields in which drug competition is high, the main pharmaceutical companies involved in the anti-HIV fight agreed to form a consortium whereby they could exchange information on their respective products and sponsor clinical trials using a combination of drugs belonging to different companies. One of us (Luc Montagnier) was permitted to attend the first meetings of this consortium as a consultant for a participating Italian company. It was an interesting, albeit short, experience, as his 'Pasteurian' hat became too visible. In any event, it was the beginning of a new era in which many patients, even those with very low CD4 cell counts and opportunistic infections, and often with Kaposi's sarcoma or lymphomas, experienced a dramatic recovery.

In the first years of triple antiretroviral therapy, the clinical world was so enthusiastic that some physicians claimed that further research on HIV was unnecessary. Others prematurely predicted cures for HIV infection. Both of us, having had extensive experience with HIV, knew that this malignant virus harboured many tricks. There are now multi-resistant strains of HIV circulating in exposed people. Moreover, side effects remain problematic. Even though the enzymatic inhibitors have high specificity, they can interfere with the metabolism of the host. Nucleoside RT inhibitors have some effects on the function of mitochondrial DNA polymerase III, which is also endowed with reverse transcriptase-like activity. Other inhibitors act on lipid metabolism, causing lipodystrophy and increasing the risk of cardiovascular disease. Last but not least, any interruption of this heavy regimen leads to a rebound of virus replication, indicating that there is a virus reservoir poorly accessible to the antiretroviral inhibitors. As a consequence, treatment has to be lifelong and does not result in a complete eradication of infection.

This situation is peculiar to HIV. Examples of chronic bacterial infections indicate that functional (not physical) eradication can be achieved by long-term antibiotic treatment that could eventually be terminated. This is the case with active tuberculosis, where, after triple or quadruple antibiotic therapy for a period of six to nine months, treatment can often be terminated. Relapses are rare. Similarly, chronic active hepatitis B can be cured, at least of its viral component, by antiviral treatment (3TC and other viral inhibitors plus interferon). Hepatitis B virus, like HIV, integrates its DNA into the host cellular DNA. DNA integration may, therefore, not be the main cause of triple antiretroviral therapy failure in HIV infection. Though this remains uncertain, we think it more likely that the main difference between AIDS and these other infectious diseases is the profound immune suppression induced by HIV. After the reduction of plasma viral load to undetectable levels, the restoration of the immune system is slow and incomplete, as demonstrated by the CD4 cell count, the partial thymic recovery and the persistence of the apoptotic death of lymphocytes.

It is therefore essential to implement additional treatments aimed at boosting the immune response against residual virus so that the latter will be kept to low, harmless levels, even after interruption of antiretroviral therapy. Nature gives us a good example: about 5% of HIV-infected individuals do not show any sign of immune depression or disease because they have mounted strong immune defences against the virus. We would like to see 100% of HIV-infected patients achieve a similar status. This goal might be reached by a second round of combination therapy following HAART, but a more biological one, for example antioxidants and active immunization against viral components. This vaccine therapy might include the main viral proteins involved in induction of immune suppression: Tat, Nef, and a modified surface glycoprotein able to induce cellular and humoral immunity against the most conserved regions of these proteins. The efficacy limits of this complex but innocuous treatment are easily measured using the lack of virus rebound after the interruption of antiretroviral therapy. Furthermore, the development of a preventive vaccine might benefit from knowledge gained from the most efficient therapeutic immunization formula. Meanwhile, advances in the science of HIV medicine will certainly occur; new generations of inhibitors such as integrase, fusion, and receptor binding are already being tested. Although very expensive, they offer an alternative solution when the virus has become resistant to more classical inhibitors.

In conclusion, the success of HAART has been a great scientific and medical achievement, saving the lives of millions of patients. Its success was built on an impressive foundation of basic knowledge of animal retroviruses and HTLV and, later, on the excellent collaboration between academic laboratories and pharmaceutical companies with the active contribution of patients. It joins the HIV antibody test as one of the two most important practical advances made against HIV/AIDS to date. However, the pandemic continues its deadly course.

In developed countries, young people are less responsive to prevention campaigns, sometimes wrongly believing that HIV is a curable disease, and the emergence of multi-resistant strains is a real danger there. In developing countries, there are still millions of patients who have no access to existing treatments, despite a drastic reduction in their cost. The difficulty of sustained treatments, the lack of adequate infrastructures and trained health workers, and low living standards are all strong impediments to treatment.

Highly active medical research programmes are still required in order to find treatments with limited duration and develop an effective preventive vaccine. After 10 years of practice with HAART, this book provides a timely analysis of the gains we have and have not achieved, as well as suggestions for future directions.

Luc Montagnier
Robert Gallo

Acknowledgements

A Decade of HAART: The Development and Global Impact of Highly Active Antiretroviral Therapy reflects the contributions of innumerable individuals and institutions, both named and unnamed, who are a part of the history of the first decade of HIV treatment following the advent of highly active antiretroviral therapy (HAART). The idea for this book arose during the course of an email exchange with my fellow co-editor, John G. Bartlett, in designing a conference that the International Association of Physicians in AIDS Care (IAPAC) would host in late 2006 entitled, not surprisingly, 'Decade of HAART: Historical Perspectives and Future Directions'. 'I think it will be important to give some substantial attention to the events that set the stage for what has become one of the most dramatic successes of medical care in the past 50 years,' he wrote in response to a query about how we should structure the conference, for which he served as Co-Chair. Given this pioneering physician's significance as one of the architects of HAART, I knew he was right on target in suggesting that its history should be memorialized—a suggestion with which Oxford University Press, through our Commissioning Editor, Georgia Pinteau, also concurred when they agreed to publish *A Decade of HAART*.

I wish to thank the more than 70 authors from 20 countries who, despite their hectic work schedules, contributed thematic chapters, country case studies and cohort reviews that make *A Decade of HAART* a robust book. I am also deeply grateful to my co-editors, John G. Bartlett, Amin Ghaziani and Alan Whiteside, for committing their time and expertise to provide the editorial leadership without which such a book project would perish. By taking a multidisciplinary approach—a clinician (Bartlett), a sociologist (Ghaziani), an economist (Whiteside) and a public health specialist (Zuniga)—we have endeavoured to ensure that the book takes a multidimensional look at all facets of the pre- and post-HAART era rather than relate its history in strictly biological terms.

During the course of its development and production, my fellow co-editors and I counted on the dedication and hard work of three consecutive managing editors: Lisa McKamy, Jeff Danielski and Lynn-Marie Holland (in that chronological order). While I am grateful to all three individuals for their invaluable assistance, it is to the latter that I assign the greatest credit for helping to transform 29 individual chapters into a comprehensive book that spans more than a decade of time from 1981 (the discovery of HIV) through to 1996 (the advent of HAART).

Finally, I wish to acknowledge the financial contributions that made *A Decade of HAART* possible. These included educational grants from the US National Institutes of Health (NIH), as well as Abbott Laboratories, Bristol-Myers Squibb, Gilead Sciences, Merck & Co., and Pfizer Inc, in support of the aforementioned 'Decade of HAART' conference, as well as support from the Health Economics and HIV/AIDS Research Division (HEARD) of the University of KwaZulu-Natal, in Durban, South Africa, which, along with IAPAC, helped to subsidize the editorial services required to complete a book of this scope.

José M. Zuniga
January 2008

Contents

List of Contributors

Jintanat Ananworanich
South-East Asia Research Collaboration
with Hawaii (SEARCH),
Bangkok, Thailand

John G. Barlett
Professor, Johns Hopkins University
School of Medicine,
Baltimore, USA

Eduard J. Beck
Senior Technical Officer,
Evaluation Department (EVA),
UNAIDS, Geneva,
Switzerland;
becke@unaids.org

Peter Bendix
GHESKIO Center, Port-au-Prince,
Haiti

John T. Brooks
National Center for HIV/STD and
TB Prevention (NCHSTP), CDC,
Atlanta, USA

Julia Carney
Research Assistant, Division of Social
Medicine and Health Inequalities,
Brigham and Women's Hospital,
Boston, USA

Sanchai Chasombat
Department of Disease Control,
Ministry of Public Health,
Bangkok,Thailand

Ray Y. Chen
Medical Officer, Division of AIDS,
National Institute of Allergy
and Infectious Diseases,
US National Institutes of Health,
Beijing, China

Benjamin H. Chi
Centre for Infectious Diseases Research
in Zambia (CIDRZ),
University of Alabama at Birmingham, USA;
benjamin.chi@cidrz.org

Bonaventura Clotet
Hospital Universitari Germans Trias I Pujol,
Badalona, Spain

David A. Cooper
Director, National Centre in HIV
Epidemiology and Clinical Research,
University of New South Wales,
Australia

Dominique Costagliola
INSERM, Paris, France;
dcostagliola@noos.fr

Mario Roberto Dal Poz
Department of Human Resources for Health,
World Health Organization, Geneva,
Switzerland;
dalpozm@who.int

Roger Detels
UCLA School of Public Health,
Deptartment of Epidemiology,
Los Angeles, USA

Arry Dieudonne
School of Medicine, University of Medicine
and Dentistry of New Jersey, Newark, USA;
dieudar@umdnj.edu

Cledy Eliana dos Santos
Ministry of Health, Rio de Janeiro,
Brazil

Norbert Dreesch
Technical Officer,
Department of Human Resources for Health,
World Health Organization,
Geneva, Switzerland

Siddharth Dube
UNAIDS, Geneva, Switzerland

Julian Fleet
UNAIDS, Geneva, Switzerland;
fleetj@unaids.org

Lieve Fransen
Head of Unit in the Directorate-General for
Development, European Commission,
and Vice-Chair of the Global Fund to Fight
AIDS, Tuberculosis and Malaria,
Brussels, Belgium

Federica Fregonese
Paediatrics Clinical Research Unit,
Department of Paediatrics,
University of Padova, Padua, Italy

Robert Gallo
Director, Institute of Human Virology,
Baltimore, USA

Amin Ghaziani
Cotsen Postdoctoral Fellow,
Society of Fellows, Princeton University,
Princeton, USA

Carlo Giaquinto
University of Pavia, Pavia, Italy

Kathleen Glenday
National Centre in HIV Epidemiology and
Clinical Research, University of
New South Wales, Sydney, Australia

Huldrych F. Günthard
Division of Infectious Diseases and Hospital
Epidemiology, University Hospital,
Zurich, Switzerland

Anthony D. Harries
Technical Assistant, HIV Unit,
Ministry of Health, Lilongwe, Malawi;
Senior Technical Assistant, Family Health
International; and Honorary Professor,
London School of Hygiene and Tropical
Medicine, London, UK

Bernard Hirschel
Associate Professor of Medicine,
University of Geneva, Medical School,
Geneva, Switzerland;
bernard.hirschel@hcuge.ch

Mark Holodniy
Professor of Medicine, Department of
Veterans Affairs and Division of Infectious
Diseases & Geographic Medicine,
Stanford University, Stanford, USA;
holodniy@stanford.edu

Lisa Jacobson
Johns Hopkins University,
Bloomberg School of Public Health,
Baltimore, USA

Hans Jaeger
KIS – Curatorium for Immunodificiency
Munich, Germany

Kelita Kamoto
HIV Unit, Ministry of Health,
Lilongwe, Malawi

Michel D. Kazatchkine
Ambassador for HIV/AIDS and
Infectious Diseases, Ministry of Foreign
Affairs, Paris, France;
michel.kazatchkine@diplomatie.gouv.fr

Ole Kirk
EuroSIDA Coordinating Centre,
HIV Program, Copenhagen, Denmark

Serena Koenig
Division of Social Medicine, Brigham and
Women's Hospital, Boston, USA;
skoenig@partners.org

Matthew G. Law
National Centre in HIV Epidemiology
and Clinical Research, University of
New South Wales, Sydney, Australia

Selina N. Lo
Clinical Advisor, Clinton HIV/AIDS
Initiative China, Chinese CDC,
Beijing, China

Jens D. Lundgren
Copenhagen HIV Programme,
Hvidovre University Hospital, Copenhagen,
Denmark;
jens-lundgren@eacs.ws

Ma Ye
National HIV/STD Control and Prevention,
Bejing, China

Simon D. Makombe
HIV Unit, Ministry of Health,
Lilongwe, Malawi

Joseph Margolick
Johns Hopkins University,
Bloomberg School of Public Health,
Baltimore, USA

Des Martin
Specialist, Clinical Virology, Kimera Solutions,
Edenvale, South Africa

Renato Maserati
HIV/AIDS Outpatient Clinic,
Infectious Diseases Department,
IRCCS Policlinico San Matteo Hospital
Foundation, Pavia, Italy;
maserati@smatteo.pv.it

James A. McIntyre
Chris Hani Baragwanath Hospital,
Perinatal HIV Research Unit,
University of Witwatersrand,
Johannesburg, South Africa

Amanda Mocroft
EuroSIDA Statistical Centre,
Royal Free and University College Medical
School, London, UK

Luc Montagnier
Director, Institut Pasteur,
Paris, France

Anne C. Moorman
National Center for HIV/STD and
TB Prevention (NCHSTP), CDC,
Atlanta, USA

Stephanie Nixon
Health Economics and HIV/AIDS Research
Division (HEARD), University of
KwaZulu-Natal, Durban, South Africa

James M. Oleske
School of Medicine, University of Medicine
and Dentistry of New Jersey, Newark, USA

Frank J. Palella, Jr.
Feinberg School of Medicine,
Division of Infectious Diseases,
Northwestern University, Chicago, USA;
f-palella@northwestern.edu

Jean William Pape
Weill Medical College of Cornell University,
GHESKIO Center, Haiti

Roger Paredes
Partners AIDS Research Center,
Cambridge, USA;
rparedes@irsicaixa.es

Kathy Petoumenos
National Centre in HIV Epidemiology and
Clinical Research, University of
New South Wales, Sydney, Australia;
kpetoumenos@nchecr.unsw.edu.au

John Phair
Feinberg School of Medicine,
Division of Infectious Diseases,
Northwestern University, Chicago,
USA; j-phair@northwestern.edu

Praphan Phanuphak
Director, Thai Red Cross Programme
on AIDS, Bangkok, Thailand;
praphan.p@chula.ac.th

Peter Piot
Director General, UNAIDS,
Geneva, Switzerland

Celso Ferreira Ramos-Filho
Associate Professor, School of Medicine,
Federal University of Rio de Janeiro,
Rio de Janeiro, Brazil;
laveran@ig.com.br

Charles Rinaldo
University of Pittsburgh,
Pittsburg, USA

Kiat Ruxrungtham
Department of Medicine, Chulalongkom
University, Bangkok, Thailand;
rkiat@chula.ac.th

Mauro Schechter
Federal University of Rio de Janeiro,
Rio de Janeiro, Brazil;
maurosch@hucff.ufrj.br

Erik J. Schouten
HIV Coordinator, Ministry of Health,
Lilongwe, Malawi;
eschouten@mw.msh.org

Renslow Sherer
Infectious Diseases, University of
Chicago Hospitals, Chicago, USA;
rsherer@projecthope.org

Moses Sinkala
Catholic Medical Missions Board,
Lusaka, Zambia

Papa Salif Sow
Department of Infectious Diseases,
University of Dakar Fann Hospital,
Dakar, Senegal;
salifsow@sentoo.sn

Suely Hiromi Tuboi
Epidemiologist, Projeto Praça Onze,
Federal University of Rio de Janeiro,
Rio de Janeiro, Brazil

Dingie van Rensberg
Centre for Health Systems Research and
Development, University of the Free State,
Bloemfontein, South Africa

Nina Veenstra
Senior Research Fellow, Health Economics
and HIV/AIDS Research Division (HEARD),
University of KwaZulu-Natal, Durban,
South Africa;
veenstran@ukza.ac.za

Rochelle P. Walensky
Division of Infectious Diseases,
Massachusetts General Hospital,
Boston, USA

Alan Whiteside, D. Econ
Director, Health Economics and HIV/AIDS
Research Division (HEARD), University of
KwaZulu-Natal,
Durban, South Africa

Eva Wolf
MUC Research GmbH,
Munich, Germany;
ewo@muresearch.de

Marcelo J. Wolff
University of Chile School of Medicine,
Fundacion Arriaran,
Santiago, Chile;
mwolff@vtr.net

Robin Wood
Principal Investigator, The Desmond
Tutu HIV Centre, Institute of Infectious
Disease and Molecular Medicine,
Cape Town, South Africa;
robin.wood@hiv-research.org.za

Zhang Fu-Jie
Director, Treatment and Care Division,
National Center for AIDS/STD Control and
Prevention, Beijing, China;
treatment@chinaaids.cntreatment@chinaaids.cn

José M. Zuniga
President and CEO, International
Association of Physicians in AIDS
Care (IAPAC), Chicago, USA;
jzuniga@iapac.org

List of Figures

List of Tables

List of Acronyms and Abbreviations

3TC	lamivudine
ABC	abacavir
ACP	AIDS Control Programme, Uganda
ACTG	AIDS Clinical Trials Group (of NIH, USA)
ACT UP	AIDS Coalition to Unleash Power, USA
ADA	American Dental Association
ADA	Americans with Disabilities Act
ADAP	AIDS drug assistance programme, USA
ADC	AIDS dementia complex
AFASS	acceptable, feasible, affordable, sustainable (re breastfeeding)
AHOD	Australian HIV Observational Database
AIDS	acquired immunodeficiency syndrome (NB not redefined each chapter)
ALT	alanine aminotransferase
AMA	American Medical Association
AMF	AIDS Medical Foundation
AmFAR	American Foundation for AIDS Research
ANAC	Association of Nurses in AIDS Care
ANC	antenatal clinic
ANRS	*Agence Nationale de Recherche sur le SIDA*, France
AP	Associated Press
API	active pharmaceutical ingredients
APV	amprenavir
ARDFP	antiretroviral drug-free period
ARL	AIDS-related lymphoma
ART	antiretroviral therapy
ARV	antiretroviral
ASHM	Australian Society for HIV Medicine
ATC	Access to Care [programme], Thailand
ATV	atazanavir
ATV/r	atazanavir/ritonavir
AUC	area under the curve
AZT	azidothymidine (zidovudine). See also ZDV.
bDNA	branched DNA (assay)
BHIVA	British HIV Association

BID	twice daily (*Bis In Die*)
BMI	body mass index
CAMACS	Center for Analysis of the MACS (see also MACS), USA
CARE	[Ryan White] Comprehensive AIDS Resources Emergency [Act], USA; National MPTCT support programme, Thailand
CASCADE	Concerted Action on SeroConversion to AIDS and Death in Europe [study]
CBO	community-based organization
CDC	US Centers for Disease Control (and Prevention)
CEG	CISIH Clinical Epidemiology Group, France
CHAI	Clinton HIV/AIDS Initiative
CHAVI	Center for HIV-AIDS Vaccine Immunology
China CARES	China Comprehensive AIDS Response [programme]
China CDC	Chinese Center for Disease Control and Prevention
CHW	community health worker
CI	confidence interval
CIDS	Chilean Infectious Disease Society
CIN	cervical intraepithelial neoplasia
CISIH	*Centres d'Information et de Soins de l'Immunidéficience Humaine*, France
CME	continuing medical education
CM	cryptococcal meningitis
CMV	cytomegalovirus
CNIL	*Commission nationale de l'informatique et des libertés personelles*, France
CNS	central nervous system
COA	*Centro Operativo AIDS*, Italy
COHERE	Collaboration of Observational HIV Epidemiological Research in Europe [study]
CONASIDA	Ministry of Health Commission on AIDS, Chile

CPT	cotrimoxazole preventive therapy		ENF	enfuvirtide (see also T20)
CREST	Can Resistance Testing Enhance Selection of Therapy [study], Australia		EQ-5D	EuroQol (study)
			ETV	etravirine (see also TMC-125)
CRF	circulating recombinant form; case report form		EU	European Union
			fAPV	fosamprenavir
CSF	cerebrospinal fluid		fAPV/r	fosamprenavir/ritonavir
CRN	(HIV/AIDS) Clinical Research Network, Thailand		FBO	faith-based organization
			FDA	US Food and Drug Administration
CROI	Conference on retroviruses and opportunistic infections		FDC	fixed dose combination
CT	computerized tomography		FFS	fees for service
CTL	cytotoxic T-lymphocyte		FHDH	French Hospital Database on HIV, France
CTX	cotrimoxazole		FHI	Family Health International
CVD	cardiovascular disease		FOPH	Federal Office of Public Health, Switzerland
D:A:D	Data collection of Adverse events of anti-HIV Drugs [study]		FPD	former plasma donor
d4T	stavudine		FRAMS	Fat Redistribution and Metabolic Change in HIV Infection study
DAGNAE	*Deutsche Arbeitsgemeinschaft niedergelassener Ärzte in der Versorgung HIV-Infizierter e.V., Germany*		FRS	fat redistribution syndrome
			FSW	female sex worker
			FTC	emtricitabine
DAIG	*Deutsche AIDS Gesellschaft, Germany*		FTE	full-time equivalent [staff]
			FXB	François Xavier Bagnoud Center for Health and Human Rights
DALY	disability adjusted life year		GDP	gross domestic product
DATASUS	MOH central database, Brazil		GHESKIO	*Groupe Haitien d'Étude du Sarcome de Kaposi et des Infections Opportunistes*
DBS	dried blood spot			
ddC	zalcitabine		GI	gastrointestinal
ddI	didanosine		GIPA	greater involvement of people with HIV/AIDS
DEXA	Dual Energy X-Ray Absortiometry			
DHHS	US Department of Health and Human Services		Global Fund	Global Fund to Fight AIDS, Tuberculosis and Malaria
DLV	delavirdine		GMHC	Gay Men's Health Crisis, USA
DM	diabetes mellitus		GNI	gross national income
DOT	directly observed therapy		GNP	gross national product
DOTS	directly observed treatment, short-course		GPA	Global Programme on AIDS
			GPO	Government Pharmaceutical Organization, Thailand
DRV	darunavir			
DRV/r	darunavir/ritonavir		GTZ	German Technical Cooperation Agency
EAP	Expanded Access Programme, Chile; Early Access Programme, Italy		HAART	highly active antiretroviral therapy
			HAD	HIV-associated dementia
EBV	Epstein-Barr virus		HBV	hepatitis B virus
EC	oesophageal candidiasis		HCV	hepatitis C virus
EFV	efavirenz		HDL	high density lipoprotein
ELISA	enzyme-linked immunosorbant assay		HDL-C	high density lipoprotein cholesterol
ELV	elvitegravir		HDI	human development index
EMA	Eligible Metropolitan Area, USA		HGC	hard gel capsule
EMEA	European Agency for the Evaluation of Medicinal Products			

HHV8	human herpes virus 8
HIV	human immunodeficiency virus (NB not redefined each chapter)
HIVDR	HIV drug resistance
HIVNAT	HIV Netherlands-Australia-Thailand [Research Collaboration]
HIV RNA	HIV ribonucleic acid (NB definition not stated in text)
HL	Hodgkin's lymphoma
HOMER	HAART Observational Medical Evaluation and Research [cohort]
HOPS	HIV Outpatient Study, USA
HPLC	high-performance liquid chromatography
HPV	human papilloma virus
HR	hazard ratio; human resource
HRH	human resources for health
HSIL	high-grade squamous intraepithelial lesion
HTA	arterial hypertension (high blood pressure)
HTLV	human T-cell lymphotrophic virus
HUI3, HUI2	Health Utilities Index Mark 2 and Mark 3
IAPAC	International Association of Physicians in AIDS Care, USA
IAS	International AIDS Society
IATEC	International Antiviral Therapy Evaluation Centre, Netherlands
ICAAC	Interscience Conference on Antimicrobial Agents and Chemotherapy
ICAB	Italian Community Advisory Board
ICASA	International Conference on AIDS and STIs in Africa
ICH GCP	International Conference on Harmonisation/WHO Good Clinical Practice [standards]
ICONA	Italian Cohort Naive for Antiretrovirals
ID	infectious disease
IDSA	Infectious Diseases Society of America
IDU	injection drug use/user
IDV	indinavir
IDV/r	indinavir/ritonavir
IEC	information, education and communication [programme]
IFN	interferon
IHE	*l'Institut Haitien de l'Enfance*, Haiti

IL-2	interleukin 2
IMEA	*Institut de Médecine et d'Épidémiologie Appliquée*, France
IMF	International Monetary Fund
ININ	integrase inhibitor
INSERM	*Institut National de la Santé et de la Recherche Médicale*, France
IOM	Institute of Medicine, USA
IQR	interquartile range
IRIS	immune reconstitution inflammatory syndrome
ISAARV	Highly Active Antiretroviral Therapy Initiative, Senegal
ISS	*Istituto Superiore di Sanità*, Italy
ITN	insecticide-treated [bed] nets
ITT	intent-to-treat
IVDU	intravenous drug use
JAMA	Journal of the American Medical Association
KS	Kaposi's sarcoma
KSHV	Kaposi's sarcoma-associated herpes virus
LAV	lymphadenopathy-associated virus
LDL	low-density lipoprotein
LPV	lopinavir
LPV/r	lopinavir/ritonavir
LYG	life years gained
M&E	monitoring and evaluation
MAC	mycobacterium avium complex
MACS	Multicenter AIDS Cohort Study
MATEC	Midwest AIDS Training and Education Center, USA
MCMD	minor cognitive motor disorder
MDG	Millennium Development Goal
MDR	multi-drug resistant
MGUS	monoclonal gammopathy of unknown significance
MHS	mental health status
MI	myocardial infarction
MIU	million International Units
MoCHiV	Swiss Mother+Child HIV (Cohort Study)
MOH	Ministry of Health
MOS-HIV	Medical Outcomes Study HIV
MOPH	Ministry of Public Health, Thailand
MRI	magnetic resonance imagery
MRV	maraviroc

MS	metabolic syndrome
MSF	Médecins Sans Frontières
MSM	men who have sex with men
MTCT	mother-to-child transmission
NAM	nucleoside analogue mutations
NAP	National AIDS Program, Brazil
NAPC	National AIDS Prevention Committee, Senegal
NAPHA	National Access to Antiretroviral Programme for People Living with HIV/AIDS, Thailand
NARF	National AIDS Research Foundation of Los Angeles
NARL	National AIDS Reference Laboratory, China
NASBA	nucleic acid sequence-based amplification
NATAP	Brazilian National STD and AIDS Program
NCAIDS	National Center for AIDS/STD Prevention and Control, China
NCHECR	National Centre in HIV Epidemiology and Clinical Research, Australia
NCI	US National Cancer Institute
NFV	nelfinavir
NGO	non-governmental organization
NHL	non-Hodgkin's lymphoma
NHS	National Health System/ Service
NIAID	US National Institute of Allergy and Infectious Diseases
NIH	US National Institutes of Health
NNRTI	non-nucleoside reverse transcriptase inhibitor
NRC	National Research Council
NRTI	nucleoside reverse transcriptase inhibitor
NtRTI	nucleotide reverse transcriptase inhibitor
NVP	nevirapine
OBT	optimized background treatment
OC	oesophageal candidiasis
ODA	overseas development assistance
OI	opportunistic infection
OPTIMA	Options in Management with Antiretrovirals (study)
OR	operational research; odds ratio
OS	overall survival
PAP	Papanicolao [smear]

PCNSL	primary central nervous system lymphoma
PCP	*Pneumocystis carinii* pneumonia
PCR	polymerase chain reaction
PEG-IFN	pegylated interferon
PENTA	Paediatric European Network for the Treatment of AIDS
PEP	post-exposure prophylaxis
PEPFAR	US President's Emergency Plan for AIDS Relief
PHAEDRA	Primary HIV and Early Disease Research: American (cohort)
PHC	primary healthcare
PHS	physical health status
PI	protease inhibitor
PIH	Partners in Health
PJP	*Pneumocystis jirovecci* pneumonia
PLATO	Pursuing Later Treatment Options (collaboration)
PLG	panleucogated assay
PLWHA	people living with HIV/AIDS
PMMA	polymethyl-methacrylate
PMTCT	prevention of mother-to-child transmission
PPAR	peroxisome proliferator-activated receptors
PPD	purified protein derivative
PPP	public-private partnership; purchasing power parity
PRO	protease
PT	proficiency testing
pVL	plasma viral load
PY	patient-year(s)
QALY	quality adjusted life year
QOL	quality of life
QT	interval between Q wave and T wave
R&D	research and development
RAL	raltegravir
RBV	ribavirin
RENAGENO	*Rede Nacional de Genotipagem* (National Network for Genotyping), Brazil
RH	relative hazard
RKI	Robert Koch Institute, Germany
RPR	rapid plasma regain
RPV	rilpivirine
RT	reverse transcriptase

RTI	reverse transcriptase inhibitor	TB	tuberculosis
RTV	ritonavir	TC	total cholesterol
SAE	serious adverse events	TCM	traditional Chinese medicine
SAHIVS	Southern African HIV Clinicians Society	TDF	tenofovir
SAMA	South African Medical Association	TDM	therapeutic drug monitoring
SARS	severe acute respiratory syndrome	TG	triglycerides
sd	single dose (e.g. sdNVP)	THF	thymic humoral factor
SD	standard deviation	TMC-125	etravirine (see also ETV)
SERT	*Servizio di Tossicodipendenze*, Italy	TPV	tipranavir
SFDA	State Food and Drug Administration, China	TPV/r	tipranavir/ritonavir
SG	standard gamble	TRC-ARC	Thai Red Cross AIDS Research Centre
SGC	soft gel capsules	TRIPS	Agreement on Trade-Related Aspects of Intellectual Property Rights
SHCS	Swiss HIV Cohort Study	TTO	time trade-off
SHW	substitute health worker	UC	Universal Coverage [Programme], Thailand
SIG	special interest group, South Africa	UCLA	University of California, Los Angeles
S/LS	sensitive/ less sensitive [assay]	UN	United Nations
SMART	Strategies for Management of Antiretroviral Therapy [study]	UNAIDS	Joint United Nations Programme on HIV/AIDS
SNSF	Swiss National Science Federation	UNGASS	United Nations General Assembly Special Session [on HIV/AIDS]
SOC	system organ class	UNHRC	United Nations Human Rights Commission
SPA	Special Programme on AIDS	UNICEF	United Nations Children's Fund
SQV	saquinavir	UPI	United Press International
SQV/r	saquinavir/ritonavir	USAID	United States Agency for International Development
SSA	Social Security Administration, USA		
SSO	Social Security Office, Thailand	VA	Veterans Administration, USA; US Dept of Veterans Affairs
STARHS	standardized algorithm for recent HIV seroconversion	VAS	visual analogue scale
STD	sexually transmitted disease	VCT	voluntary counselling and testing
STI	structured treatment interruption; sexually transmitted infection	VCV	vicriviroc
SUS	*Sistema Único de Saúde* (Unified Health System), Brazil	VDRL	Vertical Disease Research Laboratory, Chile
T20	enfuvirtide (see also ENF)	WHA	World Health Assembly
TAC	Treatment Action Campaign, South Africa	WHO	World Health Organization
		WOWO	week-on/week-off [therapy]
TAG	Treatment Action Group, USA	WTO	World Trade Organization
TAM	Thymidine analogue-associated mutation	XDR	extensively drug resistant
TASO	The AIDS Support Organization, Uganda	ZDV	zidovudine. See also AZT.

Part 1

A decade of HAART: trials, tribulations and successes

Chapter 1

Introduction

José M. Zuniga*, Alan Whiteside, Amin Ghaziani
and John G. Bartlett

For an epidemic that would explode to claim millions of lives, AIDS surfaced very quietly in the United States, with a small notice on 5 June 1981 in a weekly newsletter published by the US Centers for Disease Control (CDC) in Atlanta, alerting physicians to five unusual cases of pneumonia that had been diagnosed, without identifiable cause, in Los Angeles residents over the previous few months [1]. All five patients were homosexual men, and they presented with *Pneumocystis carinii* pneumonia (PCP), a lung infection usually seen only in severely malnourished children or in adults undergoing intensive chemotherapy. Until they developed PCP, however, these men were well-nourished, vigorous adults whose immune systems should have protected them from the infection.

Within the year, similar cases were reported throughout the United States, Western Europe and then the rest of the world. Apparently healthy adults were suddenly presenting in clinics with rare infections and malignancies that healthy people should not get. In the United States, most were from New York, California, Florida and Texas—and not all were homosexual men. Men and women who injected intravenous drugs were also becoming sick, as were haemophiliacs, the male *and* female sexual partners of individuals in these risk groups, immigrants from Africa and the Caribbean, and some of the infant children born to women at risk [2–7]. All these varied people had one thing in common: almost absent levels of CD4 cells that maintain cell-mediated immunity. Their defective immune systems left them vulnerable to a unique menu of opportunistic infections (OIs), and led many to their graves.

For the next 14 years, HIV made its global advance, assaulted by a handful of drugs that were only transiently effective. Much like all pathogens, HIV was undeterred by race, gender or socio-economic class, observing no border, political ideology or religious belief, and leaving in its wake human devastation that eventually reached a scale not witnessed since the avian influenza pandemic of 1918–20. From an initial five cases sprang an AIDS pandemic that, by December 1995, officially affected a total of 1.2 million people, though this was a mere fraction of the 6 million adults and children the World Health Organization (WHO) estimated had been infected with HIV since the beginning of the pandemic [8]. There was progress on the clinical front with trimethoprim-sulfamethoxazole for PCP prophylaxis, macrolides for prophylaxis against mycobacterium avium complex (MAC), azidothymidine (AZT) monotherapy for HIV treatment, AZT to prevent perinatal HIV transmission, and a multitude of drugs to treat virtually all OIs [9–13]. Nevertheless, the disease was inevitably progressive, and although some patients deteriorated more slowly than others, nearly all patients died. Indeed, AIDS became, for example, the leading cause of death in 1995 among Americans aged 25 to 44 [14].

*Corresponding author.

We have journeyed far from those early dark days of the AIDS pandemic—from a time in which HIV-positive patients had limited treatment options to an era in which more than 20 antiretroviral drugs are approved for combination highly active antiretroviral therapy (HAART). A little over a decade ago, at the XI International AIDS Conference in 1996, under Vancouver's cerulean skies, more than 15,000 physicians, researchers, allied health professionals and patient-activists gathered to hail the advent of HAART. Six months earlier, researchers had disclosed that a triple-antiretroviral drug combination including a protease inhibitor (PI) and two nucleoside reverse transcriptase inhibitors (NRTIs)—indinavir (IDV)/AZT/didanosine (ddI)—banished detectable circulating virus from 85% of a small cohort studied for 24 weeks [15]. A month before the conference, researchers announced groundbreaking data on the impact of viral load measurements on the natural history of HIV [16]; measuring viral load subsequently became the preferred method through which to assess HAART's therapeutic benefit (in weeks, even days, versus months or years). Furthermore, timed to coincide with the conference, a group of AIDS investigators published the first clinical recommendations for when to initiate HAART, which antiretroviral regimen to start with, and when to switch antiretroviral drugs [17]. The excitement reached a fever pitch when, two years following the gloomy IX International AIDS Conference in Berlin (whose mood could at best be described as Stygian), a number of PI-containing antiretroviral regimens—nelfinavir (NFV)/AZT/lamivudine (3TC), NFV/stavudine (d4T), ritonavir (RTV)/saquinavir (SQV), RTV/AZT/zalcitabine (ddC) and IDV/AZT/3TC—chalked up impressive clinical gains [18–22]. But it was not all pretty: IDV had to be taken thrice daily and caused kidney stones, RTV tasted like a mixture of kerosene and cherry juice, and 96% of SQV wound up in the toilet due to poor absorption.

Out of a necessity to stem the tide of devastation wrought by HIV disease, the boundaries of clinical research and practice have been pushed over the past 10 years to make the treatment easier, less toxic and more potent. Clinical trial design has also become standardized using a viral load measurement of 50 copies/mL as the ultimate goal. The US Food and Drug Administration (FDA) then recognized viral load as a surrogate for clinical efficacy; this was the first time a microbiological end point was ever accepted by the regulatory agency as proof of effectiveness. The clinical benefit of HAART was almost immediately apparent. Most clinics quickly showed a 60–80% decrease in mortality rates, hospitalizations and/or AIDS-defining OIs. The total benefit of this treatment longevity is now estimated at 13 years of life when HAART is started at a CD4 count of 87 cells/mm^3, and 24 years when initiated at a CD4 count of 310 cells/mm^3 [23,24]. This progress is expected to continue with the recent approval of two new antiretroviral drugs from two new classes—the integrase inhibitor raltegravir (RAL) and the CCR5 antagonist maraviroc (MRV)—and the anticipated addition of new drugs from existing antiretroviral drug classes (non-nucleoside reverse transcriptase inhibitors [NNRTIs], fusion inhibitors, NRTIs and PIs) as well as future drug classes making their way through the development pipeline.

Still, 25 years since the first report of HIV, the Lazarus-like effect of HAART to improve the prognosis of HIV-infected patients has not reached far beyond the industrialized world, despite recent political will, an influx of resources and bilateral and international efforts. In resource-limited settings in Africa, Asia and South America, where 90% of people living with HIV/AIDS reside, access to HAART continues to be limited. It is estimated that one million HIV-infected individuals currently receive HAART in low- and middle-income countries, which represents 15% of the 6.5 million people the WHO classifies as urgently in need of HAART [25]. The challenges that lie ahead for the next decade of HAART will thus be faced not just by researchers in their laboratories (e.g. identifying new viral targets) and by clinicians and allied health professionals at their patients' bedsides (e.g. managing drug resistance), but by a global community committed to waging a robust war against a virus with the ability to spread with devastating rapidity. Indeed, another transparent challenge is prevention, which, despite many efforts, has not worked in either the developed or developing world, as evidenced by the 40,000 new HIV infections in the United States every year for the past 15 years, and the 14,000 new HIV infections daily worldwide (95% of them in developing countries) [26,27].

In September 2006, on the decade anniversary of HAART, the International Association of Physicians in AIDS Care (IAPAC) convened an historic symposium entitled, 'Decade of HAART.' This Oxford University Press book, for which we are honored to serve as co-editors as well as contributing authors, represents an expanded version of the symposium's already broad agenda. We are privileged to count among our distinguished contributing authors some of the world's most renowned minds in the fields of HIV economics, medicine, public policy, sociology and research. Together, they have helped us complete a comprehensive review of our collective progress since the 'Dark Ages' of a world ravaged by a disease without any antiretroviral drugs. Physicians and researchers from 13 high, mid- and low human development index countries write about the obstacles faced and overcome, lessons learned, and challenges that lie ahead in HAART delivery. Principal investigators from 8 observational cohorts offer insights into HAART's impact over the past decade. And last but by no means least, experts from various disciplines round out the book by sharing their respective experiences, thus allowing a unique vantage point from which to critique the past decade of HAART as well as define future directions.

We present *A Decade of HAART: The Development and Global Impact of Highly Active Antiretroviral Therapy* with the hope that by illuminating the successes achieved over the past 25 years since the discovery of HIV, as well as the last 10 years of HAART delivery, this book contributes to forward momentum in the global battle against HIV/AIDS. Our ultimate wish is that we may some day soon look back on how humanity identified, contained, cured and eradicated the scourge of HIV disease.

References

1. US Centers for Disease Control (CDC). (1981). *Pneumocystis* Pneumonia–Los Angeles. *MMWR Weekly* **30**:1–3.
2. Masur H, Michelis MA, Greene JB, *et al.* (1981). An outbreak of community acquired *Pneumocystis carinii* pneumonia: Initial manifestation of cellular immune dysfunction. *New Engl J Med* **305**:1431–1438.
3. US Centers for Disease Control (CDC). (1982). Epidemiologic notes and reports of *Pneumocystis carinii* pneumonia among persons with hemophilia A. *MMWR Weekly* **31**:365–367.
4. US Centers for Disease Control (CDC). (1983). Epidemiologic notes and reports of immunodeficiency among female sexual partners of males with Acquired Immune Deficiency Syndrome (AIDS) – New York. *MMWR Weekly* **31**:697–698.
5. Clumeck N, Sonnet J, Taelman H, *et al.* (1984). Acquired Immune Deficiency Syndrome in African patients. *New Engl J Med* **310**:492–497.
6. US Centers for Disease Control (CDC). (1982).Opportunistic infections and Kaposi's sarcoma among Haitians in the United States. *MMWR Weekly* **31**:353–353; 360–361.
7. US Centers for Disease Control (CDC). (1982).Unexplained immunodeficiency and opportunistic infections in infants – New York, New Jersey, California. *MMWR Weekly* **31**:665–667.
8. Joint United Nations Programme on HIV/AIDS (UNAIDS). (2005). *AIDS Epidemic Update.* Geneva: UNAIDS.
9. Kovacs JA, Masur H. (1992). Prophylaxis for *Pneumocystis carinii* pneumonia in patients infected with human immunodeficiency virus. *Clin Infect Dis* **14**:1005–1009.

10. Nightingale SD, Cal SX, Peterson DM, *et al.* (1992). Primary prophylaxis with fluconazole against systemic fungal infections in HIV-positive patients. *AIDS* **6**:191–194.

11. Ocular Complications of AIDS Research Group with the AIDS Clinical Trials Group. (1992). Mortality in patients treated with either foscarnet or ganciclovir for cytomegalovirus retinitis. *N Engl J Med* **326**:213–220.

12. Fischl MA, Richman DA, Grieco MH, *et al.* (1997). The efficacy of azidothymidine (AZT) in the treatment of patients with AIDS-related complex: A double-blind placebo-controlled trial. *N Engl J Med* **317**:185–191.

13. Connor EM, Sperling RS, Gelder RD, *et al.* (1994). Pediatric AIDS Clinical Trials Group Protocol 076 Study Group. Reduction of maternal-infant transmission of human immunodeficiency syndrome type 1 with zidovudine treatment. *N Engl J Med* **331**:1173–1180.

14. US Centers for Disease Control (CDC). (1996). Update: Mortality Attributable to HIV Infection Among Persons Aged 25–44 Years – United States. *MMWR Weekly* **45**:121–125.

15. Massari F, Conant M, Mellors J, *et al.* (1996). A phase II open-label randomized study of the triple combination of indinavir, zidovudine (ZDV), and didanosine (ddI) versus indinavir alone and zidovudine/didanosine in antiretroviral-naïve patients. 3rd Conference on Retroviruses and Opportunistic Infections, 28 January–1 February 1996, Washington, DC. [Abstract 200]

16. Mellors JW, Munoz A, Giorgi JV, *et al.* (1997). Plasma viral load and CD4 + lymphocytes as prognostic markers of HIV-1 infection. *Ann Intern Med* **126**:946–954.

17. Carpenter CC, Fischl MA, Hammer SM, *et al.* (1996). Antiretroviral therapy for HIV infection in 1996. Recommendations of an international panel. International AIDS Society-USA. *JAMA* **276**:146–154.

18. Markowitz M, Cao Y, Hurley A, *et al.* (1996). Triple therapy with AZT and 3TC in combination with nelfinavir mesylate in 12 antiretroviral-naive subjects chronically infected with HIV-1. XI International AIDS Conference, 7–12 July 1996, Vancouver, Canada. [Abstract LB.B.6031]

19. Gathe J Jr, Burkhardt B, Hawley P, *et al.* (1996). A randomized, phase II study of VIRACEPT, a novel HIV protease inhibitor, used in combination with stavudine (d4T) vs. stavudine (d4T) alone. XI International AIDS Conference, 7–12 July 1996, Vancouver, Canada. [Abstract Mo.B.413]

20. Cameron DW, Sun E, Markowitz M, *et al.* (1996). Combination use of ritonavir and saquinavir in HIV-infected patients: preliminary safety and activity data. XI International AIDS Conference, 7–12 July 1996, Vancouver, Canada. [Abstract Th.B.934]

21. Mathez D, Bagnarelli P, Truchis de P, *et al.* (1996). A triple combination of Ritonavir + AZT + ddC as a first line treatment of patients with AIDS: Update. XI International AIDS Conference, 7–12 July 1996, Vancouver, Canada. [Abstract Mo.B.175]

22. Gulick R, Mellors J, Havlir D, *et al.* (1996). Potent and sustained antiretroviral activity of indinavir (IDV), zidovudine (ZDV) and lamivudine (3TC). XI International AIDS Conference, 7–12 July 1996, Vancouver, Canada. [Abstract Th.B.931]

23. Walensky RP, Paltiel AD, Losina E, *et al.* (2006). The survival benefits of AIDS treatment in the United States. *J Infect Dis* **194**:11–19.

24. Schackman BR, Gebo KA, Walensky RP. (2006). The lifetime cost of current human immunodeficiency virus care in the United States. *Med Care* **44**:990–997.

25. World Health Organization. (2005). *Progress on Global Access to HIV Antiretroviral Therapy. An Update on '3 by 5.'* Geneva: World Health Organization.

26. Fauci AS. (2007). A Decade of HAART: Historical perspectives, successes and failures, and future considerations. Decade of HAART symposium, 25–26 September 2006, San Francisco, USA. [Keynote Address]

27. Joint United Nations Programme on HIV/AIDS (UNAIDS). (2006). *Report on the Global HIV Epidemic 2006.* Geneva: UNAIDS.

Chapter 2

A world ravaged by a disease without HAART

José M. Zuniga* and Amin Ghaziani

Introduction

Before 5 June 1981, no one could have factored the human immunodeficiency virus, or HIV, into the calculus of death. Indeed, it arrived just as biomedical science offered itself cautious congratulations for having the final conquest of infectious diseases within sight. The first hints of this microbe's gathering fury struck with publication of a brief epidemiological account entitled, '*Pneumocystis* Pneumonia – Los Angeles', which appeared in a weekly US Centers for Disease Control (CDC) morbidity and mortality report [1]. The report described five homosexual men, ranging in age from 29 to 36 years, who had presented over the previous eight months with *Pneumocystis carinii* pneumonia (PCP), a pulmonary infection 'almost exclusively limited to severely immunosuppressed patients' [1]. Virtually every case of PCP previously reported had occurred in patients with immunity suppressed for organ transplantation, or by chemotherapy. Three of the men were also infected with oesophageal candidiasis, or thrush. All five were given standard courses of antifungal drugs and pentamidine, but, as of the report's publication, two had already died. Following descriptions of the individual cases, the authors concluded:

> The diagnosis of *Pneumocystis* pneumonia was confirmed for all [five] patients ante-mortem by closed or open lung biopsy. The patients did not know each other and had no known common contacts or knowledge of sexual partners who had had similar illnesses. Two of the [five] reported having frequent homosexual contacts with various partners. All [five] reported using inhalant drugs, and [one] reported [injection] drug abuse. [1]

The unusual appearance of PCP in otherwise healthy, young, homosexual men was accompanied by a similar incidence in the same population of a more aggressive variety of Kaposi's sarcoma (KS), caused by the human herpes virus 8 (HHV8). This was historically very rare, found mainly in older men of Mediterranean, Jewish or African origin [2]. A second CDC *Morbidity & Mortality Weekly Report,* published on 4 July 1981, reported on a cluster of KS cases among 26 homosexual men in New York City [3]. Michael Gottlieb, an immunologist at the University of California, Los Angeles (UCLA) and a co-author of the CDC's first report, began to connect the dots. Gottlieb had treated some of the first mysterious cases of PCP, all in formerly healthy young homosexual men. These CDC reports were the medical world's introduction to an infectious disease that would come to be known as the acquired immunodeficiency syndrome, or AIDS, and earn the distinction of becoming one of the most destructive pandemics in recorded history. As Gottlieb told *Time* magazine in 1985: 'I knew I was witnessing medical history, but I had no comprehension of what this illness would become' [4].

*Corresponding author.

Social stigma and the politics of AIDS in the West

Neither KS nor PCP was medically unfamiliar. What was puzzling was their seeming concentration in self-identified homosexual men. By 1980, this prompted the media and some medical circles to alternately refer to the mysterious illness as 'the gay disease', 'the gay cancer', or 'the gay plague' [5]. These early labels reflected lack of information that, according to journalist Randy Shilts (who himself died of AIDS in February 1994), catalyzed 'a dizzying array of [additional] acronyms … as possible monikers for an epidemic that, though 10 months old, remained unnamed' [6]. The CDC offered its variant, GRID, or Gay Related Immune Deficiency, which mistakenly connected the syndrome with homosexuality and thus selectively stigmatized homosexual men [6]. Some in the medical community preferred ACIDS, for Acquired Community Immune Deficiency Syndrome, while others used CAIDS, for Community Acquired Immune Deficiency Syndrome. As Shilts noted in his chronicle of the early AIDS epidemic in the United States entitled *And the Band Played On*, 'The 'community'… was a polite way of saying gay; the doctors couldn't let go of the notion that one identified this disease by whom it hit rather than what it did … By now, somebody was dying almost every day in America from an epidemic that still did not have a name' [6].

A fear of AIDS and homosexuals grew simultaneously. Public opinion amplified problems of discrimination, stigma and homophobia [7]. Some conservative zealots proclaimed AIDS to be 'God's punishment for gays' [6]. In a scathing *Washington Times* editorial published on 27 May 1983, conservative political commentator (and one-time US presidential candidate) Patrick Buchanan viciously chimed in, 'The poor homosexuals; they have declared war upon nature, and now nature is exacting an awful retribution' [8]. The rhetoric around homosexuality's link to AIDS grew even more vitriolic when movie screen idol Rock Hudson announced that he was HIV-positive. Hudson was diagnosed in June 1984; however, it was not until a year later, while he was in Paris for treatment with the experimental drug HPA-23 (which ultimately proved ineffective), that he disclosed his HIV serostatus and revealed he was a homosexual [9]. Yet, even in the face of a public pronouncement that he was living with a disease whose prognosis was terminal, and despite fellow actors (and friends) Doris Day and Elizabeth Taylor rallying to his side, reaction in some quarters of American society was scathing, largely reflected in a plethora of homophobic, moralizing jokes [9].

Given that the media were, for the most part, still ignoring AIDS, viewing it as a phenomenon limited in scope, unnewsworthy and of no real interest to a more general audience, Hudson's public battle with HIV was a watershed event in the history of the fight against AIDS. Overnight, HIV shifted from a disease that some nameless individuals occasionally contracted to something that visibly sapped the life of a once-beloved movie star. Hudson died on 2 October 1985.

The moral hysteria of AIDS within the American context can only be viewed against a backdrop of national homophobia [10]. This explains reactions such as that of William F. Buckley, the most respected of moderate conservatives, who, in 1986 in the *New York Times*, called for mandatory HIV testing and the forcible tattooing of HIV-infected homosexual men 'on the buttocks, to prevent the victimization of other homosexuals' as a 'crucial step in combating the AIDS epidemic' [11]. Many measures commonly suggested to deal with HIV-infected individuals in the 1980s were consistent with a definition of homosexual men as outsiders [7]. Indeed, through at least the beginning of 1983, it was 'virtually an article of faith among homosexuals that they would somehow end up in a concentration camp.' [12].

The early cultural coupling of AIDS with homosexuality made it possible for the US government to ignore the disease and not fund prevention or research programmes [13]. It was not until June 1987—six years into the epidemic—that US President Ronald Reagan held a press conference in which he used the word 'AIDS' for the first time in a public speech, although he did not honour those who were disproportionately dying; never did he use the word 'gay' [5]. Lesbian and gay history books have immortalized Reagan as an unresponsive president 'that did nothing during his eight years' [14], a time frame circumscribed by angry activist chants of 'History will recall, Reagan did least of all' [5].

This translated into the chronic underfunding of AIDS research. For example, the CDC and the US National Institutes of Health (NIH) were routinely denied additional funding for their work on AIDS. Between June 1981 and May 1982, the CDC spent less than US$1 million on AIDS, but US$9 million on Legionnaire's Disease [15]. At that point, more than 1000 of the 2000 AIDS cases reported in the United States had resulted in death; there were fewer than 50 deaths from Legionnaire's Disease [15].

Reagan's refusal to speak publicly about AIDS for the first six years of the epidemic, the lack of information about the disease and its transmission, the proliferation of hateful stereotypes and condemning public opinion, can be better understood in the context of growing neoconservativism. Reagan's landslide election and re-election victories, in 1980 and 1984 respectively, signified an expansion of the political power of his evangelical Christian constituency. His administration's politics of neglect—what some historians have termed 'an official conspiracy of silence'—was fuelled by the ascendancy of the New Right, which castigated homosexuals for undermining American 'family values' and social order [16].

The Reagan administration's legacy on HIV/AIDS provides a window to assess the social impact of HIV. While the potent combination of antiretroviral drugs that would become known as highly active antiretroviral therapy (HAART) is today capable of transforming HIV into a manageable disease, there is no preventive or curative vaccine for AIDS, and prior to the introduction of HAART in 1996, an HIV-positive diagnosis was considered a death sentence [17]. Moreover, the groups most commonly affected by HIV transmission—in terms of public morality at least—are generally considered 'deviant'. Writing in 1988, philosopher and social critic Susan Sontag observed:

> To get AIDS is precisely to be revealed, in the majority of cases so far, as a member of a certain 'risk group,' a community of pariahs. The illness flushes out an identity that might have remained hidden from neighbors, job mates, family, and friends …. Those like hemophiliacs and blood-transfusion recipients, who cannot by any stretch of the blaming faculty be considered responsible for their illness, may be as ruthlessly ostracized by frightened people, and potentially represent a greater threat because, unlike the already stigmatized, they are not as easy to identify …. Every feared epidemic disease, but especially those associated with sexual license, generates a preoccupying distinction between the disease's putative carriers (which usually means the poor and, in this part of the world, people with darker skins) and those defined – health professionals and other bureaucrats do the defining – as 'the general population.' AIDS has revived similar phobias and fears of contamination among this disease's version of the general population: white heterosexuals who do not inject themselves with drugs or have sexual relations with those who do [18].

HIV is therefore not simply the story of a virus. Its meanings extend beyond medicine and epidemiology to shape the social, cultural and political landscape as well. Powerful metaphors around the epidemic have often linked HIV to marginalized groups, which has exacerbated societal silence and promoted slow intervention.

Yet another 'plague' unfolds on the African continent

Although rich in land and natural resources, the 46 countries (including Madagascar) that make up the African continent, each with its own cultural and social traditions, had been ravaged in ways no other continent had seen, by droughts, famine, communicable diseases such as cholera, endemic diseases such as malaria, and dictatorial regimes [19]. According to most of the available epidemiological data, a new plague was added as early as the mid-1970s, and possibly even two decades earlier [20]. But it was not until the early 1980s that what would become known as HIV was discovered in a geographical band stretching from West Africa to the Indian Ocean. At this early point, the countries north of the Sahara and those in the southern cone of the continent remained unscathed. By 1987, however, the epidemic began its southward trek, eventually leading to some of the most explosive epidemics in southern Africa (e.g. Botswana and Swaziland, with the highest HIV prevalence rates in the world at 38% and 33% respectively) [21].

Unlike the West, which enjoyed robust economies and stable health and social services infrastructures, in the 1970s and 1980s—the timeframe in which AIDS originated and exploded in Africa—much of the continent was suffering with intractable poverty, crippling droughts and rampant malnutrition [19]. In addition, civil wars and cross-border conflicts contributed to famines, massive refugee flows and epidemics of various communicable diseases [19]. These and other cultural, socio-economic and political factors such as gender inequality, economic disparities and lack of political will facilitated the unchecked spread of HIV/AIDS and impeded a concentrated, remedial effort [22].

Also slowing the pace of progress was distrust of the West stemming from the history that preceded AIDS, particularly colonialism [23]. Early in his country's AIDS epidemic, Kenyan President Daniel arap Moi condemned the theory that AIDS originated in Africa, describing such Western assertions as 'a new form of hate campaign' [24]. Almost a decade later, South African President Thabo Mbeki would make almost the same argument, articulating his disbelief that a virus of African origin could kill so many of that continent's citizens. According to sociologist Deborah Posel, understanding Mbeki and Moi's collective mindset requires thinking about their beliefs within 'a background dominated by racist theories concerning the African sexual body which has been in common currency since the beginning of colonization' [25].

Distrust of the West and its medical and scientific technologies extends beyond the African continent. During a speech delivered at the African-American Summit in 1989, Nation of Islam leader Louis Farrakhan posited that 'the spread of international AIDS was an attempt by the US government to decimate the population of central Africa', a theory he reiterated on ABC television's *20/20* when he asked and answered his own rhetorical question: 'Do you know where the AIDS virus was developed? Right outside of Washington [DC]. It is my feeling that the US government is deliberately spreading AIDS' [26,27]. A 1999 study to explore whether African Americans believed that 'HIV/AIDS is a man-made virus that the federal government made to kill and wipe out [African Americans]' found that 27% thought as much, and another 23% were undecided [28].

An etiological escape into the unknown

By the end of 1981, many clinicians, including Gerald Friedland, an infectious disease specialist then practising in New York City, were witnessing the spread of the puzzling illness beyond homosexual men [29]. Friedland, who had treated infectious diseases in Africa, the Middle East and the United States for 15 years, was asked to consult on three cases of PCP among young men admitted to Montefiore Hospital. All denied being homosexual. It turned out they were heterosexual injection drug users (IDUs). Resistance to the idea that the illness could affect heterosexuals persisted, however. It took a full decade and public announcements that two prominent heterosexuals had acquired HIV—tennis player Arthur Ashe, Jr. and basketball player

Earvin 'Magic' Johnson—for the mainstream to grudgingly accept that, unlike the developing world where the disease affects the poor in general and women specifically, HIV's assault could in fact reach beyond homosexuality [30,31].

The fatal consequences of this new illness, the lack of understanding of its transmission, the marginal status of affected populations, as well as a resurgence of political conservatism in the United States, combined to create a situation in which medical uncertainties metamorphosed into politically saturated debates. Influenced by patients' self-reports of narcotics use, causal investigations focused on the common practice among young, homosexual partygoers of using inhaled amyl or butyl nitrate ('poppers') and other recreational drugs [32]. Within a year, as PCP and KS arose in non-homosexual populations, including haemophiliacs, Haitian immigrants and injection heroin users—the 'Four H's', as, when added to 'homosexuals', these populations came to be known—suspicions shifted to an infectious agent, and studies began looking at possible candidates, including cytomegalovirus (CMV) and the Epstein-Barr virus (EBV) [33].

Meanwhile, the search for the etiology of the illness continued across continents, leading to two momentous but contradictory (and controversial) announcements in 1983 and 1984. In a paper published in the 20 May 1983 issue of *Science*, virologist Luc Montagnier and his research team at the Pasteur Institute in Paris announced they had isolated a T-lymphotropic retrovirus they called lymphadenopathy-associated virus (LAV) that could be the cause of AIDS [34]. Samples of LAV culture were subsequently shared with the CDC, and within a year, US Secretary of Health and Human Services Margaret Heckler announced that a US National Cancer Institute (NCI) team had identified the causal viral agent. Led by biomedical researcher Robert Gallo, who in 1974 identified the first retrovirus in humans, the team named it human T-lymphotropic virus type III (HTLV-III) [35]. Subsequent investigations determined that LAV and HTLV-III were the same virus and that Gallo's HTLV-III was probably produced from the LAV culture sent from France the year before [36]. In 1986, the International Committee on the Taxonomy of Viruses settled on the name 'human immunodeficiency virus' [37], although the international scientific and diplomatic showdown over credit for discovery of the virus—and over royalties from sales of assays developed to detect the presence of antibodies to the virus—was not brought to a close until 1987. Its resolution was a profit-sharing arrangement between the Pasteur Institute and the US Department of Health and Human Services (DHHS) for the first serologic test for HIV, formally referred to as the Enzyme-Linked ImmunoSorbant Assay (ELISA), which the US Food and Drug Administration (FDA) approved in 1985 [38].

The name 'AIDS' was in wide use in both the public and scientific domains by 1982. In that same year, the CDC defined AIDS as 'a disease, at least moderately predictive of a defect in cell-mediated immunity, occurring in a person with no known cause for diminished resistance to that disease. Such diseases include KS, PCP, and serious [opportunistic infections (OIs)]' [39]. The CDC published an AIDS surveillance case definition in 1986 [40] that was later revised in 1987 to include 23 clinical conditions in three clinical categories:

♦ Category A, consisting of documented asymptomatic HIV infection, persistent generalized lymphadenopathy, and/or acute (primary) HIV infection with accompanying illness or history of acute HIV infection;

♦ Category B, consisting of symptomatic conditions either attributed to HIV infection or indicative of a defect in cell-mediated immunity, or considered by a clinician to have a clinical course or to require management that is complicated by HIV infection; and

♦ Category C, which includes the 23 clinical conditions listed in the AIDS surveillance case definition [41].

A further modification in 1993 added three more clinical conditions (pulmonary tuberculosis (TB), recurrent pneumonia and invasive cervical cancer), and expanded the 1986 definition to include HIV-infected individuals with CD4 counts of less than 200 cells/mm^3 or a CD4 percentage of less than 14% [42]. The CDC estimated that the addition of CD4 criteria could increase the number of AIDS cases reported in 1993 by as much as 75%. Researchers noted that this increase would include significant numbers of women, IDUs and people who had yet to develop AIDS-related symptoms. They also observed that the '[s]urvival of patients meeting the 1993 case definition is significantly longer than that of patients meeting the 1987 case definition', a fact that had profound implications for the economics of HIV/AIDS [43].

As the formalities of establishing its etiology and defining its clinical conditions proceeded at a seemingly glacial pace, HIV was beginning to leave a global footprint on every continent and across every demographic group. This reflected Nobel laureate Anatole France's dictum that 'nature is indifferent' [44], and sociologist Elizabeth Armstrong's notion that 'viruses do not respect social identity boundaries' [45].

From 1981 to 1996, the impact of HIV and AIDS was felt most acutely at individual and community levels. According to surgeon and medical historian Sherwin B Nuland, 'no matter the cultural and societal implications of AIDS, certain of its clinical and scientific manifestations must be understood before the full tragedy unfolds of how it kills its victim' [46]. One such 'victim' was Ismail Garcia, a patient that Mary Defoe first met when she was completing her medical internship at Yale-New Haven Hospital in Connecticut [47]. Infected by injecting heroin with an HIV-tainted needle, Garcia was diagnosed in February 1990 and, by January 1991, was among the countless numbers of patients with thrush and PCP. His CD4 count was 120 cells/mm^3. In January 1992, Garcia presented with worse symptoms, whose origin was determined as *Cryptococcus neoformans*, and his CD4 count dropped to 5 cells/mm^3. That summer, in response to reports of lethargy and confusion, a CT scan revealed a protozoan called *Toxoplasma gondii*, and he was diagnosed and treated for toxoplasmosis. Any gains were short-lived. By November 1992, Defoe stood at Garcia's bedside as he drew his last breath.

The human impact of HIV was similar in the developing world, although they did not have the benefit of similar resources with which to offer any therapeutic interventions. Pulitzer Prize-winning journalist Mark Schoofs, in his seminal eight-part series entitled *AIDS: The Agony of Africa*, described how a young Zimbabwean's family was decimated in the early 1990s. The case vividly illustrates the early history of HIV and its impact on families, friends and communities:

> They didn't call Arthur Chinaka out of the classroom. The principal and Arthur's uncle Simon waited until the day's exams were done before breaking the news: Arthur's father, his body wracked with pneumonia, had finally died of AIDS. They were worried that Arthur would panic, but at 17 years old, he didn't. He still had two days of tests, so while his father lay in the morgue, Arthur finished his exams. That happened in 1990. Then, in 1992, Arthur's uncle Edward died of AIDS. In 1994, his uncle Richard died of AIDS. In 1996, his uncle Alex died of AIDS. All of them are buried on the homestead where they grew up and where their parents and Arthur still live, a collection of thatch-roofed huts in the mountains near Mutare, by Zimbabwe's border with Mozambique. But HIV [hadn't] finished with this family. In April [1999], a fourth uncle lay coughing in his hut, and the virus had blinded Arthur's aunt Eunice, leaving her so thin and weak she couldn't walk without help. By September [1999] both were dead [48].

This was the natural history of HIV disease at that time, its impact reflecting the appalling patho-physiology of a disease that destroyed the very cells of the immune system whose job it is to coordinate the body's defences against invasion.

No continent left untouched

To categorize a disease as a 'pandemic', the World Health Organization (WHO) requires that it meet three conditions: first, it must emerge as a disease new to the population; second, its causative agent must infect humans and cause serious illness; and third, its causative agent must spread easily among humans [49]. Shortly after its onset, AIDS met those conditions, and by the mid-1980s, it became clear that its causative agent, HIV, had spread, largely unnoticed, throughout most of the world. In November 1983, the WHO hosted the first meeting to assess the virus's global impact. This commenced global surveillance of a pandemic known to be unfolding in Australia, Canada, Haiti, the United States and Zaire, as well as 15 Western European countries, seven Latin American countries and, potentially, Japan [50].

The first cases of HIV and AIDS in Western Europe involved two risk factors: homosexual or bisexual behaviour and injection drug use. By 1985, the majority (63%) of European adult cases were attributed to transmission among homosexual men [51]. In Denmark, West Germany and the United Kingdom, the majority of HIV diagnoses were among homosexual men. In contrast, by 1992, only 42% of the reported adult cases were due to this risk factor. The proportion of European AIDS cases infected through injection drug use increased from 5% in 1985 to 36% in the early 1990s [51]. In Spain and Italy, the major form of HIV transmission was established as injection drug use. However, data from Belgium and France suggested another AIDS epidemic occurring mainly in immigrants from Central Africa [52]. Examples of this second epidemic included a number of previously healthy African patients who were hospitalized in Belgium with cryptosporidiosis, KS, PCP and/or other AIDS-defining illnesses. These African patients all had immune deficiency similar to that of HIV-infected patients in the United States. There was, however, no history of blood transfusion, homosexuality or intravenous drug use. In light of such reports, European and American scientists would intensify their search for AIDS in Central Africa.

In Latin America and the Caribbean, the spread of HIV began in the early 1980s, predominantly among homosexual and bisexual men as well as in IDUs residing in large cities. While the spread appeared slower in this region, epidemiologists debunked this conclusion, regarding it to be based on unreliable data. Still, 12 countries in the region had HIV prevalence rates of 1% or more among pregnant women [51]. In several countries forming the poverty-stricken Caribbean Basin, adult HIV prevalence rates were soon surpassed only by rates in sub-Saharan Africa, making this the second most-affected region in the world [51].

South and South-East Asia were similarly affected in the mid- to late 1980s. By the early 1990s, India and Thailand accounted for the majority of reported HIV infections. In India, high levels of HIV prevalence were found among sex workers tested in Mumbai [51]. In Bangkok, prevalence among IDUs increased from less than 1% in late 1987 to almost 50% in 1990 [51]. By 1993, even the socially reserved People's Republic of China, with its iron grip on 'bad news', reported elevated rates of HIV infection. For example, Chinese authorities reported that 30% of IDUs in Yunnan Province were infected with HIV, an increase from the previously reported 10% [51].

For a number of years after the onset of the global AIDS pandemic, most countries in Eastern Europe and Central Asia appeared to have been spared by HIV/AIDS [53]. But between 1995 and 1998, former socialist economies of Eastern Europe and Central Asia saw their HIV infection rates climb almost sixfold, mostly among IDUs [51]. In countries such as Belarus and Ukraine, new infections jumped from virtually zero in 1995 to almost 20,000 a year from 1996 onward, with almost 80% involving injection drug use [51]. Following these rapid increases in Belarus and Ukraine in the mid-1990s, the epidemic would next explode in other countries in the region, including Latvia, Kazakhstan, Moldova and the Russian Federation.

A world caught off-guard

There have been other viruses with a human toll similar to that of HIV. For example, the WHO estimates that various influenza strains have been responsible for up to 5 million serious illnesses and as many as 500,000 deaths worldwide [54]. The 1918 Spanish influenza pandemic infected 20% of the world's population and killed between 50 and 100 million people [55]. But unlike other deadly pandemics, the HIV pandemic blossomed within a context of sexual politics and human rights. Until the appearance of HIV, the public health establishment was convinced that the threat of bacterial and viral disease was waning, and medical science seemed at liberty to conquer arthritis, cancer, cardiovascular disease and stroke. Hubris may have blinded many to the early warning signs of the looming AIDS threat, along with more basic biomedical challenges such as the emergence of drug resistant strains of bacteria [56]. As medical ethicist Stephen Genius argues, 'The medical community at times displays a lethargic and lackluster response to important scientific and epidemiological data that challenges prevailing conventional wisdom or that elucidates existing medical miscalculations' [57].

Scientists today theorize that HIV was endemic in a different form among Central African primates in which it was not a pathogen and therefore caused no disease [58]. Some hypothesize that blood from an infected primate may have come into contact with a skin or membrane wound in one or more inhabitants of a local village, who then gradually infected others in their immediate surroundings [58]. Due to sparse interactions among communities, the disease would have spread slowly from its hypothetical village of origin. Enter globalization and cultural change. Increased travel and urbanization accelerated the rate of new HIV infections. So, too, did the innovation of relatively inexpensive and accessible air travel, allowing HIV to cross regional, national and international borders [59]. This aspect of HIV transmission was popularized in *And the Band Played On*, in which Shilts referenced Gatean Dugas, the infamous 'Patient Zero' [6]. An HIV-infected flight attendant, Dugas figured in a 1984 CDC study as the likely source of infection of hundreds of other HIV-infected homosexual men [60]. US epidemiologist William Darrow, one of the 1984 CDC study collaborators, later clarified that Dugas had been referred to as 'Patient O', for 'Out of California', but that colleagues had misread the abbreviation, and the term 'Patient Zero' had given the mistaken impression that Dugas was the single individual responsible for introducing HIV to North America [61].

In the developed world, an early association of this new infectious disease with homosexual men, IDUs and dark-skinned immigrants combined with ominous epidemiological predictions to feed public ignorance regarding virus transmission. As late as 1991, a survey by the University of California at Davis found that a 'significant minority' of Americans held beliefs about HIV transmission that were at odds with established scientific consensus: 18.5% of respondents believed that infection was likely from kissing on the cheek; 47.85% believed that sharing a drinking glass could spread the virus; public toilets, coughing and sneezing, and insect bites were thought to transmit HIV by 34.3%, 45.4% and 50.1%, respectively [62]. In 1987, evolutionary biologist Stephen J Gould warned in *The New York Times* that AIDS could ultimately kill up to one quarter of the world's population [63]. There were also a number of fear-inspiring media accounts. In the early 1980s the major news wire services, including the Associated Press (AP) and United Press International (UPI), were skittish about using terminology such as anal and oral sex, which made accurate coverage of HIV transmission difficult. On 5 May 1982, UPI reported, 'The mysterious and deadly AIDS disease may be transmitted by routine close contact in a family household,' which was followed the next day by this AP lead: 'A study showing children may catch the deadly immune deficiency disease AIDS from their families could mean the general population is at greater risk' [64]. These stories were based on an article appearing in the *Journal of the American Medical Association* [65], though numerous paediatricians were available at the time to offer alternative—and more reasonable—explanations for why children born to high-risk mothers might have contracted the virus. These incidents were not isolated to the United States. Throughout the early and mid-1980s, UK newspapers such as *The Daily Telegraph* ran articles labelling AIDS 'the gay plague' [66]. Within a few years, as data reflecting the African origin of HIV were published, France, Germany, the United Kingdom and other countries with large African immigrant populations saw a disturbing slant in media coverage of AIDS, exposing an underlying link between HIV, racism and xenophobia [67].

Shortly after 1983, researchers concluded that an individual could only acquire the virus directly through the bloodstream or through sexual contact with mucosal membranes of an infected person [60]. There were no diagnosed HIV or AIDS cases among friends and family members of infected individuals who were not themselves IDUs or in sexual contact with infected individuals, and the CDC announced in 1983 that transmission via airborne and casual physical contact did not appear likely [68]. To allay healthcare professionals' concerns about providing services to HIV-infected patients, the US Public Health Service published a set of 'universal precautions' in 1983, which, although routinely updated, remain the gold standard for preventing occupational exposure to HIV [69]. Additional work by the CDC and other epidemiological institutions over the next several years plotted the estimated risks of HIV acquisition by exposure route (Table 2.1) [70].

In spite of this scientific consensus, pseudoscientific accounts of HIV transmission persisted. As described earlier, former US President Reagan made his first public statement about AIDS six years into the epidemic [5]. In response to a question about whether he would send a hypothetical child of his own to school with an HIV-infected child, he responded: 'I'm glad I'm not faced with that problem today,' and then added, 'It is true that some medical sources had said that this cannot be communicated in any way other than the ones we already know and which would not involve a child being in the school. And yet medicine has not come forth unequivocally and said, "This we know for a fact, that it is safe". And until they do, I think we just have to do the best

Table 2.1 Estimated per act risk for acquisition of HIV by exposure route

Exposure route	Estimated infections per 10,000 exposures to an infected source
Blood transfusion	9000
Childbirth	2500
Needle-sharing IDU	67
Receptive anal intercourse*	50
Percutaneous needle stick	30
Receptive penile-vaginal intercourse*	10
Insertive anal intercourse*	6.5
Insertive penile-vaginal intercourse*	5
Receptive oral intercourse*	1
Insertive oral intercourse*	0.5

* Assuming no condom use

Source: [70]

we can with this problem' [5]. Reagan's insinuation that infection by casual contact might still be a real threat came four years *after* his own CDC labelled such a hypothesis unlikely, and only three weeks after the agency issued a report advising that 'casual person-to-person contact as would occur among schoolchildren appears to pose no risk' [71].

Awakening to an 'existential' challenge

As previously discussed, the spread of AIDS in Africa began much earlier than in the industrialized world. Peter Piot, the clinician who discovered the Ebola virus in Zaire in 1976, and is now Executive Director of the Joint United Nations Programme on HIV/AIDS (UNAIDS), was among the first to witness its impact. As he noted in a *Washington Post* article on 5 July 2000: 'There were hardly any young adults there [at the 2,000-bed Mama Yemo Hospital in Kinshasa] except for traffic accidents in orthopaedic wards. Suddenly, boom, I walked in and saw all these young men and women, emaciated, dying' [72]. While the then 34-year-old Piot and other idealistic young health professionals were witnessing AIDS first-hand in developing countries, it was the onset of the HIV epidemic in the United States that finally gave a name to a phenomenon clinicians had been observing for some time.

Sero-archaeological tests identified HIV infection in individuals who had died in the early 1950s in Western Africa, and significant numbers of unexplained cases of severe wasting, diarrhoea, PCP and KS had begun to occur in Kinshasa in the mid-1970s [73,74]. It took a decade for HIV to spread throughout the sub-Saharan region. In 1985, an article entitled, 'Slim Disease: A New Disease in Uganda and its Association with HTLV-III Infection,' appeared in *The Lancet*. It recounted a wasting condition (currently known as wasting syndrome) observed since 1982 that primarily affected promiscuous heterosexuals [75]. In 1983, Piot was in Kinshasa leading a CDC/NIH team investigating an increase in reported AIDS cases. Western scientists and politicians did not take the team's finding—that heterosexual contact was the primary vector of HIV transmission—seriously [76]. Piot and his research colleagues had their manuscript submissions rejected by a dozen medical journals. Peer reviewers asserted the team must have overlooked alternate paths of transmission. At the first International AIDS Conference two years later in Atlanta, 'people came up to us and said this is nonsense,' Piot recalled. 'Denial has been a characteristic of this epidemic at all levels' [72]. Joe McCormick, a CDC epidemiologist and Piot's colleague in the Kinshasa investigation, asked the Reagan administration for funding to return to Zaire to conduct a larger study. According to Laurie Garrett, a former *Newsday* reporter and author of *The Coming Plague*, political appointees turned McCormick down, refusing to believe his finding that 'AIDS can be, and is, a heterosexual disease' [77].

There have been a number of reasons hypothesized for Africa's high prevalence of HIV and AIDS relative to Western countries, including endemic poverty and lack of education; widespread sexually transmitted infections (STIs), which increase the risk of transmitting and contracting HIV; widespread patterns of migrant labour; economic and social disempowerment of women, resulting in women being unable to demand that their sexual partners practise safer sex; large age disparities between sexual partners, leading to an intergenerational transfer of HIV uncommon in the West; and a tradition in some African countries of polygamy [58]. There is also growing evidence that other core factors may include concurrency of sexual partners and male circumcision [78, 79].

In the early years of the epidemic, official action from within Africa to combat AIDS was insufficient relative to the scale of the problem, as many African governments were either corrupt and ineffective at delivering services or were beset by political, economic and/or health crises (including epidemics of cholera, malaria and TB, and therefore lacked implementation resources. In 1983, Mobutu Sese Seko, then President of Zaire (now the Democratic Republic of Congo), banned any mention of the disease [80]. In the late 1980s, Kenya's President Moi gave orders that HIV-infected patients be quarantined, though the plan was never carried out [81]. Senior government officials in Côte d'Ivoire, Malawi and Zimbabwe ignored or were instructed not to discuss the issue, though Zimbabwe, in 1985, was the first developing country to mandate blood screening prior to transfusion [82–84]. In South Africa, while the government established working groups and an official advisory panel in the early 1980s to gather information and address the concerns of the white homosexual community, the apartheid regime did little to address the problem among Malawian migrant workers, which could have mitigated its impact in the majority black South African population [85].

Uganda and Senegal set examples at the other end of the spectrum. Uganda's President Yuweri Museveni, having taken power at the head of his National Resistance Army in 1986, was jolted into action when he discovered that 18 of 50 soldiers he sent to Cuba for training in the wake of his successful military campaign were HIV-positive [86]. Soon after, he established the AIDS Control Programme (ACP) to draft policies and coordinate blood screening, condom distribution and the promotion of safer sex and abstinence. The ACP developed a five-year plan, presented at the WHO's World Health Assembly (WHA) in 1987, which earned Uganda pledges of more than US$20 million from international donors. This policy approach dramatically decreased their HIV infection rates. Between 1990 and 2000, HIV prevalence in adults nationwide was estimated to have dropped from 14% to 8% [87].

Senegal and other countries in francophone Africa benefited from the fact that most infections there were HIV-2, a less virulent strain than the HIV-1 that plagues Western and other African countries [88]. Senegal had additional advantages in countering HIV, including a French tradition of regulating and inspecting the sex industry, a national STI programme that had been in effect well before the appearance of HIV, Islamic moral prohibitions against sexual promiscuity, and widespread male circumcision [89]. Combined with a government committed to public education, blood supply monitoring and community outreach, these characteristics prevented HIV prevalence rates in Senegal from reaching even 2% of the adult population [89].

A commitment by international institutions to confront the African AIDS pandemic was slow to materialize. The WHO was reluctant to throw its influence behind a full-throttle AIDS campaign, not only because it believed the disease to be a problem of industrialized countries, but also because its leadership was already committed to expanding primary care in the region and battling endemic diseases such as malaria and TB that were killing millions each year [90]. However, by 1986, the scope of the threat posed by HIV infection was coming into focus, and the WHO proposed what would later become known as the Global Programme on AIDS (GPA). Clinician and human rights advocate Jonathan Mann was the GPA's first Executive Director.

Under Mann's leadership, the GPA, which was the precursor to UNAIDS established in 1996, saw its budget increase from US$1 million to more than US$100 million annually. It focused on preventing new infections through screening blood supplies, clinical and counselling training for healthcare professionals and the establishment of public education programmes to discourage prejudice and stigmatization of HIV-infected people [91]. Mann resigned in 1990 in protest against the failure of the United Nations and governments worldwide to respond to the burgeoning AIDS pandemic. Throughout his tenure at GPA and in the years that followed, he devoted much of his time and energy to structuring AIDS as a human rights issue, founding several human rights-focused, non-governmental institutions including the François Xavier Bagnoud Center for Health and Human Rights. He and his wife and fellow AIDS researcher Mary-Lou Clements-Mann, died tragically in the 1998 crash of Swissair flight 111 [92].

Prevention and vaccine focal points

Prior to the advent of HAART in 1996, AIDS activism and many of the clinical community's efforts in the industrialized world were focused on prevention. The earliest programmes dedicated to behavioural interventions sprang up within the homosexual communities in New York City and San Francisco in an attempt to educate their constituents about symptoms, treatment and risk-reduction through safer-sex practices. Government-sponsored and grass-roots efforts proliferated after the identification of HIV as the causal agent. Research by the CDC indicates, '[b]ehavioral interventions were observed to substantially reduce HIV risk while remaining cost effective or cost saving for a wide range of populations at high risk' [93].

Prevention took a step forward in 1985 when the FDA approved the first commercial serologic test to detect HIV antibodies—the aforementioned ELISA [94]. The test was put to use throughout the United States in blood banks, health departments and other clinical settings, and by the end of 1985, more than 79,000 Americans had been tested. The FDA approved a second test, the Western blot test kit, in 1987 [94].

Preventive vaccine research remained mired in technical challenges, despite assurances in 1984 by the Reagan Administration's Secretary of Health and Human Services that a vaccine would be available within two years [95]. The most salient characteristic of HIV, its remarkable capacity for generating 10^9–10^{10} virions every day coupled with a high mutation rate of approximately 3×10^{-5} per nucleotide base per cycle of replication [33], is responsible for the scientific barrier to preventive vaccine development. In fact, after 10 to 20 years of infection, the HIV in a patient's body will have mutated at a rate about equal to the average mutation rate of human beings over the course of the past few million years [33]. The theory underlying vaccination is that exposing the human adaptive immune system to the infectious agent will enable it to learn and recognize appropriate defences. However, HIV specifically targets and destroys human immune response itself and mutates too quickly to be recognized by a host immune system that has been exposed to genetically distinct variations [33]. The NIH began the first clinical trial of a preventive HIV vaccine in 1987, when 138 uninfected volunteers with a history of high-risk behaviours received the gp160 subunit candidate vaccine [95]. Although the volunteers experienced no serious adverse effects, gp160 proved ineffective at preventing HIV infection. Dozens of other vaccine strategies have been tested since 1987, but none has been successful to date [96].

The 'dark ages' of HIV/AIDS treatment

In the 'dark ages' of HIV treatment, the first efforts at combating the disease focused on treating each OI with chemical agents already in use. For example, the over 50% of HIV-infected patients who typically developed PCP were treated with pentamidine, or a combination of sulfamethoxazole and trimethoprim, while patients developing fungal infections such as thrush and cryptococcal meningitis were prescribed fluconazole [97–99]. These interventions offered relief from pain and discomfort associated with the OIs, and they were able to prolong life by a few months. But it was soon obvious to clinicians, researchers and patients that scattershot tactics focusing on remediating the separate consequences of immune suppression were not the right approach. Some hope was generated by peptides such as thymic humoral factor (THF), which had been shown in laboratory tests to create immune responses in mice that had been genetically engineered to have no natural immune system functions [100]. This strategy, however, proved ineffective when applied to HIV-infected patients.

The search for drug therapies that would cure AIDS or stall immune dysfunction was a difficult undertaking that required immense financial and scientific resources.

Pharmaceutical companies were reluctant to enter the search for a drug to treat HIV because profits from the market for such a drug were unlikely to offset the required research and development costs [101]. Consequently, the first promising clinical trial of an experimental antiretroviral drug began in February 1986 and was undertaken by an NCI team headed by US researcher Sam Broder [102]. The team first tested azidothymidine, also known as AZT, which had been synthesized in the 1960s under an NIH grant as an anti-cancer agent. While it failed to show efficacy against cancer growth, UK pharmaceutical giant Burroughs Wellcome purchased its rights and intended to test it for use against the herpes virus [103]. Although AZT also proved ineffective against herpes, it did appear to block the conversion of HIV RNA into viral DNA *in vitro*, blocking integration of viral DNA into the cell DNA of the host [102].

Early laboratory success led to the initiation of the first AZT phase II clinical trial (officially known as BW 002) in 1986 [104]. This was a double-blind study consisting of 282 patients with AIDS or advanced HIV disease, in which 145 patients were treated with AZT, and the remaining 137 received a placebo. When interim data were analyzed in September 1986 (approximately six months after the trial began), only one patient who had received AZT had died, compared with 19 patients in the control group. Twenty-four patients in the AZT experimental arm had developed OIs, compared with 45 placebo recipients. Azidothymidine recipients also demonstrated improved body weight, better scores on a key clinical measure of patient fitness and increased CD4 counts. When the stunning interim results of the BW 002 clinical trial were released, the trial was shut down by the US National Institute of Allergy and Infectious Diseases (NIAID) data and safety monitoring board, which cited ethical prohibitions against continued use of placebos in clinical trials with demonstrable effects [105]. The demand for effective antiretroviral drugs and the growing intensity of civil society's attacks on the US government for dragging its feet led the FDA to approve AZT in January 1987, a mere six months after the regulatory process had begun, a record in the agency's history [106].

Many scientists and clinicians criticized the premature termination of the BW 002 clinical trial, claiming that the observation period was too short to determine whether the positive effects were durable or whether the potential toxicities outweighed the benefits. There were also unanswered questions about the clinical utility of the drug, such as when to initiate its use. All trial participants had already contracted HIV or had advanced disease symptoms, so the question was, 'what would be the consequences for asymptomatic individuals who insisted on beginning therapy early?' Nonetheless, the world was ready for some good news in the fight against HIV and AIDS, and objections of the few were drowned out by the hopeful clamour of more sanguine researchers who were themselves becoming a new breed of AIDS activists.

Among these researcher-activists was Mathilde Krim, then a research scientist at the Sloan-Kettering Institute for Cancer Research in New York City. In 1983, she co-founded the AIDS Medical Foundation (AMF), a research organization that would, two years later, merge with the National AIDS Research Foundation of Los Angeles (NARF) to form the American Foundation for AIDS Research, or AmFAR. Within a year of the merger, AmFAR, whose celebrity spokesperson was Academy award-winning actress Elizabeth Taylor, awarded US$1.5 million in research grants [6]. Within the span of a decade, AmFAR awarded over US$77 million in grants to more than 1600 research projects worldwide for biomedical research around the CCR5 co-receptor (which would yield a new class of antiretroviral drugs known as CCR5 antagonists), the viral enzyme protease (which would herald the protease inhibitor (PI) class of antiretroviral drugs) and HIV DNA candidate vaccines (which would jump-start pharmaceutical company engagement in the development and testing of more than a dozen candidate vaccines by 2007) [107].

Civil society Acts Up and commemorates

The FDA's approval of AZT catalyzed community-based AIDS activism. In March 1987, author and playwright Larry Kramer and a group of activists from New York City's Lesbian and Gay Community Service Center formed the AIDS Coalition to Unleash Power, or ACT UP [108]. These pioneering activists coalesced out of frustration with the unwillingness of other civil society groups to engage in confrontational political organizing against a federal government they viewed as unconcerned with the fate of people living with HIV/AIDS. Like many other groups, ACT UP advocated education and AIDS prevention efforts, federally funded needle exchange sites and condom distribution programmes. But 'life during wartime' was saturated with a sense of urgency that motivated ACT UP to do more, and do it more aggressively [108]. The group became best known for its carnival-style cultural politics of street theatre and civil disobedience. Its many accomplishments include efforts at forcing the FDA to shorten its approval process for experimental AIDS drugs, eliminating placebo-controlled AIDS drug studies altogether and confronting pharmaceutical companies over high prices of AIDS drugs already on the market. ACT UP held its first demonstration on Wall Street on 24 March 1987 in protest against Burroughs Wellcome's decision to price a year's worth of AZT for one person at approximately US$10,000 [108]. Other activist groups followed suit, borrowing the tactic of civil disobedience from the African American civil rights movement to garner media attention and shame the federal government and industry into getting 'Drugs into Bodies'. According to one study by the National Research Council (NRC), their efforts were remarkably successful:

> Advocacy groups made the FDA their prime focus, and from 1987 to 1989 they steadily and forcefully challenged the FDA to widen and speed the availability of drugs for AIDS. In addition, the Reagan administration, with its general philosophy of deregulation, became a sympathetic (if ironic) partner in the push toward greater consumer choice in AIDS drugs. Together, patient activism, a political climate favoring deregulation, and the exigency of an epidemic disease drove the most dramatic changes in drug regulation since the Kefauver-Harris legislation [a bill requiring drug manufacturers to provide proof of the efficacy and safety of their drugs before FDA approval] of 1962 [109].

Shortly after 1000 ACT UP demonstrators shut down operations at the FDA, the regulatory agency announced it was decreasing the drug approval timeline by two years [94]. Other ACT UP actions included sit-ins targeting Burroughs Wellcome, possibly leading to a 20% price reduction for AZT in 1989, and disruption of academic, industry and media events [92]. Among the activists' other achievements was persuading the FDA to codify the ambiguous 'compassionate use of drugs' provision that would allow limited numbers of HIV-infected patients to receive drugs that had shown efficacy in the pre-approval (but post-phase I) stage of investigation [110]. This concession by the FDA eventually led to the acceptance of another activist demand, namely the establishment of the 'parallel track' concept, whereby any drug that was proven effective in a phase I (non-human) trial and safe in a truncated phase II trial could be widely distributed [94]. The unprecedented success of the AIDS activist community in integrating itself into the policy and scientific decision-making processes is nowhere more apparent than in the formal establishment of the Community Constituency Group as a committee of the US AIDS Clinical Trials Group (ACTG) in 1990, which gave activists input into all aspects of the regulatory process, including actual clinical trial design [111].

In addition to their efforts to alter the research and treatment landscape, AIDS activists became entrenched in political movements to force the US government to take action to protect HIV-infected individuals from discrimination and to improve the quality and availability of care for low-income, under- or uninsured individuals and families affected by HIV. Activism succeeded in ensuring the inclusion of HIV/AIDS as a disability under the Americans with

Disabilities Act (ADA), a comprehensive law passed in 1990 that eliminated employment discrimination on the basis of disability [112]. The second victory came that same year when the US Congress enacted the Ryan White Comprehensive AIDS Resources Emergency (CARE) Act, which established the United States' largest federally funded social safety-net programme after Medicaid and Medicare. The programme was named after Ryan White, a haemophiliac diagnosed with HIV at age 13, whose courageous struggle against AIDS-related discrimination educated the nation about the persistent stigma and discrimination suffered by people living with HIV/AIDS [113]. He died on 8 April 1990. Yet his legacy continues through the Ryan White CARE Act, which today funds programmes that deliver care and support services to more than 500,000 HIV-infected individuals each year [113].

People were still dying despite such gains. In February 1987, San Francisco activists Cleve Jones and Joseph Durant made the first two fabric panels of the AIDS Memorial Quilt. Approximately the dimensions of a human grave, each 3 x 6-foot panel commemorated an individual who had died of AIDS-related complications. Inspired in November 1985, 'when the number of San Franciscans dead from AIDS reached 1,000,' Jones reminisced:

> So many had died, and there'd been no memorial .... If there was an obituary, and often there was not, it would describe the cause of death as cancer. The slate was wiped clean, as if this person had never been. Close friends were erased; lovers were never identified. Every one of us, whether friend or family, felt the empty echo of loss and grief and saw no way to express it. We were on the wrong side of a cultural canyon. I wanted to change all that, and believed that when we unfolded thousands of quilts on the National Mall, the stony walls of Congress would come tumbling down and the nation would awaken—that our quilt, my quilt, would crash through the fear and indifference. [5]

The AIDS Memorial Quilt had its inaugural display on the US Capitol at the 1987 National March on Washington for Lesbian and Gay Rights [114]. According to the NAMES Project Foundation, which is responsible for its maintenance, 20 years later, in 2007, the quilt contained more than 44,000 memorial panels [115]. The last display of the quilt in its entirety—which was also the first time an American president visited it—took place on the Mall in Washington, DC in October 1996 [116]. Under the auspices of the Dutch-based Global Quilt, an international version of the quilt has toured Africa, Asia, Eastern Europe, the Caribbean and South America since 1992 [117].

As commemoration continued internationally, the world experienced an increase in new HIV infections, which produced a need for emergency social services resembling those provided by relief agencies in the aftermath of natural disasters or prolonged wars. Activist groups worldwide, such as the Treatment Action Campaign (TAC) in South Africa, raised global awareness and forced action [118]. This impact mirrored the safety net of critical services, volunteer-supported community-based organizations (CBOs) such as the Gay Men's Health Crisis (GMHC) in New York City and Deutsche AIDS-Hilfe in Berlin, which helped people living with HIV/AIDS maintain and improve their health and independence [119,120]. In San Francisco, CBOs developed early to care for the sick and the dying. Within the first few years of the city's HIV epidemic, civil society groups constructed a collaborative network of city and state agencies, hospitals and healthcare providers at whose helm were many CBO leaders. This complex network became known as 'the San Francisco model' of AIDS care and has long been considered a successful approach to community mobilization [119]. Similarly, The AIDS Support Organisation (TASO) was founded in 1987 to help Ugandans confront the stigma, ignorance and discrimination associated with an HIV diagnosis [121]. Its members were either HIV-infected or affected because their loved ones were HIV-positive. In addition to offering psychological and social support, TASO visits HIV-infected people in their homes, transports them to the hospital when needed, and provides food and other material support. Much like the 'San Francisco model,' TASO's work would be replicated in the coming years throughout sub-Saharan Africa.

The health professions rally against AIDS and advocate social justice

The role of the physician as an activist for social justice is not a novel one. For example, Rudolf Virchow, a German physician who is regarded as the founder of the medical disciplines of cellular and comparative pathology, became an activist to promote the democratic revolutions sweeping across Europe in the late 1800s, with a special emphasis on yet another new medical discipline—social medicine—which focused on the fact that disease is never purely biological, but often socially derived [122]. And in the United States of the late nineteenth to early twentieth centuries, physicians such as Charles Victor Roman, an African American ophthalmologist (and the first editor of the *Journal of the American Medical Association* (1909–1916)), engaged in social activism against racial prejudice by stressing the contributions of African Americans to American civilization and maintaining that 'racial solidarity and not amalgamation is the desired and desirable goal of the American Negro' [123]. So, too, did HIV/AIDS-treating physicians—first in the United States and subsequently internationally—take up social activism in the face of HIV/AIDS. Taking their cue from community activists who had rallied for their HIV-positive friends and loved ones (and often also for themselves), in the mid-1980s groups of medical professionals began to formally organize themselves into associations and societies. Among their ranks were individuals who tended to patients 'by day' and 'by night' engaged in civil disobedience and/or behind-the-scenes activism.

The first organization to rally the health professions was the Physicians Association for AIDS Care (PAAC), which was incorporated in 1987 and brought together more than 500 physicians at its peak, including Paul J Cimoch, who was then seeing Florida's first AIDS cases at the University of Miami (and subsequently in private practice in Fort Lauderdale, Florida). Cimoch served as the second President of PAAC (1991–1993), and he remembers that prior to the Association's creation, 'We were pretty much on our own' [124]. This non-profit organization, whose mission was to educate physicians at a time when HIV treatment options were limited, was the precursor to the International Association of Physicians in AIDS Care (IAPAC). IAPAC itself was incorporated as a non-profit in 1995 (a year before the advent of HAART) and today represents more than 13,000 physicians in 103 countries [125]. Throughout its five-year history, PAAC delivered pre-HAART-era education about quality of life considerations (e.g. nutrition, pain management), therapeutic interventions against OIs and other complications of HIV disease [124]. It also tackled contentious public policy issues. For instance, PAAC engaged in a public confrontation in 1991 with the American Medical Association (AMA) and the American Dental Association (ADA), both of which were proposing the imposition of sanctions against HIV-infected healthcare workers [126] after a CDC investigation conducted earlier that year determined that an HIV-positive Florida dentist had probably transmitted HIV to three of his patients, all of whom were unaware of their serostatus [127]. The CDC would ultimately resolve the dispute by issuing less restrictive guidelines stating that HIV-positive clinicians and dentists should secure permission from local panels of experts before continuing to perform certain procedures. [128]

Similarly, the non-profit Association of Nurses in AIDS Care (ANAC) was founded in 1987 to promote professional development among nurses working in HIV/AIDS as well as to marshal the nursing profession's resources to advocate for the rights of all people affected by the disease [129]. The International AIDS Society (IAS) was founded a year later to host the biennial international AIDS conferences, which have become a global forum for the exchange of ideas, knowledge and research, as well as serving as a network for all professionals and paraprofessionals working in various aspects of HIV advocacy, care, research, prevention and treatment [130].

Fear, confusion and limited clinical benefit mark the pre-HAART era

For Wafaa El-Sadr, an infectious disease specialist at the Veterans' Hospital in New York City who was among that city's first physician-activists, the mid-1980s were 'really scary. We had no clue what we were doing, and in retrospect we made a lot of mistakes. ... We used medications in the wrong doses; we used stuff that there was better treatment for. We didn't anticipate things. We were just reacting. There was nothing you could anticipate, no way in which you could see a clear path for that patient. You just didn't know what the heck was going on' [29].

Treatment confusion persisted in spite of the excitement produced by the first AZT trial and the sophistication of AIDS activists. Results from follow-up studies suggested that optimism concerning AZT monotherapy was premature. In 1989, the first major ACTG trial (ACTG 019) focused on asymptomatic individuals with CD4 counts of less than 500 cells/mm^3. It found no survival benefits in either AZT experimental group (one receiving 1,500 mg/day, the other 500 mg/day) compared with placebo recipients, although AZT was associated with a decrease in the rate of HIV progression [131]. European and Australian research confirmed these findings, particularly the Concorde study [132]. Ironically, the success achieved by activists in making AZT more widely available contributed to a movement against the drug because more patients were experiencing its side effects, including nausea, headaches, anaemia and bone marrow suppression. Side effect severity would lead some within the AIDS movement to repudiate its use altogether and to actually blame the drug for AIDS-associated mortality [133].

Azidothymidine's limited benefit for people with 'full-blown AIDS' was still preferable to the lack of effective therapy that had prevailed before. And the 1996 ACTG 076 study had major implications for prevention of mother-to-child transmission (MTCT) of HIV [134]. According to an NIH press release, 'The first publication from ACTG 076 analyzed data from 363 mother-infant pairs in which at least one culture of the infant's blood had been performed, and demonstrated that the AZT regimen reduced mother-to-infant transmission by approximately two-thirds, with minimal short-term toxic effects' [135].

Research and development of other antiretroviral drugs continued. Lessons learned from AZT advanced this effort, including recognition of drug resistance after the first AZT-resistant strain of HIV was identified in 1989 [136]. Two trials, Delta and ACTG 175, showed the combination of AZT plus two other experimental nucleoside reverse transcriptase inhibitors (NRTIs), didanosine (ddI) or zalcitabine (ddC), were more effective than AZT monotherapy in delaying disease progression and prolonging life [137,138]. By November 1995, besides AZT, the FDA had approved ddI, ddC and two other NRTIs, stavudine (d4T) and lamivudine (3TC), all with approval times of less than eight months [94]. Having a wider array of antiretroviral drugs was helpful for patients who experienced drug intolerance, although later studies determined that NRTI-only regimens did not typically result in high levels of viral suppression, exacerbating the emerging problem of drug resistance [139].

The year 1993 often marks one of the low points in the fight against HIV/AIDS. Reports from the IX International AIDS Conference in Berlin were almost universally dismal, with one delegate describing the atmosphere as having been 'permeated' by 'therapeutic nihilism' [140]. Although multiple drugs had either been tested or were being tested—including AZT, ddI, ddC, tat inhibitors, compound Q, peptide T, dextran sulfate and AL721—all demonstrated little or no benefit [140]. However, research was presented on the penultimate day of the conference showing that a PI, which represented a new class of antiretroviral drug, 'markedly inhibited replication of the HIV-1 isolates *in vitro*, regardless of the susceptibility of the isolates to [AZT] or [ddI]' [141]. HIV-infected patients would have to wait until FDA approval of the first PI, saquinavir (SQV), in December 1995 before the path to optimal 'combination therapy' became clear. Thus, 1993 was a watershed year that would usher in HAART. Although complex and difficult to personalize based on individual side effects and resistance concerns, combination therapy would quickly represent a lifeline for many HIV-infected patients marooned on a therapeutic island with too few options to keep them alive.

Breakthroughs on the road to HAART

With the advent and through the evolution of HAART, researchers wrestled with the kinetics of HIV: the length of the virus' half-life, how often it reproduced and whether viral load decreased significantly following initial infection, as assays then available seemed to indicate. These questions had to be answered for scientists to avoid ineffective or harmful treatment models. There was also uncertainty regarding how to measure the progression of HIV disease and which measures had the most predictive value for the future course of an individual's infection.

A breakthrough came in 1995 with the publication in the British journal *Nature* of a paper entitled, 'Rapid Turnover of Plasma Virions and CD4 Lymphocytes in HIV-1 Infection,' co-authored by *Time Magazine*'s 1995 Man of the Year, David Ho, and his colleagues from the Aaron Diamond AIDS Research Center in New York City [142]. Ho learned about HIV's lifecycle by treating study participants with a PI to decrease virus production within a short time. He thus established a baseline against which to compare and measure the rate of subsequent virus replication. Applying the new technology of polymerase chain reaction (PCR) testing, Ho then measured rates of HIV replication and mutation and found large quantities of heretofore undetected virus could be identified in certain reservoirs, including lymph nodes, spinal fluid, plasma and peripheral blood mononuclear cells [142]. This research had enormous implications for therapeutic approaches to HIV disease and laid the foundation for combination therapy. Ho summarized his study's finding in a 1997 paper also published in *Nature*: 'The continuous high-level replication of the virus is the principal engine driving the pathogenesis of this viral infection. This new paradigm has in turn allowed us to formulate therapeutic strategies to effectively control HIV-1 in infected persons' [143].

John Mellors and researchers at the University of Pittsburg published a paper the following year in the *Annals of Internal Medicine* that confirmed this new approach. They argued that viral load testing, which had become available in 1995, was the strongest indicator of the effects of antiretroviral therapy [144]. This meant that accurate monitoring and therapeutic adjustment could now be carried out over the course of a few days, as compared with the months or years that were required when the sole laboratory method available was measuring declines in CD4 counts.

HAART heralds the extension and enhancement of life with HIV

For the first time in the history of the HIV epidemic in the United States, the CDC heralded a decrease in deaths among Americans living with AIDS. In its 2 February 1996 announcement, the CDC stated the decline was due to the slowing of the epidemic overall and to improved treatment options over the years [145]. Clinical documentation would soon follow in the United States and Western Europe, with population-based studies showing a 60–80% reduction in new AIDS-defining conditions, hospitalizations and deaths [146,147]. While it was too soon to determine the impact PIs would have on these trends, many clinicians and researchers predicted that this new class of antiretroviral drugs would lengthen the lifespan of HIV-infected patients.

The CDC also announced that the estimated number of Americans diagnosed with AIDS each year was continuing to slow, with an increase of only 2% in 1995. Such announcements bespoke the success of community-based prevention efforts [145].

As the death toll from AIDS and the spread of HIV receded in the United States and other industrialized countries, the same was not true in the rest of the world, especially the sub-Saharan African region. As a result of poverty, conflict, violence against women and girls, a lack of appropriate education, high-risk behaviour, gender inequality and a number of other factors, AIDS was fast on its way to undermining economic and human development efforts and exacerbating pre-existing endemic problems [148]. Callisto Madavo, the World Bank's Vice President for Africa, accurately predicted in 1998 that life expectancy in more than a dozen sub-Saharan African countries would be 17 years shorter because of AIDS [149]. Within the span of 18 years, the sub-Saharan African region would be home to two-thirds of the world's HIV-infected people (though only 10% of the world's population lives south of the Sahara Desert), as well as 12 million children orphaned by AIDS [150].

The year 1996 also witnessed seismic developments in the field of HIV/AIDS research that offered an opportunity to preserve health and life for many HIV-infected patients, *except* for the 90% of HIV-infected people in the developing world for whom such new therapeutic approaches were out of reach [151]. Several studies published that year—and many presented at the XI International AIDS Conference held in Vancouver that year—indicated that a new means of combating HIV infection might hold virus levels down below those seen with long-term non-progressors. This enabled researchers to maintain hope that new treatment strategies, properly applied on a large enough population, could alter the natural history of HIV disease, keeping hundreds of thousands of HIV-infected patients healthy longer and extending their lives.

Evidence that this might be possible began to emerge in February 1996 with the new PI ritonavir (RTV). When added to an antiretroviral regimen with an NRTI backbone, one six-month study showed that RTV cut rates of progression to AIDS and death by half [152]. Such dramatic, albeit short-term, effects on survival had not been seen with an antiretroviral drug since AZT in 1987. As AIDS activist Mark Harrington pointed out:

> Considering the barbaric state of the art of managing AIDS in 1987, compared with the far more sophisticated prevention and treatment of opportunistic complications prevalent in the mid-1990s, the impact of the [RTV] study was even more dramatic, demonstrating that potent new agents could rapidly prove clinical efficacy, and that antiretroviral therapy was still effective in patients with advanced symptoms [153].

The RTV study marked the end of an era. By mid-1996, once RTV and other PIs such as SQV and indinavir (IDV) were on the market, studies comparing PIs to a background of NRTIs would become outmoded [131]. At the same time, more studies confirmed that plasma HIV RNA levels were the most powerful surrogate markers for antiretroviral therapy effect, and that changes in plasma RNA levels could be used for initiating and switching antiretroviral regimens [154]. A new class of antiretroviral drugs, the non-nucleoside reverse transcriptase inhibitors (NNRTIs), was added to the anti-HIV repertoire in June 1996 with the FDA-approved release of nevirapine (NVP) [94].

The developments unveiled at the XI International AIDS Conference produced a new paradigm for treating HIV. With single antiretroviral drugs, HIV developed single or multiple protein mutations, which rendered those drugs inactive [155]. With two or three potent antiretroviral drugs simultaneously applied in a treatment-naïve patient, the results were consistently superior: viral levels were driven so low that drug resistance was delayed, if not prevented altogether [146]. Six individual studies of different antiretroviral regimens in varying patient populations were presented in Vancouver, and they all demonstrated that plasma viral RNA levels could be reduced to undetectable levels within three months in virtually all patients able to adhere to their regimens [156–162]. The studies ranged from combinations of three NRTIs (AZT, ddI and NVP) to those of two PIs (RTV and SQV), from newly infected patients to those with CD4 counts over 50 cells/mm^3, and from treatment-naïve patients to those with extensive prior exposure.

These breakthroughs were universally celebrated. They did, however, pose questions for clinical researchers and public health practitioners. The former confronted the issue of eliminating viral reservoirs and immune recovery from HIV-induced dysfunction and lymphoid destruction [163]. On a public health level, assuring access to and information about HAART posed an incredible challenge, even in the developed world, and chances of extending HAART's use in the developing world appeared slender given the lack of global commitment to providing universal healthcare that existed at that time [164]. Still, after so many years of fighting a 'losing battle' against an insidious virus that had, by December 1996, infected an estimated 21 million adults and 800,000 children worldwide [165], many combat-weary foot soldiers celebrated the advent of HAART as a milestone in medicine and a potential 'silver bullet' to stem the tide of suffering and death caused by HIV/AIDS in the pre-HAART era.

References

1. CDC. (1981). *Pneumocystis* Pneumonia – Los Angeles. *Morbidity & Mortality Weekly Report* **30**:1–3; 250–252.
2. Mayer K, Pfizer H, eds. (2005). *The AIDS Pandemic*. San Diego: Elsevier Academic Press.
3. CDC. (1981). Kaposi's Sarcoma and Pneumocystis Pneumonia among homosexual men – New York City and California. *Morbidity & Mortality Weekly Report* **30**:305–308.
4. Wallis C. (2005). AIDS: A Growing Threat. *Time Magazine*, April 18, 2005.
5. Jones C, Dawson J. (2000). *Stitching a Revolution: The Making of an Activist*. New York: HarperSanFrancisco.
6. Shilts R. (1987). *And the Band Played On: Politics, People, and the AIDS Epidemic*. New York: St. Martin's Press.
7. Padgug RA. (1989). Gay Villain, Gay Hero: Homosexuality and the Social Construction of AIDS. In: Peiss K, Simmons C, eds. *Passion and Power: Sexuality in History*. Philadelphia: Temple University Press. p293–313.
8. Buchanan P. (1983). Nature's Retribution. *Washington Times*, May 27, 1983.
9. Van J. (1985). Hudson AIDS Case Turns Spotlight on Drug Approval Process. *Chicago Tribune*, August 4, 1985.
10. Blumenfeld WJ, ed. (1992). *Homophobia: How We All Pay the Price*. Boston: Beacon Press.
11. Buckley WF. (1986). Crucial Steps in Combating the AIDS Epidemic: Identify All Carriers. *New York Times*, March 18, 1986.
12. Kaiser C. (1997). *The Gay Metropolis: The Landmark History of Gay Life in America Since World War II*. New York: Harcourt Brace.
13. Schlager N, ed. (1998). *Gay and Lesbian Almanac*. Detroit and New York: St. James Press.
14. Marcus E. (2002). *Making Gay History: The Half-Century Fight for Lesbian and Gay Equal Rights*. New York: Perennial.
15. Rimmerman CM. (1998). US Congress. In: Smith RA, ed. *The Encyclopedia of AIDS: A Social, Political, Cultural, and Scientific Record of the HIV Epidemic*. Chicago: Fitzroy Dearborn Publishers.
16. Adam, BD. (1995). *The Rise of the Gay and Lesbian Movement*. New York: Twayne Publishers.
17. Fauci AS. (1996). Immunopathogenic mechanisms of HIV infection. *Annals of Internal Medicine* **124**:654–663.
18. Sontag S. (1988). *AIDS and its Metaphors*. New York: Farrar, Straus, and Giroux.
19. Reader J. (1999). *Africa: A Biography of the Continent*. New York: Vintage.

20. Caraë M. (2006). Twenty Years of Intervention and Controversy. In: Denis P, Becker C, eds. *The HIV/AIDS Epidemic in Sub-Saharan Africa in a Historical Perspective.* Louvain-la-Neuve: Academia-Bruylant and Paris: Karthala (joint publication). p29–40.

21. Quinn TC. (1996). Global burden of the HIV pandemic. *Lancet* **348**:99–105.

22. Barnett T, Blaike P. (1992). *AIDS in Africa: Its Present and Future Impact.* New York, London: Guilford Press.

23. Comaroff J. (1993). The Diseased Heart of Africa: Medicine, Colionialism, and the Black Body. In: Lindenbaum S, Lock M, eds. *Knowledge, Power, and Practice: The Anthropology of Medicine and Everyday Life.* Berkeley: University of California Press. p305–329.

24. Shah S. (2006). *The Body Hunters: Testing New Drugs on the World's Poorest Patients.* New York: The New Press.

25. Posel B. (2004). Politiques de la Vie et Politisation de la Sexualité: Lectures de la Controverse sur le Sida. In: Fassin D, ed. *Afflictions: L'Afrique du Sud, de l'apartheid au sida.* Paris: Karthala. p 44–74.

26. Richburg K. (1997). Out of America: A Black Man Confronts Africa. New York: Basic Books.

27. Harris SB. (1995). The AIDS heresies: A case study in skepticisms taken too far. *Skeptic* **3**:42–58.

28. Klonoff EA, Landrine H. (1999). Do blacks believe that HIV/AIDS is a government conspiracy against them? *Preventive Medicine* **28**:451–457.

29. Bayer R, Oppenheimer GM. (2000). AIDS *Doctors: Voices from the Epidemic, An Oral History.* New York: Oxford University Press.

30. Rhoden WC. (1992). An emotional Ashe says that he has AIDS. *New York Times,* April 9, 1992.

31. Stevenson RW. (1991). Magic Johnson ends his career, saying he has AIDS infection. *New York Times,* November 8, 1991.

32. Goedert JJ, Neuland CY, Wallen WC. (1982). Amyl nitrate may alter T lymphocytes in homosexual men. *Lancet* **1**:412–416.

33. Levy JA. (1994). *HIV and the Pathogenesis of AIDS.* Washington, DC: ASM Press.

34. Barre-Sinoussi F, Chermann JC, Rey F, et al. (1983). Isolation of a T-lymphotropic retrovirus from a patient at risk for acquired immune deficiency syndrome (AIDS). *Science* **220**:868–871.

35. Gallo RC, Sarin PS, Glemann EP, et al. (1983). Isolation of human T-cell leukemia virus in acquired immune deficiency syndrome (AIDS). *Science* **220**:865–867.

36. Crewsdon J. (2002). *Science Fictions, a Scientific Mystery, a Massive Cover-Up, and the Dark Legacy of Robert Gallo.* London: Little, Brown and Company.

37. Montagnier L. (2000). *Virus.* New York: WW Norton & Company.

38. Palca J. (1987). Settlement on AIDS finally reached between US and Pasteur. *Nature* **326**:533.

39. CDC. (1982). Current Trends Update on Acquired Immune Deficiency Syndrome (AIDS) – United States. *Morbidity and Mortality Weekly Report* **31**:507–508; 513–514.

40. CDC. (1985). Revision of the Case Definition of Acquired Immune Deficiency Syndrome for National Reporting – United States. *Morbidity and Mortality Weekly Report* **34**:373.

41. CDC. (1987). Revision of the CDC Surveillance Case Definition for Acquired Immunodeficiency Syndrome. *Morbidity and Mortality Weekly Report* **36**:S1.

42 CDC. (1992). 1993 Revised Classification System for HIV Infection and Expanded Surveillance Case Definition for AIDS Among Adolescents and Adults. *Morbidity and Mortality Weekly Report* **41**:1–19.

43. CDC. (1994). Update: Trends in AIDS Diagnosis and Reporting Under the Expanded Surveillance Definition for Adolescents and Adults – United States, 1993. *Morbidity and Mortality Weekly Report* **43**:826.

44. France A, ed., Boyd E, transl. (1922). *The Opinions of Anatole France.* New York: Alfred A Knopf.

45. Armstrong EA. (2002). *Forging Gay Identities: Organizing Sexuality in San Francisco, 1950–1994.* Chicago and London: The University of Chicago Press.

46. Nuland SB. (1994). *How We Die: Reflections on Life's Final Chapter*. New York: Alfred A Knopf.

47. Carpenter B, ed. (1997). *AIDS: Reflections ... Responses*. New York: American Foundation for AIDS Research.

48. Schoofs M. (1999). AIDS: The Agony of Africa. (Part 1: The Virus Creates a Generation of Orphans). *The Village Voice*, November 3-9, 1999.

49. WHO. *Avian influenza, frequently asked questions*. Available at http://www.who.int/csr/disease/avian_influenza/avian_faqs/en/index.html (accessed on June 6 2007).

50. WHO. (1983). *Acquired Immune Deficiency Syndrome Emergencies. Report of a WHO Meeting, 22–25 November 1983*. Geneva: WHO.

51. WHO. (2003). *A History of the HIV/AIDS Epidemic with Emphasis on Africa. Report from the Workshop on HIV/AIDS and Adult Mortality in Developing Countries, New York, 8–13 September 2003*. Geneva: WHO.

52. Clumeck N, Mascart-Lemone F, de Maubeuge J, *et al.* (1983). Acquired immune deficiency syndrome in Black Africans. *Lancet* **1**:642.

53 Atani L, Caraë M, Brunet JB, *et al.* (2000). Social change and HIV in the former USSR: The making of a new epidemic. *Social Sciences and Medicine* **50**:1547–1556.

54. WHO. (2003). *Fact Sheet No. 211 – Influenza. Revised March 2003*. Geneva: WHO.

55. Kolata G. (2001). *Flu: The Story of the Great Influenza Pandemic*. New York: Touchstone.

56. Shnayerson M, Plotkin MJ. (2002). *The Killers Within: The Deadly Rise of Drug-Resistant Bacteria*. London: Little, Brown and Company.

57. Genius G. (2006). Diagnosis: Contemporary medical hubris; Rx: A tincture of humility. *Journal of Evaluation in Clinical Practice* **12**:24–30.

58. Iliffe J. (2006). *The African AIDS Epidemic: A History*. Athens, Ohio: Ohio University Press.

59. Patton C. (2002). *Globalizing AIDS*. Minneapolis: University of Minnesota Press.

60. Auerbach DM, Darrow WW, Jaffe HW, Curran JW. (1984). Cluster of cases of the acquired immune deficiency syndrome – patients linked by sexual contact. *American Journal of Medicine* **76**:487–492.

61. *Gaetan Dugas and the Cluster Study in The AIDS Epidemic in San Francisco: The Medical Response, 1981–1984*, Volume 1. Online Archive of California, California Digital Library, University of California. Available at http://content.cdlib.org/xtf/view?docId=kt2m3n98v1&doc.view= content&chunk.id=d0e1592&toc.depth=1&brand=oac&anchor.id= (accessed on 6 June 2007)

62. Herek GM, Capitanio JP. (1993). A second decade of stigma: Public reactions to AIDS in the United States, 1990–1991. *American Journal of Public Health* **83**:574–577.

63. Gould SJ. (1987). The Terrifying Normalcy of AIDS. *The New York Times Magazine*, April 19, 1987.

64. Kinsella J. (1989). *Covering the Plague: AIDS and the American Media*. New Brunswick, New Jersey: Rutgers University Press.

65. Rosner F, Giron JA. (1983). Immune deficiency syndrome in children. *Journal of the American Medical Association* **250**:3046.

66. Berridge V. (1992). AIDS, the Media, and Health Policy. In: Aggleton P, Davies P, Hart G, eds. *AIDS: Rights, Risk, and Reason*. London: Falmer Press. p13–27.

67. Kitzinger J, Miller D. (1992). 'African AIDS': The Media and Audience Beliefs. In: Aggleton P, Davies P, Hart G, eds. *AIDS: Rights, Risk, and Reason*. London: Falmer Press. p 28–52.

68. CDC. (1983). Current Trends in Acquired Immunodeficiency Syndrome (AIDS): Update – United States. *Morbidity and Mortality Weekly Report* **32**:309–311.

69. CDC. (1983). Prevention of Acquired Immune Deficiency Syndrome (AIDS): Report of Inter-Agency Recommendations. *Morbidity and Mortality Weekly Report* **32**:101–103.

70. Smith DK, Grohskopf LA, Black RJ, *et al.* (2005). Antiretroviral postexposure prophylaxis after sexual, injection-drug use, or other nonoccupational exposure to HIV in the United States: recommendations from the US Department of Health and Human Services. *Mortality and Morbidity Weekly Report* **54**:1–20.

71. CDC. (1985). Current Trends in Education and Foster Care of Children Infected with Human T-Lymphotropic Virus Type III/Lymphadenopathy-Associated Virus. *Morbidity and Mortality Weekly Report* **34**:518–519.

72. Gelman B. (2000). The Belated Global Response to AIDS in Africa. *Washington Post*, July 5, 2000.

73. Zhu T, Korber B, Nahinias AJ, *et al.* (1998). African HIV-1 Sequence from 1959 and Implications for the Origin of the Epidemic. *Nature* **391**:594.

74. Kalish ML, Robbins KE, Pieniazek D, *et al.* (2004). Recombinant Viruses and Early Global HIV-1 Epidemic. *Emerging Infectious Diseases* **10**:1227–1234.

75. Serwadda D, Mugerwa RD, Swankambo NK, *et al.* (1985). Slim disease: A new disease in Uganda and its association with the HTLV-III infection. *Lancet* **2**:849–852.

76. Piot P, Quinn TC, Taelman H, *et al.* (1984). Acquired Immune Deficiency Syndrome in a heterosexual population in Zaire. *Lancet* **2**:65–69.

77. Garrett L. (1994). *The Coming Plague: Newly Emerging Diseases in a World Out of Balance.* New York: Farrar, Straus, and Giroux.

78. Halperin D, Epstein H. (2004). Concurrent sexual partnerships help to explain Africa's high HIV prevalence: Implications for prevention. *Lancet* **363**:4–6.

79. Weiss HA, Quigley M, Hayes RJ. (2000). Male circumcision and risk of HIV infection in sub-Saharan Africa: A systematic review and meta-analysis. *AIDS* **14**:2361–2370.

80. Schoepf BG. (2004). *Gender, Sex, and Power: A Social History of AIDS in Mobutu's Zaire.* Malden, Massachusetts: Blackwell.

81. Ndinga-Muvumba A. (2006). Aligning HIV/AIDS and Security: The United Nations and Africa. In: Adejabo A, Scanlon H, eds. *Dialogue of the Deaf: Essays on Africa and the United Nations.* Johannesburg, South Africa: Fanele. p 1–16.

82. Toungara JM. (2001). Ethnicity and political crisis in Côte d'Ivoire. *Journal of Democracy* **12**:6–72.

83. Lwanda JL. (2003). Politics, Culture, and Medicine: An Unholy Trinity? Historical Continuities and Ruptures in the HIV/AIDS Story in Malawi. In: Kalipeni E, Craddock S, Oppong J, Ghosh H, eds. *HIV and AIDS in Africa: Beyond Epidemiology.* Oxford: Blackwell Publishing. p29–42.

84. Price-Smith A, Daly JL. (2004). *Downward Spiral: HIV/AIDS, State Capacity, and Political Conflict in Zimbabwe.* Washington, DC: US Institute of Peace.

85. Riviere P. (2002). South Africa's AIDS Apartheid. *LeMonde Diplomatique*, August 1, 2002.

86. Bond GC, Vincent J. (1997). AIDS in Uganda: The First Decade. In: Bond GC, Kreniske J, Susser I, Vincent J, eds. *AIDS in Africa and the Caribbean.* Boulder, Colorado: Westview Press. p85–97.

87. Parkhurst JO, Ssengooba F, Serwadda D. (2006). Uganda. In: Beck EJ, Mays N, Whiteside A, Zuniga JM, eds. *The HIV Pandemic: Local and Global Implications.* Oxford: Oxford University Press. p255–269.

88. Boyd N. (1990). Fighting AIDS in francophone African countries. *Canadian Medical Association Journal* **143**:257–258.

89. Simms S, Salif Sow P, Sy E. (2006). Senegal. In: Beck EJ, Mays N, Whiteside A, Zuniga JM, eds. *The HIV Pandemic: Local and Global Implications.* Oxford: Oxford University Press. p228–239.

90. Wachter RM. (1991). *The Fragile Coalition.* New York: St. Martin's Press.

91. van Praag E, Dehne KL, Chandra-Mouli V. (2006). The UN Response to the HIV Pandemic. In: Beck EJ, Mays N, Whiteside A, Zuniga JM, eds. *The HIV Pandemic: Local and Global Implications.* Oxford: Oxford University Press. p593–505.

92. Voelker R. (1998). Tragic Loss of Leaders in AIDS and Public Health. *Journal of the American Medical Association* **280**:1037.

93. CDC. (2006). Evolution of HIV/AIDS Prevention Programs – United States, 1981–2006. *Morbidity and Mortality Weekly Report* **55**:597–603.

94. FDA. *HIV/AIDS Historical Timeline.* Available at http://www.fda.gov/oashi/aids/miles81.html (accessed on 6 June 2007).

95. Cohen J. (2001). *Shots in the Dark: The Wayward Search for an AIDS Vaccine.* New York and London: WW Norton & Company.

96. Berkley S. (1998). HIV vaccine development for the world: An idea whose time has come? *AIDS Research and Human Retroviruses* 14:S191–S196.

97. Masur H. (1992). Drug therapy: Prevention and treatment of pneumocystis pneumonia. *New England Journal of Medicine* 327:1853.

98. Pons V, Greenspan D, Debruin M, *et al.*, on behalf of the Multicenter Study Group. (1993). Therapy for oropharyngeal candidiasis in HIV-infected patients: A randomized, prospective multicenter study of oral fluconazole versus clotrimazole troches. *Journal of Acquired Immune Deficiency Syndrome* 6:1311–1316.

99. Saag MS, Powderly WG, Cloud GA, *et al.*, on behalf of the NIAID Mycoses Study Group and the AIDS Clinical Trials Group. (1992). Comparison of amphotericin B with fluconazole in the treatment of acute AIDS-associated cryptococcal meningitis. *New England Journal of Medicine* 326:83–89.

100. Beall G. (1990). A double-blinded, placebo-controlled trial of thymostimulin in symptomatic HIV-infected patients. *AIDS* 4:679–681.

101. Arno PS, Feiden K. (1992). *Against the Odds: The Story of AIDS Drug Development, Politics, and Profits.* New York: Harper Collins.

102. Mitsuya H, Weinhold K, Furman P, *et al.* (1985). 3'-Azido-3'-deoxythymidine (BW A509U): An antiviral agent that inhibits the infectivity and cytopathic effect of human T-lymphotropic virus type III/lymphadenopathy-associated virus *in vitro*. *Proceedings of the National Academy of Sciences USA* 82:7096–7100.

103. Epstein S. (1996). *Impure Science: AIDS, Activism, and the Politics of Knowledge.* California: University of California Press.

104. Fischl MA, Richman DD, Grieco MH, *et al.* (1997). The efficacy of azidothymidine (AZT) in the treatment of patients with AIDS and AIDS-related complex: A double-blind placebo-controlled trial. *New England Journal of Medicine* 317:185–191.

105. Idänpään-Heikkilä JE, Fluss S. (2006). Emerging international norms for clinical testing: good clinical trial practice. In: Santoro M, Gorrie TM, eds. *Ethics and the Pharmaceutical Industry.* Cambridge: Cambridge University Press. p37–48.

106. Jonsen A, Stryker J, eds. (1993). *The Social Impact of AIDS in the United States.* Washington, DC: National Academy Press.

107. AmFAR. (2006). *Annual Report.* Available at http://www.amfar.org (accessed on 6 June 2007).

108. Gould DB. (2002). Life During Wartime: Emotions and the Development of ACT UP. *Mobilization* 7:177–200.

109. Smith R, Siplon P. (2006). *Drugs Into Bodies.* Westport, Connecticut: Praeger.

110. FDA News Release. (1988). *Making drugs available for life-threatening diseases. FDA News Release, October 19, 1988.* Rockville, Maryland: United States Food and Drug Administration.

111. Barr D. (1991). Policy: Monitoring the ACTG. *Gay Men's Health Crisis Treatment Issues* 5. Available at: http://www.aidsinfobbs.org/periodicals/gmhcissues/55/txt

112. Ghaziani A. (2004). Anticipatory and actualized identities: A cultural analysis of the transition from AIDS disability to work. *Sociological Quarterly* 45:273–301.

113. Fetter B, Morgan D, Levi J. (2006). The United States of America. In: Beck EJ, Mays N, Whiteside A, Zuniga JM, eds. *The HIV Pandemic: Local and Global Implications.* Oxford: Oxford University Press. p577–589.

114. Ghaziani, A. (in press). *The Dividends of Dissent: How Conflict and Culture Work in Lesbian and Gay Marches on Washington.* Chicago: The University of Chicago Press.

115. NAMES Project Foundation. (2006). *Annual Report 2006.* Atlanta: NAMES Project Foundation.

116. Morse R. (1996). AIDS quilt final fold. *San Francisco Chronicle,* October 11, 1996.

117. *Global Quilt website*. Available at http://www.globalquilt.org/ (accessed on 6 June 2007).

118. Kauffman KD, Lindauer DL, eds. (2004). *AIDS and South Africa: The Social Expression of a Pandemic*. New York: Palgrave Macmillan.

119. Bayer R. (1991). *Private Acts, Social Consequences*. New Brunswick, New Jersey: Rutgers University Press.

120. *Berliner AIDS-Hilfe*. Available at http://berlin.aidshilfe.de/ (accessed on 6 June 2007).

121. Putzel J. (2004). The politics of action on AIDS: A case study of Uganda. *Public Administration and Development* 24:19–30.

122. Geiger HJ. (1996). A Life in Social Medicine. In: Bassuk EL, ed. *The Doctor-Activist: Physicians Fighting for Social Change*. New York: Plenum. p11–27.

123. Cobb WM. (1953). Dr. Charles Victor Roman. *Journal of the National Medical Association* 45:301–305.

124. Private Communication with Paul J Cimoch, 30 August 2007.

125. Nary G. (1995). From the Editor. *Journal of the International Association of Physicians in AIDS Care* 1:5.

126. [no author listed]. (1991). PAAC challenges AMA/ADA sanctions against HIV-infected healthcare workers. *Boletín de la Asociación Médica de Puerto Rico* 83:172.

127. Altman LK. (1991). US drafts guidelines for doctors with AIDS. *Washington Post*, April 5, 1991.

128. CDC. (1991). Recommendations for Preventing Transmission of Human Immunodeficiency Virus and Hepatitis B Virus to Patients During Exposure-Prone Invasive Procedures. *Morbidity and Mortality Weekly Report* 40:1–9.

129. Blanchfield JC, O'Brien AM.(1990). The Association of Nurses in AIDS Care (ANAC). IV International AIDS Conference, 20–23 June 1990. Stockholm. [Abstract SD863]

130. *IAS History*. Available at: http://www.iasociety.org/Default.aspx?pageId=67 (accessed on 29 August 2007).

131. Volberding PA, Lagakos SW, Koch MA, *et al.* (1990). Zidovudine in asymptomatic human immuno deficiency virus infection: A controlled trial in persons with fewer than 500 CD4-positive cells per cubic millimeter. *New England Journal of Medicine* 322:941.

132. Concorde Coordinating Committee. (1994). Concorde: MRC/ANRS randomized double-blind controlled trial of immediate and deferred zidovudine in symptom-free HIV infection. *Lancet* 343:871–881.

133. Frieberg P. (2000). Name dropping in San Francisco: ACT Up chapter changes moniker to distinguish from other group. *The Washington Blade*, March 31, 2000.

134. Connor EM, Sperling RS, Gelber R, *et al.* (1994). Reduction of maternal-infant transmission of Human Immunodeficiency Virus type 1 with zidovudine treatment. *New England Journal of Medicine* 331:1173–1180.

135. NIH. (1996). *New ACTG 076 Analysis Emphasizes Importance of Offering AZT Therapy to All HIV-Infected Pregnant Women: NIH News Release*. Bethesda, MD: NIH.

136. Larder BA, Darby G, Richman DD. (1989). HIV with reduced sensitivity to zidovudine (AZT) isolated during prolonged therapy. *Science* 243:1731–1734.

137. [No authors listed]. (1996). Delta: A randomized double-blind controlled trial comparing combina-tions of ziodvudine plus didanosine or zalcitabine with zidovudine alone in HIV-infected individuals. *Lancet* 348:283–291.

138. Hammer SM, Katzenstein DA, Hughes MD, *et al.* (1996). A trial comparing nucleoside monotherapy with combination therapy in HIV-infected adults with CD4 counts from 200 to 500 cubic millimeter. *New England Journal of Medicine* 335:1081–1090.

139. Manfredi R, Calza L, Chiodo F. (2001). Dual nucleoside analogue treatment in the era of highly active antiretroviral therapy (HAART): a single-centre cross-sectional survey. *Journal of Antimicrobial Chemotherapy* 48:299–302.

140. Bartlett JG. (2001). *HIV: Twenty Years in Review*. Available at: http://www.hopkins-aids.edu/ publications/report/july01_6.html (accessed on 6 June 2007).

141. D'Aquila RT, Johnson VA, Welles Seth L, *et al.* (1995). Zidovudine resistance and HIV-1 disease progression during antiretroviral therapy. *Annals of Internal Medicine* **122**:401–408.

142. Ho DD, Neumann AU, Perelson AS, *et al.* (1995). Rapid turnover of plasma virions and CD4 lymphocytes in HIV-1 infection. *Nature* **373**:123–126.

143. Ho DD. (1997). Dynamics of HIV-1 replication in vivo. *Journal of Clinical Investigation* **99**:2565–2567.

144. Mellors JW, Munoz A, Giorgi JV, *et al.* (1997). Plasma viral load and CD4+ lymphocytes as prognostic markers of HIV-1 infection. *Ann Intern Med* **126**:355–363.

145. CDC. (1997). Update: Trends in AIDS Incidence, Deaths, and Prevalence – United States, 1996. *Morbidity and Mortality Weekly Report* **46**:861–867.

146. Palella F, Delaney KM, Moorman AC, *et al.* (1998). Declining morbidity and mortality among patients with advanced human immunodeficiency virus infection. *New England Journal of Medicine* **338**:853–860.

147. Mocroft A, Vella S, Benfield TL, *et al.* (1998). Changing patterns of mortality across Europe in patients infected with HIV-1. EuroSIDA Study Group. *Lancet* **352**:1725–1730.

148. Decosas J. (1996). HIV and development. *AIDS* **10**:S69–S74.

149. Madavo C. (1998). AIDS, Development, and the Vital Role of Government. XII International AIDS Conference, 28 June–3 July 1998, Geneva, Switzerland. [Plenary Address]

150. Baggaley RC, Needham D. (1997). Africa's emerging AIDS-orphans crisis. *Canadian Medical Association Journal* **156**:873–875.

151. Editorial. (1998). Looking forward to the back of HIV. *Nature Medicine* **4**:867–868.

152. Cameron B, Heath-Chiozzi M, Kravcik S, *et al.* Prolongation of life and prevention of AIDS in advanced HIV immunodeficiency with ritonavir. 3rd Conference on Retroviruses and Opportunistic Infections, 28 January–1 February 1996, Washington, DC, USA. [Abstract LB6a]

153. Harrington M. (1996). *An extraordinary year for basic and clinical research on AIDS.* Available at http://www.thebody.com/content/art1417.html#OAR (accessed on 29 August 2007).

154. Saag MS, Holodiny M, Kuritzkes DR, *et al.* (1996). HIV viral load markers in clinical practice. *Nature Medicine* **2**:425–429.

155. Daar ES. (2003). Antiretroviral resistance in clinical practice. *Journal of the International Association of Physicians in AIDS Care* **2**:4–18.

156. Cameron DW, Sun E, Markowitz M, *et al.* (1996). Combination use of ritonavir and saquinavir in HIV-infected patients: preliminary safety and activity data. XI International AIDS Conference, 7–12 July 1996, Vancouver, Canada. [Abstract Th.B.934]

157. Hirschel BJ, Rutschmann O, Fathi M, *et al.* (1996). Treatment of advanced HIV infection with ritonavir plus saquinavir. XI International AIDS Conference, 7–12 July 1996, Vancouver, Canada. [Abstract LB.B.6030]

158. Gulick RM, Mellors J, Havlir D, *et al.* (1996). Potent and sustained antiretroviral activity of indinavir, zidovudine and lamivudine. XI International AIDS Conference, 7–12 July 1996, Vancouver, Canada. [Abstract Th.B.931]

159. Mathez D, Bagnarelli P, De Truchis. P, *et al.* (1996). A triple combination of ritonavir plus AZT plus ddC as a first line treatment of patients with AIDS: Update. XI International AIDS Conference, 7–12 July 1996, Vancouver, Canada. [Abstract Mo.B.175]

160. Baruch A, Mastrodonato-Delora P, Schnipper E, Salgo M. (1996). Efficacy and safety of triple combination therapy with Invirase (saquinavir/SQV/HIV protease inhibitor), Epivir (3TC/lamivudine) and Retrovir (ZDV/zidovudine) in HIV-infected patients. XI International AIDS Conference, 7–12 July 1996, Vancouver, Canada. [Abstract Mo.B.172]

161. Markowitz M, Cao Y, Hurley A, *et al.* (1996). Triple therapy with AZT, 3TC, and ritonavir in 12 subjects newly infected with HIV-1. XI International AIDS Conference, 7–12 July1996, Vancouver, Canada. [Abstract Th.B.933]

162. Myers MW, Montaner JG. (1996). A randomized, double-blinded comparative trial of the effects of zidovudine, didanosine and nevirapine combinations in antiviral-naive, AIDS-free, HIV-infected patients with CD4 counts between 200–600 cells/mm^3. XI International AIDS Conference, 7–12 July 1996, Vancouver, Canada. [Abstract Mo.B.294]

163. Mascolini M. (1996). Antiviral update from Vancouver. *Journal of the International Association of Physicians in AIDS Care* 2:29–56.

164. Coovadia HM. (1998). Healthcare resource challenges to the world community. Keynote Address. *Journal of the International Association of Physicians in AIDS Care* 4:20–22, 26.

165. WHO. (1997). HIV/AIDS: The global epidemic, December 1996. *WHO Weekly Epidemiological Record* 72:17–24.

Chapter 3

Turning the world on its ear: defining milestones on the road to HAART

Michel D. Kazatchkine* and Lieve Fransen

It was 15 years into the epidemic before an antiretroviral treatment capable of suppressing viral replication and reversing HIV-associated immunodeficiency became available. Highly active antiretroviral therapy (HAART) was initially only available in industrialized countries; it took almost 10 more years before HAART became accepted as a necessity to address the AIDS crisis in the developing world [1]. In this chapter, we look back at some of the milestones on the road to HAART in the developed and developing world, recognizing the remarkable progress that has been achieved. We also acknowledge that the accumulated short-term experience may be neither sufficient nor appropriate when facing the long-term challenges raised by the epidemic, and the need for effective large-scale access to prevention, treatment and care for all those in need worldwide.

Milestones on the road to HAART in North America, Europe and Australia

AIDS is the area in modern medicine that has witnessed the most rapid and dramatic progress in therapy. This is shown by the short period that separates the identification of HIV as the causal agent of AIDS in 1983 and the advent of HAART in 1996.

The demonstration of the strong antiviral effects of azidothymidine (AZT) in 1986 gave rise to a great deal of hope among infected people, activists, physicians and caregivers. The years 1986–90, however, brought frustration and disarray for all. Despite progress in the treatment and prophylaxis of opportunistic infections (OIs) with improved use of, and widespread access to, cotrimoxazole, ganciclovir, foscarnet and fluconazole, AIDS-related mortality remained largely unaffected during this period. Cytomegalovirus (CMV) retinitis and infections with atypical mycobacteria, the neurological manifestations of advanced HIV disease and the AIDS wasting syndrome, remained the primary concern in AIDS care and the main causes of death. Monotherapy with AZT failed to show clinical efficacy in the Concorde trial [2]. The DELTA and ACTG 175 trials then demonstrated that dual combination therapy, with two nucleoside reverse transcriptase inhibitors (NRTIs), was more effective on disease progression and death than monotherapy, and showed that the combination of two drugs was well tolerated [3]. However, the clinical limitations of dual NRTI regimens and their lack of significant efficacy on mortality soon became apparent in the early 1990s.

*Corresponding author.

The breakthrough came in February 1996 with the first demonstration of a significant decrease in AIDS-related mortality in patients who received the then-experimental protease inhibitor (PI) ritonavir (RTV) in addition to a dual NRTI regimen [4], and with the dramatic results on viral load and CD4 counts shown in controlled studies of triple drug regimens (including the PI indinavir (IDV)), as compared with dual therapy [5]. The year 1996 also witnessed the fast-track approval of IDV, RTV and another PI, saquinavir (SQV), by regulatory agencies in the United States and Europe. There was enthusiasm and excitement during the XI International AIDS Conference held that year in Vancouver, where the expression 'highly active antiretroviral therapy', or HAART, was born. The benefit from triple combination therapies that contained a PI rapidly became apparent. It was suggested that treatment should 'hit hard and early' [6]. Most patients who met clinical criteria for HAART in the United States, Europe and Australia started treatment between 1996 and 1998. Nevirapine, the first non-nucleoside reverse transcriptase inhibitor (NNRTI), was approved later in 1996, so that three classes of antiretroviral drugs had become available on the market by the end of that year. This breakthrough represented new hope for the millions of people infected and affected by HIV/AIDS, as reflected in the slogan, 'one world, one hope', coined in Vancouver. It soon became clear, however, that at a price of US$10,000 for one year of treatment, hope would not translate into reality for most people infected in the developing world.

In the years immediately following this breakthrough, the early virologic, immunologic and clinical efficacy of HAART was shown to persist and improve [7,8]. AIDS-associated morbidity and mortality decreased by more than 85% in the United States and Europe between 1995 and 1998, and the incidence of AIDS decreased more than 10-fold in Europe [9]. Successful treatment was documented to be associated with immune reconstitution. In addition to an increase in peripheral blood CD4 T-cell numbers that could reach levels observed in healthy seronegative individuals, the generation of a new, naïve CD4 T-cell repertoire was demonstrated. This translated clinically into a restored ability of treated patients to respond appropriately to pathogens and thus to discontinue primary and secondary OI prophylaxis.

The issues of concern that next arose in patients receiving HAART included: virologic and immunologic failure; uneven adherence patterns and HIV drug resistance, lipodystrophy and metabolic toxicities; when and how to start treatment; how and when to switch to second- and third-line treatment; and the inability of HAART to eradicate the virus and to prevent the generation of viral reservoirs. These issues are discussed in detail elsewhere in this book. For the purpose of this chapter on the milestones to effective treatment, it is sufficient to remind ourselves that the advent of HAART showed that the immunodeficiency associated with HIV is reversible. Since the clinical manifestations of AIDS are a direct consequence of HIV-induced immunodeficiency, reversion of immunodeficiency with HAART provides a strong enough basis to advocate expanded access to antiretroviral treatment for all of those in need worldwide.

Milestones on the road to HAART in developing countries

The first call for large-scale access to treatment for AIDS patients in the developing world came from President Jacques Chirac of France and his Minister of Health, Bernard Kouchner, at the International Conference on AIDS and STIs in Africa (ICASA) held in Abidjan in 1997 [10]. Brazil, by that time, was already committing to a significant nationwide effort on prevention and treatment. However, despite the advocacy of many non-governmental organizations (NGOs) in Africa, Latin America, Europe and the United States, only small 'pilot' antiretroviral treatment programmes were being initiated in developing countries. These were often outside national frameworks and strategies designed for a broad access to prevention and treatment.

Little was achieved in terms of access to treatment until the XIII International AIDS Conference in Durban in 2000, which called for 'breaking the silence' four years after the generous 'one world, one hope' theme of the Vancouver conference. The Durban conference sent the strong message to the world that scale-up efforts for antiretroviral treatment were failing and that the inequity between the rich and the poor with regard to access to antiretroviral treatment was deepening. This message resonated in an address delivered by South African Justice Edward Cameron, himself HIV-positive: 'I stand before you because I am able to purchase health. I am here because I can pay for life itself. To me this seems a shocking and monstrous inequity that, simply because of relative affluence, I should be living when others have died [11].' A few months later, the world's attention focused on the pharmaceutical industry's legal attempt to prevent the South African government from issuing licenses for the production of generic versions of branded antiretroviral drugs (an effort which would fail and ultimately, because of public outrage, force the pharmaceutical industry to take a new approach to pricing their products in most of the developing world).

As a result of the growing inequality in accessing treatment, civil society and certain voices in both the North and the South called for more affordable drug prices. Some NGOs criticized the Agreement on Trade-Related Aspects of Intellectual Property Rights (TRIPS Agreement) as one of the causes of high prices and limited access to patented drugs among the poor. The pharmaceutical industry argued that the aim of patent protection is to provide incentives for research into and development of new products and to ensure publication and disclosure of innovation for the benefit of the public, as well as to recover the costs of investments in new products. The European Commission initiated a first dialogue with industry, NGOs and the United Nations (UN) to assess the implementation of intellectual property rights agreements and examine possible action, including differential pricing. The road to tiered prices for patented drugs had been opened through the 'Drug Access Initiative', which was jointly launched between the Joint United Nations Programme on HIV/AIDS (UNAIDS) and the manufacturers of several patented drugs. In September 2000, at a high-level round table meeting held in Brussels, a new strategy was agreed to by all stakeholders to accelerate access and affordability of key pharmaceuticals, while increasing research and development (R&D) investments for new products, including vaccines and microbicides [12]. An agreement was reached on tiered prices for patented drugs. The Indian generic manufacturer CIPLA announced the availability of a first-line antiretroviral regimen at an annual cost of only US$350 per patient. The European Union stressed the importance of increasing prevention efforts as access to treatment increases.

The prices of first-line antiretroviral regimens decreased by more than 90% in low- and middle-income countries between 2000 and 2002. This allowed triple combination therapy to become available in poor countries at approximately US$300 per patient-year. There were two reasons for such a dramatic decrease. The first was the pharmaceutical industry policy of differential prices, charging high prices to markets in developed countries and low prices in developing countries; the other determinant was generic competition. Low marginal costs explain why generic manufacturers are able to provide substitutes to branded products at low prices. Using its own manufacturing capacity to produce generic versions of eight antiretroviral drugs, Brazil has been able to offer free treatment to more than 200,000 HIV-positive people in need, and the Indian generic industry has provided first-line treatment to a large number of nationally and internationally funded programmes.

In Abuja in 2001, African heads of state committed to significantly increase the budgets devoted to health and their national efforts to fight HIV, and the UN Secretary-General, Kofi Annan, called for the creation of a US$7–10 billion fund to fight HIV/AIDS [13]. The UN Human Rights Commission (UNHCR) stated that access to treatment is an essential component of the right to health. Soon after, the UN General Assembly met in its first special session on HIV/AIDS and committed to '... make every effort to provide ... the highest attainable standard of treatment of HIV/AIDS, including the effective use of quality-controlled antiretroviral therapy' [14]. Representatives from governments of both rich and poor countries, NGOs and the private sector met for the first time in Brussels with the specific mandate to set up a global fund for the scale-up of prevention and treatment efforts against three of the world's deadliest diseases: AIDS, malaria and tuberculosis. They formed a transitional working group and governance structure, and their work yielded the final model of the Global Fund to Fight AIDS, Tuberculosis and Malaria (Global Fund) in January 2002. With a Board of Directors in which all stakeholders are represented as voting members, an independent evaluation panel that selects the most relevant and strongest programmes among those submitted on a regular basis, a policy of performance-based disbursement, and transparency, the Global Fund has established a new model of multilateral governance and intervention in health. By June 2006, the portfolio of grants supported by the Global Fund had resulted in 550,000 people receiving antiretroviral therapy, provided HIV counselling and testing to 6 million people, brought tuberculosis treatment to 1.5 million people and trained 1.5 million additional service deliverers to fight the three pandemics [15].

Also in 2002, the World Health Organization (WHO) included 10 antiretroviral drugs in its Essential Medicines List, and provided a set of internationally agreed guidelines for antiretroviral treatment in resource-limited settings [16].

Early in 2003, US President George W Bush launched the US President's Emergency Plan for AIDS Relief (PEPFAR), endowed with US$15 billion over five years, the largest commitment of any country to fight the epidemic. PEPFAR has allowed for major progress in access to antiretroviral treatment, particularly in the 15 'target' countries on which the programme is focusing [17]. Between PEPFAR and the Global Fund, antiretroviral treatment for 1.2 million patients was being supported in developing countries at the end of 2006.

The rapid increase in the number of people receiving treatment in low- and middle-income countries over the last three years followed the call by the WHO and UNAIDS, in 2003, for 3 million people in the developing world to be receiving treatment by 2005 (the '3 by 5 initiative'). Although it significantly missed its mark (only 1 million were on treatment as of December 2006), this time-delimited initiative contributed significantly to the mobilization of the international community and affected countries in favor of scaling up antiretroviral therapy [18].

In 2006, following strong statements at the G8 summit in Gleneagles, Scotland, in 2005, the UN General Assembly committed to 'pursue all necessary efforts to scale up ... nationally-driven responses ... towards the goal of universal access to comprehensive prevention programs, treatment, care and support by 2010' [19]. The world had realized the urgent need for treatment in parallel with prevention to respond to the AIDS crisis. It was also clear that large-scale antiretroviral treatment programmes were feasible in resource-constrained settings.

Many consider that this occurred far too late in the history of the HIV pandemic. Yet many people, including scientists at the forefront of the fight against AIDS, had long remained opposed to antiretroviral treatment scale-up. They argued that if resources were limited, they should primarily be devoted to prevention; that antiretroviral treatment was too expensive and had not demonstrated cost-efficacy; that the tolerance and effectiveness of treatment in resource-limited settings were unknown; that health infrastructures were insufficient to allow for treatment scale-up; that moving too fast with treatment in the developing world could lead to treatment failure and a 'second wave' of drug resistant HIV; and finally, that scaling up therapy raised considerable ethical concerns, since antiretroviral treatment could not be brought rapidly to all those in need.

Between 2003 and 2005, empirical evidence showed that, despite the difficulties encountered, none of the above contentions should prevent initiation or scaling up of antiretroviral treatment in emerging and developing countries [20]. At the end of 2006, the WHO and UNAIDS reported that over 2 million people were receiving treatment in low- and middle-income countries, more than 10 times the number who were on treatment in 2002. Strong evidence has now been gathered on the feasibility, tolerance and effectiveness of antiretroviral treatment in resource-limited settings, and data are becoming available on the impact of treatment on mortality in high-prevalence settings [21] as well as the restored economic productivity of workers in such settings following initiation of antiretroviral treatment programmes.

Prevention and treatment have clearly been shown to be mutually reinforcing within an integrated approach to care. The availability of antiretroviral treatment and the prevention of mother-to-child transmission of the virus has been documented as an incentive to testing. Many of the countries that have been successful in decreasing the number of new infections or in keeping the prevalence of HIV infection low, including Brazil, Thailand, Cambodia, Ghana and Senegal, are also countries that were among the first to initiate large-scale antiretroviral treatment programmes. Clearly, reduction in new infections is to be achieved by combining primary and secondary prevention with antiretroviral treatment programmes. Recently developed population-based models indicate that free treatment access on a global scale could curb the growth of the epidemic. In the United States and Europe, where HAART is widely available, there have been reports of a decreased awareness of HIV risk in the general population and decreased adherence to safer-sex practices among men having sex with men. In the developing world, however, there is evidence of a lower likelihood of risky behaviour in treated patients, and of a positive impact of antiretroviral treatment on the motivation for testing and disclosure [22].

HAART has been shown to be affordable and cost-effective in developed countries [23] and in middle-income countries such as Brazil and South Africa. A recent World Bank study demonstrated that the national treatment of HIV/AIDS in Thailand is also affordable and cost-effective [24]. It further indicated that Thailand's success with prevention is the main reason the country can afford universal access to antiretroviral treatment today, and is an essential condition of the country's continued ability to afford treatment in the future, emphasizing the need for enhanced preventive efforts in other settings where antiretroviral therapy (ART) becomes available. The epidemiological model designed by Salomon et al. further indicates the importance of integrating prevention and treatment [25]: ART can enable more effective prevention, and prevention is effective in reducing new infections and makes treatment affordable.

Modelling of the macroeconomic impact of HIV has also recently shown that scaling up access to ART should limit the loss in gross domestic product (GDP) due to HIV in a number of African countries. This is provided that investment in treatment scale-up is large enough, and that large-scale treatment programmes are implemented early enough, before the AIDS shock has driven the economy beyond an irreversible no-development epidemiological trap [26].

The effectiveness and tolerance of ART in resource-poor settings has now been shown in all regions of the developing world where expanded access is needed. The ART-LINC meta-analysis of over 20 cohorts in the developing world has shown a mean mortality of 5.8% one year after initiation of ART, as compared with 1.6% mortality in developed world cohorts, a remarkable result given that treatment is often initiated at significantly more advanced stages of the disease in developing countries [27]. In contrast to predictions by some, the available evidence clearly indicates that good adherence is attained in resource-limited settings [28, 29].

Out-of-pocket expenses for treatment remain the main obstacle to adherence in poor countries. Based on this fact, the WHO has been building its advocacy for free access to ART at the end-user's level. Consistent with the high rates of adherence reported in developing world cohorts is the encouraging evidence of low rates of resistance in ART-treated patients in poor countries. Therefore, fear of the emergence of drug resistance should not be taken as an argument to prevent expansion of ART in the developing world [30].

Challenges ahead

As mentioned above, the increase in access to ART in the developing world has been remarkable in the last three years. Yet ART coverage is only of approximately 25% of the estimated needs, and major challenges lie ahead.

The first challenge deals with resources. The last five years have witnessed a significant increase in international and domestic resources for AIDS programmes, from less than US$1 billion/year to over US$8 billion/year [31]. Main players have been the European countries, the US PEPFAR initiative, the World Bank, the Global Fund and the governments of developing and emerging countries that now contribute one-third of global resources for AIDS. Of note, however, is the fact that resources devoted to health have increased less in the last four years than the mean overall amount that has become available for development.

First-line antiretroviral regimens are now priced at less than US$1/day in most developing countries. However, an estimated 10% of treated patients each year will need to switch to more sophisticated 'second-line' regimens because of acquired viral resistance or drug-related toxicities. The cost of these drugs currently remains four times that of first-line regimens in low-income countries and 10 times that of first-line regimens in middle-income countries. The TRIPS Agreement, which was amended during a series of global trade negotiations held in Doha in 2003, allows for countries to use a patent without the owner's consent in the case of a 'national emergency', for which HIV certainly qualifies. However, a number of constraints, including those dependent on bilateral trade agreements, have prevented developing countries from using the flexibilities introduced in Doha to their advantage. Thus, if decreases in prices do not soon extend to second-line drugs, AIDS programmes will face tragic choices between maintaining long-term access to ART for currently treated patients and initiating therapy for an increasing number of new patients in need. One recent initiative in this regard is the UNITAID International Drug Purchase Facility supported by Brazil, Chile, France, Norway and the United Kingdom that aims to use its purchasing power based on long-term funding commitments to lower prices.

The second challenge is that of the scarcity of trained healthcare workers in health services and health providers [32, 33]. It is estimated that today, 1 million more health professionals are needed in Africa to provide basic health services alone. Initial scale-up of ART has relied on existing health infrastructures and healthcare personnel, mainly concentrated in capital cities and large urban areas, but the availability of qualified personnel continuously diminishes, in part because of 'brain drain' and AIDS mortality. Further scale-up will not occur without massive efforts to increase healthcare manpower, and without innovative ways of dividing labour between physicians, nurses, social workers and a health workforce originating from NGOs. It will also fail to reach universal access without reforms aimed at decentralization of healthcare supply in peripheral and rural settings.

The third challenge is the need to accelerate the adoption of prevention behaviours and methods by those who have been exposed to HIV. The growth of the epidemic will not be curbed as long as the incidence of new HIV infections exceeds the number of people accessing treatment, and while the majority of infected people remain ignorant of their HIV status. The field of HIV prevention needs new tools, including microbicides, adult male circumcision and vaccines. Increasing the effectiveness of prevention also depends on the capacity of treatment programmes to provide the opportunity to break the chain of HIV transmission by disseminating preventive tools among HIV-positive people and their personal and social environments.

The lives of treated people in developing countries largely rely on foreign aid. In most African countries, over half of healthcare expenditure for AIDS treatment is directly funded by international donors. This trend will persist and may increase if the funding needs of US$20 billion/year for an expanded response to AIDS are to be met in the coming years. The fourth and toughest challenge is thus that of long-term sustainability of appropriate levels of funding. Sustainability cannot solely rely on the countries that have so far fuelled an unprecedented transfer of resources for AIDS to developing countries. Long-term funding mechanisms are needed at both international and national levels. The International Funding Facility recently proposed by the United Kingdom to guarantee loans for access to vaccines on financial markets, and the airline ticket contribution implemented by France (to which 18 additional countries have now committed), pioneer innovative approaches to sustainability of international funding. At the national level, out-of-pocket payment by households remains the major source of funding for healthcare in most developing countries. Sustainability will imply that a growing share of healthcare expenditures will be funded through health insurance and prepayment schemes.

Conclusion

A decade of experience has been gained and numerous obstacles overcome since the advent of HAART. This therapeutic intervention has saved countless lives and, equally important, allowed people living with HIV/AIDS (PLWHA) to lead healthier, more productive lives where access to HIV/AIDS care, treatment and support services is unimpeded by socio-economic or other factors. However, myriad challenges lie ahead. We thus require ongoing advocacy, political will and resources to ensure that the progress made in the HAART era translates into continuous benefit for the 40 million men, women and children who are today living with HIV/AIDS worldwide.

References

1. Schwartlander B, Grubb I, Perriens J. (2006). The ten-year struggle to provide antiretroviral treatment to people with HIV in the developing world. *Lancet* **368**:541–46.
2. Concorde Trial. (1994). MRC/ANRS randomized double-blind controlled trial of immediate and deferred zidovudine in symptom-free HIV infection. *Lancet* **343**:871–81.
3. Delta Trial. (1996). A randomized double-blind controlled trial comparing combinations of zidovudine plus didanosine or zalcitabine with zidovudine alone in HIV-infected individuals. *Lancet* **348**:283–91.
4. Cameron DW, Health-Chiozzi M, Danner S, *et al*. (1998). Randomised placebo-controlled trial of ritonavir in advanced HIV-1 disease. *Lancet* **351**:543–9.
5. Hammer SM, Katzenstein DA, Hughes MD, *et al*. (1996). A trial comparing nucleoside monotherapy with combination therapy in HIV-infected adults with CD4-cell counts from 200 to 500 per cubic millimeter. AIDS Clinical Trials Group Study 175 Study Team. *N Eng J Med* **335**:1081–90.
6. Ho DD. (1995). Time to hit HIV, early and hard. *N Engl J Med* **333**:450–1.
7. Gulick RM, Mellors JW, Havlir D, *et al*. (2000). Three-year suppression of HIV viremia with indinavir, zidovudine and lamivudine. *Ann Intern Med* **133**: 35–9.
8. Hogg RS, Heath KV, Yip B, *et al*. (1998). Improved survival among HIV-infected individuals following initiation of anti-retroviral therapy. *JAMA* **27**:450–54.

9. Mocroft A, Ledergerberg B, Katlama C, *et al.* (2003). Decline in the AIDS and death rates in the EuroSIDA study : an observational study. *Lancet* **362**:22–29.

10. Chirac J. (1997). *Address to the 10th International Conference on STD/AIDS in Africa*, Abidjan, Côte d'Ivoire,7 December 1997.

11. Cameron, E. (2000). The Deafening Silence of AIDS. *Health and Human Rights* **5**:7–24.

12. European Commission, Directorate General for Development. (2001). *Programme for action: accelerated action on HIV/AIDS, malaria and tuberculosis in the context of poverty reduction*. Brussels: European Commission.

13. UN Secretary General. (2001). *Secretary General proposes Global Fund for fight against HIV/AIDS and other infectious diseases*. New York: United Nations. Available at http:://www.un.org/News/Press/docs/2001/SGSM7779R1.doc.htm (accessed on 8 February 2007).

14. United Nations General Assembly. (2001). *Declaration of Commitment on HIV/AIDS: "Global crisis, Global action"*. New York: United Nations.

15. Global Fund. (2006). Investing in Impact: Mid-Year Results Report. Available at http//www.theglobal-fund.org/en/media_centerspublications/key_publications/#investinginimpact (accessed on 1 May 2008).

16. World Health Organization. (2002). *Scaling up antiretroviral therapy in resource-limited settings: guidelines for a public health approach*. Geneva: WHO.

17. US Department of State. (2005). *The President's Emergency Plan for AIDS Relief, 5 year strategy*. Washington DC, USA: US Department of State. Available at http://www.state.gov/documents/organization/48746.pdf (accessed on 8 February 2007).

18. World Health Organization. (2003). *The WHO strategy: treating 3 million by 2005-making it happen*. Geneva: WHO/UNAIDS.

19. United Nations General Assembly. (2006). *High-level meeting on AIDS uniting the world against AIDS, political declaration*. New York: United Nations. Available at http://www.un.org/ga/aidsmeeting2006 (accessed on 8 February 2007).

20. Moatti JP, Ndoye I, Hammer S, *et al.* (2003). Antiretroviral treatment for HIV infections in developing countries: an attainable new paradigm. *Nature Medicine* **94**: 1449–52.

21. Stroneburner R, Montagu D, Pervilhac C, *et al.* (2006). Declines in adult HIV mortality in Botswana, 2003–2005: evidence for an impact of antiretroviral therapy programs. XVI International AIDS Conference, Toronto, 13–18 August 2006. [Late breaker abstract Thlb 0507]

22. Agence nationale de recherches sur le SIDA (ANRS), Joint United Nations Programme on HIV/AIDS (UNAIDS), World Health Organization (WHO). (2004). *The Senegalese antiretroviral drug access initiative: an economic social behavioural analysis*. Available at http:www.popline.org/docs/1518/275756.html (accessed on 26 March 2008).

23. Freedberg KA., Losina E, Weinstein MC, *et al.* (2001). The Cost Effectiveness of Combination Antiretroviral Therapy of HIV Disease. *N Eng J Med* **344**:824–31.

24. Revenga A, Over M., Masaki E, *et al.* (2006). *The economics of effective AIDS treatment: evaluating policy options for Thailand*. Washington, DC, USA: World Bank.

25. Salomon JA, Hogan DR, Stover J, *et al.* (2005). Integrating HIV prevention and treatment : from slogans to impact. *PloS Med* **2**:e16.

26. Ventelou B., Moatti JP, Videau Y, *et al.* (2008). Time is costly: modeling the macroeconomic impact of scaling-up access to antiretroviral treatment for HIV/AIDS in sub-Saharan Africa. *AIDS* **22**: 107–13.

27. The ARTLINC and ART-CC groups. (2006). Mortality of HIV-infected patients in the first year of antiretroviral therapy: comparison between low-income and high-income countries. *Lancet* **367**:817–24.

28. Laniece I, Ciss M, Delainte E, *et al.* (2003). Adherence to HAART and its principal determinants in a cohort of Senegalese adults. *AIDS* **17, suppl.3**:S103–108.

29. Mills E, Nachega J, Singh S, *et al.* (2006). Adherence to antiretroviral therapy in Africa versus North America: a comparative meta-analysis. *JAMA* **296**:679–90.

30. Kuritzkes D, Lange J, Zwedie D. (2003). World Bank meeting concludes: resistance should not prevent distribution of antiretroviral therapy to poor countries. *Nature Med* **9**:1343–44.

31. UNAIDS. (2005). *Resource needs for an expanded response to AIDS in low-and middle-income countries.* Geneva: UNAIDS. Available at *http://data.unaids.org/publications/irc-pub06/resourceneedsreport_en.pdf* (accessed on 8 February 2007).

32. European Commission, Directorate General for Development. (2006). *A European program for action to tackle the critical shortage of health workers in developing countries 2007–2013.* Brussels: European Commission.

33. World Health Organization. (2006). *Working together for health. The world health report 2006.* Geneva: WHO.

Chapter 4

The outcome and impact of 10 years of HAART

Eduard J. Beck* and Rochelle P. Walensky

The HIV pandemic

The estimated number of people living with HIV infection in 2007 was 33.2 million (range 30.6–36.1 million), of whom 93% were adults over 15 years of age and 46% were women [1]. Worldwide, an estimated 2.5 million (range 1.8–4.1 million) new HIV infections occurred in 2007, 84% of which were in adults, an annual rate that has not changed substantially since 2001. In 2007 an estimated 2.1 million deaths (range 1.9–2.4 million) were attributable to HIV infection or AIDS, a decrease from 3.9 million (range 3.3–5.8 million) in 2001 [1].

Geographically, sub-Saharan Africa remains the region with the largest number of people living with HIV infection (Tables 4.1a and 4.1b). The total number infected in sub-Saharan Africa in 2007 was estimated at 22.5 million, equivalent to an HIV prevalence of 5.0%, compared with 1.3 million in the United States, or a prevalence of 0.6%, and 760,000 in Western Europe, a prevalence of 0.3%. While in some sub-Saharan African countries HIV prevalence has decreased, in others it continues to rise, especially in southern Africa. Increasing numbers of people living with HIV infection have been observed in every continent and region of the world [1].

Human immunodeficiency virus infection was first recognized as a disease entity in 1981 with the diagnosis of AIDS in homosexual males in the United States [2]. The virus itself was not identified and isolated until 1983, and ELISA antibody tests to demonstrate the presence of HIV infection were not developed and marketed until 1985. The II International AIDS Conference held in Paris in June 1986 highlighted the worldwide extent of the pandemic, including continents and countries beyond North America and Europe, particularly Africa.

Evolution of antiretroviral therapy

In 1987, six years after the first documented cases of AIDS [2], zidovudine (ZDV) was approved by the US Food and Drug Administration (FDA) for use in the treatment of AIDS. Zidovudine initially produced promising results in symptomatic patients, showing improved short-term outcomes and decreased rates of mortality and opportunistic infections (OIs) [3]. However, its impact proved transient when used alone [4]. In asymptomatic patients, it improved CD4 counts but did little to reduce clinical progression to AIDS; median survival from AIDS was only increased by a year [5]. Other nucleoside reverse transcriptase inhibitors (NRTIs) received FDA approval in 1992. Combination therapy with two NRTIs reduced clinical progression and improved survival in both antiretroviral-naïve and experienced patients compared with the sequential use of single drugs [6,7].

*Corresponding author.

Table 4.1.a Regional HIV and AIDS statistics, 2001 and 2007

	Adults & children living with HIV		Adults & children newly infected with HIV	
	2007	2001	2007	2001
Sub-Saharan Africa	22.5 million [20.9 – 24.3 million]	20.9 million [19.7 – 23.6 million]	1.7 million [1.4 – 2.4 million]	2.2 million [1.7 – 2.7 million]
Middle East & North Africa	380 000 [270 000 – 500 000]	300 000 [220 000 – 400 000]	35 000 [16 000 – 65 000]	41 000 [17 000 – 58 000]
South and South-East Asia	4.0 million [3.3 – 5.1 million]	3.5 million [2.9 – 4.5 million]	340 000 [180 000 – 740 000]	450 000 [150 000 – 800 000]
Latin America	1.6 million [1.4 – 1.9 million]	1.3 million [1.2 – 1.6 million]	100 000 [47 000 – 220 000]	130 000 [56 000 – 220 000]
Caribbean	230 000 [210 000 – 270 000]	190 000 [180 000 – 250 000]	17 000 [15 000 – 23 000]	20 000 [17 000 – 25 000]
Eastern Europe & Central Asia	1.6 million [1.2 – 2.1 million]	630 000 [490 000 – 1.1 million]	150 000 [70 000 – 290 000]	230 000 [98 000 – 340 000]
Western & Central Europe	760 000 [600 000 – 1.1 million]	620 000 [500 000 – 870 000]	31 000 [19 000 – 86 000]	32 000 [19 000 – 76 000]
North America	1.3 million [480 000 – 1.9 million]	1.1 million [390 000 – 1.6 million]	46 000 [38 000 – 68 000]	44 000 [40 000 – 63 000]
Oceania	75 000 [53 000 – 120 000}	26 000 [19 000 – 39 000]	14 000 [11 000 – 26 000]	38 000 [3000 – 56000]
TOTAL	33.2 million [30.6 – 36.1 million]	29.0 million [26.9 – 32.4 million]	2.5 million [1.8 – 4.1 million]	3.2 million [2.1 – 4.4 million]

Source: http://data.unaids.org/pub/EPISlides/2007/2007_epiudate_report_fullpresentation_en.ppt#385,5,Slide 5.

Table 4.1.b Regional HIV and AIDS statistics, 2001 and 2007

| | Adult prevalence (%) | | Adult and child deaths due to AIDS | |
	2007	2001	2007	2001
Sub-Saharan Africa	5.0% [4.6% – 5.5%]	5.8% [5.5% – 6.6%]	1.6 million [1.5 – 20 million]	1.4 million [1.3 – 1.9 million]
Middle East & North Africa	0.3% [0.2% – 0.4%]	0.3% [0.2% – 0.4%]	25 000 [20 000 – 34 000]	22 000 [11000 – 39 000]
South and South-East Asia	0.3% [0.2% – 0.4%]	0.3% [0.2% – 0.4%]	270 000 [230 000 – 380 00]	170 000 [120 000 – 220 000]
East Asia	0.1% [<0.2%]	<0.1% [<0.2%]	32 000 [28 000 – 49 000]	12 000 [82 00 – 17 000]
Latin America	0.5% [0.4% – 0.6%]	0.4% [0.3% – 0.5%]	58 000 [49 000 – 91 000]	51 000 [44 000 – 100 000]
Caribbean	1.0% [0.9% – 1.2%]	1.0% [0.9% – 1.2%]	11 000 [9800 – 18 000]	14 000 [13 000 – 21 000]
Eastern Europe & Central Asia	0.9% [0.7% – 1.2%]	0.4% [0.3% – 0.6%]	55 000 [42 000 – 88 000]	8000 [5500 – 14 000]
Western & Central Europe	0.3% [0.2% – 0.4%]	0.2% [0.1% – 0.3%]	12 000 [<15 000]	10 000 [<15 000]
North America	0.6% [0.5% – 0.9%]	0.6% [0.4% – 0.8%]	21 000 [18 000 – 31 000]	21 000 [18 000 – 31 000]
Oceania	0.4% [0.3% – 0.7%]	0.2% [0.1% – 0.3%]	1200 [<500 – 2700]	<500 [1100]
TOTAL	0.8% [0.7% – 0.9%]	0.8% [0.7% – 0.9%]	2.1 million [1.9 – 2.4 million]	3.9 million [3.3 – 5.8 million]

Source: http://data.unaids.org/pub/EPISlides/2007/2007_epiudate_report_fullpresentation_en.ppt#385,5,Slide 6.

In 1995, saquinavir (SQV) was the first of a new class of drugs, the protease inhibitors (PIs), approved by the FDA. Saquinavir was quickly followed by the approval of the more tolerable and effective indinavir (IDV) in March 1996. Nevirapine (NVP) was the first of a third class of drugs, the non-nucleoside reverse transcriptase inhibitors (NNRTIs), approved by the FDA in June 1996. Based on the success of treating people with two drugs, trials to treat people concurrently with three drugs were commenced [8]. The term 'highly active antiretroviral therapy (HAART)' was coined for combination regimens with three or more drugs from at least two antiretroviral drug classes. Since 1996, therapy has involved the sequential use of three or more antiretroviral regimens for first-, second-, third-line or salvage therapy. 'First-line' refers to the first set combination of antiretroviral drugs that patients are started on, while 'salvage' therapy refers to the combinations of drugs with which patients are treated after they have failed their third or more lines of antiretroviral therapy (ART). At all stages, the aim is to optimize regimens, even when high levels of viral resistance have emerged.

The global response to the epidemic

In the 1980s, to combat the then newly recognized HIV pandemic, the United Nations (UN) formed the Special Programme on AIDS (SPA), which evolved into the World Health Organization's (WHO) Global Programme on AIDS (GPA). Initially, GPA's approach was primarily focused on disease control, 'in the same spirit that WHO has addressed smallpox eradication' [9]. National control programmes were established, with emphasis on 'technologies' like 'value-free information, condoms and drugs to treat sexually transmitted infections' [10].

Though valuable, such programmes could not, in isolation, address the social diversity and complexity of the HIV epidemic as it manifested around the world. In the 1990s, increased emphasis was placed on changes in individual risk as a broad resolution, but soon tensions emerged regarding the competing needs surrounding behaviour change, supportive environments and individual versus community-based approaches [10]. In 1996, the Joint United Nations Programme on HIV/AIDS (UNAIDS) was created to synergize the response by the various UN organizations, and in 2000, WHO established its Department of HIV/AIDS, whose key role was to ensure that relevant interventions were available and affordable to middle- and lower-income countries [10].

Although the need to complement prevention programmes with appropriate treatment and care of HIV-infected individuals was recognized early on in the pandemic [11], only recently has the global containment strategy been focused on combining effective prevention with comprehensive treatment, care and support programmes [12]. The scaling up of such HIV services to millions of HIV-infected people has now become a major policy strategy among national and international organizations around the world.

The WHO's commitment towards scaling up access to treatment was publicly expressed by Gro Harlem Brundtland, WHO's Director-General at the time of the XIV World AIDS Conference held in 2002 in Barcelona [13], and was primarily aimed at scaling up HIV treatment with affordable antiretroviral drugs in middle- and low-income countries. The aim of the WHO/UNAIDS '3 by 5' initiative was to provide ART for 3 million HIV-infected individuals—half of those estimated to be in need of ART worldwide—by the end of 2005 [14]. This programme was complemented by initiatives such as the US President's Emergency Plan for AIDS Relief (PEPFAR), the Global Fund to Fight AIDS, Tuberculosis and Malaria (Global Fund) and other multilateral and bilateral programmes [15–18]. While '3 by 5' fell short of its ambitious goal, these programmes have ensured that access to ART has expanded dramatically, from 240,000 people in 2001 to more than 2 million people in low- and middle-income countries by

December 2006. HIV treatment coverage, however, still varies considerably within and between regions [19].

The momentum generated through these initiatives led to the 2005 G8 meeting endorsing the principle of providing 'universal free ART by 2010' [20]. Given that the process of scaling up HIV treatment and care services reiterated the importance of successful prevention services, the G8 declaration was transformed into the country-led 'Universal Access' programme unanimously endorsed by United Nations (UN) member states in the 2006 Political Declaration on HIV/AIDS [21]. The focus of universal access is to enable middle- and lower-income countries to scale up HIV prevention, treatment, care and support services, while the onus is on individual countries to set their own ambitious yet realistic 2010 targets [20, 21].

Criteria for a successful HIV intervention

For the long-term success of any HIV intervention, it must be biomedically, economically, socially and politically sustainable, and strengthen local health services [22]. Once introduced, such prevention and treatment programmes should be assessed in terms of their effectiveness, efficiency, equity of coverage and acceptability to both users and providers [23]. 'Effectiveness' in this context refers to the outcome of interventions in routine clinical care; 'efficiency' focuses on the resources required to achieve a certain outcome; 'equity' considers who benefits from the intervention; and 'acceptability' refers to both the acceptability of the intervention to users and providers and to the improvements in quality of life it achieves [23]. While applicable to all countries, the need to critically monitor and evaluate these criteria is more urgent in middle- and low-income countries where infection rates are higher and resources more limited [23].

Effectiveness

Outcomes related to ART should be evaluated both in terms of efficacy and effectiveness. 'Efficacy' refers to the extent to which a specific intervention, procedure, regimen or service produces a beneficial effect under controlled conditions [23,24]. Randomized controlled trials are theoretically best suited to evaluate efficacy. These trials are designed to examine the outcome of an intervention between groups that are in all ways similar and differ only in the intervention under consideration.

In contrast, 'effectiveness' evaluates the outcome of a specific intervention when introduced into a programme or routine service [23,24]. Through observational studies, epidemiological modelling and cost-effectiveness analyses, these operational research methods evaluate the effectiveness of an intervention within the context of local conditions that could affect the implementation of the intervention [22,23,25].

Individual outcomes and population impact of antiretroviral therapy

In the United States, the HIV-related mortality rate increased rapidly for both men and women during the late 1980s and early 1990s, reaching a peak in the mid-1990s. The rate then decreased sharply after the introduction of combination ART, levelled off and, by 2003, was at 25% of the rate observed in the mid-1990s [26]. The decline in mortality observed in the United States was seen in all racial and transmission groups. It dropped from 29.4 per 100 person-years in 1995 to 8.8 per 100 person-years in 1997 and then to 1.3 per 100 person-years in 2004 [27]. In high-income countries, non HIV-related causes of death became more numerous; hepatic disease was the only cause for which HIV-mortality has increased over time [27]. By 2003, the mean survival period from the time of HIV infection was over 21 years, and for those diagnosed with AIDS, mean survival was over 13 years in the United States [28, 29]. Similar reductions in clinical progression and improved survival, which can be attributed to ART, have been observed in other high-income countries, including Canada, Singapore and the United Kingdom [30–33]. In the United States, these individual survival benefits exceed those for other chronic diseases, including post-myocardial infarction and certain types of breast cancer. It has been estimated that the introduction of HAART has accounted for over 3 million years of life saved in the United States alone [29].

Survival benefits from ART have also been observed in middle-income countries like Brazil and South Africa [34–37]. In Brazil, where the National AIDS Program provides free ART at the point of service delivery, over half of patients diagnosed with AIDS were receiving treatment by 2003. Median survival for Brazilian AIDS patients was 5.1 months in 1989 [37], which increased to 18 months by 1995 and to 58 months by 1996, when effective therapy became available [35].

Cohort studies have demonstrated the effectiveness of ART in low-income countries. However, compared with high-income countries, patients in low-income countries had a higher mortality rate in the six months after starting therapy, and it remained higher even after one year according to data published in 2006 [38]. In high-income countries, after one year the mortality of people living with HIV and who started ART was 1.8% (95% confidence intervals (CI):1.5–2.2) compared with 2.3% (95% CI:1.5–3.2) for those who were passively followed up and 6.4% (95% CI:5.1–7.7) for those with active follow-up [38]. These higher mortality rates are thought to be multifactorial in origin and related to the fact that people in low-income countries had, on average, lower baseline CD4 counts and more advanced clinical disease when starting ART. A greater number of people in low-income countries also had co-morbidities and immune reconstitution disease, especially those people with tuberculosis (TB) [38].

When applied to resource-limited settings, individual survival benefits associated with ART range from four to ten years [34,36,39]. This comparatively small projected benefit in middle- and lower-income countries may be due, in part, to the type of drugs used, less sophisticated disease-monitoring laboratory tests and more limited options when first-line treatment regimens fail. Thus, in resource-limited settings, there are both smaller individual survival benefits and fewer individuals receiving therapy compared with those eligible. However, at a population level, cumulative assessments of years of life saved in resource-limited settings would still be likely to exceed those in the United States because of the magnitude of the epidemics in these countries and the absolute number of patients receiving therapy, even if the coverage is suboptimal. Studies examining the impact of alternative ART scale-up strategies suggest that nearly one million South African deaths might be averted by 2010 with improved coverage [40].

Efficiency

The increasing cost of treating people living with HIV has become an issue in high-, middle- and lower-income countries. The most effective way to reduce healthcare costs in general, however, is by *not* treating people with chronic diseases and simply allowing them to die. If a society accepts that healthcare is ultimately a collective social responsibility that should not be available only to those who can afford to pay for it, then considerations of the cost and cost-effectiveness of interventions come into play. In chronic conditions like HIV infection, starting ART generally implies a lifetime commitment. As HIV survival improves, an increasing number of people with HIV infection will continue to require therapy for longer periods of time. If the annual number of new HIV infections does not decrease, an increasing number of people will require prolonged ART, resulting in higher cumulative healthcare costs [41].

Increasing costs are an issue in all countries, but especially for middle- and lower-income countries, which need to rapidly scale up HIV services in the face of limited economic resources and already overburdened healthcare systems. In any healthcare system, costs should include the direct cost of healthcare for providing services, the indirect costs and the programme costs [23]. Indirect costs include travel and time costs incurred while seeking care, time and other costs to household members, funeral and orphan costs, as well as productivity gains or losses through changes in health status.

Treatment costs

In high-income countries, combination ART has shifted HIV-related care from a predominantly inpatient- to a largely outpatient-based service, with drug costs now the main cost driver among non-terminally ill patients [28]. In the late 1980s, the cost of ZDV monotherapy in the United Kingdom accounted for 28% of the estimated annual care costs of a patient of US$23,000 [42]. By the mid-1990s, 40% of the estimated US$20,000 annual treatment and care costs in the United States was spent on antiretroviral drugs [43].

In Canada, the costs of ART for patients without AIDS increased from 66% of the US$4,300 annual inpatient and outpatient care costs for the period 1991–5 to 84% of US$9,400 for the period 1997–2001 [25]. Over the same time periods, combination ART costs for patients with AIDS increased from 29% of US$9,100 to 72% of US$11,800, respectively [30]. In the United Kingdom in 2002, 70–75% of annual inpatient and outpatient costs for first-, second- or third-line therapy were spent on antiretroviral drugs, with annual inpatient and outpatient costs varying between US$18,300 and US$29,600 [33].

A 2004 US-based cost analysis reported that the undiscounted lifetime cost of one person living with HIV infection was US$618,900 [28]. This study also projected that ART costs accounted for 38% of treatment and care costs when the CD4 count was less than 50 cells/mm^3, and 77% when the CD4 count was greater than 300 cells/mm^3.

There is relatively little published information on the cost of HIV services in middle- or lower-income countries. A literature review performed up to the year 2000 [44] revealed that costing studies had only been published from five middle- or lower-income countries, while an updated literature review for the years 2000–5 identified an additional 12 published costing studies from middle- or lower-income countries [45]. A recent South African study estimated that 54% of the US$1,300 annual inpatient and outpatient hospital costs for a person with WHO stages 1–3 disease was spent on combination ART, compared with 48% of US$1,500 for those with WHO stage 4 disease [34]. Cost issues related to acute illness and end-of-life care are, however, very different in settings with limited treatment and care services, where many patients may die untreated or at home.

Over the last five years, reductions in the price of certain antiretroviral drugs have been observed for middle- and lower-income countries. This trend is due, in part, to both the reduction of prices charged by pharmaceutical companies and the increased use of less expensive generic drugs [46]. As the South African study demonstrated, lowering antiretroviral drug costs has a profound effect on annual inpatient and outpatient costs [34]. However, the current lowest annual cost of US$150 per patient for first-line ART is still beyond what the public sector in many middle- and most lower-income countries can afford [46]. Costs of second-line regimens are considerably higher and continue to be a major concern for patients who fail first-line therapy [47].

Indirect costs of HIV care

In the late 1990s, the estimated indirect costs of treatment and care of HIV-infected individuals in the United Kingdom ranged between 45% and 124% of the direct HIV treatment and care costs [48]. A recent study in the United States estimated that the total lifetime cost of the 40,000 annual incident HIV infections was US$62 billion. Productivity losses accounted for US$54 billion, or 85% of this total, while medical care accounted for US$8 billion, or 15% [49]. Productivity losses also loomed large in a study of the Swiss HIV cohort, with the mean annual productivity loss per patient estimated to be US$15,500 [50].

In resource-limited settings, indirect costs also have a large impact on HIV care. One study of the private sectors in South Africa and Botswana noted that each new HIV infection among employees costs a company between 0.5 and 3.6 times the annual salary of the affected worker [51]. In addition, orphan care places a substantial burden on already economically stretched households. For example, in a study of family health in Botswana, 37% of respondents were providing orphan care, half of whom reported financial strain associated with that care [52].

Cost-effectiveness of ART

In order to determine the efficiency of interventions or services, costs can be linked to individual outcome measures, through cost-effectiveness, cost-minimization, cost-utility or cost-benefit studies. In 'cost-effectiveness' studies, costs are evaluated with biological or clinical outcomes such as life years gained (LYG) for treatment, or infections averted for prevention interventions. For 'cost-minimization' studies, the effectiveness of the interventions being compared is similar, but the resources required to achieve a particular outcome may differ. In 'cost-utility' studies, biological outcomes are converted into disability adjusted life years (DALYs) or quality adjusted life years (QALYs), which weight life expectancy with a value of the quality of disability or life, respectively. 'Cost-benefit' studies translate biological outcomes into monetary ones, allowing for the overall analysis to be expressed in monetary terms [23].

The cut-off point for what constitutes a 'cost-effective' intervention requires the implicit acceptance of a threshold of what a society is willing to pay for another year of life or other outcome. These thresholds vary among countries [53].

A recent review of published studies on the cost-effectiveness of HIV-related interventions [54] evaluated antiretroviral drug studies published during the period 1994–2004. In Canada, combination ART was found to be cost-effective for people who did not yet have AIDS, with an incremental cost of US$14,600 per LYG, and US$12,800 per LYG for people with AIDS [30]. Similar findings have been reported from the United States [55–57], Switzerland [58], Singapore [32], the United Kingdom [59,60] and other countries [54].

Most of these cost-effectiveness studies evaluated clinical progression between stages of HIV infection, using either US Centers for Disease Control and Prevention (CDC) or WHO classifications [61,62]. Only recently have studies started to compare different antiretroviral regimens for progression between different lines of therapy. In one UK study, it was observed that NNRTI-containing regimens were cost-effective compared with PI-containing regimens for first-, second- or third-line therapy [33].

Until 2004, most published cost-effectiveness studies [54] were set in the United States or Europe, and only a few specifically examined sub-Saharan Africa or Asia; none was identified from Latin America. One recently published study on the cost-effectiveness of antiretroviral therapy in South Africa estimated that for people with WHO stage 1, 2 or 3 disease, the incremental cost was US$680–1,600 per LYG at annual antiretroviral therapy costs of US$181 and US$730, respectively. For people with AIDS (WHO stage 4), combination ART was cost-saving, regardless of whether the annual price was US$180 or US$730 [34]. Another study set in Côte d'Ivoire reported the cost-effectiveness of three antiretroviral drugs with co-trimoxazole prophylaxis to be US$620 per LYG if CD4 monitoring was unavailable and US$1,180 per LYG with CD4 testing capacity [39]. Studies performed in resource-limited settings have to date relied on outcomes or costs generated from multiple sources or from computer models because of insufficient data from a single source on both effectiveness and costs [54].

Equity

'Equity' in healthcare relates to who benefits from available services. The underpinning philosophy is that healthcare is not just an individual's responsibility, but rather one shared among members of a community or society. Equity in providing a service can be assessed within the context of a particular disease or assessed across different diseases. The former relates to questions like, 'among those with HIV infection, who should be and who is receiving ART?', whereas the latter relates to questions like, 'should services be provided for people with HIV infection or should services be provided for people with malaria?'. While healthcare professionals have tried to devise systematic methods to address these questions, ultimately the answers are largely driven by socio-economic and cultural determinants.

Antiretroviral drugs worldwide are in limited supply [63]. To address questions like 'among those with HIV infection, who should receive ART?', a number of different perspectives and settings might be considered. Some of the criteria by which equity and distribution of resources are assessed include age, gender, ethnic group, socio-economic background, stage and severity of HIV infection, occupation and geography. The latter may include urban or rural comparisons as well as differences between high-, middle- and lower-income countries.

ART coverage in high-income countries

Even in high-income countries, where combination ART is comparatively widely available, coverage varies among ethnic populations and geographical areas. In the United States, ART is funded through a variety of organizations, which include private insurance, Medicaid, the Department of Defense and Veterans Affairs and state-funded AIDS drug assistance programmes (ADAPs) [64]. States receive funds for ADAPs from Title II of the federal Ryan White CARE Act. Upon receipt of these funds, individual states decide how they are managed, administered and distributed [65]. As such, drug formularies, eligibility criteria and individual coverage among states are not uniform, leading to reported differences in both coverage and treatment outcomes depending on state of residence [66]. As states are now faced with more expensive treatments required for more patients who are living longer, ADAPs are meeting with increasing restrictions in order to remain within budget [67], with some eligible patients reportedly dying while waiting to be started on ART [68].

The trade-offs of using alternative eligibility criteria for ART, such as improved outcomes associated with severity or CD4-based criteria, as opposed to a 'first come, first served' approach, have been examined [69]. However, this highlights other ethical problems. For example, because individuals' CD4 counts change over time, a patient's place in the queue for starting ART may change. Some patients eligible for treatment under current conditions might become ineligible under CD4-based criteria. The ADAP example highlights that even healthcare systems with relatively good resources are struggling to find the most appropriate solutions to optimally fund and deliver HIV-related healthcare.

ART coverage in lower- and middle-income countries

Despite recent price reductions, antiretroviral drug costs continue to place a large economic strain on middle- and lower-income countries [46,63]. Antiretroviral drug coverage rates vary between and within global regions, countries and communities [19]. For instance, coverage of those clinically eligible for ART ranges from as high as 90% in Botswana to 3% in the Central African Republic [19].

What are the criteria for deciding who will receive ART? In accordance with their public health approach, the WHO has recommended using ART on the basis of both WHO clinical stage and CD4 count. Current guidelines recommend antiretroviral therapy if CD4 counts are lower than 200 cells/mm^3 in WHO stage 1, 2 and 3 [70]. In Brazil, people with CD4 counts lower than 350 cells/mm^3 are considered to be eligible for ART [71]. A current debate is whether the CD4 threshold should be raised to 350 cells/mm^3 globally. Apart from biomedical reasons for using the 200 cells/mm^3 thereshold, raising CD4 count treatment thresholds to 350 cells/mm^3 has resource implications. For example, in South Africa, where the current treatment coverage rate is 18% [19], changing WHO guidelines to start ART at a CD4 threshold of 350 cells/mm^3 would increase the proportion of HIV-infected patients eligible for therapy to 56% [72].

Even with a CD4 treatment threshold of 200 cells/mm^3, CD4 criteria alone remain insufficient because demand still exceeds the global supply of antiretroviral drugs and there are infrastructure limitations to the provision of adequate care. Therefore, allocation of antiretroviral therapy often uses additional criteria. Strategies might be evaluated along various dimensions in terms of their overall outcomes, but none of these criteria will perform optimally along all scales [73]. Other suggested allocation criteria include giving priority: to mothers in order to prevent mother-to-child transmission of HIV, thereby diminishing the need for orphan support by increasing survival of mothers; to skilled workers in order to promote economic growth and maintain social welfare; to the most at-risk populations, thereby diminishing transmissibility as a part of public health prevention efforts; or to patients with a demonstrated commitment to treatment adherence who will benefit most from therapy. For example, a recent South African study reported that one in seven nurses and nursing students is infected with HIV. This led to a statement requesting ART to be targeted specifically to nurses. 'You want to make sure they get priority so that they can deliver services to other people' [74]. Apart from healthcare workers, it has also been suggested that teachers should be targeted as a priority group [75].

Another study noted that access to ART is greatest in urban settings and sought to evaluate the impact of drug distribution according to geographical areas [76]. The findings of this study suggested that drug allocation strategies focusing on urban settings provide the largest epidemiological transmission benefit, avert the greatest number of AIDS deaths and generate the lowest levels of resistance. However, if implemented, urban ART distribution could increase existing disparities in healthcare resources between urban and rural communities. Thus, in situations where healthcare resources are limited, tensions exist between offering treatment to those in greatest individual need and offering it to those through whom long-term outcomes or population impact might be maximized.

Acceptability

Even if programmes are effective, efficient and available, their successful integration into any society will only be realized if they are acceptable to those who both receive and provide the service. If an intervention is unacceptable to those who are meant to benefit from it, it will be underutilized and result in suboptimal outcomes. Similarly, if service providers consider the intervention to be unacceptable, services cannot be maximized [23].

As well as monitoring objective dimensions such as 'waiting times' or 'hotel standards' of the hospital or clinic, acceptability involves 'a cognitive evaluation of an emotional reaction to health care' [77]. Dimensions of patient satisfaction that have been identified include the expressive qualities of staff, technical competence, accessibility, facilities, cost, outcomes and continuity of care [78]. The importance of acceptability is illustrated by the reported links between patient satisfaction and comprehension of information received from the physician, re-attendance at the clinic, adherence to medical advice and the more limited and explicit use of alternative therapies [78].

Another aspect of patient satisfaction involves the extent to which the quality of life of those using the intervention or service is actually improved through the intervention. This can be documented through the use of quality of life questionnaires and can involve general or HIV-specific questionnaires, or both [79–82].

Acceptability might also be evaluated in terms of the tolerability of prescribed treatment regimens. In 1996, when combination ART was first introduced into routine clinical care in high-income countries, drug regimens often required that patients take up to 30 tablets per day [83]. The frequency of doses was often dictated by time of day and proximity to meals; some required drinking copious amounts of water to prevent toxicity [84,85]. Such inconveniences led to lower adherence rates and consequently poorer rates of viral suppression [86]. The increase in the number of available antiretroviral drugs, paralleled by improved bioavailability patterns and lower toxicity profiles, now allows patients to take tablets once or twice daily with fewer side effects [87,88]. Similarly, the number of fixed-dose combinations containing two or three antiretroviral drugs in one tablet is increasing, leading to improved patient adherence and treatment outcomes [29,70]. Maintaining high levels of drug adherence is very important in terms of delaying, let alone preventing, the spread of antiretroviral drug resistance [89].

Drug toxicity from ART regimens still remains a concern. Adverse effects from drugs include hypersensitivity reactions, lipodystrophy, lactic acidosis and premature myocardial disease [90]. Toxicity trade-offs have evolved over time. In 1996, when the alternative to combination ART was death from AIDS, frequent renal stones associated with the PI IDV were considered acceptable. Now, with improved treatment options and outcomes, IDV is rarely used, having been replaced with more expensive PIs that have better bioavailability and toxicity profiles. However, even with these new drugs, around 50% of patients who fail first-, second- or third-line therapy do so because of adverse drug effects [33].

Drugs developed relatively early, which often have more adverse effects, are usually less expensive and therefore more affordable in resource-limited settings [91]. Recent formulations are relatively expensive, while generic drugs are more likely to be earlier drugs, which have lost their patent protection. Thus, while WHO promotes a 'public health approach' to providing ART to middle- and lower-income countries [92], some of the drugs recommended are not only cheaper but also more likely to have more metabolic adverse effects. Many compounds that now comprise first-line regimens favoured in high-income countries are not recommended for middle- or lower-income countries because of their higher prices [70,90]. Ethical debates continue about the expected higher rates of drug toxicity in such settings because of drug costs.

The success of treatment and care also relies on the availability of providers to deliver services. This point has been raised in the United States, where funding through the Ryan White CARE Act has not kept pace with an increasing number of people living with HIV and an increased demand for services. Stretched budgets for service providers, reduced access to care in underfunded clinical sites and overworked healthcare providers, many of whom are poorly paid, may result in insufficient physicians available to care for HIV-infected patients [93].

These considerations are even more applicable to resource-limited countries trying to scale up HIV services. The staffing problems associated with scale-up of HIV services were recently summarized as follows [75]:

- years of neglecting to plan for human resources in light of aging populations and the increased volume of long-term care needs in high-income countries;
- recruitment of care personnel from middle- and lower-income countries as a rapid and highly cost-effective solution to human resource shortages in high-income countries, leading to a net outflow of human resources from poor countries with continuing high levels of population growth and associated care and prevention needs, including for HIV;
- massive impact of HIV on an already overburdened health workforce;

- low morale caused by poor working conditions and lack of incentives to stay in the health workforce; and
- years of seeing ever-swelling numbers of people living with HIV filling up more and more hospital beds without any sign of a cure.

Solutions to these problems need to involve developing different healthcare roles among different types of staff. Apart from defining new roles for existing service providers, new providers are required within a continuum of care covering prevention and treatment. This includes direct participation by people living with HIV, their families and other community members. It will also require adjusting education and training systems to include community members [75].

At the international level, stakeholders will need to collaborate to find ways to support these developments. There is thus a great need to rethink the current models of care, who the caregivers should be and what roles different professional staff and community members should play. Dealing successfully with the HIV pandemic calls for innovative, socially responsible and flexible approaches to human resources development and use [75].

Future perspectives

With the introduction of ART involving three or more drugs, HIV infection has been transformed into a treatable, chronic condition for those with access to therapy [94]. With the introduction of a fourth class of drugs, the fusion inhibitors, the number of available antiretroviral drugs at the time of writing is 30. In addition, there are currently two newly developed drug classes—the integrase inhibitors and the CCR5/CXCR4 entry inhibitors—both of which will soon become part of the HIV treatment armamentarium. These drugs will be especially valuable for patients who might have previously exhausted all other treatment options and in whom the addition of two drug classes together may work more effectively than just one.

However, big challenges remain. As more chemotherapeutic agents become available for the effective management of patients with HIV infection, they can only prove useful if they reach those in need. Access to care remains a problem, even in high-income countries. Racial and ethnic minorities and other most at-risk and vulnerable populations continue to carry relatively high rates of HIV infection. These groups also often display lower antiretroviral therapy survival benefits. Recent data suggest that some groups in the United States lose up to six years of life, compared with more privileged groups [95, 96].

In resource-limited settings, access to care is an even more urgent problem. With only 35% of those estimated worldwide to be in need of treatment now receiving first-line therapy, its availability must be expanded. But as more patients are initiated on ART, most, if not all, will eventually fail their first-line therapy and need to start second-line, and ultimately third-line or salvage options. In some countries, ART programmes have been scaled up, but these will need to be expanded in those countries where ART scale-up has not been so rapid. Increased and sustained resources will be required to enable these countries to continue to do so.

One of the most salient lessons to be learned from the success of ART scale-up in middle- and lower-income countries is that, in order to contain and overcome the HIV pandemic, the number of people infected with HIV per year needs to be sharply reduced. Universal access provides an opportunity for countries to scale up prevention, treatment, care and support services. For this to be successfully implemented in many countries, strengthening of healthcare systems is required. However, long-term sustainability of these efforts within countries involves numerous elements: a single, multisectoral strategic response agreed upon by, and implemented through, national and international stakeholders, including public and private healthcare sectors; adequate funding for HIV therapeutic and preventive services; strong multisectoral collaboration; decentralization of the response where required; strong civil society involvement through community-based and civil society organizations; and political will and accountability. These efforts must be informed by robust and contemporary strategic information based on an integrated surveillance and monitoring and evaluation framework [22].

References

1. UNAIDS/WHO. (2007). *AIDS Epidemic Update 2007*. Available at http://www.unaids.org/en/HIV_data/ 2007EpiUpdate/default.asp (Accessed 26 November 2007).

2. US Centers for Disease Control and Prevention. (1981). *Pneumocystis* Pneumonia – Los Angeles. *MMWR* **30**:250–252.

3. Fischl MA, Richman DD, Grieco MH, *et al*. (1987). The efficacy of azidothymidine (AZT) in the treatment of patients with AIDS and AIDS-related complex. A double-blind, placebo-controlled trial. *N Engl J Med* **317**:185–191.

4. Dournon E, Matheron S, Rozenbaum W, *et al*. (1988). Effects of zidovudine in 365 consecutive patients with AIDS or AIDS-related complex. *Lancet* **2**:1297–1302.

5. Volberding PA, Lagakos SW, Grimes JM, *et al*. (1995). A comparison of immediate with deferred zidovudine therapy for asymptomatic HIV-infected adults with CD4 cell counts of 500 or more per cubic millimeter. AIDS Clinical Trials Group. *N Engl J Med* **333**:401–407.

6. Delta Trial. (1996). A randomised double-blind controlled trial comparing combinations of zidovudine plus didanosine or zalcitabine with zidovudine alone in HIV-infected individuals. Delta Coordinating Committee. *Lancet* **348**:283–291.

7. Carpenter CC, Fischl MA, Hammer SM, *et al*. (1996). Antiretroviral therapy for HIV infection in 1996. Recommendations of an international panel. International AIDS Society-USA. *JAMA* **276**:146–154.

8. Cameron DW, Heath-Chiozzi M, Danner S, *et al*. (1998). Randomised placebo-controlled trial of ritonavir in advanced HIV-1 disease. The Advanced HIV Disease Ritonavir Study Group. *Lancet* **351**:543–549.

9. WHO Special Programme on AIDS. (1987). *Progress Report No. 1, WHO/SPA/GEN 87.1*. Geneva: WHO.

10. Van Praag E, Dehne KL, Chandra-Mouli V. (2006). The UN response to the HIV pandemic. In: Beck EJ, Mays N, Whiteside A, Zuniga JM, eds. *The HIV Pandemic: local and global implications*. Oxford: Oxford University Press. p593–606.

11. Beck EJ. (1991). HIV infection and intervention: the first decade. *AIDS Care* **3**:295–302.

12. Piot P, Zewdie D, Turmen T. (2002). HIV/AIDS prevention and treatment. *Lancet* **360**:86; author reply 87–88.

13. Brundlandt G. (2002). International Collaboration In Scaling Up The Response to AIDS. 14th World AIDS Conference, 7–12 July 2002, Barcelona, Spain. Available at http://www.who.int/director-general/ speeches/2002/english/20020709_InternationalCollaborationScalingUptheRResponsetoAIDS.html (Accessed 30 July 2007).

14. WHO. (2006). *Progress in scaling up access to HIV treatment in low and middle income countries*. Geneva: WHO. Available at http://www.who.int/hiv/toronto2006/FS_Treatment_en.pdf (Accessed 8 May 2007).

15. USAID. *The US President's Emergency Plan for AIDS Relief: Fact Sheets*. Available at http://www.usaid.gov/our_work/global_health/aids/pepfarfact.html (Accessed 8 May 2007).

16. Clinton Foundation Programs. *HIV/AIDS Initiative*. Available at http://www.clintonfoundation.org/ cf-pgm-hs-ai-home.htm (Accessed 8 May 2007).

17. DFID. *HIV/AIDS Strategy*. Available at http://www.dfid.gov.uk/pubs/files/hiv-isp.pdf (Accessed 8 May 2007).

18. Ministère des Affaires Étrangères, France. (2005). *Stratégie sectorielle: lutte contre le sida*. Available at http://www.diplomatie.gouv.fr/fr/thematiques_830/aide-au-developpement_1060/politique-francaise_3024/strategies-gouvernementales_5156/strategies-sectorielles-cicid_4570/strategie-sectorielle-lutte-contre-sida-mai-2005_13087.html?artsuite=0 (Accessed 8 May 2007).

19. WHO. (2007). *Towards Universal Access: Scaling up priority HIV/AIDS interventions on the health sector. Progress Report.* Available at http://www.who.int/hiv/mediacentre/univeral_access_progress_report_en. pdf (Accessed 8 May 2007).

20. Anonymous (2005). *The Gleneagles Communiqué.* Available at http://www.fco.gov.uk/Files/kfile/PostG8_Gleneagles_Communique.pdf (Accessed 8 May 2007).

21. UNAIDS. (2006). *Towards Universal Access: assessment by the Joint United Nations programme on HIV/AIDS on scaling up HIV prevention, treatment, care and support. UN General Assembly document A/60/737.* New York, NY: UNAIDS.

22. Beck EJ, Mays N. (2006). Some Lessons Learned. In: Beck EJ, Mays N, Whiteside A, Zuniga JM, eds. *The HIV Pandemic: local and global implications.* Oxford: Oxford University Press. p757–776.

23. Beck EJ, Miners AH. (2001). Effectiveness and efficiency in the delivery of HIV services: economic and related considerations. In: Gazzard B, Johnson M, Miles A, eds. *The effective management of HIV/AIDS. UK Key Advances in Clinical Practice.* London: Aesculapius Medical Press. p113–138.

24. Last J, ed. (1988). *A Dictionary of Epidemiology.* 2nd Edition. Oxford: Oxford University Press.

25. Winston W. (1991). *Operations Research: Applications and Algorithms.* 2nd Edition. Boston: PWS-Kent Publishing Company.

26. US Centers for Disease Control and Prevention. (2005). World AIDS Day: December 1, 2005. *MMWR* **54**:1188.

27. Palella FJ Jr, Deloria-Knoll M, Chmiel JS, *et al.* (2003). Survival benefit of initiating antiretroviral therapy in HIV-infected persons in different CD4+ cell strata. *Ann Intern Med* **138**:620–626.

28. Schackman BR, Gebo KA, Walensky RP, *et al.* (2006). The lifetime cost of current human immunodeficiency virus care in the United States. *Med Care* **44**:990–997.

29. Walensky RP, Paltiel AD, Losina E, *et al.* (2006). The survival benefits of AIDS treatment in the United States. *J Infect Dis* **194**:11–19.

30. Beck EJ, Mandalia S, Gaudreault M, *et al.* (2004). The cost-effectiveness of highly active antiretroviral therapy, Canada 1991–2001. *AIDS* **18**:2411–2418.

31. Lima VD, Hogg RS, Harrigan PR, *et al.* (2007). Continued improvement in survival among HIV-infected individuals with newer forms of highly active antiretroviral therapy. *AIDS* **21**:685–692.

32. Paton NI, Chapman CA, Sangeetha S, Mandalia S, Bellamy R, Beck EJ. (2006). Cost and cost-effectiveness of antiretroviral therapy for HIV infection in Singapore. *Int J STD AIDS* **17**:699–705.

33. Beck EJ, Mandalia S, Brettle R, *et al.*(2006). Cost-effectiveness of NNRTI compared with PI containing regimens for first-, second- and third-line HAART regimens in UK NPMS-HHC clinics 1996–2002. XVI International AIDS Conference, 13–18 August 2006, Toronto, Canada. [Abstract TuPe 0073]

34. Badri M, Maartens G, Mandalia S, *et al.* (2006). Cost-effectiveness of highly active antiretroviral therapy in South Africa. *PLoS Med* **3**:e4.

35. Marins JR, Jamal LF, Chen SY, *et al.* (2003). Dramatic improvement in survival among adult Brazilian AIDS patients. *AIDS* **17**:1675–1682.

36. Cleary SM, McIntyre D, Boulle AM. (2006). The cost-effectiveness of Antiretroviral Treatment in Khayelitsha, South Africa – a primary data analysis. *Cost Eff Resour Alloc* **4**:20.

37. Chequer P, Hearst N, Hudes ES, *et al.* (1992). Determinants of survival in adult Brazilian AIDS patients, 1982–1989. The Brazilian State AIDS Program Co-Ordinators. *AIDS* **6**:483–487.

38. Braitstein P, Brinkhof MW, Dabis F, *et al.* (2006). Mortality of HIV-1-infected patients in the first year of antiretroviral therapy: comparison between low-income and high-income countries. *Lancet* **367**:817–824.

39. Goldie SJ, Yazdanpanah Y, Losina E, *et al.* (2006). Cost-effectiveness of HIV treatment in resource-poor settings – the case of Côte d'Ivoire. *N Engl J Med* **355**:1141–1153.

40. Walensky RP, Wood R, Losina E, *et al.* Waiting for ART in South Africa: Deaths Averted with a More Aggressive Scale-up. XIV Conference on Retroviruses and Opportunistic Infections, 25–28 February 2007, Los Angeles, CA, USA. [Abstract 549]

41. US Centers for Disease Control and Prevention. (2003). Advancing HIV Prevention: New Strategies for a Changing Epidemic – United States, 2003. *MMWR* **52**:329–332.

42. Beck EJ, Kupek EJ, Petrou S, *et al.* (1996). Survival and the use and costs of hospital services for London AIDS patients treated with AZT. *Int J STD AIDS* **7**:507–512.

43. Bozzette SA, Joyce G, McCaffrey DF, *et al.* (2001). Expenditures for the care of HIV-infected patients in the era of highly active antiretroviral therapy. *N Engl J Med* **344**:817–823.

44. Beck EJ, Miners AH, Tolley K. (2001). The cost of HIV treatment and care. A global review. *Pharmacoeconomics* **19**:13–39.

45. Beck EJ, Blandford J, Boulle A, *et al.* (2006). Essential Information for Countries to Monitor & Evaluate the Economic Aspects of HIV Service Provision: proceedings from a workshop. WHO/TDR Generic Tools Workshop, 16–18 January 2006, Geneva, Switzerland. Available at http://www.who.int/hiv/events/GenericToolsWorkshop.pdf (Accessed 8 May 2007).

46. Fleet J, N'Daw B. (2006). Trade, Intellectual Property and Access to Affordable HIV Medications. In: Beck EJ, Mays N, Whiteside A, Zuniga JM, eds. *The HIV Pandemic: local and global implications*. Oxford: Oxford University Press. p660–673.

47. Spiritindia.com. (2007). *Abbott reduces price of Kaletra, Aluvia in developing countries*. Available at http://www.spiritindia.com/health-care-news-articles-8231.html (Accessed 8 May 2007).

48. Mullins CD, Whitelaw G, Cooke JL, Beck EJ. (2000). Indirect cost of HIV infection in England. *Clin Ther* **22**:1333–1345.

49. Hutchinson AB, Farnham PG, Dean HD, *et al.* (2006). The economic burden of HIV in the United States in the era of highly active antiretroviral therapy: evidence of continuing racial and ethnic differences. *J Acquir Immune Defic Syndr* **43**:451–457.

50. Sendi P, Schellenberg F, Ungsedhapand C, *et al.* (2004). Productivity costs and determinants of productivity in HIV-infected patients. *Clin Ther* **26**:791–800.

51. Rosen S, Vincent JR, MacLeod W, Fox M, Thea DM, Simon JL. (2004). The cost of HIV/AIDS to businesses in southern Africa. *AIDS* **18**:317–324.

52. Miller CM, Gruskin S, Subramanian SV, Rajaraman D, Heymann SJ. (2006). Orphan care in Botswana's working households: growing responsibilities in the absence of adequate support. *Am J Public Health* **96**:1429–1435.

53. Garber A. (2000). Advances in Cost-effectiveness Analysis of Health Interventions. In: Culyer A, Newhouse J, eds. *Handbook of Health Economics*. Vol 1A, Chapter 4. Amsterdam: Elsevier. p181–221.

54. Harling G, Wood R, Beck EJ. (2005). Efficiency of interventions in HIV Infection, 1994–2004. *Dis Manag Health Out* **13**:371–394.

55. Freedberg KA, Losina E, Weinstein MC, *et al.* (2001). The cost effectiveness of combination antiretroviral therapy for HIV disease. *N Engl J Med* **344**:824–831.

56. Schackman BR, Freedberg KA, Weinstein MC, *et al.* (2002). Cost-effectiveness implications of the timing of antiretroviral therapy in HIV-infected adults. *Arch Intern Med* **162**:2478–2486.

57. Schackman BR, Goldie SJ, Freedberg KA, Losina E, Brazier J, Weinstein MC. (2002). Comparison of health state utilities using community and patient preference weights derived from a survey of patients with HIV/AIDS. *Med Decis Making* **22**:27–38.

58. Sendi PP, Bucher HC, Harr T, *et al.* (1999). Cost effectiveness of highly active antiretroviral therapy in HIV-infected patients. Swiss HIV Cohort Study. *AIDS* **13**:1115–1122.

59. Miners AH, Sabin CA, Trueman P, *et al.* (2001). Assessing the cost-effectiveness of HAART for adults with HIV in England. *HIV Med* **2**:52–58.

60. Trueman P, Youle M, Sabin CA, Miners AH, Beck EJ. (2000). The cost-effectiveness of triple nucleoside analogue therapy antiretroviral regimens in the treatment of HIV in the United Kingdom. *HIV Clin Trials* **1**:27–35.

61. US Centers for Disease Control and Prevention. (1992). 1993 Revised Classification System for HIV Infection and Expanded Surveillance Case Definition for AIDS Among Adolescents and Adults.

MMWR **41**(RR-17). Available at http://www.cdc.gov/MMWR/preview/MMWRhtml/0018871.htm (Accessed 26 March 2008).

62. WHO. (2006). *WHO Case Definition of HIV Surveillance and Revised Clinical Staging and Immunological Classification of HIV-Related Disease in Adults and Children.* Available at http://www.who.int/hiv/pub/guidelines/WHO%20HIV%20Staging.pdf (Accessed 8 May 2007).

63. Pinheiro E, Vasan A, Kim JY, Lee E, Guimier JM, Perriens J. (2006). Examining the production costs of antiretroviral drugs. *AIDS* **20**:1745–1752.

64. Beck EJ, Morgan D. (2003). HIV Service Provision for Ethnic Minorities: people of African descent in the UK and US. In: Erwin J, Peters B, Smith D, Myers H, eds. *Ethnicity and HIV.* Atlanta: International Medical Press. p121–140.

65. Walensky RP, Paltiel AD, Freedberg KA. (2002). AIDS Drug Assistance Programs: highlighting inequities in human immunodeficiency virus-infection health care in the United States. *Clin Infect Dis* **35**:606–610.

66. Schackman BR, Freedberg KA, Goldie SJ, Weinstein MC, Swartz K. (2005). Budget impact of Medicaid Section 1115 demonstrations for early HIV treatment. *Health Care Financ Rev* **26**:67–80.

67. NASTAD. *The ADAP Watch.* Available at http://www.nastad.org/Docs/highlight/20061214_NASTAD_ADAP_Watch_121206.pdf (Accessed 8 May 2007).

68. Kaiser Family Foundation. *HIV/AIDS Advocacy Group Calls for Emergency ADAP Funds To End Waiting Lists in South Carolina.* Available at http://www.kaisernetwork.org/daily_reports/rep_index.cfm?hint=1&DR_ID=40955 (Accessed 8 May 2007).

69. Linas BP, Zheng H, Losina E, *et al.* (2006). Optimizing resource allocation in United States AIDS drug assistance programs. *Clin Infect Dis* **43**:1357–1364.

70. WHO. *Revision of Antiretroviral Therapy for HIV Infection in Adults and Adolescents: recommendations for a public health approach.* Available at http://www.who.int/hiv/pub/guidelines/artadultguidelines.pdf (Accessed 8 May 2007).

71. Ministério da Saúde, Brazil. *Recomendações para Terapia Anti-Retroviral em Adultos e Adolescentes Infectados pelo HIV 2004.* Available at http://www.aids.gov.br/final/biblioteca/adulto_2004/consenso.doc (Accessed 8 May 2007).

72. Auvert B, Males S, Puren A, Taljaard D, Carael M, Williams B. (2004). Can highly active antiretroviral therapy reduce the spread of HIV? A study in a township of South Africa. *J Acquir Immune Defic Syndr* **36**:613–621.

73. Rosen S, Sanne I, Collier A, Simon JL. (2005). Rationing antiretroviral therapy for HIV/AIDS in Africa: choices and consequences. *PLoS Med* **2**:e303.

74. Shisana O. CDC News. (2007). CDC HIV/STD/TB Prevention News Update 22 February 2007. Available at http://listmanager.aspensys.com/read/messages?id=49582 (Accessed 8 May 2008).

75. Dreesch N, Dal Poz M, Gedik G, Adams O, Evans T. (2006). Developing Human Resources for the HIV Pandemic. In: Beck EJ, Mays N, Whiteside A, Zuniga JM, eds. *The HIV Pandemic: local and global implications.* Oxford: Oxford University Press. p688–705.

76. Wilson DP, Kahn J, Blower SM. (2006). Predicting the epidemiological impact of antiretroviral allocation strategies in KwaZulu-Natal: the effect of the urban-rural divide. *Proc Natl Acad Sci USA* **103**:14228–14233.

77. Fitzpatrick R. (1993). Scope and measurement of satisfaction. In: Fitzpatrick R, Hopkins A, eds. *A measurement of patients' satisfaction with their care.* London: Royal College of Physicians. p1–17.

78. Beck EJ, Griffith R, Fitzpatrick R, *et al.* (1999). Patient satisfaction with HIV service provision in NPMS hospitals: the development of a standard satisfaction questionnaire. *AIDS Care* **11**:331–343.

79. Ware J, Snow K, Kosinski M, Gandek B. (1993). *SF-36 Health Survey Manual and Interpretation Guide.* Boston: The Health Institute, New England Medical Center.

80. Ware J, Snow K, Kosinski M, Gandek B. (1994). *SF-36 Physical and Mental Health Summary Scales: a user's manual.* Boston: The Health Institute, New England Medical Center.

81. Wu AW, Hays RD, Kelly S, Malitz F, Bozzette SA. (1997). Applications of the Medical Outcomes Study health-related quality of life measures in HIV/AIDS. *Qual Life Res* **6**:531–554.

82. Singer J, Thorne A, Khorasheh S, *et al.* (2000). Symptomatic and health status outcomes in the Canadian randomized MAC treatment trial (CTN010). Canadian HIV Trials Network Protocol 010 Study Group. *Int J STD AIDS* **11**:212–219.

83. Von Bargen J, Moorman A, Holmberg S. (1998). How many pills do patients with HIV infection take? *JAMA* **280**:29.

84. Mueller BU, Sleasman J, Nelson RP Jr, *et al.* (1998). A phase I/II study of the protease inhibitor indinavir in children with HIV infection. *Pediatrics* **102**:101–109.

85. Lesho EP, Gey DC. (2003). Managing issues related to antiretroviral therapy. *Am Fam Physician* **68**:675–686.

86. Nilsson Schönnesson L, Williams ML, Ross MW, Bratt G, Keel B. (2007). Factors associated with suboptimal antiretroviral therapy adherence to dose, schedule, and dietary instructions. *AIDS Behav* **11**:175–183.

87. Haubrich R, Berger D, Chiliade P, *et al.* (2007). Week 24 efficacy and safety of TMC114/ritonavir in treatment-experienced HIV patients. *AIDS* **21**:F11–18.

88. Jayaweera DT, Kolber MA, Brill M, *et al.* (2004). Effectiveness and tolerability of a once-daily amprenavir/ritonavir-containing highly active antiretroviral therapy regimen in antiretroviral-naïve patients at risk for nonadherence: 48-week results after 24 weeks of directly observed therapy. *HIV Med* **5**:364–370.

89. Bennett DE. (2006). The requirement for surveillance of HIV drug resistance within antiretroviral rollout in the developing world. *Curr Opin Infect Dis* **19**:607–614.

90. US Department of Health and Human Services. (2006). *Guidelines for the Use of Antiretroviral Agents in HIV-1-Infected Adults and Adolescents.* Available at aidsinfo.nih.gov/contentfiles/AdultandAdolescentGL.pdf (Accessed 8 May 2007).

91. Médecins sans Frontières. (2006). *Untangling the Web of Price Reductions: a pricing guide for the purchase of ARVs for developing countries.* Available at http://www.accessmed-msf.org/documents/untanglingtheweb%209.pdf (Accessed 8 May 2007).

92. Grubb I, Perriëns J, Schwartländer B. (2003). *A Public Health Approach to Antiretroviral Treatment: overcoming constraints.* Geneva: WHO. Available at http://www.who.int/hiv/pub/prev_care/en/PublicHealthApproach_E.pdf (Accessed 8 May 2007).

93. National Institutes of Health. (2006). *Opportunities for Improving HIV Diagnosis, Prevention and Access to Care in the U.S. – Day2: Where do Americans Access Care? Considerations for Testing and Planning for Additional HIV-Infected People in the Health Care System.* Available at http://kaisernetwork.org/health_cast/uploaded_files/1130-nih-access_transcript1.pdf (Accessed 8 May 2008).

94. Vermund SH. (2006). Millions of life-years saved with potent antiretroviral drugs in the United States: a celebration, with challenges. *J Infect Dis* **194**:1–5.

95. US Centers for Disease Control and Prevention. (2007). Racial/Ethnic Disparities in Diagnoses of HIV/AIDS – 33 States, 2001–2005. *MMWR* **56**:189–193.

96. Losina E, Schackman BR, Sadownik S, *et al.* (2007). Disparities in Survival Attributable to Suboptimal HIV Care in the US: Influence of Gender and Race/Ethnicity. XIV Conference on Retroviruses and Opportunistic Infections, 25–28 February 2007, Los Angeles, CA, USA. [Abstract 142]

Chapter 5

HAART in HIV-infected children: one decade later

Arry Dieudonne*, James A. McIntyre, Federica Fregonese, Carlo Giaquinto and James M. Oleske

History

The HIV epidemic has entered its second decade since the initial cases of an unusual syndrome of immunodeficiency in children were described and soon recognized as part of the syndrome seen in adults. There have been considerable advances, especially in the last 10 years, in the management of paediatric HIV infection. These have included the development and availability of HIV DNA polymerase chain reaction (PCR) assays, the use of ultrasensitive P_{24} antigen $(UP_{24}$ Ag) and dried blood spot (DBS) DNA PCR for early diagnosis in resource-constrained countries, the advent of new classes of antiretroviral drugs for use in combination therapy and better monitoring tools—in particular, HIV RNA PCR (viral load) and HIV genotype and phenotype.

With these advances, the prevalence of HIV infection in infants through significant interruption in perinatal HIV transmission has been reduced, and the epidemiology of paediatric HIV infection in the United States and Western European countries has changed from an acutely fatal disease to a chronic, treatable illness. While this epidemic was first described in the Western hemisphere, it soon became clear that it was turning into a global problem. New challenges include the changing care required for children surviving with HIV infection into adulthood, while striving to translate the HIV care and prevention advances in the United States and developed hemispheres to the rest of the world.

As, through monitoring, we have learned more about the relationship between clinical symptoms, immune status and viral load, the clinical and laboratory definition of HIV infection has undergone several revisions, and guidelines for antiretroviral therapy and medical management of paediatric HIV infection are updated on a regular basis. The World Health Organization (WHO) guidelines addressing diagnosis, care and treatment are being adapted by developing countries based on their needs and their resources. This chapter will provide an overview of paediatric HIV management in the population entering adulthood after a decade of highly active antiretroviral therapy (HAART). It will not address in detail many health and social issues of adolescents who acquired HIV infection through adult behaviours. It is hoped that the achievements noted in this review of HIV infection in children will serve as the roadmap for the treatment of all children, regardless of geography or means.

* Corresponding author.

Prevention of mother-to-child transmission of HIV

Vertical transmission from mother to child is the predominant source of HIV-1/HIV-2 acquisition in children. The prevention of mother-to-child transmission (PMTCT) of HIV represents one of the most successful interventions in the history of the HIV epidemic to date. Although there has been significant progress in developing and implementing treatment strategies and in service provision, an estimated 530,000 children were infected with HIV worldwide in 2006, mainly through mother-to-child transmission (MTCT) [1], and the 2001 United Nations (UN) General Assembly's goal of a 50% reduction in the proportion of infants infected with HIV by 2010 remains out of reach.

Following the first descriptions of paediatric AIDS and of MTCT in the mid-1980s [2,3], evidence accumulated on the factors influencing the risk of transmission, the timing of transmission and the additional risk of infection through breastfeeding [4]. Three major preventive interventions became obvious from this work: the use of antiretroviral therapy (ART) to reduce the risk of PMTCT, the use of elective caesarean section delivery in HIV-positive mothers and the avoidance of breastfeeding. Ten years passed before the first results of a randomized trial of an antiretroviral intervention showed the potential to reduce the risk of HIV transmission from mothers to babies. The ACTG 076 study, published in 1994 [5], rapidly changed practice in well-resourced settings and had a remarkable effect on the rates of transmission from mother to child.

In the decade after 1994, as the availability of antiretroviral drugs and access to treatment for pregnant women increased, the numbers of infants perinatally infected with HIV dropped substantially in the United States and Europe (Figure 5.1) [6]. The initial zidovudine (ZDV)-only PMTCT regimens gave way first to dual therapy and later to triple combination HAART in pregnant women. The transmission rates dropped concomitantly to less than 2% in those well-resourced settings where the full gamut of interventions was available. In these settings, the dual approach of starting ongoing HAART in pregnancy (for those women who qualify for it), and using HAART through the pregnancy and stopping post-partum for those with higher CD4 counts, combined with the avoidance of breastfeeding, has become standard management in pregnancy [7,8].

Although it cannot be claimed that paediatric HIV has been eliminated, with fewer than 200 HIV-infected children now born annually in the United States, the goal has almost been reached there.

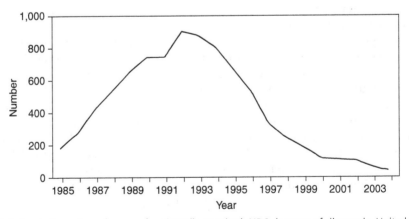

Fig. 5.1 Estimated number of cases of perinatally acquired AIDS, by year of diagnosis, United States 1985–2004.

Notes: Data adjusted for reporting delays and for estimated proportional redistribution of cases in persons reported without an identifed risk factor.

Source: [6]

Further attention is needed to identify and treat those women in vulnerable circumstances who do not currently access antenatal care, or who do so too late to benefit from these interventions. In Europe, much of the HIV epidemic in pregnant women in recent years has been seen among marginalized immigrant populations [9], and similar issues complicate the delivery of PMTCT care there.

PMTCT in low-resource settings

The remarkable advances in reducing MTCT in well-resourced settings have unfortunately not yet been replicated in low-resource settings. In contrast to the United States or Europe, where one child a day is born with HIV, close to 1800 children are infected daily in Africa and Asia. According to United Nations Children's Fund (UNICEF) estimates, a child dies every minute of every day from HIV infection, and most of these deaths are the result of MTCT [10].

Following the results of the ACTG 076 study, a number of trials were undertaken in low-resource countries to investigate the effect of shorter, more feasible and less expensive ART regimens to reduce MTCT. These studies, initially using short courses of ZDV alone [11], ZDV and lamivudine (3TC) [12], and nevirapine (NVP) [13,14], all showed a range of effectiveness in reducing transmission. In the HIVNET 012 study, administering a single dose of NVP to mothers at the onset of labour and a dose to infants within 72 hours of birth reduced the risk of transmission in a Ugandan cohort by 50% [13]. This provided evidence for a regimen that was safe, affordable, feasible and potentially accessible for women in high-prevalence, low-resource countries. The reduction in transmission achievable with either the short course regimens of ZDV, ZDV and 3TC, or NVP is limited, with most studies reporting transmission at six weeks of around 10–15% [14]; the addition of intrapartum and infant NVP doses to a short antenatal regimen of ZDV and 3TC in Côte d'Ivoire showed a transmission rate of 5% [15]. A study in Thailand, using a combination of ZDV from 28 weeks of pregnancy together with a single dose of NVP to mother and baby, demonstrated transmission rates of 2% or less [16,17], equivalent to the rates seen with triple-therapy prophylaxis. The use of this more effective regimen would further reduce global transmission rates.

Notwithstanding these successes, some concern has arisen over the use of NVP alone or in non-suppressive combination regimens: non-nucleoside reverse transcriptase inhibitor (NNRTI) resistance, which requires only one point mutation in the viral codon, is common in NVP use, arising rapidly following even a single dose. A number of reports have now demonstrated this in around 20–60% of mothers and more than half the children receiving single-dose NVP (sdNVP) in different settings, with the risk of resistance being higher with clade C virus, higher viral load and lower CD4 counts [18,19]. More sensitive assays for the K103N and Y181C resistance mutations have shown that resistant virus is present, at least in small proportions, in closer to 80% of these women [20]. The levels of resistant variants have been shown to drop over time, with a return to wild-type virus as the predominant virus [21].

The major concern about this resistance is that it could have a negative impact on future antiretroviral therapy for mothers. Although this question has not yet been definitively answered, and randomized trials are in progress, observational studies have suggested that future treatment is not markedly affected by perinatal prophylaxis. Although the full implications of NNRTI resistance are not known, the avoidance of selecting an NNRTI for perinatal prophylaxis would appear to be the best option. NVP has a long half-life and is detectable in plasma for up to 21 days after its single-dose use in mothers [22], resulting in effective monotherapy with a drug that has a low barrier for selection of viruses resistant to NNRTIs. While the full implications of mutations selected as a consequence of sdNVP administration to mothers are under investigation, strategies that could prevent this selection in the first place would appear to be the best option. For example, the addition of four or seven days of the co-formulation of ZDV and 3TC (marketed as Combivir®) for mothers, starting with the intrapartum NVP dose, has been shown to reduce the risk of resistance detectable by population sequencing from approximately 60% to almost 10% [23]. Using the more sensitive allele-specific PCR in a sub-sample from this study showed a reduction in the proportion of women with resistant variants from 71% to 25%, with a lower frequency of resistant variants in the treated group [24]. The use of a ZDV/3TC 'tail cover' has now been included in WHO's PMTCT guidelines [17].

Breastfeeding

Transmission of HIV through breast milk is a major contributor to infection in infants, accounting for more than 300,000 of the 530,000 estimated transmissions each year in areas of the world with the highest maternal HIV infection rates [25]. The reduction in MTCT achieved through antiretroviral strategies can be completely negated by the effect of breastfeeding. Complete avoidance of breastfeeding removes this risk, and this strategy has contributed to the near-eradication of paediatric HIV in high-resource settings. This situation is much more difficult in lower-resource countries. The WHO recommends that breastfeeding be avoided where replacement feeding is 'acceptable, feasible, affordable, sustainable' [26]—the so-called AFASS criteria. This is the standard of care for women in the United States and Europe and is widely practised in some areas of Asia, such as Thailand. In Africa, while possible for some women, for many others it is not currently feasible, and replacement feeding carries a high risk of morbidity for the baby. In these settings, exclusive breastfeeding carries a lower risk of HIV transmission than 'mixed feeding' and is recommended [25].

Exclusive breastfeeding, where no other food or water is given to the child, is uncommon in most settings, and mixed feeding is the norm. If it is to be successful, the promotion and support of exclusive breastfeeding requires staff and strategies that do not currently exist in most places. The WHO's guidelines initially recommend exclusive breastfeeding for the first three to six months of the baby's life, with rapid weaning at that point, followed by the use of alternative foods [26]. The additional risk of transmission from breast milk between the ages of six weeks and six months was found to be around 1% per month in several studies [25]. This approach has to be balanced against the risk of severe morbidity or mortality from replacement feeding in unsafe circumstances; it may carry risks if the criteria of acceptability, feasibility, affordability and safety set by the WHO are not met [27]. Updated recommendations now suggest that it may be safer in these circumstances to continue to breastfeed, despite the increased HIV transmission risk [28].

An alternative approach to reducing transmission via breast milk would be the use of antiretroviral prophylaxis to breastfed infants or the provision of HAART to breastfeeding mothers. Such an approach has biological plausibility; ART has been shown to reduce the viral load in breast milk [29], and several trials, both observational and randomized, are in progress. If this strategy proves successful, it could provide another option to retain the benefits of breastfeeding where access to antiretroviral drugs is available. Long-term toxicities, however, have been described in women with normal CD4 counts who are given NVP-containing HAART. Antiretroviral therapy given for several months during pregnancy and six months postpartum before being discontinued, but subsequently restarted at the time of decrease in CD4 counts, could be associated with potentially fatal side effects as demonstrated in treatment interruption trials [30]. Effective ways to make either exclusive replacement feeding or exclusive breastfeeding safer are key to achieving further reductions in MTCT.

Public health implications of PMTCT

The introduction, in 2000, of NVP-based PMTCT programmes in low-resource settings provided prophylaxis to more than a million mothers and infants by 2006 [31]. Unfortunately, even this level of scale-up is not enough. In 2006, the Joint United Nations Programme on HIV/AIDS (UNAIDS) estimated that less than 8% of all pregnant women globally, and less than 6% in sub-Saharan Africa, had access to HIV diagnosis and prevention services, and that only 9% of HIV-infected women received an antiretroviral regimen for PMTCT. The lack of access is reflected in the estimates of transmission: rates of 26% are estimated in the 33 most affected countries, a 10-fold higher rate than that now seen in the developed world [1]. Although the antenatal ZDV with intrapartum NVP regimen has become the first-line recommendation in the WHO's PMTCT guidelines for low-resource settings [17], few country programmes have yet been able to extend beyond the sdNVP regimen. With the increasing access to antiretroviral therapy in low-resource settings, the provision of PMTCT services needs to be seen more as an integral part of care and treatment for HIV-infected women during and after delivery. Increased access to antiretroviral drugs sets a new imperative to identify pregnant women in need of HAART and initiate treatment as soon as possible during the pregnancy. The use of effective ART in these women will both benefit their own health and be the best prophylaxis against MTCT of HIV. The 2006 WHO guidelines recommend, in line with most other national and international guidelines, that a pregnant woman with CD4 counts less than 200 cells/mm^3, or with WHO clinical stage 3 or 4 disease, begin and continue HAART. In addition, the guidelines recommend starting HAART in pregnant women with CD4 counts between 200 and 350 cells/mm^3, where possible.

The implementation of these recommendations is proving difficult to achieve in many settings where treatment programmes have only recently been established and the capacity to expand is limited. In high-prevalence HIV settings such as much of southern Africa, a third (or more) of pregnant women are infected, and of these, close to 20% will have CD4 counts of less than 200 cells/mm^3 and half will have counts of less than 350 cells/mm^3. This represents a significant number of women immediately in need of ART and underscores the urgency for rapid expansion of sustainable treatment programmes.

Given the lower efficacy of most of the short-course regimens, the concerns about NVP resistance and the increasing availability of antiretroviral drugs, there are increasing calls for the use of HAART in all pregnant women, including those in low-resource settings, as the most effective and appropriate PMTCT regimen [31]. Favourable reports of HAART used in Mozambique and elsewhere in Africa have demonstrated the potential for such use [32]. However, major logistical and clinical issues remain as barriers to the use of HAART for MTCT prophylaxis. One example is the choice of regimen in settings where drug choices are limited and protease inhibitors (PIs) are generally reserved for second-line therapy, particularly for women with high CD4 counts, in whom NVP-based regimens are currently discouraged given the increased risk of hepatotoxicity [33]. Since there is little capacity in many African programmes to provide HAART even for those pregnant women with low CD4 counts, and a huge unmet need for even the simplest of PMTCT regimens, the approach outlined in the 2006 version of the WHO's PMTCT guidelines may be most appropriate at present. The WHO guidelines recommend starting or continuing HAART for those women who require treatment for their own health, with a suggested CD4 count entry point of 350 cells/mm^3, and an effective short-course regimen of ZDV with intrapartum NVP for mothers who do not yet qualify for HAART. As treatment access programmes increase in scale and scope, moving to more intensive HAART regimens for PMTCT will become more feasible and should remain a longer-term goal in order to provide mothers in these settings with the same level of comprehensive HIV treatment and care as they would receive in the developed world.

Antiretroviral management

Treatment of HIV infection has evolved over the last 20 years. Prior to the availability of antiretroviral drugs, care was mostly focused on prevention and management of HIV-related complications and provision of palliative care. Treatment in the early 1990s consisted of a single drug, usually ZDV, and significant clinical and immunologic benefits were demonstrated in many studies [34]. Subsequently, dual nucleoside reverse transcriptase inhibitor (NRTI) treatment showed better clinical, immunologic and virologic outcomes than monotherapy [35]. The introduction of PI-containing regimens including at least three drugs has been associated with enhanced survival, reduction in opportunistic infections (OIs) and other complications of HIV infection, improved growth and neurocognitive function, and improved quality of life in children [36]. European (Paediatric European Network for the Treatment of AIDS (PENTA)), US (Department of Health and Human Services (DHHS)) and WHO guidelines for prevention of HIV and treatment in children with HIV are available and regularly updated (see Tables 5.1 and 5.2).

European and US guidelines focus on treatment and monitoring tools available for children in the industrialized countries, while WHO guidelines have a public health approach for resource-constrained settings [37–40] (see Figure 5.2). The use of prophylaxis for OIs and childhood immunization has played an important role in the decreased incidence of infections in the paediatric population [41]. In developed countries, with the advent of HAART, the morbidity and mortality in HIV-infected children and adolescents under 13 years of age has changed tremendously [42,43]. However, the natural history of paediatric HIV disease is not much altered in resource-poor countries.

The most stringent questions still open and in constant development are: 'what is the best moment to start ART?' and, 'which combinations are the most suitable for children?' Short- and long-term toxicities associated with antiretroviral drugs have become a new challenge and are well recognized in children [44]. HIV drug resistance may be seen in treatment-naïve children who have become infected with HIV despite maternal/infant ART [45,46]. Monitoring of children on ART in resource-constrained settings is still problematic and challenging.

Despite greater antiretroviral drug availability in developed and less-developed countries, the choice of a regimen in treatment-naïve and treatment-experienced children remains complex. It is generally recommended that the management of HIV infection should be directed by, or be in consultation with, a specialist in paediatric and adolescent HIV infection. Some specific issues need to be addressed before starting ART, as described below.

Adherence

Adherence is defined as the engaged and active participation of an informed patient and/or family in a treatment plan. Treatment with HAART has dramatically changed prognosis and life expectancy of HIV-infected children, but it has the important limitation of needing an optimal adherence in order to be efficacious over time, adherence that is particularly difficult to achieve for a lifelong, complex treatment with serious side effects. Focusing on adherence is critical for maximizing the effectiveness of ART and preventing HIV drug resistance.

Several factors, such as lack of paediatric formulation, the taste of the antiretroviral drugs, high pill burden and frequent dosing make adherence a major challenge. In addition, the child's developmental level and the severity of the disease may affect his or her ability to take the medication and the caregiver's ability to administer them. Lack of adherence to prescribed regimens, resulting in sub-therapeutic levels of antiretroviral drug, may lead to the development of resistance [47]. Therefore, as with adults, ensuring adherence to therapy has become the cornerstone of HIV management in infants, children and adolescents. Strategies should be developed to increase the

Table 5.1 Criteria for when to start treatment: PENTA, CDC and WHO guidelines

Age	Criteria[c]	PENTA	CDC	WHO
≤ 12 months	Clinical	**CDC stage B or C**[a]	CDC stage A or B or C[a]	**WHO stage 3 or 4**
	Immunologic	**CD4<30%**	CD4<25%	**CD4<25% or <1500 cells/mm³ TLC*<4000 cells/mm³**
	Virologic	*>1,000,000 copies/mm³*	Not considered	Not considered
13 months– ≤ 4 years	Clinical	**CDC stage C**	CDC stage B or C	**WHO stage 4 WHO stage 3 (excluded TB, LIP**, OHL***, TCP**[b]****)**
	Immunologic	**CD4<20%**	CD4<20%	**CD4<20% or<750 cells/mm³ (<3 years); 15% or <350 cells/mm³ (3–4 years) TLC<3000 cells/mm³ (<3 years); <2500 cells/mm³ (3–4 years)**
	Virologic	*>250,000 copies/mm³*	*>100,000 copies/mm³*	Not considered
5–12 years	Clinical	**CDC stage C**	CDC stage B or C	**WHO stage 4 WHO stage 3 (excluded TB, LIP, OHL, TCP**[b]**)**
	Immunologic	**CD4<15%**	CD4<15%	**CD4<15% or<350 cells/mm³ (<5 years); <15% or<200 cells/mm³ (>5 years) TLC<2500 cells/mm³ (<5 years); <2000 cells/mm³ (>5 years)**
	Virologic	*>250,000 copies/mm³*	*>100,000 copies/mm³*	Not considered
>12 years	Clinical	**CDC stage C**	CDC stage B or C	**WHO stage 4 WHO stage 3 (excluded TB, LIP, OHL, TCP**[b]**)**
	Immunologic	**CD4 <350 cells/mm³**	**CD4 <200 cells/mm³** [c]*201–350 cells/mm³*	**CD4 <15% or <200 cells/mm³ TLC <2000 cells/mm³**
	Virologic	Not considered	*>*[c]*100,000 copies/mm³*	Not considered

Bold type: highly recommended

Italics: consider treatment

[a] Some experts recommend treating all children <12 months.

[b] Only if CD4 available.

[c] Just one criterion

* total lymphocyte count

** lymphocytic interstitial pneumonitis

*** oral hairy leukoplakia

**** thrombocytopenia

Sources: Modified from [38–40]

education of infected children and adolescents, as well as their caregivers, over several visits, to accommodate the administration of drugs and to increase medication adherence.

Several factors make adherence in children more challenging than it is for adults, as infants and children are dependent on their caregivers for administration of medication. Special and individual adjustments are necessary in many cases, from choosing an appropriate regimen to scheduling

Table 5.2 How to start antiretroviral therapy: PENTA, CDC and WHO guidelines

PENTA			NRTI+ NNRTI or PI	
◆ Preferred treatment	ABC + 3TC ZDV + 3TC or FTC or ddI ddI + 3TC		NVP (<3 years) EFV (>3 years)	LPV/r ATV*/r or fAPV/r
CDC			**NRTI + NNRTI or PI**	
◆ Preferred treatment	ZDV + 3TC or FTC or ddI ddI + 3TC or FTC		NVP (<3 years) EFV (>3 years)	LPV/r
◆ Alternative	ABC + 3TC or ZDV or FTC or d4T d4T + 3TC or FTC			Nelfinavir
WHO			**NRTI + NNRTI**	
◆ Preferred treatment	ABC + 3TC ZDV + 3TC d4T + 3TC		NVP (<3 years) EFV (>3 years)	
◆ Alternative	ZDV + 3TC + ABC			

* adolescent

Combinations not recommended: d4T + ZDV; 3TC + FTC

Sources: modified from [38–40].

administration and the suitability of a formulation. Adherence problems with adolescents are patient-, family- and environment-specific and should be dealt with on an individual basis. Treatment regimens for adolescents must balance the goal of prescribing a maximally potent antiretroviral regimen with a realistic assessment of existing and potential support systems to facilitate adherence [34]. Multiple methods to reinforce and assess adherence have been developed over the last ten years, including the use of electronic monitoring devices, home visits, inpatient and outpatient directly observed therapy (DOT), quantitative self-reporting of missed doses by caregivers, children and adolescents, family support and education [48–50]. Each of these has yielded different results and revealed its limitations.

Viral load response to a new regimen is often the most accurate indication of adherence, but it may be a less valuable measure in children with long treatment histories and multi-drug resistant virus [39]. In resource-limited settings where the HIV viral load measurement is not routinely available for treatment monitoring, increase in CD4 count and absence of clinical symptoms are the main tools for assessing treatment efficacy. Despite the awareness that suboptimal adherence is key for treatment failure, simple and effective tools for measuring adherence, as well as randomized clinical trials on efficacy and feasibility of interventions to improve adherence, are lacking [48–50].

The WHO guidelines recommend including interventions to promote adherence in ART programmes that extend access to adolescents and children. Activities such as workshops to train children and caregivers in taking pills, home visits, peer counselling sessions and children's camps need to be implemented and evaluated to provide the essential background necessary to designing more complete guidelines on the management of HAART in children and adolescents. Problems of non-adherence have also been described in children with other illnesses, including life-threatening conditions such as cancer and renal transplants [51]. Experience gleaned from treating such conditions could provide strategies that are applicable to the management of HIV infection in children.

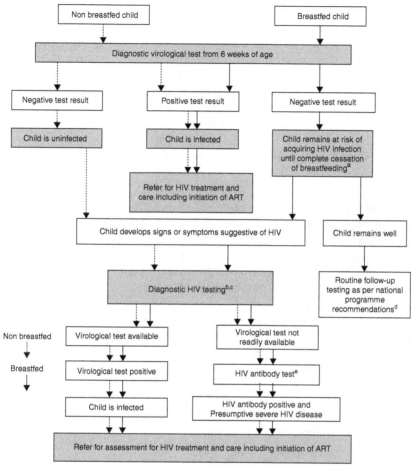

Fig. 5.2 Establishing presence of HIV infection in HIV-exposed children under 18 months old in resource-limited settings to facilitate ART and HIV care.

Notes:

[a] The risk of HIV transmission remains if breastfeeding continues beyond 18 months of age.

[b] Infants over 9 months old can be tested initially with HIV antibody test, as these who are HIV Ab negative are not usually HIV-infected, although still at risk of acquiring infection if still breastfeeding.

[c] In children older than 18 months antibody testing is definitive.

[d] Usually HIV antibody testing from 9–18 months of age.

[e] Where virological testing is not readily available HIV antibody testing should be performed, it may be necessary to make a presumptive clinical diagnosis of severe HIV disease in HIV seropositive children. Confirmation of diagnosis should be sought as soon as posiible.

Source: [38]

Antiretroviral drugs for paediatric use

As of July 2007, 22 different antiretroviral drugs were available in industrialized countries for use in adults and adolescents, but only 13 of these had been approved for management of HIV infection in infants, children and adolescents under 13 years of age. Furthermore, few of them were widely available in resource-constrained settings (Figure 5.2). Such drugs are divided into four major classes: NRTIs, NNRTIs, PIs and fusion inhibitors. Antiretroviral drugs with other viral targets—integrase, entry and maturation inhibitors—are under development. A few are currently undergoing testing and clinical trials, including phase III studies, and are available for use on a compassionate basis for adolescents and young adults when indicated. More complete descriptions of these antiretroviral drugs are provided elsewhere in this book.

An additional barrier to the proper treatment of HIV-infected children is that not all antiretroviral drugs are available in either liquid formulation or in tablet or capsule formulation with dosing suitable for use in children. However, many drugs are now available in combinations of two or three drugs in one tablet, and once- or twice-daily dosing has become the rule in treatment regimens for adolescents, adults and children who can swallow pills. This has decreased the pill burden and consequently improved adherence to medication to some extent.

HAART

The availability of HAART has markedly reduced the morbidity and the mortality of HIV-infected infants, children and adolescents under the age of 13 in the United States and Europe. Aggressive combination therapy with at least three antiretroviral drugs from at least two drug classes is strongly and universally recommended for initial treatment of infants, children and adolescents and is found to be effective in decreasing the viral burden, preserving the immune function and delaying disease progression [37,39,40].

Monotherapy with the currently available drugs is not recommended to treat HIV infection. Use of ZDV or a single dose of NVP is appropriate only in HIV-exposed infants to prevent perinatal transmission. PMTCT programmes have been using antiretroviral drugs in different ways to prevent transmission. Examples include short course versus long course, monotherapy, single-dose therapy or a short course of dual therapy, according to each country's national recommendations and the WHO's PMTCT guidelines. It is usually recommended to discontinue those interventions if the HIV-exposed infant is found to be infected, and to perform proper assessment of whether ART should be initiated.

The goals of ART for HIV-infected children include:

+ reducing HIV-related mortality and morbidity;
+ restoring and preserving immune function;
+ maximally and durably suppressing viral replication;
+ minimizing drug-related toxicities;
+ maintaining normal physical growth and neurocognitive development; and
+ improving quality of life [39].

Early initiation of ART in asymptomatic HIV-infected patients versus delaying therapy until the onset of clinical or immunologic symptoms is an issue that continues to generate considerable controversy among HIV experts. Multiple retrospective data have shown the virologic, immunologic and clinical benefits of early ART in infants with HIV infection [52–54], while delaying therapy until the patient becomes symptomatic may result in reduced evolution of drug-resistant virus due to a lack of drug selection pressure, greater adherence to the therapeutic regimen and reduced or delayed adverse effects of the treatment regimen [39]. However, the rates of virologic failure when ART is started early in life may be higher than when started later. Incomplete viral suppression can lead to the development of drug resistance and compromise future options [55]. Although all published guidelines for both resource-rich and resource-constrained settings have recommended the use and selection of combination ART, the choice of drugs for initiation of therapy varies widely based on virologic, immunologic and clinical criteria for initiation of therapy, drug availability, drug sequencing and preservation for future options [37,39,40].

In resource-constrained settings, ART is usually initiated with a combination of two NRTIs and one NNRTI. Protease inhibitors are not used on a large scale and are reserved for future treatment when virologic failure is present [37]. In more developed countries, a regimen consisting of two NRTIs and one NNRTI or one PI is routinely recommended for initiation of therapy [39,40,56]. Alternative regimens are suggested in some special circumstances and are based on drug availability. They can be very complex, since drug combinations are not recommended where there are insufficient data concerning their toxicity or potency [37,39,40]. Adolescents older than 13 may benefit from some regimens used in the adult HIV population.

Adherence assessment and monitoring are based on available resources to maximize the benefits of antiretroviral regimens and to decrease the risk of developing drug resistance and the likelihood of virologic failure. T-lymphocyte subsets, quantitative HIV DNA PCR (viral load) tests, a complete blood count and a comprehensive metabolic panel are used to assess efficacy of a regimen and detect drug toxicities. Since laboratory testing, including HIV viral load monitoring, has not been used on a large scale in resource-limited settings due to lack of availability, for these populations clinical improvement, weight gain, CD4 count and basic laboratory tests are relied upon to assess the response to a regimen.

Changing treatment regimens and resistance testing

Immunologic and virologic considerations before changing therapy are integral parts of therapy monitoring. However, before choosing a new regimen, it is important to distinguish between the need to change therapy due to drug failure versus drug toxicity or poor adherence to the present regimen (See Table 5.3). Antiretroviral resistance testing, where it is available, is now part of clinical management in children as well as adults. If an actual regimen fails to reduce plasma HIV RNA to below detection levels by the most sensitive assay available, then genotypic/phenotypic resistance studies should be considered. Phenotypic resistance assays are the most direct method for determining drug resistance of isolates, measuring the 50% or 90% inhibitory concentrations

Table 5.3 How to switch to second-line treatment after first-line failure: PENTA, CDC and WHO guidelines

First-line combination	Second-line treatment		
	WHO	**CDC**	**PENTA**
NRTI			
- ZDV/d4T + 3TC or FTC	ABC + ddI	Consider genotype	Consider genotype
- ZDV/d4T + ddI[2]	ABC + 3TC or FTC	results	results [1]
- ZDV + ABC[2]	ddI + 3TC or FTC		
- ABC + 3TC or FTC	ZDV + ddI		
- ABC + ddI[2]	ZDV+ 3TC or FTC		
- ZDV + 3TC + ABC	NVP o EFV + ddI + PI		
NNRTI			
- NVP or EFV	Ritonavir-boosted PI	Ritonavir-boosted PI	Ritonavir-boosted PI
PI			
- LPV/r or other	NVP or EFV	NVP or EFV[3]	NVP or EFV[3]

[1] If genotype resistance results are not available, consider WHO recommendations;

[2] Second choice combination;

[3] Consider a second-generation PI (DRV or TPV) if resistance profile shows susceptibility.

Sources: modified from [38–40].

of a drug against the virus *in vitro* and detecting the effects of resistance interactions between various drug-selected mutations. However, they require specialized laboratories, are expensive and take several weeks to complete. Also, the results may lag behind genotypic changes and the results may be strain-specific.

Genotypic resistance assays detect actual viral genome mutations. They are rapid and inexpensive with potential for high sensitivity. Their analysis can be quite comprehensive but, at this time, difficult to interpret. Genotypic assays, while helping the clinician in his or her decision to choose a regimen, have their own limitations, since minor quasi-species may not be detected. Interaction between mutations is not described, and correlation with phenotypic resistance is not universal. Expert clinical interpretation is advised to determine the clinical applications of these resistance assays [39,57]. The most recent US guidelines recommend the systematic use of resistance testing prior to initiation of ART for HIV-infected infants whose mothers have received antiretroviral drugs for prophylaxis or treatment during pregnancy [39].

The evidence of long-term virologic or immunologic benefits of using resistance testing needs to be further assessed, as to date there have been few studies in children assessing test significance and no consensus has yet been reached [58]. Changing a regimen, in itself cumbersome, is even more challenging in resource-constrained settings given the restricted drug choice and limited availability of viral load and resistance testing. A change in the regimen backbone is usually suggested if no PI-based second line is available, and is based on clinical criteria and CD4 count [37]. Protease inhibitors are not used in the initiation of ART and are usually spared for future options.

Adverse drug events

Some basic principles should be observed when clinicians face adverse events potentially secondary to antiretroviral drugs. The first step is to try to determine if the adverse event is attributable to antiretroviral and other drugs, to progressive HIV infection itself, or to other infections that may complicate the course of HIV infection. One example is the development of neutropenia in a child on prophylaxis for *Pneumocystis carinii* pneumonia (PCP) and an antiretroviral regimen that includes ZDV. That episode of neutropenia may be secondary to ZDV, to cotrimoxazole (trimethoprim-sulfamethoxazole (TMP-SMX)), to the HIV infection itself, or to a co-infection. The decision about therapy management should be taken based on the severity grade of the event. Life-threatening events (grade 4), for example a hypersensitivity reaction due to abacavir (ABC), require an immediate suspension of the suspected associated drug. For less severe events, the differential diagnosis should be clarified before a decision on stopping or continuing therapy is made. Grades of severity of abnormal laboratory tests and adverse clinical events that may reflect common and potentially severe drug toxicities are described in most up to date published guidelines [37,39,40]. As a rule, attempts should be made to continue ART at effective doses, especially when future options and drug availability are limited, except in the presence of severe (grade 4) or life-threatening toxicities, in which circumstances therapy should be stopped [37,39,40]. Toxicities for each antiretroviral drug must be known and explained in layman's terms to the child's parent or guardian.

Close monitoring and evaluation are recommended for lower-grade toxicities. For moderately severe toxicities (grades 2 and 3), specific interventions should be considered, such as use of erythropoietin for the treatment of anaemia, granulocyte colony stimulating factor for the treatment of neutropenia, or switching to another antiretroviral drug [59,60]. In the presence of renal disease, dose reduction should be considered for agents for which a range of effective dosages has been documented.

If there is a need to discontinue ART for an extended period of time, it is recommended that all antiretroviral drugs be stopped in a way that minimizes the risk of selection of drug-resistant mutations, either by stopping all drugs simultaneously if the combination contains all short half-life drugs (NRTIs and PIs), or by staggering the discontinuation of treatment if the regimen contains agents with a long half-life (NNRTIs and 3TC) [61]. This approach attempts to minimize the risk of developing drug resistance in the face of suboptimal drug plasma level exposure and the potential for increased viral replication.

The decline in opportunistic diseases and the increasingly recognized need for long-term therapy with drug combinations create the potential for long-term side effects. Despite our improved knowledge of HIV pathogenesis and therapy, there is no existing consensus regarding how best to use the drugs and decrease the risk of side effects. Mitochondrial dysfunctions (primarily seen with the NRTI drugs), lactic acidosis, hepatic toxicity and pancreatitis have been described. Lipodystrophy and other metabolic disturbances in patients taking antiretroviral drugs have been well documented and are major causes for decreased adherence to regimens because of their negative impact on self-image in HIV-infected adolescents and young adults [62,63].

Discontinuation of ART may occur in some special circumstances, such as the presence of serious life-threatening toxicities, acute illnesses, lack of available medication, or deliberate discontinuation. In such cases, all therapy should be stopped simultaneously in order to avoid exposure to suboptimal therapy. A major concern in these situations arises when drugs with long half-lives are used, as this results in functional monotherapy with the drug with the longest half-life [39]. Since long-term structured treatment interruptions to reduce toxicities and costs have not been extensively studied in children, there are no data to support this strategy, and it should be considered only in a clinical trial setting.

While improving the immune function and CD4 count in HIV-infected children, ART leads to an increased risk of an inflammatory response. This paradoxical inflammatory response is referred to as immune reconstitution inflammatory syndrome (IRIS), or immune reconstitution (restoration) disease, and has been reported in both adult and paediatric HIV populations [64,65]. It can occur following ART initiation due to worsening of an existing active, latent, or occult OI, where infectious pathogens that were not previously recognized by the immune system now evoke an immune response. There are no randomized controlled trials assessing the timing and the treatment of IRIS. According to a limited number of published reports and expert opinion, most cases in the adult population occur in the first two to three months of treatment. Antiretroviral therapy should be continued during this time while managing the acute disease. The use of anti-inflammatory agents based on the severity of the condition is suggested and may be considered.

Adolescence and HIV infection

Most children who benefited from HAART in the mid-1990s are now in adolescence or young adulthood. They are familiar with the routine of chronic medical care and the challenges of taking complex drug regimens, and they may have a long history of inadequate adherence to treatment. Choosing a regimen in the presence of multi-drug resistance has become a real challenge in the management of this treatment-experienced population. Despite the absence of paediatric data, the use of fusion inhibitors and other drugs such as ritonavir (RTV)-boosted tipranavir (TPV) and darunavir (DRV), and the compassionate use of integrase and entry inhibitors, is becoming more accepted. Ongoing studies of such treatments in adults and adolescents will be of benefit to the HIV-infected paediatric population.

Several studies have identified pill burden, lifestyle issues, denial and fear of their HIV infection, misinformation about HIV and distrust of the medical establishment as major barriers to complete adherence [66]. Perinatally infected youth share the same issues with those adolescents who have acquired HIV infection through their high-risk behaviours. Regardless of the mode of acquisition, HIV-infected adolescents and young adults may suffer from low self-esteem, may have unstructured and chaotic lifestyles and concomitant illnesses and may cope poorly with their illness due to a lack of familial and social support [39]. Multi-drug resistance, depression, alcohol abuse, poor school attendance and advanced HIV disease stage all correlate with non-adherence [67]. Adolescents and young adults with HIV infection may also be sexually active; safer-sex techniques for prevention of HIV transmission should be discussed [68] and partners' notification encouraged. In addition, antiretroviral regimen selection should take into account the possibility of pregnancy. Efavirenz (EFV)-containing regimens should be avoided in adolescent girls who are trying to conceive or who are not using effective contraception, because of the potential for teratogenicity with foetal exposure to EFV in the first trimester [39,69]. Pregnancy should not prevent adolescents from benefiting from the optimal therapeutic regimens, although timing and initiation of treatment may be different for pregnant women than for non-pregnant female adolescents. It is recommended to follow the appropriate PMTCT guidelines.

Paediatric and adolescent patients may benefit from the establishment of formal programmes to introduce them into the adult care setting. Transitioning adolescents with any chronic health condition to the adult care system is far from easy. Transition is a multifaceted, active process that addresses the medical, psychosocial, educational or vocational needs of adolescents as they move from the child-focused to the adult-focused healthcare system [39,69]. The longstanding relationship between paediatric care providers and their patients and families does not facilitate a smooth transition. Adolescent patients may feel they are being abandoned when transferred to the adult care model, with its busier clinic settings and an unfamiliar provider. A multidisciplinary approach with input from the paediatric and adolescent healthcare providers, including nurses, social workers and mental health professionals, can be of great help in such a situation.

Social issues in the delivery of care

The epidemiological data on paediatric HIV disease make it clear that, worldwide, there has been a disproportionate impact upon the poor and people of colour. The healthcare needs of these populations have traditionally been underserved, and previous contact with public agencies may dispose them toward distrust and discourage them from seeking timely medical care. Often, one of the first relationships of trust that affected families develop is with the healthcare providers who treat their children. Healthcare professionals should attempt to establish a partnership with the family rather than reinforce the more traditional role of passivity and dependence. The conditions of poverty, including inadequate housing, may interfere with the delivery of optimal healthcare.

Mothers are typically the strongest advocates for their children, but this advocacy may be hindered by the fact that the mothers of HIV-infected children are often single parents and poor. In some cases, symptomatic HIV infection or drug use may interfere with a mother's ability to care properly for her child; more often, however, mothers are assertive in seeking care for their children, even if they are neglecting their own care needs. The general shortage of openings in drug treatment programmes is especially severe for women who are HIV-infected, pregnant, or who have children. All of these socio-economic conditions have to be addressed in designing effective healthcare systems for families with HIV infection. Similar difficulties are encountered by HIV-infected adolescents, who traditionally have not received adequate healthcare.

Families can also benefit from psychosocial support in dealing with many aspects of an HIV diagnosis in a child. The diagnosis may be the first evidence that a parent is infected and may give rise to guilt or anger, leading to further disruption of the family unit. Apparently resolved emotional issues may require periodic re-examination, as, for example, when parents are repeatedly confronted by the differences between a child who is developmentally delayed and his or her healthy peers [70].

Decisions about the disclosure of an HIV diagnosis may arise on multiple occasions as different audiences—family, friends, siblings of the infected child, the child himself, day care workers, school nurses and teachers—are encountered. Many parents choose to disclose the diagnosis on a need-to-know basis. However, children and their siblings often find it less stressful to know the diagnosis than to be left in the dark about something unnamed but apparent. Counselling may help parents decide whether and how to disclose the diagnosis, which should be done in a developmentally appropriate way. Clinical experience suggests that, under the proper circumstances, it is beneficial for children with normal cognitive development to have the opportunity to discuss aspects of their illness with trusted adults [71].

The issue of disclosure of diagnosis is particularly pressing as perinatally infected children live into mid- and late adolescence. Uninfected but HIV-affected siblings often have mental health needs as well, especially when they face the eventual loss of siblings and of one or both parents. The failure to deal successfully with psychosocial issues may prevent families from seeking out optimal medical care for their children.

Conclusion

The HIV epidemic has been a challenge to worldwide health resources and has unfortunately reversed the trends towards improved infant mortality rates, enhanced longevity and the structural and social stability of all areas of the globe. The response to the epidemic, most evident in the developed world, has resulted in strategies to prevent perinatal transmission from mothers to infants and to improve the quality and duration of life in those infected with HIV, either perinatally or by other means of transmission, using HAART. The gains made in the developed world in the treatment and control of HIV and its associated, complicating opportunistic diseases must be channelled to the vast majority of the world's population in resource-poor

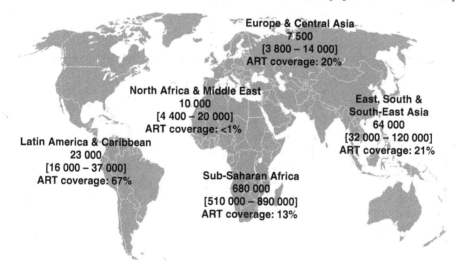

Fig. 5.3 Number of children in need of antiretroviral therapy in low- and middle-income countries and percentage coverage of ART for children in 2008.

Sources: UNICEF. (2006). *Children and AIDS: A Stocking*. New York: UNICEF.

WHO. (2007). *Towards universal access: scaling up priority HIV/AIDS interventions in the health sector: progress report*, April 2007. Geneva: World Health Organization.

countries that bear the brunt of HIV/AIDS (see Figure 5.3). This includes the severe complications attendant to the immune suppression caused by HIV, the increased mortality from endemic infections such as malaria, as well as the resurgence in multi-drug resistant tuberculosis (TB), which poses a threat in even the wealthiest regions of the world. In resource-poor countries, where the majority of HIV-infected individuals live, most have not been diagnosed, much less treated. These parts of the world, in which the majority of the world's population resides, are unable to provide nutritional, economic, educational and health stability, thus profoundly limiting the potential and future of their children. The well-being of all societies will depend on our meeting this obligation and goal.

The negative consequences of our failure to meet the WHO's objective of worldwide control of HIV/AIDS must be forestalled, but this will require sometimes complex approaches and vast resources. There may also be some simpler approaches that could be critical in the control of HIV but have not initially been accepted, such as the recommendation to new mothers to have their infant sons circumcised, a decision which might, over time, lead to the reduction and control of this tragic epidemic that has so disproportionately impacted women and children in this, its third decade.

References

1. UNAIDS. (2006). *2006 Report on The Global AIDS Epidemic*. Geneva: UNAIDS.

2. Oleske J, Minnefor A, Cooper R, *et al*. (1983). Immune deficiency syndrome in children. *JAMA* **249:**2345–2349.

3. Cowan MJ, Hellmann D, Chudwin D, Wara DW, Chang RS, Amman AJ. (1984). Maternal transmission of acquired immune deficiency syndrome. *Pediatrics* **73:**382–6.

4. Mofenson LM. (1997). Mother-child HIV-1 transmission: Timing and determinants. *Obstet Gynecol Clin North Amer* **24:**759–84.

5. Connor EM, Sperling RS, Gelber R, *et al*. (1994). Reduction of maternal-infant transmission of human immunodeficiency virus type 1 with zidovudine treatment. Pediatric AIDS Clinical Trials Group Protocol 076 Study Group. *N Engl J Med* **331:**1173–80.

6. US Centers for Disease Control and Prevention (CDC). (2006). Achievements in Public Health: Reduction in Perinatal Transmission of HIV Infection: United States 1985–2005. *MMRW weekly report* **55:**592–597. Available at http://www.cdc.gov/mmwr/preview/mmwrhtml/mm5521a3.htm#fig. (Accessed 10 November 2007).

7. US Public Health Service. (2006). *Public Health Service Task Force Recommendations for Use of Antiretroviral Drugs in Pregnant HIV-1 Infected Women for Maternal Health and Interventions to Reduce Perinatal HIV-1 Transmission in the United States – October 12 2006*. Available at http://www.aidsinfo.nih.gov/guidelines/ (Accessed 12 October 2006).

8. The British HIV Association. (2005). *Guidelines for the management of HIV infection in pregnant women and the prevention of mother-to-child transmission of HIV*. London: The British HIV Association.

9. Floridia M, Tamburrini E, Bucceri A, *et al*. (2007). Pregnancy outcomes and antiretroviral treatment in a national cohort of pregnant women with HIV: overall rates and differences according to nationality. *BJOG* **114:**896–900.

10. The United Nations Children's Fund (UNICEF). (2005). *A Call To Action: Children, the missing face to AIDS. The Global Campaign on Children and AIDS*. New York: UNICEF.

11. Shaffer N, Chuachoowong R, Mock PA, *et al*. (1999). Short-course zidovudine for perinatal HIV-1 transmission in Bangkok, Thailand: A randomized controlled trial. Bangkok Collaborative perinatal HIV Transmission Study Group. *Lancet* **353:**773–80.

12. The Petra Study Team. (2002). Efficacy of three short-course regimens of zidovudine and lamivudine in preventing early and late transmission of HIV-1 from mother-to-child in Tanzania, South Africa, and Uganda (Petra study): randomized, double-blind, placebo-controlled trial. *Lancet* **359:**1178–86.

13. Guay LA, Musoke P, Fleming T, *et al.* (1999). Intrapartum and neonatal single-dose nevirapine compared with zidovudine for prevention of mother-to-child transmission of HIV-1 in Kampala, Uganda: HIVNET 012 randomized trial. *Lancet* **354:**795–802.

14. Moodley D, Moodley J, Coovadia H, *et al.* (2003). A multicenter randomized controlled trial of nevirapine versus a combination of zidovudine and lamivudine to reduce intrapartum and early postpartum mother-to-child transmission of human immunodeficiency virus-1. *J Infect Dis* **187:**725–35.

15. Dabis F, Bequet L, Ekouevi DK, *et al.* (2005). Field efficacy of zidovudine, lamivudine and single-dose nevirapine to prevent peripartum HIV transmission. *AIDS* **19:**309–18.

16. Lallemant M, Jourdain G, Le Coeur S, *et al.* (2004). Single-dose perinatal nevirapine plus standard zidovudine to prevent mother-to-child transmission of HIV-1 in Thailand. *N Engl J Med* **351:**217–28.

17. World Health Organization. (2006). *Antiretroviral drugs for treating pregnant women and preventing HIV infection in infants in resource-limited settings: towards universal access. Recommendations for a public health approach.* Geneva: World Health Organization.

18. Eshleman SH, Hoover DR, Chen S, *et al.* (2005). Nevirapine (NVP) resistance in women with HIV-1 subtype C, compared with subtypes A and D, after the administration of single-dose NVP. *J Infect Dis* **192:**30–6.

19. Martinson NA, Morris L, Gray G, *et al.*(2007). Selection and persistence of viral resistance in HIV-infected children after exposure to single-dose nevirapine. *J Acquir Immune Defic Syndr* **44:**148–53.

20. Palmer S, Boltz V, Martinson N, *et al.* (2006). Persistence of nevirapine-resistant HIV-1 in women after single-dose nevirapine therapy for prevention of maternal-to-fetal HIV-1 transmission. *Proc Natl Acad Sci USA* **103:**7094–9.

21. Flys TS, Donnell D, Mwatha A, *et al.* (2007). Persistence of K103N-containing HIV-1 variants after single-dose nevirapine for prevention of HIV mother-to-child transmission. *J Infect Dis* **195:**711–5.

22. Cressey TR, Jourdain G, Lallement MJ, *et al.* (2005). Persistence of nevirapine exposure during the postpartum period after intrapartum single-dose nevirapine in addition to zidovudine prophylaxis for the prevention of mother-to-child transmission of HIV. *J Acquir Immune Defic Syndr* **38:**283–8.

23. McIntyre J, Martinson N, Boltz V, *et al.* (2004). Addition of short course Combivir (CBV) to single dose Viramune (sdNVP) for prevention of mother-to-child transmission of HIV-1 can significantly decrease the subsequent development of maternal NNRTI-resistant virus. XV International AIDS Conference, 11–16 July 2004, Bangkok, Thailand. [Abstract LbOrB09]

24. Palmer S, Boltz F, Maldarelli N, *et al.* (2006). Addition of short course combivir to single dose nevirapine reduces the selection of nevirapine-resistant HIV-1 with in frequent emergence of 3TC-resistant variants. 14th Conference on Retroviruses and Opportunistic Infections (CROI), 25–28 February 2006, Los Angeles CA. [Abstract 763]

25. Holmes WR, Savage F. (2007). Exclusive breastfeeding and HIV. *Lancet* **369:**1065–6.

26. World Health Organization. (2006). *HIV and Infant Feeding. Technical Consultation on behalf of the Inter-Agency Task Team (IATT) on Prevention of HIV infections in pregnant women, mothers and their infants. 25–27 October 2006. Concensus Statement.* Geneva: World Health Organization.

27. Coovadia HM, Rollins NC, Bland RM, *et al.* (2007). Mother-to-child transmission of HIV-1 infection during exclusive breastfeeding in the first 6 months of life: an intervention cohort study. *Lancet* **369:**1107–16.

28. Sinkala M, Kuhn L, Kankasa C, *et al.* (2007). Early cessation of breastfeeding at 4 months on HIV-free survival of infants born to HIV-infected mothers in Zambia: The Zambia exclusive breastfeeding Study. 14th Conference on Retroviruses and Opportunistic Infections (CROI), 25–28 February 2007, Los Angeles CA, USA. [Abstract 74]

29. Shapiro RL, Ndung'u T, Lockman S, *et al.* (2005). Highly active antiretroviral therapy started during pregnancy or postpartum suppresses HIV-1 RNA, but not DNA, in breast milk. *J Infect Dis* **192:**713–9.

30. El-Sadr WM, Lundgren JD, Neaton JD, *et al.* (2006). CD$_4$+ count-guided Interruption of antiretroviral treatment. *N Engl J Med* **355**:2283–96.

31. Chersich MF, Gray GE. (2005). Progress and Emerging Challenges in Preventing Mother-to-Child Transmission. *Curr Infect Dis Rep* **7**:393–400.

32. Palombi L, Germano P, Liotta G, *et al.* (2005). HAART in Pregnancy: Safety, Effectiveness Infections. Conference on Retroviruses and Opportunistic Infections (CROI), 22–25 February 2005, Boston, MA, USA. [Abstract 67]

33. Leith J, Piliero P, Storfer S, Mayers D, Hinzmann R. (2005). Appropriate Use of Nevirapine for Long-Term Therapy. *J infect. Dis* **192**:545–6.

34. McKinney RE, Maha MA, Connor EM, *et al.* (1991). A multicenter trial of oral zidovudine in children with advanced human immunodeficiency virus disease. The protocol 043 Study group. *N Engl J Med* **324**:1018–25.

35. Paediatric European Network for Treatment of AIDS (PENTA). (1998). A randomized double-blind trial of the addition of lamivudine or matching placebo to current nucleoside analogue reverse transcriptase inhibitor therapy in HIV-infected children: the PENTA trial. *AIDS* **12**:F151–60.

36. McConnell MS, Byers RH, Frederick T, *et al.* (2005). Trends in antiretroviral therapy use and survival rates for a large cohort of HIV-infected children and adolescents in the US, 1989–2001. *J Acquir Immune Defic Syndr* **38**:488–94.

37. World Health Organization (WHO). (2006). *Guidelines for Cotrimoxazole prophylaxis for HI-related infections in Children, Adolescents and Adults in resource-limited settings: Recommendations for a public health approach.* Geneva: WHO.

38. World Health Organization (WHO). (2006). *Antiretroviral drugs for the therapy of HIV infection in infants and children in resource-limited settings. Recommendations for a public health approach.* Geneva: WHO.

39. US Centers for Disease Control and Prevention. (2006). *Guidelines for the use of antiretroviral agents in pediatric HIV infection.* Available at www.aidsinfo.nih.gov (Accessed July 2007).

40. Sharland M, Blanche S, Castelli G, Ramos J, Gibb DM. (2004). PENTA guidelines for the use of antiretroviral therapy, 2004. *HIV Med* **5**(suppl 2):61–86.

41. Selik RM, Lindegren ML. (2003). Changes in death reported with HIV infection among US children less than 13 years old, 1987–1999. *Pediatric Infect Dis J* **22**:635.

42. Luzuriaga K, Sullivan J. (2001). The changing faces of pediatric HIV-1 infection. *N Engl J Med* **345**:1568–1569.

43. Gonzales TM, Ramos A Jr, Granado JM, *et al.* (2005). Effectiveness of antiretroviral therapy in HIV-1 infected children (a crossectional study). *An Pediatr (Barc)* **62**:32–7.

44. Leonard EG, McComsey GA. (2003). Metabolic complications of antiretroviral therapy in children. *Pediatr Infect Dis J* **22**:77–84.

45. Johnson VA, Petropoulos CJ, Woods CR, *et al.* (2001). Vertical transmission of multi-drug resistant human immunodeficiency virus type 1 (HIV-1) and continued evolution of drug resistance in an HIV-1 infected infant. *J Infec Dis* **18**: 1688–93.

46. Cohan D, Feakins C, Wara D, *et al.* (2005). Perinatal transmission of multidrug- resistant HIV-1 despite viral suppression on an enfuvirtide-based treatment regimen. *AIDS* **19**:989–90.

47. Williams A, Friedland G. (1997). Adherence, Compliance and HAART. *AIDS Clin Care* **9**:51–54, 58.

48. Rueda S, Park-Wyllie LY, Bayoumi AM, *et al.* (2007). Patient support and education for promoting adherence to highly active antiretroviral therapy for HIV/AIDS. *Cochrane Database of Syst Rev* **3**:CD00142.

49. Williams AB, Fennie KP, Bova CA, *et al.* (2006). Home visits to improve adherence to highly active antiretroviral therapy: a randomized control trial. *J Acquir Immune Defic Syndr* **42**:314–21.

50. Parsons GN, Siberry GK, Parsons JK, *et al.* (2006). Multidisciplinary inpatient directly observed therapy for HIV-1 infected children and adolescents failing HAART: A retrospective study. *AIDS Patient Care STDS* 20:275–84.

51. Matsui DM. (1997). Drug compliance in pediatrics clinical and research issues. *Pediatr Clin North Am* 44:1–14.

52. Chiappini E, Galli L, Tovo PA, *et al.* (2006). Virologic, immunologic, and clinical benefits from early combined antiretroviral therapy in infants with perinatal HIV-1 infection. *AIDS.*20:207–15.

53. Newell ML, Patel D, Goetghebuer T, Thorne C. (2006). European Collaborative Study. CD4 cell response in children with vertically acquired HIV infection: is it associated with age at initiation? *J Infec Dis* 193:954–62.

54. Hainaut M, Peltier CA, Gérard M, Marissens D, Zissis G, Levy J. (2000). Effectiveness of antiretroviral therapy initiated before the age of 2 months in infants vertically infected with the human immunodeficiency virus type 1. *Euro J Pediatr* 159:778–82.

55. Walker AS, Doerholt K, Sharland M, *et al.* (2004). Response to highly antiretroviral therapy varies with age: the UK and Ireland Collaborative HIV Paediatric Study. *AIDS* 18:1915–24.

56. Verweel G, Saavedra-Lozano J, van Rossum AMC, *et al.*(2006). Initiating Highly Active Antiretroviral Therapy in Human Immunodeficiency Virus Type 1-Infected Children in Europe and the United States: Comparing Clinical Practice to Guidelines and Literature Evidence. *Pediatr Infect Dis J* 25: 987–994.

57. Hanna GJ, D'Aguila RT. (2001). Clinical use of phenotypic and genotypic drug resistance testing to monitor antiretroviral chemotherapy. *Clin Infect Dis* 32:774–82.

58. Green H, Gibb DM, Compagnucci A, *et al.* (2006). A randomized controlled trial of genotypic HIV drug resistance testing in HIV-1-infected children: the PERA (PENTA 8) trial. *Antivir Ther* 11:857–67.

59. Hermans P, Rosenbaum W, Jou A, *et al.* (1996). Filgrastin to treat neutropenia and support myelosuppressive medication dosing in HIV infection, G-CSF 92105 Study Group. *AIDS* 10:1627–33.

60. Volberding P. (2000). Consensus statement: anemia in HIV infection – current trends, treatment options, and practice strategies. *Clin Ther* 22:1004–1020; discussion 1003.

61. Lallemant M, Burger D, Lyall H. (2006*)*. Pharmacokinetic and virological evaluations after stopping NNRTIs in children: a sub study of the PENTA 11 (TICCH) trial. XVI International AIDS Conference, 13–18 August 2006, Toronto, Canada. [Abstract MOPE0206]

62. Nwaobasi E, Oleske JM. (2006). Toxicities of antiretroviral therapy in children. *AIDS Read* 16:537–40.

63. Leonard EG, McComsey GA. (2003). Metabolic complications of antiretroviral therapy in children. *Pediatr Infect Dis J* 22:77–84.

64. Puthanakit T, Oberdofer P, Akarathum N, *et al.* (2006). Immune reconstitution syndrome after highly active antiretroviral therapy in children with HIV infection. *Pediatr Infect Dis J* 25:645–8.

65. Nuttall JJC, Wilmshurst JM, Ndondo AP, *et al.* (2004). Progressive multifocal leukoencephalopathy after initiation of highly active antiretroviral therapy: a case of immune inflammatory syndrome. *Pediatr Infect Dis J* 23:683–4.

66. American Academy of Pediatrics, American Academy of Family Physicians, American College of Physicians, American Society of Internal Medicine. (2002). A consensus statement on health care transitions for young adults with special health care needs. *Pediatrics* 110:1304–6.

67. Reddington C, Cohen J, Baldillo A, *et al.* (2000). Adherence to medication regimens among children with human immunodeficiency virus infection. *Pediatr Infect Dis J* 19:1148–53.

68. Ezeanolue E, Wodi PA, Patel R, *et al.* (2005). Sexual behaviors and procreation intentions of adolescents and young adults with perinatally acquired HIV infection: Experience of an urban tertiary center. *Journal of Adolescent Health* 38:719–25.

69. US Centers for Disease control and Prevention, Perinatal HIV Guidelines Working Group. (2007). *Public Health Service Task Force recommendations for use of antiretroviral drugs in pregnant HIV-infected women for maternal health and interventions to reduce perinatal HIV transmission in the United States.* Available at http://aidsinfo.nih.gov/ContentFiles/PerinatalGL.pdf (Accessed 10 November 2007).

70 Oleske JM, Ruben-Hale A. (1995). Enhancing supportive care and promoting quality of life: *clinical practice* guidelines. *Pediatr AIDS HIV Infect Fetus Adolesc* **6:**187–203.

71. Lewis SY, Haiken HJ, Hoyt LG. (1994). Living beyond the odds: A psychosocial perspective of long-term survivors of pediatric HIV infection. *J Dev Behav Pediatr* **15:**S12–17.

Part 2

HAART in high human development countries

Chapter 6

Country review: Australia

Kathleen Glenday, Kathy Petoumenos*,
Matthew G. Law and David A. Cooper

Introduction

The first diagnosed case of HIV infection in Australia was reported in 1982. Since then, this country's HIV epidemic has predominantly affected gay and other homosexually active men. By 1985, the annual number of newly diagnosed cases of HIV infection temporarily peaked, followed by a steady decrease over the next 15 years [1]. AIDS diagnoses would peak again almost a decade later in 1994.

Antiretroviral therapy for people living with HIV/AIDS (PLWHA) became available in 1988, with the release of zidovudine (ZDV) onto the Australian pharmaceutical market. Following the availability of other antiretroviral drugs, dual therapy became available in Australia in 1991, and highly active antiretroviral therapy (HAART) became available in 1996.

In 1989, the first National HIV/AIDS Strategy was released by the Commonwealth of Australia's Department of Community Services and Health. In the early days of the HIV epidemic, Australia was at the forefront of HIV prevention. Timely mobilization and action among affected or at-risk communities, particularly the gay community and sex workers, alongside harm-reduction strategies such as needle and syringe programmes, have been core factors in the success of Australia's response to HIV/AIDS. In light of recent increases in newly acquired cases of HIV infection and the increased lifespan and subsequent chronic healthcare needs of PLWHA, a major focus of the fifth National HIV/AIDS Strategy released by the Australian government's Department of Health and Ageing in 2005 was the revitalization of Australia's response to the HIV epidemic.

Epidemiology of HIV infection in Australia

Newly diagnosed HIV infection and AIDS are notifiable conditions in all state and territory health jurisdictions in Australia. All cases of diagnosed HIV infection or AIDS are reported through the state and territory health authorities to the national HIV/AIDS surveillance centre. At the end of 2005, the cumulative number of HIV infections diagnosed in Australia was over 22,300, with an estimated 15,300 people living with HIV infection nationally [1]. Approximately 9870 AIDS diagnoses and 6670 deaths following AIDS had been reported in Australia at this time.

Following a long-term decline, the annual number of new HIV diagnoses in Australia has gradually increased over the past five years, from 656 cases in 2000 to around 930 in 2005. Among these new diagnoses, an increasing number were in people who had acquired HIV infection within the previous year. The proportion of new AIDS cases classified as late HIV infection diagnosis, defined as HIV diagnosis within three months of AIDS diagnosis, has increased from 18%

* Corresponding author.

in 1996 to 54% in 2005 among women, and from 19% in 1996 to 47% in 2005 among men [1]. The increase in late HIV diagnosis in 2001–5 compared to 1996–2000 has been seen across all exposure categories, particularly injecting drug users (IDUs) (Figure 6.1).

In Australia, HIV transmission continues to occur mainly through sexual contact between gay and other homosexually active men. The majority of newly diagnosed and newly acquired cases of HIV infection (over 60% and 80%, respectively) during 1996–2000 and 2001–5 were attributed to male homosexual contact (Figure 6.2) [1,2]. Heterosexual contact was the second most common route of HIV transmission, accounting for one in five newly diagnosed infections and almost 10% of newly acquired infections during the same two periods [1,2]. Injecting drug use, male homosexual contact together with injecting drug use and other routes of transmission were less common exposure categories among newly diagnosed infections between 2001 and 2005 (4%, 4% and 9%, respectively) [1]. Mother-to-child transmission (MTCT) accounted for 0.2–1.1% of newly diagnosed HIV infections annually between 1996 and 2000 [2], and ≥0.1% between 2001 and 2005 [1].

The vast majority of HIV infection in Australia involves HIV-1 subtype B [3]; however, HIV-1 subtype CRF01_AE has been shown to be common among a population of Vietnamese IDUs in Melbourne [4].

Gay and other homosexually active men

The HIV epidemic in Australia since the 1980s has predominantly affected gay and other homosexually active men. There is some evidence of increased HIV transmission rates between 2003 and 2005 among gay and other sexually active men who attended metropolitan health clinics in Australia, with rates of newly acquired HIV infection doubling among people aged less than 25 years (0.8% to 1.6%) and tripling among those aged 25 years or more (0.5% to 1.5%) [1]. Recent data from the Health in Men cohort, a study that recruited HIV-negative men in Sydney

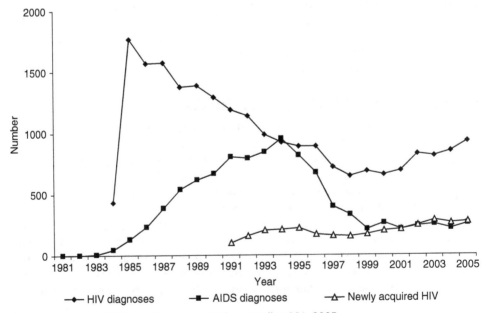

Fig. 6.1 Diagnoses of HIV infection[a] and AIDS in Australia,1981–2005.
[a] HIV diagnoses adjusted for multiple reporting. AIDS diagnoses adjusted for reporting delays.
Source: [1].

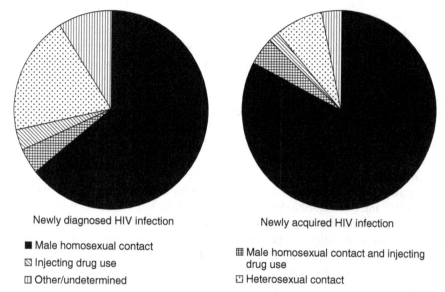

Newly diagnosed HIV infection   Newly acquired HIV infection

■ Male homosexual contact
◨ Injecting drug use
▦ Other/undetermined

▦ Male homosexual contact and injecting
   drug use
◫ Heterosexual contact

Fig. 6.2 Newly diagnosed and newly acquired HIV infection, 2001–2005, by exposure category.
Source: [1].

between 2001 and 2004, found an incidence rate of HIV seroconversion of 0.94 per 100 person-years among this group [5].

There has been considerable epidemiological and social research investigating the risk behaviours of gay and other homosexually active men in Australia. In order to explore trends in the prevalence of important sexual risk factors over time, the baseline data from four studies of gay and other homosexually active men in Sydney, conducted between 1986 and 2003, were compared. These studies included the Social Aspects of AIDS study (1986–7 data), the Sydney Men and Sexual Health study (1993–5), the Positive Health cohort study (2001–2) and the Health in Men cohort (2001–3), which all used similar methods, including detailed interviews with men who identified as homosexual or reported sex with at least one man during the previous five years. There was a decreasing trend between 1986–7 and 2001–3 in the proportion of HIV-positive men reporting sex in the previous six months with casual partners[6]. In contrast, there was an increasing trend in the proportion of HIV-negative men reporting sex in the previous six months with casual partners, and an increasing number of casual partners, over the same time period. There was an overall decrease between 1986–7 and 2001–3 in unprotected anal intercourse with ejaculation among men who were HIV-negative, while there was an overall increase in unprotected anal intercourse with ejaculation among HIV-positive men. Some of this is likely to represent sex with other HIV-positive men.

Aboriginal and Torres Strait Islander populations

Since 1985, 'Indigenous Australian' (i.e. Aboriginal and/or Torres Strait Islander) status of all newly diagnosed cases of HIV/AIDS has been routinely reported to the national HIV/AIDS surveillance system in Australia by five of the eight state/territory health authorities, with the other authorities reporting these data by 1998 [7]. Despite similar rates of HIV diagnosis per capita among indigenous and non-indigenous populations, the distribution of HIV exposure has continued to differ by indigenous status over the past decade. In contrast to HIV exposure in non-indigenous populations, there has been a reduction in the proportion of newly diagnosed HIV infections attributed to male homosexual contact among indigenous populations, from 50% in 1993–2000 to 34% in 2001–5 [1,2]. In the period 1992–8, there were greater proportions of women affected, heterosexual exposure and rural people affected, and a younger age of HIV/AIDS diagnoses among indigenous compared to non-indigenous populations [7]. Heterosexual contact accounted for approximately double the proportion of new HIV diagnoses among indigenous compared to non-indigenous populations in Australia between 1993 and 2000 (36% versus 16%) and between 2001 and 2005 (38% versus 19%) [1,2]. Injecting drug use has increasingly been attributed as the route of HIV transmission among indigenous populations, increasing from 6% in the period 1993–2000 to 18% in 2001–5.

In contrast to the gradual increase in newly diagnosed HIV infection among the non-indigenous population in 2001–5 (4.2–5.2 per 100,000 population), there was a decline in newly diagnosed HIV infection among the indigenous population in 2002–5 (7.1–4.5 per 100,000 population) [1]. While the rate of AIDS diagnosis remained stable at around 1.1 per 100,000 population among non-indigenous people in 2001–5, there was considerable fluctuation among indigenous people, ranging from 2.3–3.9 per 100,000 population in the same period. These trends are, however, based on small numbers and may reflect localized rather than national patterns among indigenous populations.

Immigrant populations

The limited information available on HIV and AIDS among immigrant populations in Australia mostly comes from national HIV/AIDS surveillance data. In 2001–5, more than a third of the 802 cases of newly diagnosed HIV infection for which exposure was attributed to heterosexual contact were acquired through heterosexual contact in high-prevalence countries (estimated prevalence of 1% or greater) [1]. A further 21% reported heterosexual contact with a partner from a high-prevalence country. Among cases attributed to heterosexual contact that were diagnosed in Australia, country of birth was reported as Australia in 38%, sub-Saharan African countries in 26% and South-East Asian countries in 18%. In 1996–2000 and 2001–5, AIDS incidence was highest among cases born in sub-Saharan Africa (6.0 and 5.0 per 100,000 population, respectively) and South/Central America (4.8 and 2.7 per 100,000 population, respectively) [8]. While male homosexual contact accounted for 71.8% of Australian-born cases of newly diagnosed HIV infection and 69.4% of cases in people born in other industrialized countries, HIV exposure was attributed to heterosexual contact in 71.3%, 46.3% and 24.4% of cases from sub-Saharan Africa, Asia and South/Central America, respectively [8]. Late diagnosis of HIV was more common among individuals from sub-Saharan Africa (55.4%), Asia (58.7%) and South/Central America (39.0%) than among people born in Australia or other industrialized countries (31.2%) [8].

Women and children

The annual number of new HIV diagnoses among women has remained stable over the past 10 years at approximately 70–90 per year, except in 2004, when 123 women were newly diagnosed. The increasing number of HIV diagnoses among women, and in a subgroup of women who have had perinatally exposed children, has been associated with heterosexual contact in a high-prevalence country or heterosexual contact with a partner from a high-prevalence country [1]. In 2003–4, perinatal exposure to HIV occurred in 8.6 per 100,000 live births [9]. Between 1995 and 2004, 26 of 207 perinatally HIV-exposed children were diagnosed with HIV infection [9].

People who inject drugs

From 1996 to 2005, approximately 8% of HIV diagnoses in Australia were in people who reported a history of injecting drug use, over half of whom also reported male homosexual contact [1]. Information on HIV prevalence among IDUs nationally is collected via the annual Australian Needle and Syringe Program Survey. Approximately 2000 IDUs participate in the survey each year, with most providing an anonymous capillary blood specimen for HIV and hepatitis C virus (HCV) antibody testing. While HIV prevalence has remained below 2% among IDUs in Australia since 1996, the prevalence among IDUs reporting male homosexual identity ranged between 14% and 32% over the decade, with over 20% in 2005 [10, 11]. However, these prevalence rates are based on small numbers of HIV-positive cases, with fewer than 15 cases identified annually between 2001 and 2005 among the 45–80 male participants who reported homosexual identity in each of the five survey years.

Primary and newly diagnosed HIV infection in Australia

Primary HIV Infection

All patients diagnosed with HIV infection in Australia are reported to state and territorial health authorities and included on the National HIV Database. In 1991, the national HIV surveillance system was expanded to include data on the number of cases of newly acquired HIV infection, defined as newly diagnosed infection with evidence of a negative or indeterminate HIV antibody test result [12]. In the past decade, there has been a gradual increase in the total number of newly acquired infection cases reported in Australia, with just over 150 cases reported annually in 1997–8 and up to 260–285 cases annually in 2003–5 [1].

Primary HIV infection has been a focus of research in Australia since the definition of the syndrome locally [13]. More than 2000 cases of newly acquired HIV infection were recorded through the national surveillance system between 1996 and 2005, and Australia has contributed to several randomized trials and observational studies of primary HIV infection [14,15].

Immunologic and virologic markers among newly diagnosed cases of HIV infection

The National HIV Database collects CD4 count information for all cases of newly diagnosed HIV infection. Between 2001 and 2005, the national median CD4 cell count at diagnosis of HIV infection ranged from 432–455 cells/mm^3 [1]. Among males with newly diagnosed HIV infection in 2001–5 in Australia, the median CD4 count for those with newly acquired HIV infection ranged between 540 and 577cells/mm^3, compared to 360–399 cells/mm^3 among other HIV diagnoses [1]. While the numbers of newly diagnosed cases of HIV infection among women were much smaller, a similar pattern was observed. Consistent with data from the National HIV Database, a median CD4 cell of 517 cells/mm^3 (interquartile range (IQR): 411–660) and log$_{10}$ median viral load of 5.73 copies/mL (IQR: 4.82–5.88) were reported among a sample of patients with primary HIV infection recruited to a clinical trial in Australia between 2000 and 2002, prior to commencing HAART [14].

HIV drug resistance and resistance testing

The prevalence of HIV drug resistance among recently transmitted virus in Sydney fluctuated between 1992 and 2001, influenced by treatment trends [16]. During the period 1992–2000, almost a third of 130 therapy-naïve patients with primary HIV infection seen at participating clinical sites in Sydney had a mutation associated with reverse transcriptase resistance [17].

Following the introduction of protease inhibitors (PIs) in Australia in January 1996, a significant decrease in the frequency of primary nucleoside reverse transcriptase inhibitor (NRTI) resistance mutations was seen among patients with primary HIV infection (9% in 1996–2001 compared to 29.3% in 1992–5) [16]. Between 1992 and 2000, only 0.8% (n=1) were found to have a primary mutation in the protease (PR) gene [17]. While secondary PR mutations were found in 60% of the sample, no increase in PR resistance over the period 1992–2000 was observed, supporting the notion that many secondary resistance mutations in the PR gene are naturally occurring polymorphisms.

From 2001 to 2002, the CREST (Can Resistance Testing Enhance Selection of Therapy) study recruited more than 300 therapy-experienced, HIV-positive patients from 41 clinical sites in Australia and New Zealand to investigate the effect of conducting genotype—as opposed to both genotype and virtual phenotype—resistance testing on the prescription of antiretroviral drugs [18]. The CREST study also supported a national quality assurance programme for genotype testing and development of clinician familiarity with HIV-1 resistance testing at a time when such testing was not routinely available in either Australia or New Zealand. While HIV resistance test results affected antiretroviral prescribing in CREST, no additional benefit was gained from receiving the virtual phenotype resistance test results.

Although the Australasian Society for HIV Medicine (ASHM) commentary on the US Department of Health and Human Services (DHHS) Guidelines for the Use of Antiretroviral Agents in HIV-1 Infected Adults and Adolescents in 2005 [19] recommends genotypic resistance testing for all antiretroviral therapy-naïve patients prior to commencing HAART, as well as for treatment-experienced patients who have a poor virologic response to treatment, resistance testing had limited public funding in Australia in 2006.

Treatment strategies during the era of HAART in Australia

The first PI became publicly available in Australia in 1996, with widespread availability of HAART by late 1996–7. The currently preferred treatment regimens in Australia, based on the US Public Health Service Guidelines for the Use of Antiretroviral Agents in HIV-1-Infected Adults and Adolescents [19], include either: a non-nucleoside reverse transcriptase inhibitor (NNRTI)-based regimen including efavirenz (EFV), typically with lamivudine (3TC) and ZDV or emtricitabine (FTC) and tenofovir (TDF); or a PI-based regimen, including the lopinavir/ritonavir (LPV/r) co-formulation plus 3TC or FTC, plus ZDV.

Prior to 2001, guidelines for commencing antiretroviral treatment in Australia were based on measures of viral load (>10,000 copies/mL) or CD4 count (<500 cells/mm^3) [20]. However, in response to increased recognition of the toxicity associated with antiretroviral therapy, Australian guidelines now recommend delaying initiation of therapy until the patient's CD4 count is around 350 cells/mm^3 [20].

Patients are monitored at approximately three- to four-monthly intervals clinically and for CD4 count and viral load; this is publicly funded. If virologic failure is detected and confirmed, a resistance genotype is usually performed and a new regimen is selected. For patients failing on an NNRTI-based regimen, a ritonavir (RTV)-boosted PI is usually selected together with NRTIs that show sensitivity on the genotype.

For salvage therapy, consistent with guidelines, a resistance genotype is obtained and a new regimen is constructed based on sensitivity and tolerability. For patients who have failed a PI-based regimen, a PI with activity based on the genotype together with the fusion inhibitor enfuvirtide (ENF) and optimization of other background drugs are usually selected. All anti-retroviral drugs from each of the four classes are publicly funded and available.

Observational cohort treatment data in Australia

In 1999, the Australian HIV Observational Database (AHOD) was established to monitor long-term treatment and health outcomes among a cohort of HIV-positive patients nationally. The mean CD4 count at cohort entry, between 1999 and March 2006, was 492 cells/mm^3 (SD=288 cells/mm^3), and the median HIV viral load was 400 copies/mL (IQR=400–13,550 copies/mL) [21]. During any six-month period of follow-up between January 2002 and December 2005, 7–10% of the cohort was antiretroviral (ARV) therapy-naïve, and 76–84% of patients were on ARV therapy [21].

Over the past decade (to 2006), the proportion of patients receiving monotherapy has declined from 12% to 1%, and the proportion receiving dual therapy has declined from 26% to 4%[1]. A simultaneous increase in the proportion of patients in the cohort receiving combination treatment, including at least three antiretroviral drugs, was observed [22]. Consequently, there is an increasing proportion of patients who are not on any therapy, and over 70% who are on combination treatment, during any year.

From 1998 to 2000, the most common combination was three or more antiretroviral drugs, including a PI and excluding an NNRTI [22]. Between January 2001 and March 2005, the main treatment combinations (of three or more antiretroviral drugs) were NRTIs with either a PI (~40% of all patients on treatment) or NNRTI (~40% of all patients on treatment) [23]. In 2005, the five most commonly prescribed antiretroviral combinations among the AHOD cohort included: 1) 3TC, abacavir (ABC) and nevirapine (NVP); 2) the co-formulated Combivir® (which combines ZDV and 3TC in one pill) and NVP; 3) 3TC, TDF and NVP; 4) 3TC, TDF and EFV; and 5) Combivir® and EFV [21].

By September 2003, 63% of the 113 primary HIV-infected patients recruited to the Primary HIV and Early Disease Research: American (PHAEDRA) observational cohort since September 2002 had commenced treatment by their last follow-up visit. More patients commenced PI- (52%) compared to NNRTI- (10%) based combination antiretroviral therapy [15] during that time. Clinical site and geographical area were found to be predictive of whether the first regimen included a PI or an NNRTI.

The rate of combination antiretroviral regimen change was investigated among 596 patients recruited to the AHOD between 1999 and September 2002 who had commenced HAART after January 1997 [24]. The median treatment duration for the first combination antiretroviral regimen was 646 days. Among the 322 patients who commenced a second, and the 149 patients who progressed to a third, combination antiretroviral regimen during the study period, the median treatment durations were 623 days and 392 days, respectively.

An increasing proportion of patients among the AHOD cohort was observed to have treatment interruptions between January 1999 and June 2001 [25], and 8–14% of treatment-experienced patients were not on treatment during any six-month period between January 2002 and December 2005 [21]. However, structured treatment interruptions are no longer recommended in Australia outside of the context of clinical trials [19], following the findings of increased rates of HIV disease progression and death among patients on CD4-guided treatment interruptions in the Strategies for Management of Antiretroviral Therapy (SMART) study [26].

Clinical trials in Australia

Australian clinicians and researchers have contributed to or conducted clinical trials since the earliest days of the HIV epidemic, both locally and internationally. During the last decade, subjects of these trials have included: antiretroviral therapy, including licensure and strategies [26–39]; immunomodulatory therapies [14,40–43]; antiretroviral drug-associated toxicities and strategies to control these toxicities [44–53]; and prophylactic and therapeutic vaccines [54,55].

Despite the relatively small HIV epidemic in Australia, the HIV-positive population is one of the most intensively recruited populations into clinical trials in Australia.

Therapeutic drug monitoring

There are currently two laboratories in Australia that provide therapeutic drug monitoring services, with tests available for the following antiretroviral drugs: saquinavir (SQV), nelfinavir (NFV), indinavir (IDV), RTV, lopinavir (LPV), amprenavir (APV), atazanavir (ATV), EFV and NVP.

Impact of HAART in Australia

There is limited information regarding the early uptake of HAART in Australia. However, data from the Sydney Men and Sexual Health Study suggested that uptake of HAART increased rapidly from 12% in January–June 1996 to 40% in July–December 1996, and to 57% and 72% in the first and second halves of 1997, respectively, among a population of HIV-positive, homosexually active men in Sydney [56]. Over three-quarters of patients under follow-up in the AHOD cohort were on antiretroviral treatment during any six-month period between 2002 and 2005 [21]. Almost all of the patients on treatment were receiving three or more antiretroviral drugs by the end of the first decade of HAART.

Viraemia

Viral load testing first became available in Australia in 1996, and since that time there have been a number of commercially available tests. While the lower limit of detection was initially 400 copies/mL, the latest viral load tests have an analytical range of <40 to 10,000,000 copies/mL. There are currently a number of real-time polymerase chain reaction (PCR) tests becoming available in Australia.

The proportion of HIV-positive patients with an undetectable viral load (<400 copies/mL) increased from 15% in 1996 (retrospective data) to over 50% in 2005 in patients under follow-up in the AHOD [21]. Among those on treatment during any six-month period in 2002–5, there was an increase in the proportion with an undetectable viral load from 75% in January–June 2002 to 88% in July–December 2005 [21]. In comparison, the proportion with an undetectable viral load remained relatively stable at 11–14% among patients who were off treatment during any six-month period in 2002–5 [21]. Median CD4 count also differed between the on- and off-treatment groups in 2002–5, ranging from 420 to 450 cells/mm^3 in the off-treatment group and from 500 to 528 cells/mm^3 in the on-treatment group [21].

Opportunistic disease

The introduction of HAART had a profound effect on the natural history of AIDS-related opportunistic disease in Australia. Overall, there has been a decrease in AIDS-related opportunistic disease since the advent of HAART, with notable reductions in *Pneumocystis jirovecci* pneumonia (PJP) and other opportunistic infections (OIs). The number of AIDS cases with PJP decreased from 150 in 1996 to 70 in 2005 [1], despite PJP remaining the most commonly reported single AIDS-defining illness in Australia during that time [1, 21] (see Figure 6.3).

Following HAART, an increased proportion of new AIDS cases with early HIV diagnosis were diagnosed at higher levels of immune function, with the exception of those presenting with PJP [57]. In contrast, there was no change in average CD4 count at AIDS diagnosis among patients with late HIV diagnosis across the pre- and early HAART eras [57]. This is most likely to be related to the lack of antiretroviral treatment opportunity prior to AIDS in the late HIV diagnosis group.

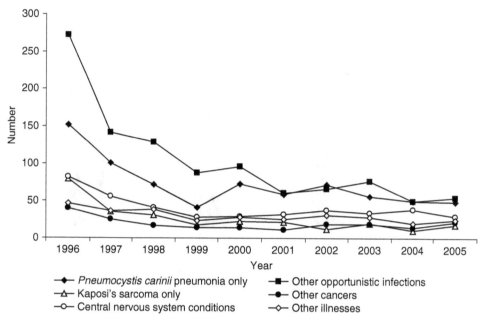

Fig. 6.3 AIDS diagnoses, 1996–2005, by AIDS-defining illness and year.
Source: [1].

AIDS dementia complex (ADC), non-Hodgkin's lymphoma and tuberculosis (TB) accounted for higher proportions of AIDS diagnoses with early HIV diagnosis in the HAART (1996–2000) compared to the pre-HAART (1993–5) era [58]. Conversely, serious cytomegalovirus (CMV) infections and cryptosporidiosis decreased among AIDS cases with early HIV diagnosis in the HAART era [58].

The profile of opportunistic disease among AIDS cases with late HIV diagnosis differed from those with early HIV diagnosis, with double the proportion presenting with PJP in the late HIV diagnosis group [58]. Tuberculosis and HIV wasting syndrome accounted for an increasing proportion of all AIDS-defining illnesses among new AIDS cases with late HIV diagnosis in the HAART era compared to the pre-HAART era [58]. The increase in TB was probably related to increased migration during the 1990s from regions with high prevalence, including sub-Saharan Africa and Asia.

Survival

Survival following AIDS diagnosis vastly improved during the first decade of HAART in Australia. In 1991, median survival time following AIDS diagnosis was 6.6 months among people diagnosed with AIDS during 1982–4 [59]. By 1999, median survival time had increased to 27.7 months among people diagnosed with AIDS in 1996 [60]. Survival at one year post-AIDS diagnosis increased from around 60% in the pre-HAART era to 80% in 1997 [9]. Similarly, there was an increase from 40% to 60% in survival two years after AIDS diagnosis over the same time period [9]. Immune function at AIDS diagnosis, measured by CD4 count, has remained a significant predictor of survival in the HAART era [58].

Despite improved survival, mortality in people with HIV in Australia has remained high in the HAART era in comparison to the general population (see Figure 6.4). A crude mortality rate of 1.58 per 100 person-years was found among patients recruited to AHOD by March 2004

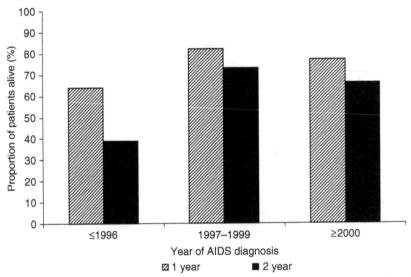

Fig. 6.4 Proportion of patients alive at one year and two years post-AIDS diagnosis, by year of AIDS diagnosis.

Source: [1].

(n=2329) [61], which was around five times higher than in the general population. Of the 105 patient deaths, 40% were directly attributed to an AIDS-defining illness, 52% of all other known causes of death were not due to an AIDS-defining illness and 8% were from causes unknown. The most common causes of death not directly associated with an AIDS-defining diagnosis in AHOD were cancer (27%), liver-related (18%), suicide/drug overdose (18%) and cardiovascular-related (15%), suggesting that deaths in the HAART era may be HIV-related but not due to classic OIs. Advanced immune deficiency (i.e. low CD4 count) was a predictor of deaths, while having not received HAART was a predictor of HIV-related mortality, and age was a predictor of mortality not due to an AIDS-defining illness [61].

Side effects of antiretroviral treatment in Australia

Australian clinicians and researchers played a significant role in documenting the original clinical descriptions of the lipodystrophy syndrome in prospective clinic-based studies [46, 50]. Lipodystrophy was found to occur in about half of patients in a highly treatment-experienced, tertiary clinic-based population in Australia in 1998–9, with 55% of these reporting both peripheral lipoatrophy and central fat accumulation [50]. Lipodystrophy research continues to be very active in Australia, with clinical research on case definitions [44], switch strategies [49], the role of thymidine analogue reverse transcriptase inhibitors (RTIs) [48] and mitochondrial toxicity having a very high priority. Indeed, Australian researchers in the MITOX study established that switching from NRTIs to ABC-based regimens had some effect in recovery of limb fat mass [49]. After 72 weeks of follow-up, mean limb fat mass had increased by 1.26 kg in the group assigned to ABC-based therapy, as compared to 0.49 kg in the group receiving NRTIs.

Australian clinicians and researchers have been involved in international collaborations investigating side effects of antiretroviral therapy and suitable prevention and treatment strategies. One such collaboration is the multi-cohort Data collection of Adverse events of anti-HIV Drugs (D:A:D) study, which includes HIV-positive patients from the United States, Europe and Australia. The D:A:D study found that patients receiving first-line, PI-containing regimens had poorer lipid profiles, including higher total cholesterol (TC), triglycerides (TG) and TC: high density lipoprotein cholesterol (HDL-C) ratios than antiretroviral-naïve patients [62]. When comparing different PI-containing regimens, RTV was associated with higher TC and TG levels and TC:HDL-C ratios in comparison to IDV, and SQV was associated with lower TC:HDL-C ratios. Patients receiving NNRTIs had higher levels of TC and low density lipoprotein cholesterol (LDL-C) than did antiretroviral-naïve patients, although there was less risk of having lower HDL-C levels than in patients receiving a single PI. On comparison of different NNRTI-containing regimens, EFV was associated with higher levels of TC and TG than NVP. An increased risk of myocardial infarction [63] and cardio- and cerebrovascular events [64] have also been associated with combination antiretroviral drug use in the multi-cohort D:A:D study.

Despite the ongoing participation of Australian clinicians and researchers in investigating the side effects of antiretroviral therapy, there has been no systematic data collection on these side effects in Australia. Systematic collection of data on antiretroviral-related toxicities among the AHOD cohort is currently in the planning phases.

While the therapeutic goals of antiretroviral therapy include achieving and maintaining viral suppression and improving patient immune function, finding an effective regimen involves taking into account underlying conditions of individual patients, concomitant medications and history of drug intolerance [19]. As per the ASHM treatment guidelines [65], switching drug classes and use of lipid-lowering agents is recommended for the treatment of hyperlipidaemia among HIV-positive patients in Australia. In the case of lipodystrophy, switching drug classes to a non-thymidine analogue NRTI-containing regimen, behavioural modification such as increasing exercise, and use of cosmetic approaches are recommended. Lifestyle modifications such as diet and exercise, switching antiretroviral drug classes and use of oral hypoglycaemic agents are recommended for HIV-positive patients presenting with diabetes. In the case of osteonecrosis, surgery is often necessary, while exercise, calcium and vitamin D supplements as well as therapy with biphosphonates are recommended for patients with osteoporosis.

HIV co-infection with hepatitis

In Australia, hepatitis B virus (HBV) is most common among immigrants from South-East Asian countries with high HBV prevalence [66]. In contrast, the HCV epidemic in Australia largely affects IDU populations [1]. While the prevalence of HCV among injecting drug users in Australia was estimated at 61% in 2005, HIV prevalence has remained less than 2% since 1996 [10, 11].

The impact of HBV and/or HCV co-infection on rate of treatment change and HIV disease outcomes has been investigated among patients in the AHOD cohort who commenced HAART after January 1997, had follow-up of more than three months and had test results for HBV surface antigen and HCV antibody. By March 2003, 4.8% (39/805) of patients had a positive HBV surface antigen test, and 12.8% (103/805) had a positive HCV antibody test [67]. The overall rate of treatment change after initiating HAART was 0.74 combinations per year. The median time before first treatment change was longest among HIV-positive patients with HBV co-infection (686 days), followed by 482 days for HIV-positive patients without HCV or HBV co-infection, 398 days for those co-infected with HCV alone and 172 days for those with HBV and HCV co-infection [67]. Co-infection with HBV and/or HCV was not found to be significantly associated with the rate of combination treatment change. Factors associated with an increased rate of change included prior AIDS-defining illness, prior exposure to dual NRTI combination antiretroviral therapy and antiretroviral treatment class.

Healthcare delivery and related expenditure

In Australia, antiretroviral drugs are prescribed by a mixture of specialist physicians in infectious diseases and clinical immunology in teaching hospitals, physicians in sexual health clinics and physicians in high-caseload general practices. Prescription of antiretrovirals requires a specialist qualification, or, for high-caseload primary care physicians, certified training is provided through ASHM. All healthcare in Australia is publicly funded through Medicare agreements between state and federal Australian governments. All licensed antiretroviral drugs are provided through the pharmaceutical benefits schedule under a special section of highly specialized drugs with limited prescriber access as described above. A capped co-payment is required, with a considerable discount for patients who are on disability support. There is currently a gap in availability of antiretroviral therapy and healthcare for tens to hundreds of people with HIV who are not Australian citizens or who do not hold residency permits. State health departments occasionally fund this gap.

Quality is assured through the requirement of antiretroviral drug prescribers to be specialist physicians or general practitioners who are certified by ASHM. The numbers of general practitioners taking up HIV medicine is dwindling because of the sliding reimbursement scheme for consultation times in general practice, which are insufficient to deliver high-quality care for complex medical disorders like HIV disease. There is little external brain drain, but overseas-trained physicians encounter numerous barriers to registration in Australia. As in all developed countries, there is currently a serious nursing shortage that is not just restricted to care of PLWHA. By contrast, HIV/AIDS is a popular and satisfying area for nurses to take up in Australia.

Total expenditure related to the Highly Specialised Drugs (S100) programme in Australia has increased gradually over the past six years, with semi-annual costs estimated at US$27 million for the period January–June 2000 and US$40 million for July–December 2005 [21]. As the death rate from HIV disease continues to decrease and the number of PLWHA steadily increases, it is anticipated that spending in this area will undergo a steady increase over the coming years.

There has been no published data quantifying direct clinical costs associated with the management of HIV infection in Australia since the pre-HAART era. In a study conducted in the second most populated state of Australia, Victoria, in 1992–3, it was found that healthcare utilization and subsequent costs increased with the severity of illness in HIV patients [68]. These costs were found to be highest in the three months prior to death. In light of the decline in AIDS-related opportunistic disease [1] and the significant proportion of non AIDS-related mortality among HIV-positive patients [61] in Australia since the introduction of HAART, it is likely that there has been a shift in health utilization and associated costs since the pre-HAART era. At the end of the first HAART era, management of HAART-related toxicities and non AIDS-related illnesses are likely to account for a growing proportion of healthcare costs in the HIV-positive population in Australia.

Conclusion

Since the 1980s, the HIV epidemic in Australia has predominantly affected gay and other homosexually active men, with very low HIV prevalence maintained among IDU and heterosexual populations. Over the past decade, HAART has been widely and freely available to people with an HIV diagnosis in Australia, and has been associated with large reductions in AIDS-related morbidity and mortality.

While Australia has enjoyed relative success in its response to the local HIV epidemic to date, recent data showing an increase HIV incidence among gay men highlight the importance of maintaining ongoing HIV prevention, harm reduction and treatment strategies. With a likely increase in non AIDS-related conditions among an aging and growing HIV-positive population, Australia will be faced with the changing chronic and complex healthcare needs of this patient group over the coming decade.

Acknowledgements

Kathleen Glenday, Matthew Law and David Cooper are supported in part by grants from the American Foundation for AIDS Research (amfAR) and the US National Institutes of Health's National Institute of Allergy and Infectious Diseases (NIAID) (Grant No. U01-AI069907). The National Centre in HIV Epidemiology and Clinical Research is funded by the Australian Government's Department of Health and Ageing, and is affiliated with the Faculty of Medicine, The University of New South Wales.

References

1. National Centre in HIV Epidemiology and Clinical Research. (2006). *HIV/AIDS, viral hepatitis and sexually transmissible infections in Australia Annual Surveillance Report 2006*. Sydney, NSW: National Centre in HIV Epidemiology and Clinical Research, The University of New South Wales; Canberra, ACT: Australian Institute of Health and Welfare.

2. National Centre in HIV Epidemiology and Clinical Research. (2001). *HIV/AIDS, viral hepatitis and sexually transmissible infections in Australia Annual Surveillance Report 2001*. Sydney, NSW: National Centre in HIV Epidemiology and Clinical Research, The University of New South Wales.

3. Oelrichs RB, Lawson VA, Coates KM, Chatfield C, Deacon NJ, McPhee DA. (2000). Rapid full-length genomic sequencing of two cytopathically heterogeneous Australian primary HIV-1 isolates. *J Biomed Sci* 7:128–35.

4. Ryan CE, Elliot JH, Middleton T, *et al.* (2004). The Molecular Epidemiology of HIV Type 1 among Vietnamese Australian Injecting Drug Users in Melbourne, Australia. *AIDS Res Hum Retroviruses* 20:1364–7.

5. Jin F, Prestage G, Mao L, *et al.* (2006). Anal sexually transmissible infections as risk factors for HIV seroconversion: data from the HIM cohort. XVI International AIDS Conference, 13–18 August 2006, Toronto, Canada. [Abstract TUAC0504]

6. Prestage G, Mao L, Fogarty A, *et al.* (2005). How has the sexual behaviour of gay men changed since the onset of AIDS: 1986–2003. *Aust N Z J Public Health* 29:530–5.

7. Guthrie JA, Dore GJ, McDonald AM, Kaldor JM. (2000). HIV and AIDS in aboriginal and Torres Strait Islander Australians: 1992–1998. The National HIV Surveillance Committee. *Med J Aust* 172:266–9.

8. Middleton M, McDonald AM, Kaldor JM. (2006). Birthplace and AIDS Incidence in Australia, 1996–2005. 18th Annual Australasian Society of HIV Medicine Conference, 11–14 October 2006, Melbourne, Australia.

9. National Centre in HIV Epidemiology and Clinical Research. (2005). *HIV/AIDS, viral hepatitis and sexually transmissible infections in Australia. Annual Surveillance Report 2005*. Sydney, NSW: National Centre in HIV Epidemiology and Clinical Research, The University of New South Wales; Canberra, ACT: Australian Institute of Health and Welfare.

10. National Centre in HIV Epidemiology and Clinical Research. (2003). *Australian Needle and Syringe Program Survey National Data Report 1995–2002*. Sydney, NSW: National Centre in HIV Epidemiology and Clinical Research, The University of NSW.

11. National Centre in HIV Epidemiology and Clinical Research. (2006). *Australian Needle and Syringe Program Survey National Data Report 2001–2005*. Sydney, NSW: National Centre in HIV Epidemiology and Clinical Research, The University of NSW.

12. McDonald AM, Gertig DM, Crofts N, Kaldor JM. (1994). A national surveillance system for newly acquired HIV infection in Australia. National HIV Surveillance Committee. *Am J Public Health* **84**:1923–8.

13. Cooper DA, Gold J, Maclean P, *et al.* (1985). Acute AIDS retrovirus infection. Definition of a clinical illness associated with seroconversion. *Lancet* **1**:537–40.

14. Bloch MT, Smith DE, Quan D, *et al.* (2006). The role of hydroxyurea in enhancing the virologic control achieved through structured treatment interruption in primary HIV infection: final results from a randomized clinical trial (Pulse). *J Acquir Immune Defic Syndr* **42**:192–202.

15. Ramacciotti T, Smith D, Johnston M, *et al.* (2004). Clinical characteristics and treatment uptake in patients newly infected with HIV identified over a 1-year period: The Phaedra Collaborative Cohort. 11th Conference on Retroviruses and Opportunistic Infections, 8–11 February 2004, San Fransisco, California, USA. [Abstract 398]

16. Ammaranond P, Cunningham P, Oelrichs R, *et al.* (2003). No increase in protease resistance and a decrease in reverse transcriptase resistance mutations in primary HIV-1 infection: 1992–2001. *AIDS* **17**:264–7.

17. Ammaranond P, Cunningham P, Oelrichs RB, *et al.* (2003). Rates of transmission of antiretroviral drug resistant strains of HIV-1. *J Clin Virol* **26**:153–61.

18. Hales G, Birch C, Crowe S, *et al.* (2006). A Randomised Trial Comparing Genotypic and Virtual Phenotypic Interpretation of HIV Drug Resistance: The CREST Study. *PLoS Clin Trials* **1**:e18.

19. DHSS Panel on Antiretroviral Guidelines for Adults and Adolescents, Office of AIDS Research Advisory Council. (2006). USA Guidelines for the Use of Antiretroviral Agents in HIV-1-Infected Adults and Adolescents: Incorporating commentary to adapt the guidelines to the Australasian setting. Available at http://www.ashm.org.au/uploads/File/aust-ARVG-2006–05.pdf

20. Australasian Society of HIV Medicine. (2004). *HIV/Viral hepatitis: a guide for primary care.* Sydney, NSW: Australasian Society of HIV Medicine.

21. National Centre in HIV Epidemiology and Clinical Research. (2006). *Australian HIV Observational Database Annual Report.* Sydney, NSW: National Centre in HIV Epidemiology and Clinical Research, The University of NSW.

22. The Australian HIV Observational Database. (2001). Time trends in antiretroviral treatment in Australia, 1997–2000. *Venereology* **14**:162–8.

23. National Centre in HIV Epidemiology and Clinical Research. (2005). *Australian HIV Observational Database Annual Report.* Sydney, NSW: National Centre in HIV Epidemiology and Clinical Research, The University of NSW.

24. The Australian HIV Observational Database. (2002). Rates of combination antiretroviral treatment change in Australia, 1997–2000. *HIV Med* **3**:28–36.

25. Petoumenos K. (2003). The role of observational data in monitoring trends in antiretroviral treatment and HIV disease stage: Results from the Australian HIV observational database. *J Clin Virol* **26**:209–22.

26. El-Sadr WM, Lundgren JD, Neaton JD, *et al.* (2006). CD4+ count-guided interruption of antiretroviral treatment. *N Engl J Med* **355**:2283–96.

27. Delta Trial. (1996). Delta: a randomised double-blind controlled trial comparing combinations of zidovudine plus didanosine or zalcitabine with zidovudine alone in HIV-infected individuals. *Lancet* **348**:283–91.

28. Amin J, Moore A, Carr A, *et al.* (2003). Combined analysis of two-year follow-up from two open-label randomized trials comparing efficacy of three nucleoside reverse transcriptase inhibitor backbones for previously untreated HIV-1 infection: OzCombo 1 and 2. *HIV Clin Trials* **4**:252–61.

29. Carr A, Chuah J, Hudson J, *et al.* (2000). A randomised, open-label comparison of three highly active antiretroviral therapy regimens including two nucleoside analogues and indinavir for previously untreated HIV-1 infection: the OzCombo1 study. *AIDS* **14**:1171–80.

30. CAESAR Coordinating Committee. (1997). Randomised trial of addition of lamivudine or lamivudine plus loviride to zidovudine-containing regimens for patients with HIV-1 infection: the CAESAR trial. *Lancet* **349**:1413–21.

31. Cooper DA, Gatell JM, Kroon S, *et al.* (1993). Zidovudine in persons with asymptomatic HIV infection and CD4+ cell counts greater than 400 per cubic millimeter. The European-Australian Collaborative Group. *N Engl J Med* **329**:297–303.

32. Feinberg JE, Hurwitz S, Cooper D, *et al.* (1998). A randomized, double-blind trial of valaciclovir prophylaxis for cytomegalovirus disease in patients with advanced human immunodeficiency virus infection. AIDS Clinical Trials Group Protocol 204/Glaxo Wellcome 123–014 International CMV Prophylaxis Study Group. *J Infect Dis* **177**:48–56.

33. French M, Amin J, Roth N, *et al.* (2002). Randomized, open-label, comparative trial to evaluate the efficacy and safety of three antiretroviral drug combinations including two nucleoside analogues and nevirapine for previously untreated HIV-1 Infection: the OzCombo 2 study. *HIV Clin Trials* **3**:177–85.

34. Kroon ED, Ungsedhapand C, Ruxrungtham K, *et al.* (2000). A randomized, double-blind trial of half versus standard dose of zidovudine plus zalcitabine in Thai HIV-1-infected patients (study HIV-NAT 001). HIV Netherlands Australia Thailand Research Collaboration. *AIDS* **14**:1349–56.

35. Ruxrungtham K, Kroon ED, Ungsedhapand C, *et al.* (2000). A randomized, dose-finding study with didanosine plus stavudine versus didanosine alone in antiviral-naive, HIV-infected Thai patients. *AIDS* **14**:1375–82.

36. Staszewski S, Keiser P, Montaner J, *et al.* (2001). Abacavir-lamivudine-zidovudine vs indinavir-lamivudine-zidovudine in antiretroviral-naive HIV-infected adults: A randomized equivalence trial. *JAMA* **285**:1155–63.

37. Yeni P, Cooper DA, Aboulker J-P, *et al.* (2006). Virological and immunological outcomes at 3 years after starting antiretroviral therapy with regimens containing non-nucleoside reverse transcriptase inhibitor, protease inhibitor, or both in INITIO: open-label randomised trial. *Lancet* **368**: 287–98.

38. Ananworanich J, Gayet-Ageron A, Le Braz M, *et al.* (2006). CD4-guided scheduled treatment interruptions compared with continuous therapy for patients infected with HIV-1: results of the Staccato randomised trial. *Lancet* **368**:459–65.

39. Ananworanich J, Nuesch R, Le Braz M, *et al.* (2003). Failures of 1 week on, 1 week off antiretroviral therapies in a randomized trial. *AIDS* **17**:F33–7.

40. Carr A, Emery S, Lloyd A, *et al.* (1998). Outpatient continuous intravenous interleukin-2 or subcutaneous, polyethylene glycol-modified interleukin-2 in human immunodeficiency virus-infected patients: a randomized, controlled, multicenter study. Australian IL-2 Study Group. *J Infect Dis* **178**:992–9.

41. Emery S, Abrams DI, Cooper DA, *et al.* (2002). The evaluation of subcutaneous proleukin (interleukin-2) in a randomized international trial: rationale, design, and methods of ESPRIT. *Control Clin Trials* **23**:198–220.

42. Losso MH, Belloso WH, Emery S, *et al.* (2000). A randomized, controlled, phase II trial comparing escalating doses of subcutaneous interleukin-2 plus antiretrovirals versus antiretrovirals alone in human immunodeficiency virus-infected patients with CD4+ cell counts >/=350/mm3. *J Infect Dis* **181**:1614–21.

43. Pett SL, Wand H, Law MG, *et al.* (2006). Evaluation of Subcutaneous Proleukin (interleukin-2) in a Randomized International Trial (ESPRIT): geographical and gender differences in the baseline characteristics of participants. *HIV Clin Trials* **7**:70–85.

44. Carr A. (2003). An objective case definition of lipodystrophy in HIV-infected adults: a case-control study. *Lancet* **361**:726–35.

45. Carr A, Samaras K, Burton S, *et al.* (1998). A syndrome of peripheral lipodystrophy, hyperlipidaemia and insulin resistance in patients receiving HIV protease inhibitors. *AIDS* **12**:F51–8.

46. Carr A, Samaras K, Thorisdottir A, Kaufmann GR, Chisholm DJ, Cooper DA. (1999). Diagnosis, prediction, and natural course of HIV-1 protease-inhibitor-associated lipodystrophy, hyperlipidaemia, and diabetes mellitus: a cohort study. *Lancet* **353**:2093–9.

47. Carr A, Workman C, Carey D, *et al.* (2004). No effect of rosiglitazone for treatment of HIV-1 lipoatrophy: randomised, double-blind, placebo-controlled trial. *Lancet* **363**:429–38.

48. Martin A, Smith D, Carr A, *et al.* (2004). Progression of lipodystrophy (LD) with continued thymidine analogue usage: long-term follow-up from a randomized clinical trial (the PIILR study). *HIV Clin Trials* **5**:192–200.

49. Martin A, Smith DE, Carr A, *et al.* (2004). Reversibility of lipoatrophy in HIV-infected patients 2 years after switching from a thymidine analogue to abacavir: the MITOX Extension Study. *AIDS* **18**:1029–36.

50. Miller J, Carr A, Emery S, *et al.* (2003). HIV lipodystrophy: prevalence, severity and correlates of risk in Australia. *HIV Med* **4**:293–301.

51. Smith DE, Carr A, Law M, *et al.* (2002). Thymidine analogue withdrawal for lipoatrophic patients on protease-sparing therapy improves lipoatrophy but compromises antiviral control: the PIILR extension study. *AIDS* **16**:2489–91.

52. Carr A, Hudson J, Chuah J, *et al.* (2001). HIV protease inhibitor substitution in patients with lipodystrophy: a randomized, controlled, open-label, multicentre study. *AIDS* **15**:1811–22.

53. Carr A, Workman C, Smith DE, *et al.* (2002). Abacavir substitution for nucleoside analogs in patients with HIV lipoatrophy: a randomized trial. *JAMA* **288**:207–15.

54. Emery S, Workman C, Puls RL, *et al.* (2005). Randomized, placebo-controlled, phase I/IIa Evaluation of the Safety and Immunogenicity of Fowlpox Virus Expressing HIV gag-pol and Interferon-g in HIV-1 Infected Subjects. *Hum Vaccin* **1**:232–8.

55. Kelleher AD, Puls RL, Bebbington M, *et al.* (2006). A randomized, placebo-controlled phase I trial of DNA prime, recombinant fowlpox virus boost prophylactic vaccine for HIV-1. *AIDS* **20**:294–7.

56. National Centre in HIV Epidemiology and Clinical Research. (1998). *HIV/AIDS and related diseases in Australia Annual Surveillance Report 1998.* Sydney, NSW: National Centre in HIV Epidemiology and Clinical Research, The University of New South Wales.

57. Law MG, de Winter L, McDonald A, Cooper DA, Kaldor JM. (1999). AIDS diagnoses at higher CD4 counts in Australia following the introduction of highly active antiretroviral treatment. *AIDS* **13**:263–9.

58. Dore GJ, Li Y, McDonald A, Ree H, Kaldor JM. (2002). Impact of highly active antiretroviral therapy on individual AIDS-defining illness incidence and survival in Australia. *J Acquir Immune Defic Syndr* **29**:388–95.

59. Luo K, Law M, Kaldor JM, McDonald AM, Cooper DA. (1995). The role of initial AIDS-defining illness in survival following AIDS. *AIDS* **9**:57–63.

60. Li Y, McDonald AM, Dore GJ, Kaldor JM. (2000). Improving survival following AIDS in Australia, 1991–1996. National HIV Surveillance Committee. *AIDS* **14**:2349–54.

61. Petoumenos K, Law MG, on behalf of the Australian HIV Observational Database. (2006). Risk factors and causes of death in the Australian HIV Observational Database. *Sex Health* **3**:103–12.

62. Fontas E, van Leth F, Sabin CA, *et al.* (2004). Lipid profiles in HIV-infected patients receiving combination antiretroviral therapy: are different antiretroviral drugs associated with different lipid profiles? *J Infect Dis* **189**:1056–74.

63. Friis-Moller N, Sabin CA, Weber R, *et al.* (2003). Combination antiretroviral therapy and the risk of myocardial infarction. *N Engl J Med* **349**:1993–2003.

64. d'Arminio A, Sabin CA, Phillips AN, *et al.* (2004). Cardio- and cerebrovascular events in HIV-infected persons. *AIDS* **18**:1811–7.

65. Australasian Society of HIV Medicine. (2003). *HIV Management in Australasia: a guide for clinical care.* Sydney, NSW: Australasian Society of HIV Medicine.

66. O'Sullivan BG, Gidding HF, Law M, Kaldor JM, Gilbert GL, Dore GJ. (2004). Estimates of chronic hepatitis B virus infection in Australia, 2000. *Aust N Z J Public Health* **28**:212–6.

67. Petoumenos K, Ringland C. (2005). Antiretroviral treatment change among HIV, hepatitis B virus and hepatitis C virus co-infected patients in the Australian HIV Observational Database. *HIV Med* **6**:155–63.

68. Hurley SF, Kaldor JM, Carlin JB, *et al.* (1995). The usage and costs of health services for HIV infection in Australia. *AIDS* **9**:777–85.

Chapter 7

Country review: Chile

Marcelo J. Wolff

Background

Chile is a middle-income South American country with a traditionally strong public healthcare network that, at the end of the first decade of highly active antiretroviral therapy (HAART), has reached universal coverage for the treatment of human immunodeficiency virus (HIV) infection, both in the public health system and the much smaller private health system. It was neither an easy nor smooth path, and the beginning was slow and late, but it is now a consolidated endeavour. The purpose of this chapter is to describe the epidemiological characteristics of HIV infection in Chile, to discuss the healthcare system and its approach to antiretroviral therapy from the advent of HAART until 2007, with a focus on the difficulties, challenges and lessons learned, and to outline the present status of the national treatment programme and the evaluation of its impact.

By 1996, Chile had a population of 14.4 million people with an annual per capita income of US$3,700 and was not considered a highly developed country, as it would be 10 years later. The country was emerging from a long period of military rule that had weakened the public health system, its reborn fragile democracy had a government committed to rebuilding the public health system, and encountering the AIDS epidemic was becoming a common occurrence in health institutions around the country. The annual rate of HIV/AIDS reported was 5 cases/100,000 people, five times higher in men than in women: 95% of cases were sexually transmitted, with 50% seen in homosexual men, 15% in bisexual men and 30% in heterosexual men and women; less than 5% of infections were due to contaminated needles used by injecting drug users (IDUs); and 1% were through perinatal exposure. Blood product transfusion as a route of transmission had all but disappeared after the introduction of mandatory blood screening 10 years before. Almost 60% of the cases were reported from the metropolitan region, which is where 40% of the population lives and includes the capital and largest city, Santiago.

Patients were mostly cared for by the public health system, which is responsible for the health of 70% of the population, including indigents. Almost half of the patients entered the healthcare system with advanced disease, that is, at the AIDS stage. The annual mortality rate associated with HIV infection was 2.6/100,000. Although not systematically evaluated, according to pilot studies it was felt that only HIV-1 infections were prevalent, a situation concordant with the lack of contact with people of African descent in the country as a whole and the infected population in particular. Sentinel studies also suggested that most, if not all, viral subtypes were Type B. Foreign immigration played no role in the epidemic, but the return of expatriates due to an improvement in the country's economic and political circumstances had a slight temporary impact in cases associated with injecting drug use.

Although there was a strong public health network throughout the country, AIDS care centres had not been established in all 28 health areas into which the country is divided, and many of those that existed were inappropriately staffed and poorly equipped. However, there was one larger centre that provided comprehensive, multiprofessional care within the public sector, and that had already studied the clinical and epidemiological characteristics of the epidemic in detail [1]. This institution, the Arriarán Foundation, also became a training centre for healthcare professionals from around the country. CD4 count monitoring and viral load testing were available in only one centre in the public health network. A Ministry of Health Commission on AIDS (CONASIDA) with regulatory as well as operative responsibilities played a leading role in prevention campaigns, medical education and the organization of AIDS care centres; it also provided the drugs then available for treatment.

Ten years later, in 2006, the epidemic had changed little, but the country had changed considerably, including its approach and commitment to care and treatment of people living with HIV and AIDS (PLWHA). The population had increased to 16.4 million, and the national annual per capita income had more than doubled to US$8,600, the highest on the American continent south of the US border [2]. Close to 1500 new HIV/AIDS cases per year had been reported in the previous three years, with an incidence rate of 7/100,000; the male:female ratio remained at 5:1. Official statistics estimated that 0.3% of the adult population—some 30,000 to 35,000 people—were HIV-infected, with two-thirds of them receiving no medical care and most unaware of their serologic status. The annual mortality rate was similar to that of a decade earlier, having decreased from a high of 3.5/100,000 in 2001, when access to HAART was low. One-third (5000) of all HIV/AIDS cases reported from 1984 to 2005 had died.

The epidemic still had the same mix of risk factors, but heterosexual transmission was steadily increasing over time, comprising up to 40% of cases [3,4]. Immigration from northern bordering countries was beginning to have an impact in terms of imported HIV and tuberculosis (TB) infections, sometimes manifesting as co-infections, with an unusually high incidence of resistance to antituberculous drugs, which was quite different from the local pattern of very low rates of mycobacterial resistance. The public healthcare system was still responsible for the care of most cases (85%), and patients were still admitted with severe immunodepression and advanced clinical disease, although with higher CD4 counts at baseline than before. A major health reform with great implications for HIV infection management was in full implementation phase. Monitoring through CD4 count, viral load and even genotyping was now available and was performed in many more centres. The annual budget for the public health system programme had gone from US$1 million to US$21 million, 90% of it allocated for direct care of patients.

Antiretroviral therapy

The provision of antiretroviral therapy in the 10-year period since the introduction of HAART in 1996 went from suboptimal in terms of both quality and access for those in need, to universal access to HAART, free of charge in the public health system, and with a small co-payment in the private health sector. This section describes how this process evolved, what institutions were involved and what results were achieved.

Free antiretroviral therapy began in 1993 in the form of zidovudine (ZDV) monotherapy provided to a fraction of patients in the public health system without detailed local guidelines about whom to select for treatment, but with a trend to favour its use in pregnant women to prevent vertical transmission. In 1996, CONASIDA initiated a programme of more potent antiretroviral treatment using two drugs, mainly ZDV and lamivudine (3TC), although didanosine (ddI) and zalcitabine (ddC) were also available. At that time, there were high expectations for better results than with monotherapy. However, mistakes were made; once again there were no clear guidelines about when to initiate therapy, many patients went from the previous single-drug regimen to dual therapy just by adding a second drug, and many asymptomatic people began therapy with CD4 counts that by present standards would not require treatment.

The main problem, which would recur for years to come, was that the supply of drugs was insufficient for the number of candidates no matter what treatment guideline was used. Given an inadequate supply of drugs, centres faced the dilemma of whom to select for treatment among patients with the same degree of need. Discrimination, either in favor of certain groups (e.g. women with children), or against them (e.g. homosexuals), was common. In addition, only those who could obtain a 'third drug' by other means were treated, since physicians were becoming aware of the birth of HAART as a major breakthrough in the treatment of AIDS. Some centres decided they just could not choose under these conditions and opted for random assignment in which one out of three candidates at the same level of need was chosen in each round of selection. Patients quickly coined the term 'HIV cocktail lottery'. Most centres, however, decided on a first-come, first-served basis until the drugs available to that centre ran out. Whatever mechanism was used, in all centres tensions among staff, between staff and patients, and even between patients ran high. Patients sat in different sections of the waiting room depending on whether they were or were not receiving treatment, and those without treatment outnumbered the others. Often, the feeling of support and solidarity that patients and their families had shared when no therapy existed—or, if it did exist, was available to very few—was lost. Sometimes HIV-infected family members or couples would share a therapeutic regimen for one. That was a stressful period for everybody, and of little benefit for those sick with HIV; moreover, it soon became apparent that patient outcomes did not change significantly under these conditions. The annual mortality rate at the Arriarán Foundation, the largest AIDS care centre in Chile, reached a peak in 1996 of 16% [5], and national statistics only pointed to increasing mortality due to AIDS [3].

Yet, despite all the negative aspects of providing what was soon recognized as suboptimal therapy to an insufficient number of patients, the process had a positive effect: it helped to establish the network of centres providing HIV care, to define their relationship to the central health authorities and to create the system for drug delivery and treatment monitoring that would become extremely valuable in the future.

A major decision in the public health system was that HIV/AIDS care would be carried out in dedicated centres and not in primary care facilities, except for diagnosis or emergencies. This was due to the level of development of the public health network and the fact that the epidemic had neither reached, nor was it expected to reach, a magnitude that might overwhelm these centres' capabilities. However, after about two years, several things happened at the local level to trigger some changes. First, research at the Arriarán Foundation showed better outcomes using dual therapy compared with no therapy in terms of reduced morbidity, hospitalizations and mortality, though these benefits were minimal and short-lived when compared with the standards of care in developed countries using triple-drug therapy, or HAART [6]. When these results were presented at an international meeting [7], the Chilean authors spent a lot of time and embarrassment explaining that the 'no-therapy' arm of their study was simply the reality in their country at the time. They expressed the hope that Chilean authorities would recognize the existing inequities and lack of ethical standards around access to antiretroviral therapy and take appropriate action. Eventually, they did.

Second, the Chilean Infectious Disease Society (CIDS) created an AIDS commission to study important issues around the HIV epidemic at global and local levels and to advise the Society about them. The growing body of evidence regarding the qualitative improvement of HIV outcomes resulting from HAART, in addition to the inequity of not providing therapy to all in need—at least for those cared for with public funds—led CIDS to publish a position paper written by its AIDS commission calling on the state to provide modern and optimal therapy to all who needed it [8]. A paper published by a foreign group that ranked all countries in the Americas in terms of the percentage of their gross national product (GNP) they would have to spend to provide HAART to their infected populations played an important role in the commission's deliberations [9]. The analysis indicated that the higher the income and the lower the rate of infection, the lower the percentage of GNP needed [9]. Chile ranked third after Canada and the United States (Figure 7.1).

Antiretroviral drugs became available in Chile on the open market to private patients, but at a cost of approximately US$1,000 a month; very few could afford it. By 1999, pressure on the government had mounted to a level that compelled a change in commitment. The Ministry of Health (MOH) modified its policy regarding AIDS, from a major focus on prevention to the more balanced approach of both prevention and care espoused by all international organizations. Antiretroviral drugs began to be distributed, but in a very restrained manner; physicians were instructed to maintain the patients on suboptimal dual therapy unless there was clinical failure. There were 750 patients in dual therapy at that time, and HAART was to be indicated mostly for new treatment-naïve patients. The health authority issued a strict guideline for

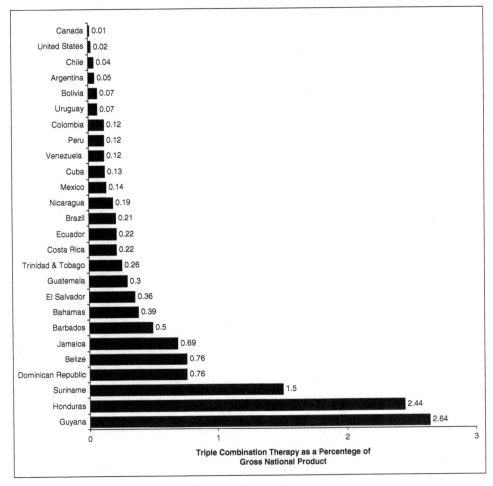

Fig. 7.1 Relative cost of antiretroviral therapy in the Americas.

Source: [9], with permission of the editors.

HAART whereby another 750 regimens were prescribed. In a few months all the dual therapy and HAART quotas were in use, with at least 1000 patients on the waiting list, which had expanded greatly due to an influx of patients from the private to the public sector in the hope of receiving free therapy. Many private sector patients could not afford to pay for HAART, since private insurers covered medications received during hospitalization but not on ambulatory basis (for all diseases, not only for HIV).

Within a short time, several problems emerged, including failure of suboptimal dual therapies documented by the then more widely available CD4 count and viral load, and failure of HAART in patients previously treated with weaker therapies, whether or not the regimen was a totally new one or had been initiated to potentiate a weaker therapy with a third drug. But again, there was not enough drug supply to satisfy the increasing demand. Unfortunately, and perhaps due to competition with many other unmet needs in healthcare, no modifications were made to this programme for two years.

The CIDS maintained its solitary voice requesting more and better treatments. Support for these appeals came not from the medical establishment, but from organizations of PLWHA with a similar but more urgent and personal demand: proper treatment now, and for all. These groups were best represented by *Vivopositivo* (Living Positive), which was the first organization to openly demand proper care without discrimination. In 2001, the government launched the Expanded Access Programme (EAP) to HAART in the public health system, aimed at providing optimal treatment for all who needed it—both children and adults—and at reaching this goal in the shortest possible time. All except a few successful dual therapies (in patients who probably never needed therapy to begin with) were changed to the newly available antiretroviral drugs, but still without the benefit of genotype testing. The gradual increase in the uptake of antiretroviral therapy was due to a rise in the budget allocated to antiretroviral drugs, but only for proprietary drugs. Negotiations with several pharmaceutical companies reduced the price of most drugs, but no generics were included in the programme until late 2006, when the MOH began buying generic nevirapine (NVP).

With this new scenario in the public health system, which was not reflected in the private health system, more and more HIV-infected people migrated to the public health system. Others were tempted to obtain the drugs they needed through a black market created by the sale of free public health system drugs by PLWHA, some of whom were willing to sell their life-saving drugs, usually quite cheaply. Many private practice patients felt a great deal of guilt about this, but would tell their physicians, if they were at all inclined to discuss the matter, that they had no other choice.

The EAP not only dealt with antiretroviral drugs, but also had a much wider scope of patient care, including what was called 'comprehensive care' and related to the organization of the network and the way it would work. By mid-2001, the public health system network of AIDS care centres was fully in place, with 32 centres around the country, at least one of which was located in each of the 28 local health districts that comprised the public health system. Each AIDS care centre was responsible for ambulatory care of patients and had variable capability for performing diagnostic and therapeutic procedures, but all had a referral hospital for admissions.

A centralized system for drug distribution was in operation, whereby forms with individualized HAART requests were first faxed to CONASIDA and then referred to members of the advisory group who verified the appropriateness of each request in accordance with the national guidelines. Each request was then approved, modified, or postponed pending additional information. The decision was sent back to CONASIDA, which instructed the pharmaceutical companies to deliver the medications directly to the pharmacies at the points of care. CD4 counts and viral load for treatment monitoring were available and paid for by central funds. Tests were performed in a few sites, mainly around the metropolitan region. Due to the reluctance of many hospitals to take care of HIV-infected patients for fear that associated higher costs would put further pressure on scarce resources, the central health authority decided to grant additional funds for drugs used to treat 'opportunistic' conditions, thus relieving the reluctance to accept patients with HIV(Figure 7.2). Over the next few years, this additional budget allocation would switch from mainly antimicrobials (antifungal, antiprotozoan and antiviral drugs) to more drugs for the metabolic complications of HAART and chemotherapy. With few adjustments, this would be the way the programme would function over the next five years.

New, comprehensive and updated guidelines, written by a group of local experts under the sponsorship of CONASIDA, were issued in 2001 [10]. Although the budget for HIV prevention and care had increased fourfold in the public health system in five years, and 10-fold for antiretroviral drugs, there was still a gap, and therapies only met 80% of need. A grant from the Global Fund to fight AIDS, Tuberculosis and Malaria (Global Fund) closed that 20% gap by mid-2003. The US$35 million, five-year grant was mainly for treatment (~ 55%) and prevention (~ 37%), but also contributed to many other important advances in the quality of the programme and its evaluation as well as support to social organizations. By 2003, the country could say it had total, free access to modern therapy in the public health system, with roughly 4500 patients receiving HAART. Proper monitoring with CD4 counts and viral load determinations was in unrestricted operation, and genotyping was available, though with restrictions. Funding for HAART, treatment monitoring, and therapy for a number of complications associated with HIV disease or its treatment was provided by the central government, thus avoiding the

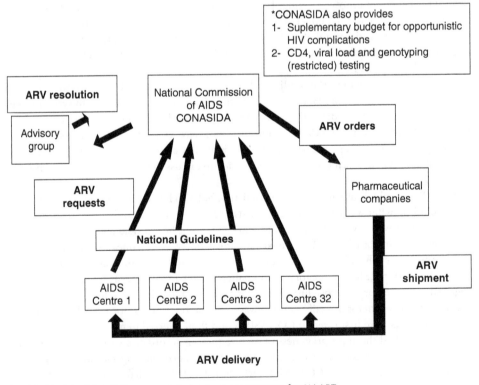

Fig. 7.2 Model of the Chilean expanded access programme for HAART.

Source: [13], with permission of the editors.

overburdening of already strained local health budgets, although each health area had to take care of all other costs, including the salaries of healthcare workers involved in the programme.

The 2001 guidelines allowed physicians to freely choose among several different pharmacologically sound regimens made up from 10 different antiretroviral drugs. Most were ZDV and 3TC in the form of the fixed-dose combination Combivir® plus NVP, indinavir (IDV), or efavirenz (EFV). The guidelines followed the usual standard recommendations for therapy indication: all symptomatic patients (except those with some CDC B symptoms or pulmonary tuberculosis (TB), where it was not considered mandatory) and asymptomatic patients with CD4 counts < 200 cells/mm³, or between 200 to 350 cells/mm3 if the viral load was high, had access to therapy. The programme became complex, involving centres all over the country with several thousand patients in treatment and directed centrally from CONASIDA, which maintained administrative, regulatory and operational roles. The health authority kept good records of the number of therapies, regimen distribution, and quantity of CD4 counts, viral load, and genotype determination performed, but had little information about the impact of the programme on morbidity and mortality. It relied on global figures, which began to show a decrease in the number of AIDS cases reported (but not in non-AIDS cases) and a stabilization in the previously increasing mortality rate. There was also virtually no information about more refined parameters such as viral response, immune recuperation, or even the total number of patients under care, including those not yet needing HAART.

A new development, again driven by CIDS' AIDS commission, would deal successfully with that need: the creation of a network of AIDS care centres in the public health system in order to standardize patient care, establish a forum to discuss common topics and needs, and follow patients in a systematic way in order to evaluate results and generate its own data with which to tailor the programme. This group was organized by physicians and other health professionals from 29 of the 32 centres and included 98% of all adult patients receiving HAART in the public health system. It was called the Chilean AIDS Group, and all participating patients approved by CONASIDA for HAART after 2001 became the Chilean AIDS Cohort (ChiAC). A proposal for funding was accepted by the Global Fund, and the project had the main goal of evaluating the impact of the Expanded Access Programme to HAART. The grant allowed the development of cohort headquarters at the Arriarán Foundation and the hiring of full-time personnel, including a nurse, a secretary and a computer supervisor; two part-time physicians were also part of the staff. ChiAC was chaired by two coordinators and had a board of directors with representatives from the major regions in the country [11].

ChiAC began enrolling patients retrospectively from 2001, when the EAP was launched, and prospectively from 2003, when the cohort began receiving funds. Protocol forms for standardized intake and follow-up were created and distributed to the centres using the same public health system network. Information was exchanged by fax or Internet. A web page was created that maintained updated information about the cohort and uploaded relevant information and links, including scientific presentations and publications derived from cohort evaluation.

After 17 years of authoritarian rule, the country's third democratic government, by then in its third year in office, began implementing what would be one of its main priorities, health reform. This wide-ranging reform of the whole healthcare system, applied first in the public health system, established that, for certain pathologies, there would be legal guarantees of proper and timely care and that health institutions, and even healthcare professionals, would be held accountable for not delivering legally guaranteed services. The list of pathologies considered either epidemiologically or strategically important began with 14 diseases, to which others were gradually added to reach a total of 54 in 2006, and with the aim of reaching 80 by 2010. HIV infection was on the list from the beginning.

In the case of HIV infection, HAART was guaranteed for children and adults who required it according to the guidelines, plus a less well-defined 'antiretroviral therapy' for pregnant women aimed at preventing vertical transmission irrespective of whether they needed it for themselves. Treatment monitoring with CD4 count, viral load and genotyping was now legally assured and no longer depended on temporary availability [12]. Between 2004 and mid-2005, this updated programme was implemented in the public health system, following which new therapeutic guidelines came into effect. These 2005 guidelines [13] contained important changes relative to those established in 2001, incorporating newer drugs (tenofovir (TDF) and atazanavir (ATV)) and withdrawing certain other drugs (stavudine (d4T) and IDV) from first-line therapy, except in special circumstances. Most importantly, information gathered by ChiAC was used to issue new national recommendations. The guidelines created the category of 'early initiation' for those with baseline CD4 counts below 100 cells/mm3 or pregnancy beyond the sixteenth week, and 'early change' for those who experienced severe toxicity to an antiretroviral regimen. For these categories, the health reform set a period of one week from drug request to drug delivery to the patient, as compared with the time frame of 37 days for all other conditions. In order to implement these changes, and especially to abide by the time frame now imposed, the number of first-line regimens was restricted, and physicians were no longer free to use whatever regimen they considered appropriate. The indications for antiretroviral therapy initiation, first-line therapeutic regimens and modifications required by initial contraindication or early toxicity to any of its components are shown in Table 7.1.

A distinct recommendation was not to initiate therapy in any asymptomatic patient with a baseline CD4 count above 250 cells/mm3, regardless of viral load. This particular point was

Table 7.1 National guidelines for antiretroviral therapy in adults under the health reform legislation supporting universal access to HIV treatment, Chile, 2005.

Indications for antiretroviral therapy:

a) All CDC C conditions (AIDS-defining events), except pulmonary tuberculosis;
b) Asymptomatic patients with CD4 <200/mm^3;
c) Patients with CD4 >200 and <250/mm^3 if:
 - Symptoms CDC B as: oropharyngeal candidiasis, weight loss, chronic diarrhoea and prolonged fever
 - CD4 decline >20 cells per month
 - Viral load >100.000 copies/mL

Time frame for initiation:

If CD4 is <100/mm^3, legal guarantee is treatment initiation within one week of request; if higher, within 37 days.

First-line therapy for first therapy:

Zidovudine plus lamivudine plus efavirenz;
If zidovudine contraindicated, replace by didanoside;
If efavirenz contraindicated, replaced by nevirapine;
If severe Kaposi's sarcoma present, replace efavirenz or nevirapine by lopinavir/ritonavir.

Early change due to toxicity:

Replace zidovudine by abacavir if anaemia develops;
Replace efavirenz by nevirapine if neuropsychiatric symptoms develop;
Replace nevirapine or efavirenz by lopinavir/ritonavir or atazanavir if severe cutaneous allergy develops.

Source: [13] (summarized).

supported by results from ChiAC (see below). Other drugs within the formulary became available under special circumstances, mainly previous therapeutic failures. Second-line regimens were not specified, since they became dependant on genotype results; this test remained restricted due to its high cost (US$400) and technical difficulties, but its indication was moved from second to first virologic failure and was not authorized for patients without therapeutic experience.

There were also guidelines for antiretroviral therapy in pregnant women with the aim of preventing vertical transmission. A previous controversy over the potency of the regimens to be used in this situation (HAART or weaker therapies) was resolved, and only HAART was recommended, even in women without need of therapy for themselves. The regimen of choice was Combivir® plus nelfinavir (NFV), with similar precautions to those of the general guidelines, but NVP use was discouraged and EFV was contraindicated.

The guidelines included recommendations for the treatment of children, which basically supported therapy in all infants under one year of age, and between one and three years of age if symptomatic with immune deterioration or with a high viral load; after that age, the adult recommendation applied. While the same regimens as in adults were recommended, there was insufficient experience with TDF and ATV at that time to recommend its use in paediatric patients.

Therapy for non-pregnant women was considered a lifelong commitment with existing drugs, with no place for programmed interruption except for temporary discontinuations due to drug toxicities, harmful interactions, or occurrence of opportunistic infections (OIs) preventing concomitant antiretroviral therapy due to immune reconstitution manifestations (e.g. TB). No blood drug level monitoring has been part of the programme.

These guidelines were part of a larger regulatory document by the MOH called the *Model for Comprehensive Care of HIV Disease*. The other important components of this recommendation, soon to be mandatory for all public health institutions, were standards for infrastructure and equipment in the public health system's AIDS care centres, as well as for the number and training of the healthcare personnel manning these centres. For the first time, institutions were mandated to have a certain level of infrastructure, equipment, and a certain number of qualified personnel according to the number of patients under care in each centre, and were no longer dependent on the willingness of each local authority to commit resources for HIV. It also stipulated that patients should be seen a minimum of four times a year.

With regard to manpower, the standard explicitly established that a centre should have 1.5 physician hours per week for every 24 patients under care, one full-time (44 hours/week) registered nurse or obstetric nurse (midwife) for every 250 patients, one half-time (22 hours/week) pharmacist and pharmacist's assistant for every 400 patients, and four hours/week of psychologist time and two hours/week of social worker time for every 100 patients (Table 7.2). Other professionals or specialists were mentioned, but not quantified in this precise way. Nevertheless, most centres were heavily understaffed by these standards. A centre like the Arriarán Foundation, with 1500 patients, should have had at least two full-time physicians or its equivalent in physician time, six full-time nurses or midwives, one full-time psychologist, one part-time social worker, and 1.5 pharmacists and pharmacist's assistants. The institution had the proper number of physicians but was short of nurses/midwives and had no pharmacist or pharmacist's assistant.

In 2005, ChiAC was recognized as a major player in the fight against AIDS in the country and obtained another grant to supplement its budget, this time through the recently created National Fund for Research in Health, a government-sponsored competitive programme to develop operational research on important clinical or epidemiological topics. With this grant, plus an expanded budget approved by the Global Fund, additional manpower was added to the ChiAC.

Table 7.2 Professional personnel requirements for AIDS care centres in the public health system recommended by the Chilean Ministry of Health within the framework of the 2005 health reform legislation.

Professional	Number of hours per week/ 100 patients	Number of patients under care required for full time position (44 hrs/week)
Physician	6.25	700
Registered nurse/ Midwife nurse	18	250
Psychologist	4	1,100
Social worker	2	2,200
Pharmacist	11	400
Pharmacist assistant	11	400

Notes: Requirement for other personnel stated but not quantified. Requirements will be mandatory within 2–3 years.

Source: [13] (summarized).

ChiAC's goal was now expanded to become a representative cohort for other countries with similar economic and epidemiological circumstances, and committed to providing the best and most accessible treatment possible for their HIV-infected population. Such countries, easily identified in Latin America, Eastern Europe and some parts of Asia, might not feel that the experiences of highly industrialized countries with universal access to therapy, or of truly underdeveloped countries with much larger rates of infection but dependent on foreign aid to undertake the task of treating their population, are applicable to their circumstances.

In mid-2005, another milestone in Chile's healthcare occurred: health reform was now applicable not only to the public health system, but also to the private health sector, which was responsible for the healthcare of close to 20% of the population. Only armed forces personnel and their dependents (5% of the population) were excluded from this reform, but generally their health system provided full coverage for most diseases. Most important was the fact that private health insurers, called *ISAPRES*, would have to provide medications for patients with the pathologies included in the reform, and with the same guarantees as in the public system. Therefore, in the case of PLWHA, they had to provide the same drugs and the same monitoring as the public formulary, all with a co-payment that could be no higher than 20% of the cost of the drugs or tests. For a first-line regimen, this co-payment was usually about US$50 a month, which was quite affordable for people who were, for the most part, actively employed. *ISAPRES* used a small, flat surcharge in the monthly dues of all enrollees to finance the whole programme, which included many other common diseases, such as diabetes, hypertension, renal insufficiency, cervical carcinoma and myocardial infarction. With this new step, the situation changed from expanded access with 100% coverage in the public health system to universal access for all. It also virtually stopped the migration of HIV-infected people from the private system to the public system and, as an added benefit, contributed markedly to putting the black market in antiretroviral drugs to an end.

The next important step was to make the offer of HIV testing mandatory for all pregnant women; those found positive would have the benefits of therapy to prevent vertical transmission.

By the end of 2003, ChiAC had enrolled around 3000 patients, and by mid-2004 this number had risen to 4365, including more than 98% of all patients receiving HAART in the public health system. Information from that population showed that 83.4% were male, the mean age was 38.3 years, 94% had acquired the infection through sexual contacts, and most cases were seen in men who have sex with men (MSM). Injecting drug use accounted for less than 3% of infections, and blood transfusion less than 1%; 58% of patients were treatment-naïve when enrolled in the EAP, 47.5% had clinical AIDS, and only 26% were asymptomatic; 80% had pre-therapy CD4 counts below 200 cells/mm3 (51.2% below 100 cells/mm3). Combivir® plus EFV was the most common regimen used, and IDV use rapidly declined [11] (Table 7.3).

Results from ChiAC's database, unpublished at the time of writing, showed the estimated cost of a first-line therapy at US$2,034 per year, and a second-line therapy (often including a ritonavir (RTV)-boosted protease inhibitor (PI)) at US$5,000 per year.

ChiAC prioritized the follow-up of treatment-naïve patients (n=2479) with their first regimen. Close to 50% of patients who initiated HAART had an AIDS-defining event. The most common were *Pneumocystis carinii* pneumonia (PCP), oesophageal candidiasis, wasting disease, TB, and various neurological conditions, in that order. Tuberculosis was seen in 10–12% of patients. After a median follow-up of 2.4 years, mortality for the whole cohort was 8.5%, with a similar percentage lost to follow-up. Actuarial survival was 92% at 1600 days; 80% of the population with that follow-up period had undetectable virus. There was a marked difference in

Table 7.3 Baseline characteristics of the Chilean AIDS Cohort (ChiAC)

Percentage of patients from the EAP followed by the ChiAC*	98%
Male	83.4%
Mean age (y)	38.3
Sexual acquisition	94%
Baseline CDC classification	
A	26.2%
B	26.3%
C	47.5% (clinical AIDS)
Baseline CD4 count	
> 200 cells/mm^3	19.8%
≤ 200 cells/mm^3	80.2%
≤100 cells/mm^3	51.2%[†]
Treatment-naïve	2479 (58.2%)
ART in naïve patients	
Background dual therapy	
Zibovudine and lamivudine	2033 (84.2%)
Stavudine and lamivudine	310 (12.5%)
Others	136 (3.3%)
Third drug	
Efavirenz[‡]	703 (39.5%)
Nevirapine	532 (29.9%)
Indinavir (single and boosted)	384 (21.6%)
Others	161 (9.0%)

* Initiating therapy as of October 31, 2003.

[†] 64.4% of those initiating with CD4 counts ≤ 200 cells/mm^3.

[‡] Dating from late 2003 and 2004. Efavirenz is part of 61.5% of new therapies.

Notes: N=4.365; EAP= Expanded Access Programme to antiretroviral therapy

Source: [11].

mortality according to baseline US Centers for Disease Control and Prevention (CDC) status, from 14.9% if AIDS was present at baseline versus 1.75% if asymptomatic at baseline. Mortality was similar in those with a baseline CD4 count between 100–200 cells/mm³ and those with CD4 counts above 200 cells/mm³ (3.5% and 3.1%, respectively), but three times higher if the baseline CD4 count was below 100 cells/mm³, and almost five times if below 50 cells/mm³ (Figure 7.3) [ChiAC database, unpublished results].

A cross-sectional study in the largest national centre, using both treatment-naïve and experienced patients with more than three months of HAART, showed that 75% had no virus detected at last count. CD4 counts had increased from a median of 151 cells/mm³ at baseline to 331 cells/mm³ at last count, with four times fewer patients in the CD4 range below 200 cells/mm³ (71% versus 18.6%) [5]. Annual mortality was at its historically lowest level of 1.2% (Figure 7.4).

At the national level, the immune recovery of the ChiAC population was seen at three ranges of baseline CD4 count: below 100, between 100 and 200, and above 200 cells/mm³, with a median of 278 cells/mm³ at three years for the group with the lowest baseline CD4 count [14]. In the national cohort, most deaths (55%) occurred in the first six months of HAART, before the therapy could exert its effect in this population which, for the most part, had begun therapy with advanced disease; only 22% of deaths occurred after the first year of treatment. A significant drop in the rate of OIs and Kaposi's sarcoma (KS) was seen in the ChiAC population, and a sub-study in one centre showed a similar drop in hospitalization over time. National statistics showed a reduction in the incidence of reported cases of AIDS despite the continuing upward trend in HIV cases not meeting the criteria for AIDS, and also, for the first time, a decrease in mortality rate due to AIDS. ChiAC also studied the pattern of toxicity of antiretroviral drugs: 26.6 % of patients required a change of their initial therapy due to toxicity, which occurred mostly (60%) in the first six months of HAART. Predominant toxicity was haematological (anaemia), consistent with the predominant use of Combivir®; 7% of patients receiving this combination required discontinuation due to anaemia, 9% discontinued NVP due to rash, and less than 1% discontinued EFV due

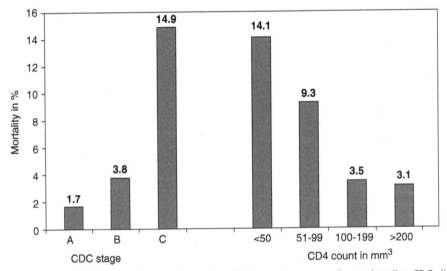

Fig. 7.3 Mortality in patients without prior antiretroviral experience according to baseline CDC clinical stage and baseline CD4 count. Median follow up time of 2.4 years; n=2479.

Source: chiAC database, unpublished results.

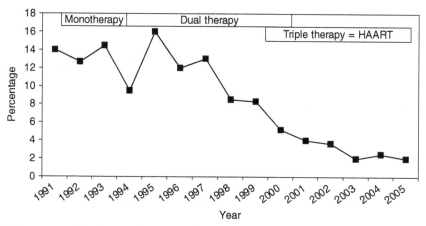

Fig. 7.4 Percentage of patients under care at the Arriarán Foundation dying annually and available type of therapy at each period, 1991–2005.

Source: [5], translated from Spanish and reproduced with permission of the editors.

to neurological toxicity [14]. The probability of remaining on the same initial regimen was 50% at five years.

Regarding co-morbidity, 8.5% of patients had positive serology for surface antigen for hepatitis B (the test had been done in more than 80% of the population); in a smaller set of patients, overrepresented by injecting drug users in whom hepatitis C serology was performed, 7.8% of cases were found to be positive. A positive Venereal Disease Research Laboratory (VDRL) test at some point during the follow-up was present in 18.5% of cases, and toxoplasma serology was positive in 36%. Tuberculin tests were reactive in 5% of cases. A survey of a representative sample of patients with the median follow-up of 2.4 years showed that 80% perceived themselves to be in good health, compared with 43% at baseline. Unemployment was reduced from 27.7% at baseline to 19.6% at the end of the follow-up period [ChIAC, unpublished data].

Genotype testing has been performed in a small number of untreated patients as a sentinel study; although mutations were present in 10 of the 60 samples, none showed high-level resistance to any of the three families of antiretroviral drugs [15]. Another study from the same group, evaluating specimens from 349 patients countrywide who failed therapy, showed that there were mutations of significant resistance in 73.3% for nucleoside transcriptase inhibitors, in 60% for non-nucleoside inhibitors, and in 22% for PIs, but less than 1% had resistance to all three groups [16]. Interestingly, 17% resistance to TDF was also found, although that drug had not been used in the country at that time [17].

In mid-2006, another survey done by ChiAC in the 32 public health system AIDS treatment centres across the country showed there to be 9635 adult patients under care, 60% of whom were in the metropolitan region. 6782 (70%) were under treatment, and 30% did not yet meet the requirements for treatment according to the latest national recommendations, but there was variable proportion of treatment/no treatment groups in the centres, with a higher percentage of treatment in larger centres located in major cities. There was a sufficient number of physicians staffing the centres (n=73), but they were unevenly distributed, with 16 centres understaffed. The most important conclusion was a continuing deficit of nurses/midwives, pharmacists and mental health professionals [ChiAC, unpublished data].

Also by mid-2006, there were around 600 privately insured patients receiving therapy under the health reform guarantees, with dozens enrolling in the programme each month. The national paediatric committee on AIDS reported that 253 HIV-infected children had been reported since 1987, of whom 25% had died, and all survivors requiring therapy (160/192) were receiving it, with similar regimens to that of adults. Almost all cases were cared for in the public health system, and the first cases of former paediatric patients being handed over to adult specialists were occurring. The rate of mother-to-child transmission under the present guidelines has been 2% since they were implemented.

Conclusion

Chile has changed considerably over the last decade. It now has a solid democracy and has experienced unprecedented economic growth. In terms of antiretroviral therapy, it has progressed from half-hearted to full commitment to the care of its PLWHA. Expanded access to antiretroviral therapy, health reform, availability of HAART and the development of the Chilean AIDS Cohort have played a synergistic role in making universal access to very effective HIV therapy a reality. All this suggests that Chile's current high ranking in human development may be well-deserved.

Acknowledgement

The author wishes to thank Donald B Louria for reviewing the manuscript and for his useful comments and suggestions and friendly editing.

References

1. Wolff M, Northland R, Segovia J, *et al.* (1995). Características clínicas e historia natural de la infección por Virus de Inmunodeficiencia Humana. *Rev Méd Chile* **123**:61–73.
2. Central Bank of Chile. (2006). *Economic indicators, second trimester 2006.* Santiago: Central Bank of Chile.
3. Government of Chile, Ministry of Health. (2005). *National Commission on AIDS. Epidemiological situation of HIV/AIDS 1984–2004.* Santiago: Chilean Ministry of Health.
4. Government of Chile, Ministry of Health. (2005). *National Commission on AIDS. Interim report of Epidemiologic situation of HIV/AIDS.* Santiago: Chilean Ministry of Health.
5. Wolff M, Alvarez P, Flores I, *et al.* (2006). Evolución de mortalidad y estado actual de una población infectada por VIH controlada en un centro multiprofesional. *Rev Méd Chile* **134**:581–588.
6. Wolff M, Diomedi A, Dabanch J, *et al.* (2001). Seguimiento prospectivo de una población infectada por VIH con y sin posibilidades de terapia antiretroviral: impacto en sobrevida y complicaciones (EFITAR). *Rev Méd Chile* **129**:886–94.
7. Wolff M, Northland R, Diomedi A, *et al.* (2001). Prospective follow-up of a cohort of HIV patients with and without access to antiretroviral therapy. Survival and complications. 8th Conference on Retrovirus and Opportunistic Infections (CROI), Chicago, USA, 4–8 February 2001. [Abstract 489]
8. Sociedad Chilena de Infectología, Comité Consultivo de SIDA, Wolff M, coordinador. (1998). Terapia anti retroviral. *Rev Méd Chile* **126**:577–81.
9. Montaner JS, Hogg RS, Weber AE, Anis AH, O'Shaughnessy MW, Schechter MT. (1998). The costs of triple-drug anti-HIV therapy for adults in the Americas. *JAMA* **279**:1263–4.
10. Government of Chile, Ministry of Health. (2001). *National Commission on AIDS. Clinical guideline. Acquired Immunodeficiency Syndrome. HIV/AIDS 2001.* Santiago: Chilean Ministry of Health.
11. Wolff M, Beltrán C, Vásquez P, *et al*, for the Chilean AIDS Group. (2005). The Chilean AIDS Cohort. A model for evaluating the impact of an expanded access programme to antiretroviral therapy in a middle-income country: Organization and preliminary results. *J Acquired Immune Defic Syndr* **40**:551.

12. Government of Chile. (2004). *Law 19,966. General regimen in guarantees in health.* Santiago: Government of Chile.

13. Government of Chile, Ministry of Health. (2005). *National Commission on AIDS. Clinical guideline. Acquired Immunodeficiency Syndrome. HIV/AIDS 2005.* Santiago: Government of Chile.

14. Arancibia J, Gallardo D, Beltrán C, Wolff M, Morales O. (2006). Grupo SIDA Chile. Evaluación de recuperación inmunológica en pacientes bajo terapia antiretroviral (TARV) pertenecientes a la Cohorte Chilena de SIDA. XXIII Congress of the Chilean Infectious Disease Society, Viña del Mar, 8–10 November 2006. [Abstract CO-43]

15. Afani A, Ayala M, Meyer A, Cabrera R, Acevedo W. (2005). Resistencia primaria a terapia antirretroviral en pacientes con infección por VIH/SIDA en Chile. *Rev Méd Chile* **133:**295–301.

16. Afani A, Beltrán C, Orellana L, Duarte P, Acevedo W, Vásquez P. (2005). Resistance to antiretroviral therapy in patients with HIV-1 infection in Chile, 2002–2004. 10th European AIDS Conference/EACS, Dublin, Ireland, 2005. [Abstract: A-007–0017–00093]

17. Afani A, Beltrán C, Orellana L, Duarte P, Acevedo W, the Chilean AIDS Group. (2006). Patterns of Resistance to tenofovir in Chilean patients infected by HIV-1. 4th Workshop on HIV Resistance, 29 March – 2 April 2006, Montecarlo, Monaco. [Abstract 48]

Chapter 8

Country review: Germany

Eva Wolf* and Hans Jaeger

Epidemiology

Prevalence and incidence of HIV infection

The HIV epidemic varies considerably between continents and countries. Compared with other European countries or with the situation worldwide, HIV prevalence and incidence in Germany have remained relatively modest during the last decade. By the end of 2006, 56,000 HIV-infected people were living in Germany, of whom 15% were female and 0.7 % were children. This reflects a prevalence of 0.07 % compared with an overall prevalence of 0.3% in Western and Central Europe. Estimated HIV incidence in Germany is approximately 3 per 100,000 inhabitants [1,2]. Epidemiological data are provided and regularly updated by the Robert Koch Institute (RKI). The RKI is the German government's central institute for surveillance and prevention of diseases, with a major focus on their epidemiological aspects and the development of corresponding public health strategies. Table 8.1 shows the RKI's most recent overview of the epidemic's scope in Germany.

HIV prevention can be considered one of the first nationwide implementations of public health policy in Germany. Since the mid-1980s, there has been a close collaboration between several federal agencies, such as the Federal Centre for Health Education, which was responsible for the national 'Don't Give AIDS a Chance' education campaign, and non-governmental organizations (NGOs) such as the *Deutsche AIDS-Stiftung* or the *Deutsche AIDS-Hilfe*, which primarily developed prevention strategies for high-risk populations like men who have sex with men (MSM). Although injecting drug use (IDU) has played a major role in the spread of HIV in several European countries—notably in France, Italy, Portugal, and Spain—most HIV infections in Germany are attributable to unsafe sex. The striking geographical differences in the IDU-associated epidemics may reflect drug use behaviour, the time of introduction of HIV, and prevention measures whose relative contributions to the spread of HIV are difficult to quantify [3].

The first AIDS cases were reported in Germany in 1982 [4]. As a consequence, a nationwide anonymous AIDS registry was established by the RKI, and this registry provided the basis for estimating the spread of HIV/AIDS in Germany. In the same year, *Der Spiegel* was the first German news magazine to report on a mysterious disease that was affecting homosexuals an ocean away in the United States [5]. One year later, approximately 100 similar suspicious cases and several deaths were noted in Germany. The *Deutsches Ärzteblatt*, Germany's equivalent to the *Journal of the American Medical Association (JAMA)*, carried the first comprehensive article on AIDS in 1983 [6].

Since 1987, laboratories have had to report all confirmed positive test results to the RKI. In 1993, the laboratory reports were supplemented by voluntary information from the treating physician, whether the respective positive tests results were from newly diagnosed HIV patients

* Corresponding author.

Table 8.1 Estimated prevalence and incidence of HIV infection in Germany

People living with HIV/AIDS in 2006	~56 000
Males	~47 000
Females	~8 500
Children	~300–500
People living with AIDS	~8 700
Modes of HIV transmission	
Homosexual contacts (MSM)	~34 000
Heterosexual contacts	~6 500
People from high prevalence countries (mostly infected by heterosexual contacts)	~7 500
Injection drug use	~6 500
Haemophiliacs infected by contaminated blood products	~550
Mother-to-child transmission	~300–500
New HIV infections in 2006	~2 700
Males	~2 200
Females	~500
Children	~20
Modes of HIV transmission in 2006 (estimates)	
Homosexual contacts (MSM)	70%
Heterosexual contacts	20%
Injection drug use	9%
Mother-to-child transmission	1%
New AIDS cases in 2006	~1 200
Males	~975
Females	~225
Children	~5
Deaths among HIV/AIDS patients in 2006	~600
Overall number of HIV infections since the beginning of the epidemic	~82 000
AIDS cases since the beginning of the epidemic	~32 500
Males	~28 100
Females	~4 400
Children	~200
Overall number of deaths since the beginning of the epidemic	~26 000

Source: Robert Koch Institute, 2006

or there had been preceding positive HIV test results. Since 2001, notifications have included demographic information as well as clinical characteristics of the patients.

HIV surveillance and prevention efforts were improved by instituting the testing of all newborns in several German regions and reporting positive screening test results from blood donors. HIV antibody screening of blood donations has been obligatory since 1985. Prior to transfusion of fresh plasma, the donor is required to be tested twice at an interval of four months. A special sentinel programme on new HIV infections and other sexually transmitted diseases (STDs) was set up by the RKI in 2002. Since then, a representative subset of HIV-specialized private practices and ambulances, as well as HIV and STD outreach clinics, must report all incident STDs.

HIV incidence reached its peak level at the beginning of the epidemic, with more than 7000 estimated new infections in 1983. In the late 1980s and early 1990s, the HIV infection rate stabilized at about 2000 new infections per year and decreased even further in the late 1990s and the beginning of the new century, with fewer than 1500 new cases in 2001. However, since 2002, HIV incidence is once again increasing, with 2600 and 2700 new infections in 2005 and 2006, respectively. A major increase (about 50%) was particularly noted in MSM. The majority of MSM with newly diagnosed HIV infection in 2006 were aged between 30 and 39 years.

These results correspond to two consecutive, nationwide German cohort studies (Prime-DAG and Ac-DAG) of people diagnosed with primary HIV infection between July 2001 and May 2004 [7]. These cohorts were initiated by the *Deutsche Arbeitsgemeinschaft niedergelassener Ärzte in der Versorgung HIV-Infizierter e.V.* (DAGNAE), the German network of physicians providing HIV treatment in private practice, in order to increase physicians' awareness concerning acute HIV infection and investigate treatment strategies and outcomes. Two hundred cases (191 males, nine females) in 35 private clinics and seven hospital outpatient departments have been reported, with the main risks for transmission being homosexual (83%) and heterosexual (8%) contact. The mean age at presentation was 35 years (range 18–62 years) [2].

The rate of injecting drug use as mode of infection decreased from >10–15 % to <5 % between 1995 and 2001, followed by a slight increase in the past few years. Along with this increase, a rise in the proportion of newly HIV-infected injection drug users (IDUs) coming from Eastern Europe was observed. Between 15% and 20% of patients who are newly diagnosed with HIV infection come from high-prevalence countries.

AIDS cases and deaths

The number of German patients diagnosed with AIDS since the beginning of the epidemic is currently estimated at 32,500. Some 26,000 HIV-infected people have died since then—one-third of the overall number of HIV infections since the beginning of the epidemic. The highest death rate occurred in 1994, with about 2000 deaths in that year [2].

Currently, approximately 15% of the people living with HIV/AIDS (PLWHA) are classified as Stage 4 under the World Health Organization (WHO) clinical staging case definition for HIV/AIDS surveillance (n=8,700). In 2006, 1,200 new patients met the criteria for AIDS, and 600 HIV-infected people died. The average age at death was 41.2 years, in line with an increase from 40.1 years before 1990 to 42.8 years after 1996. Injection drug users and immigrants generally died at a younger age (34.4 and 35.6 years, respectively) than MSM or heterosexually infected people (42.1 and 42.5 years, respectively). Due to the increased longevity of HIV-infected patients in the past decade, the number of older PLWHA is likely to continue to increase in the coming years [8].

Primary and newly diagnosed chronic HIV infection: subtypes and prevalence of resistance in Germany

Primary drug resistance

In 1997, the RKI initiated a prospective nationwide study on HIV seroconverters. The objective was to rule out the factors associated with disease progression and to evaluate the spread of HIV-drug resistant virus. So far, resistance data on 817 seroconverters are available. Primary resistance based on the Stanford University algorithm, version 4.2.1, was observed in 14% of treatment-naïve seroconverters. Resistance to non-nucleoside reverse transcriptase inhibitors (NNRTIs) has increased over time, while nucleoside reverse transcriptase inhibitor (NRTI) resistance has declined. The overall proportion of patients with primary resistance mutations has been relatively stable since 2001 [9].

HIV subtypes in HIV seroconverters

Between 1994 and 2003, the proportion of HIV-1 subtype B infection in seroconverters remained relatively constant at between 80% and 90%. Among non-B infections, primarily subtype A infections followed by CRF01_AE, CRF02_AG, C, G and complex recombinant forms have been observed [10].

Treatment strategies

CD4, RNA and clinical status at first treatment

Azidothymidine (AZT) monotherapy was introduced in Germany in 1986. Although, from today's perspective, this strategy was less than optimal, it saved many very sick patients a year of life and reduced the incidence of opportunistic infections (OIs) and tumours.

Of all the international AIDS conferences held since 1985, the IX International AIDS Conference held in Berlin in 1993 may have been the most disappointing. High hopes that had been set on the results of the Concorde Study, which was designed to show whether it was beneficial to begin AZT treatment before HIV symptoms appear, were shattered. There was a rare feeling of communal despair in a very heterogeneous group of scientists, comparable only to 2003, when data were reported at the 10th Conference on Retroviruses and Opportunistic Infections (CROI) by Harvard Medical School's Bruce Walker of a case of superinfection in a patient who had been treated very early when first acutely infected [11,12].

The 'Rule of 500'—500 mg of AZT for patients with CD4 counts less than 500 cells/mm^3—never gained momentum in Germany, unlike the 'Hit hard, hit early' axiom established by the Aaron Diamond AIDS Research Center's David Ho immediately prior to, and then during, the XI International AIDS Conference held in Vancouver in 1996. Most treatment decision-makers in Germany readily accepted the 'Hit hard, hit early' axiom. After a transitional period of two to three years, dual drug therapy, which was then the standard of care, gave way to triple drug therapy using the first rather toxic protease inhibitors (PIs) and the NNRTIs nevirapine (NVP), and later, efavirenz (EFV). Interestingly, both NNRTIs were widely prescribed over the years, even before the results of the 2NN study were released in 2003, the first head-to-head comparison of these two drugs. Sales curves for NVP and EFV moved in parallel over many years, with EFV always slightly higher than NVP (Personal communication with pharmaceutical companies; data from IMS Health, Frankfurt, Germany).

Since Ashley Haase's work showed that there is no 'point of no return' for immune reconstitution [13]—even completely destroyed lymph node architectures seem to recover—the criteria for initiation of HIV therapy have changed in Germany. The country's HIV treatment guidelines went from suggesting that anyone with a measurable viral load be treated, to treating patients whose viral load was more than 10,000 copies/mL. The current guidelines suggest that treatment initiation can be considered if 50,000 to 100,000 copies/mL are measured in an asymptomatic patient.

In the area of ritonavir (RTV)-boosted PIs, the rationale for an early start on highly active antiretroviral therapy (HAART) is hard to define. Randomized studies looking at late versus early therapy starts are planned but have not yet begun. The past five to ten years have seen a gradual delay in treatment initiation in Germany, reflecting the ever-evolving nature of treatment guidelines [14]. At the time of writing this chapter, most physicians in Germany tend to initiate HAART in asymptomatic patients if their CD4 count is between 200 and 250 cells/mm^3 and/or they have a viral load of 50,000 to 100,000 copies/mL. Opportunistic infections and tumours (e.g. Kaposi's sarcoma) have become a rare clinical feature, with the exception of some late-presenting patients.

Treatment guidelines

Over the last 10 years, many of the German HIV/AIDS-related guidelines have been developed in collaboration with Austrian AIDS scientists and are therefore called 'German-Austrian Guidelines' (Table 8.2). There are several joint committees established to constantly revise the guidelines, under the leadership of the *Deutsche AIDS Gesellschaft* (DAIG) and in close collaboration with other pertinent groups, including scientific medical societies, activists and physicians in private practice (DAGNAE). Besides adult and paediatric care, pregnancy issues—including discordant couples who wish to have a child—and guidelines for the management of needle-stick injuries are also considered in specific guidelines. In addition, scientists from both countries organize the biannual national conference on AIDS.

Preferred first-line antiretroviral regimen

There is no officially designated first-line antiretroviral regimen in Germany. Rather, clinical practice and guidelines allow significant latitude in choosing and initiating HAART. A backbone with two NRTIs combined with either an NNRTI (EFV or NVP) or a PI is most commonly used. Since RTV-boosted lopinavir (LPV) is the gold standard for PIs at the time of writing, the co-formulated LPV/r is the drug most often prescribed, followed in order of frequency of prescription by atazanavir (ATV), saquinavir (SQV) and fosamprenavir (fAPV). In terms of NRTI use, a clear switch has been observed from zidovudine (ZDV) plus lamuvudine (3TC) (co-formulated as the fixed-dose combination (FDC) known as Combivir®), to tenofovir (TDF) plus emcitritabine (FTC), known as the FDC Truvada®, and lately, since the availability of genetic tests for HLA B*5701, to Kivexa® as well.

Table 8.2 Guidelines for HIV/AIDS management in Germany

German/Austrian Guidelines for Different Situations in HIV/AIDS Management
Spanos A, Harrell FE Jr, Durack DT. (1989). Differential diagnosis of acute meningitis: an analysis of the predictive value of initial observations. *JAMA* **262**, 2700-7
DAIG, OEAG. (May 2004). German-Austrian Guidelines for Diagnosis and Treatment of HIV-discordant Couples who wish to have Children. *(www.daignet.de/ 17. html)*
Salzberger B, Marcus U, Vielhaber B, et al. (2005). German-Austrian Recommandations for the Antiretroviral Therapy of HIV-Infection (May 2004). *AIDS und HIV-Infektionen. ecomed. Landsberg a L.* **47**, XIV-1.9
Kuhlmann B, Liess H. (September 2004). Leitlinien der DAGNÄ zur Unterstützung der Adhärenz im Rahmen einer antiretroviralen Therapie bei HIV-Infektionen (based on the draft BHIVA/MSSVD Guidelines 2002). *(www.daignet.de/ 17. html)*
Arasteh K, Gölz J, Marcus U, Rockstroh J, Salzberger B, Vielhaber B. (Teilaktualisierung Stand Juni 2005). Deutsch-Österreichische Empfehlungen zur postexpositionellen Prophylaxe der HIV-Infektion. *(www.daignet.de/ 17. html)*
DAIG, OEAG. (2005). Deutsch-Österreichische Empfehlungen zur postexpositionellen Prophylaxe der HIV-Infektion. *HIV-Journal* **1**, 22-36
Mauss S, Behrens G, Walker UA. (2006). Appendix to the German-Austrian HIV Therapeutic Guidelines – Strategies for Treating Morphological and Metabolic Alterations under Antiretroviral Treatment. *Eur J Med Res* **11**, 47-57
DAIG, OEAG. (2006). German-Austrian Recommendations for HIV-therapy in Pregnancy and in HIV-exposed Newborn. *Eur J Med Res* **11**, 359-376

Current practices in switching to second-line therapy

The most common reason for switching from first-line antiretroviral drugs is toxicity, mainly gastrointestinal (GI), followed by allergies, hypersensitivity and psychological disturbances. Failure of a first regimen is much less common than it was years ago, when Trizivir® (a co-formulation of AZT, 3TC and abacavir (ABC)) was commonly prescribed as first-line therapy. Many treating physicians may choose a first-line antiretroviral regimen based on its therapeutic robustness with regard to the possible development of resistance and, increasingly, for reasons of ease and convenience for both patient and physician.

Once a regimen fails, genotypic resistance testing is carried out, and often plasma levels are measured to find the reasons for failure to completely suppress HIV replication. In the (infrequent) case of insufficient drug levels, possible interactions with other drugs are considered, or compliance counselling to improve adherence is introduced. Especially in the case of early resistance, a medication switch is used to prevent the development of cross-resistance. Based on the genotypic results, the regimen is chosen and discussed with the patient. Add-on drugs are used infrequently, except where viral load blips in a Trizivir® or PI monotherapy regimen may require them.

Salvage therapy options and the limited reservoir of salvage patients

Large HIV treatment units—those with several hundred patients or more—have been quick to adopt a successful enfuvirtide (ENF) strategy with their patients in salvage situations. Smaller units, however, have been slower to introduce ENF, often due more to opposition from physicians than to patients' fears. Several German centres carried out a cohort study on the use of ENF, which was recently published [15]. Unlike most other countries, randomized studies in Germany cannot be carried out with a prescribed medication—a major impediment to clinical research. In randomized studies, all drugs have to be procured by the sponsoring pharmaceutical companies. In the case of ENF, this has meant that, in most cases, observational data were used to describe outcomes [15]. The results compare well with the international T-20 versus Optimized Background Regimen Only (TORO) and post-TORO randomized data.

New compounds such as tipranavir (TPV), darunavir (DRV) and the new class of integrase inhibitors have somewhat reduced the prescription frequency of ENF. Mainly used in expanded access or research settings, these drugs have given new hope to patients and their physicians. However, it appears that at this time, the number of salvage patients in need of these new PIs or the integrase inhibitors is limited. It is unclear whether, as well tolerated as they seem, these drugs have the potential to evolve from their status as 'salvage' drugs to be licensed for earlier infections.

Structured therapy interruptions

Even before the publication of results from the Strategies for Management of Antiretroviral Therapies (SMART) study, structured therapy interruptions (STIs) were looked upon with some scepticism by many HIV specialists, activists and patients in Germany. Early studies conducted in Frankfurt and Paris seemed to indicate that there were advantages to STIs in salvage situations [16,17]. Waiting about eight weeks to introduce a new salvage regimen seemed, by reverting some of the resistant viruses back to wild-type, to at least temporarily improve results in those patients, many of whom had been prescribed more than 10 different antiretroviral drugs in their treatment history. Waiting longer than eight weeks was shown to be counterproductive, perhaps because the viruses were more robust when reversion to wild-type occurred.

The 'Berlin Patient', a gay man who was treated very early in his primary infection and then decided on his own to interrupt therapy, had undetectable infection for years despite receiving no further treatment [18]. This patient gave reason to believe that there might be some kind of auto-vaccination process through treatment interruption during acute infection. This principle, as elegant and attractive as it first appeared, is still in question. There has been no second or third 'Berlin (or Boston or New York, for that matter) Patient'.

Many patients and their physicians felt, and most still feel, that therapy interruption, even if immunologic or virologic improvements turned out to be false hopes, was still an advantage because it meant fewer drugs and lower costs, especially in developing countries. The results of the international SMART study published in 2006 put an end to such hopes, at least when a CD4 count of 350 cells/mm^3 is used as a starting point for interrupting therapy [18]. However, if a much higher CD4 count is used as a cut-off in patients who have had well-suppressed virus over time, the situation, as shown by the Italian Basta study, looks different and more promising for STIs [20].

An early German study over a two-year period showed no clinical disadvantage in HIV-infected patients who interrupted their therapy when compared with matched controls [20]. There was, however, a blunting of CD4 count increase of about 100 cells/mm^3 over the two years in patients who interrupted therapy between one and three times, compared with patients whose therapy was not interrupted. A clear advantage seemed to be the fact that the area under the curve (AUC) for blood lipids was significantly lower in those patients who interrupted their therapy compared with those who did not. The effect was even clearer than it was in other patients who received lipid-lowering drugs for antiretroviral drug- or HAART-induced elevated cholesterol, low-density lipoprotein (LDL) levels, or triglycerides. Unfortunately, the same effect was not seen in the SMART study.

Monotherapy

A few of the large HIV/AIDS units in Germany have, in a proof-of-principle manner or in prospective randomized studies, used PI and, in some cases, 3TC monotherapy in an estimated 100–200 patients nationwide. In Germany, the 3TC study was initiated by the Swiss HIV Cohort group, and results are still pending. The results for PI monotherapy—mainly LPV—were presented at the XVI International AIDS Conference in Toronto in 2006 as 'late breakers' [22–24] and received conflicting reviews depending on the eye of the beholder [17–19]. Our own group in Munich continues to collect information on monotherapy, not only for patients on LPV monotherapy, but also for those on SQV, ATV and fAPV monotherapy [25].

In collaboration with the Swiss HIV Cohort Study, data on 3TC monotherapy in patients who are resistant to most NRTIs (including 3TC), as well as to NNRTIs and/or PIs, have been collected. Some patients have now been on 3TC monotherapy without clinical events for more than one year, after stopping what was often their third- or fourth-line pre-treatment lasting several years. These experiences concur with the recently published randomized pilot study on HIV patients with a 3TC-resistant virus, in which 3TC monotherapy led to better immunologic and clinical outcomes than complete therapy interruption [26].

Effects of HAART

Effects of HAART on the incidence of AIDS and death rates

The number of deaths in HIV-infected patients fell from about 2000 in 1994 to 600–700 by 2006. There are no exact data concerning the drop in the incidence of AIDS. However, comparing the early 1990s with the era of HAART, the number of AIDS cases for which the RKI was notified has fallen by 60–80%. The most impressive reduction has been in the proportion of patients presenting with Kaposi's sarcoma as the first AIDS-defining disease. This trend had already started in the late 1980s, with a drop from 30% to less than 10% after 1995.

A rapid decline in the incidence of new cytomegalovirus (CMV) manifestations was reported from an HIV cohort in Cologne. The incidence of CMV disease has declined rapidly and significantly, from 7.34 cases per 100 patient-years in the pre-HAART era to 0.75 cases per 100 patient-years since the advent of HAART [27].

Effects of HAART on survival times after AIDS diagnosis

The RKI has collected survival data from more than 13,000 HIV-infected people. The median survival time after AIDS diagnosis in the early phase of the epidemic was between two and seven months. Probably due to the introduction of AZT and improved management of opportunistic infections, survival times increased to 11 months in 1989 and to 14–15 months in 1993–4. Due to the effects of HAART, survival times in the period 1998–2002 rose to between 24 and 28 months. Since 2003, the median survival time has been 50–60 months. It must be noted that survival times after AIDS diagnosis may be biased by the timing of HAART initiation; the effects of HAART on survival are more pronounced in patients who were still untreated at the time of their AIDS diagnosis [2].

HIV-related lymphoma

Response to HAART strongly predicted outcomes in a nationwide, multi-centre cohort of 203 HIV-infected patients with systemic AIDS-related lymphoma (ARL) who were diagnosed between 1990 and 2001. The only factors independently associated with prolonged survival were response to HAART (relative hazard (RH)=0.3) and complete remission (relative hazard=0.2). A previous diagnosis of AIDS (RH=1.9) and extranodal involvement (RH=2.8) were associated with poorer survival [28].

Immune recovery induced by HAART has also led to dramatic improvement in survival of patients with AIDS-associated primary central nervous system lymphoma (PCNSL). This was verified in a small, multi-centre retrospective cohort of 29 German HIV-infected patients presenting with PCNSL. Survival times in patients treated with HAART differed significantly from those receiving only cranial radiation or receiving neither cranial radiation nor HAART. The median Kaplan-Meier survival estimates were 1093, 132, and 33 days, respectively. In the multivariate regression model, HAART and cranial radiation were identified as independently associated with prolonged survival [29].

CMV disease

A better prognosis for patients with CMV disease was observed with the introduction of HAART in a retrospective study of a clinic cohort in Cologne, in which 127 HIV-infected patients diagnosed with CMV disease between 1993 and 1999 were analyzed. The median survival time in the pre-HAART era was 9.5 months; at four years of follow-up in the HAART era, the median survival had been not yet reached. A higher CD4 count and the initiation of a triple-drug combination after diagnosis of CMV disease were independently associated with prolonged survival [27].

Atypical mycobacteriosis

In a single-centre evaluation from January 1994 to December 1998, the half-year incidences of atypical mycobacterial disease decreased significantly, from 1.5–2% before 1996 to 0.5–0.6% in 1997, and to 0% in 1998, based on a total of 600–850 patients attending the centre in a six-month period. This trend paralleled a significant decline in the proportion of patients with a CD4 count <100 cells/mm^3, which was about one-third in 1994–5 and ≤10% in 1998. However, the incidence of infections with atypical mycobacteria was not significantly reduced in the severely immuno-suppressed patients [30].

Monitoring

The following section concerning monitoring of laboratory parameters is based on the June 2005 German-Austrian recommendations for antiretroviral treatment of HIV infection [14].

Viral load and CD4 count

The CD4 lymphocyte count and HIV RNA in plasma should be determined at the time of HIV diagnosis and thereafter at intervals of approximately two to three months. For viral load measurements, the most sensitive available test should be used (lower limit of detection 20–50 copies/mL). After initiation or a change of antiretroviral therapy, more frequent measurements may be necessary; however, it is not considered necessary to test at intervals shorter than four weeks. For a treatment-experienced patient with undetectable viral load, controls are recommended every two to three months. A decrease of less than $1 \log_{10}$ after four weeks, or a failure to drop below the detection limit within a maximum of six months, is regarded as an inadequate treatment response and should prompt re-evaluation of the therapeutic regimen. In the case of a confirmed rebound in viral load to low-positive values (≤ 1000 HIV RNA copies/mL), antiretroviral therapy should be re-evaluated and, if necessary, either intensified or changed [14].

Resistance testing

Genotypic resistance testing is recommended for therapeutic decisions after initial or multiple therapeutic failures. Resistance testing should be performed as long as therapy is ongoing. If infection by a resistant virus is suspected, genotyping is recommended before therapy is initiated. Since epidemiological studies on primary resistance in newly infected patients and in chronically HIV-infected treatment–naïve patients have shown a prevalence of ≥ 10–15%, it is considered justifiable to perform resistance testing before therapy is initiated [9,31]. In Germany, the costs of genotypic resistance tests have been covered by health insurance since April 2004.

Besides an adequate interpretation of genotypic resistance mutations, previous antiretroviral regimens should also be considered. Additional phenotypic testing is recommended in more complex salvage regimens and when newer antiretroviral agents are in use. For phenotyping, most samples are sent to the Institute for Clinical and Molecular Virology's National Reference Centre for Retroviruses at the University of Erlangen, which is involved in many research projects in the area of HIV drug resistance.

Therapeutic drug monitoring

Although the benefits of therapeutic drug monitoring (TDM) have not yet been completely assessed, measurement of plasma levels is considered helpful in certain clinical situations. TDM for NNRTIs and PIs is recommended in cases where:

- complex antiretroviral drug combinations and concomitant medications are known to, or are supposed to, interact;
- an active antiretroviral regimen is lacking in efficacy;
- there are signs of disrupted absorption;
- there are toxic effects; and
- liver function is impaired.

In general, the lowest drug level should be measured, although for evaluating toxic effects, the AUC should be considered. As a consequence of TDM, it is also recommended to adapt dosages when drug levels are inadequate or there are drug-related side effects.

To help estimate the potential for interactions, the German guidelines refer to various Internet-based databases, such as <http://www.hivdruginteractions.org> or <http://www.ifi-interaktions-hotline.de>. Drug interactions mainly involve the cytochrome p450 system and result from either enzyme inhibition or induction. Interactions of interest are the concomitant use of NNRTIs or PIs with antidepressants, lipid-lowering drugs like statins, tuberculostatics, or methadone.

Side effects

To best understand side effects, the specific situation of the patients concerned must be considered. When, for a period of about 18 months in the late 1990s, RTV was available only in liquid formulation, many more patients than expected adapted rather well. It had been predicted that taste intolerance for this product would be detrimental to its use, but this turned out not to be the case. Side effects have to be understood in their 'time capsule environment'. When, in the mid-1980s, very high doses of AZT led to severe anaemia, there were still patients benefiting from this therapy at the time, even though it was no longer tolerated a few years later. In the years when stavudine (d4T) was the prevailing antiretroviral compound in first-line therapy, there was not much attention paid to facial lipatrophy, although there was some concern about peripheral polyneuropathy. Several years later, no HIV/AIDS-treating physician in the developed world would prescribe d4T to their patients, although it remains one of the leading first-line drugs of choice in the developing world. Research in Germany and other countries shows that dose reduction of d4T preserves efficacy and markedly reduces toxicity [32]. And recent experience with ENF has again shown that the prescribing physicians' attitudes, rather than the patient's fears, seem to predict adherence and effective use [15].

When evaluating drug toxicity, PLWHA who have to take antiretroviral medication need to be understood in the context of their own treatment history. Patients on salvage treatment are more apt to go for potentially hard to tolerate drugs than are treatment-naïve patients who are still considering whether to begin treatment. Most physicians will try to choose a regimen for their patients that is both effective and relatively easy to tolerate, especially at the beginning of treatment.

The example of EFV

Although EFV is often not prescribed to women of childbearing age, patients with a history of psychological disorders seem to be rather good candidates for this NNRTI, in numbers greater than initially expected. Agitated, vivid dreams are manageable in these patients. However, based on the experience of pregnant women who first present when they are into their sixth to eighth week of pregnancy, willingness to prescribe EFV for younger females has diminished, mainly due to rare but severe possible side effects on foetal central nervous systems [33, 34].

How does the concern about side effects reflect on the prescribed first-line regimen in Germany? The NNRTI and PI 'factions' seem to be of comparable size. The 2006 results on long-term use of EFV may have increased the pro-NNRTI group to a certain degree (Figures 8.1 and 8.2) [35].

Other ARV regimens

By far the most commonly used NRTI backbone in German patients is the FDC Truvada®. The 2006 Predict study, together with the experiences of the British National Health Service in using genetic HLA B*5701 testing for exclusion of hypersensitivity candidates from abacavir (ABC) exposure, have helped to push for Kivexa® (ABC plus 3TC) as the second standard of care NRTI

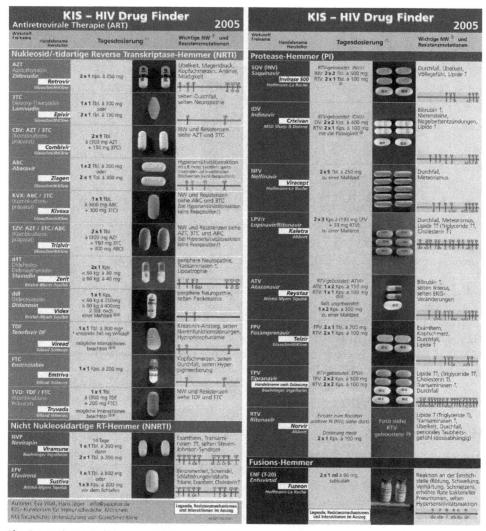

Fig. 8.1 Antiretroviral drug use in Germany, 2006.

Notes: STI=structured treatment interuption

Source: unpublished internal report of the HIV cohort of the competence network for HIV/AIDS

backbone [36]. The use of Combivir®—for many years the mainstay of NRTI treatment—is rapidly decreasing, especially in treatment-naïve patients.

The NRTIs d4T and didanosine (ddI) were very commonly used for many years, up until the late 1990s or even later. Because of facial lipoatrophy, this is no longer the case. AZT seems to be prescribed to a lesser degree nowadays, and for the same reason. For antagonistic resistance pathways, and in special cases, AZT is combined with TDF [37].

The reconstitution of subcutaneous fat is very slow after the drugs are stopped, but is nevertheless noticeable. 'Buffalo humps' and gynaecomastia are seen much less frequently than they were some five years ago. The newer RTV-boosted PIs seem to be less of a trigger for these signs of fat redistribution disorders than their older cousins. Intra- and extra-abdominal fat accumulation, though, tends to be an unwanted reality for many, if not most, patients on successful antiretroviral therapy these days. One of the first published case reports on the use of growth hormone in

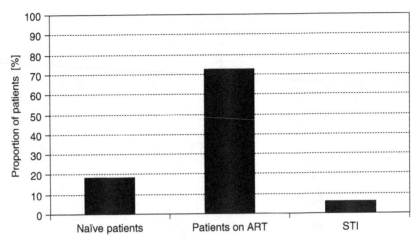

Fig. 8.2 NNRTI and PI use in Germany, 2006.

Source: Unpublished internal report of the HIV cohort of the competence network for HIV/AIDS

patients with massive intra-abdominal fat accumulation showed a clear benefit from using recombinant growth hormone in this situation [37].

A closer look at possible body changes over the years has shown that very few patients in Germany suffer from wasting syndrome, but around 15% of patients have a body mass index (BMI) of 27 or more. There are numerous limitations in the medical treatment of adipose patients. Rimonabant (Acomplia®) is licensed but not paid for by insurance in Germany. However, because of possible interactions due to common CYP 450 3A4 pathways, rimonabant is not licensed for HIV patients.

High blood lipids

The use of lipid-lowering agents in HIV-positive patients with elevated blood lipids is not very widespread in Germany so far. Some of the reasons why their use has been limited include doubts regarding the pathogenetic potential of these lipid elevations, concerns regarding interactions of lipid-lowering agents and antiretroviral drugs, and the common experience that the agreed-upon targets of lipid-lowering therapy in these patients are rarely met. Exceptions to this rule have been HIV patients suffering from coronary problems, many of whom have been treated with coated or uncoated stents. Such patients are more likely to use lipid-lowering agents as well as to comedicate with Aspirin and clopidogrel (Plavix®). When the cardiovascular risk factors of these patients are looked at, smoking seems to be more of a contributing factor than elevated blood fats [39].

Co-infection (hepatitis, tuberculosis, and malaria)

The estimated number of people with chronic hepatitis B virus (HBV) or hepatitis C virus (HCV) infections in Germany is between 400,000 and 500,000. Most cases of HCV in Germany are subtype 1. Approximately 6000 people are co-infected with HIV and HCV, and 2800 people are estimated to be co-infected with HIV and HBV [40].

HIV/HCV

There has been a bell curve in the theoretical understanding of how high CD4 cell counts need to be to effectively treat HCV co-infection. The estimate rose from 200 cells/mm^3 to about 500 cells/mm^3, and is now thought to be around 300 cells/mm^3. In any case, patients with HIV/HCV co-infection who present with very low absolute CD4 cell numbers (<200–350 cells/mm^3) will, as a rule, first be treated for their HIV infection, then for HCV.

Strategies for the treatment of hepatitis C have been modified several times over the past few years. The duration of standard treatment with pegylated interferon (PEG-IFN) alfa-2b, or PEG-IFN alfa-2a in combination with ribavirin (RBV), depends on the 12-week treatment response. If HCV RNA is not negative and has dropped by less then 2 logs, treatment should be discontinued. If HCV RNA is negative or has dropped by at least 2 logs, treatment should be continued until week 48 irrespective of genotype. Earlier recommendations to stop therapy after 24 weeks in patients with genotype 2 or 3 have been revised because of lower relapse rates with treatment durations of 48 weeks [41]. Long-term results are not as good in co-infected patients as they are in patients infected with HCV alone. Newer compounds that increase the probability of sustained virologic response are urgently needed.

It is still unclear how best to treat acute hepatitis C in HIV-infected patients. Researchers [42] at the University of Bonn suggest treating patients with asymptomatic acute hepatitis C immediately, whereas patients with symptomatic hepatitis should be followed for 12 weeks in order to await possible spontaneous clearance. Treatment is given for a period of 24 weeks with either PEG-IFN alone (for genotypes 2 and 3) or PEG-IFN plus RBV (for genotypes 1 and 4) [42]. Treatment of acute hepatitis C in HIV-infected patients has shown impressive response rates in a study coordinated at the University of Bonn. In 30 HIV-infected patients with acute HCV infection, treatment with PEG-IFN was initiated within four months of diagnosis. Treatment duration was 24 weeks, and eight patients extended treatment to 48 weeks, while treatment was discontinued early in four patients. By intention-to-treat analysis, about two-thirds of patients had sustained virologic response [43].

Around 10 patients with HIV/HCV co-infection have received liver transplants in Germany to date [44]. Their post-transplant results are comparable to those patients who received transplants with HCV monoinfection. However, post-transplant management in HIV/HCV co-infected patients is a challenge. Not only is there a need for carefully considered antiretroviral therapy, but levels of immunosuppressive drugs such as cyclosporine (Sandimmune®) as well as monitoring of renewed IFN/RBV treatment should and can be integrated. The universities of Essen and Bonn currently have the most extensive experience in Germany with regard to the new field of liver transplantation in HIV/HCV co-infected patients.

HIV/HBV

Since gay men belong to the largest risk group for HIV/AIDS in Germany, it is unsurprising that many HIV/HBV co-infections are seen. If there is HBV antigen positivity, acute active treatment is sought. The use of TDF plus 3TC or Truvada® in these patients facilitates the task of reducing HBV DNA. When Truvada® is (or has to be) stopped, the clinician should be alerted to the possibility of rare but clinically impressive flare-ups of the known hepatitis B, sometimes with deadly consequences.

Tuberculosis

Tuberculosis (TB) is rare in HIV-positive patients treated in Germany, and malaria is rarer still. Because about 15–20 % of HIV patients come from pattern II (HIV-endemic) countries, mainly sub-Saharan Africa or Thailand, the diagnosis and treatment of TB is part of the clinical patterns that patients present with. The internationally agreed-upon rules of combining antiretroviral and anti-TB drugs apply.

Healthcare delivery

The situation in Germany is different from that of many other countries insofar as about two-thirds of patients are treated and cared for on a long-term basis in private practices (*Schwerpunktpraxen*). These private practices are highly regionalized and are often, if not always, close to the patient's home. In a chronic manageable disease such as HIV, treatment within a steady physician-patient relationship—often over decades—has turned out to be very effective for clinical and cost issues. Decentralized care and responsibility for prescribing new drugs in Germany have proved beneficial for the rapid introduction of innovative technologies and new antiviral compounds. For example, the everyday use of viral load measurements has been faster in private practice than in most academic institutions (university hospitals) and public health hospitals. The fight for reimbursement of viral load measurements took about two years, during which time HIV/AIDS-treating physicians shouldered the high risk of unpaid costs (in the event that reimbursement had been decided against). This was only possible because, thanks to important AIDS conferences, knowledge of the clinical relevance of viral load monitoring permeated quickly into the treatment community.

More than 300 physicians in private practices are organized nationally within DAGNAE. This not-for-profit organization is an important national body with strong influence on shaping and establishing policy around HIV/AIDS. Constitutionally, it represents the rights of patients and collaborates with activist groups, politicians and medical, scientific and industrial structures. A second large and influential body in the field is DAIG, the German AIDS society. This society, with active input from academics, scientists and treating physicians, is responsible for discussing and deciding on HIV treatment guidelines as well as organizing the national AIDS conferences.

With support from both organizations, a national data bank, the Competence Network for HIV/AIDS, was established. It includes about 15,000 patients nationwide and is updated every six months. This database was set up after more than 18 months of intense negotiations around issues of data safety and security, and was modelled, in part, after the long-standing and very successful Swiss HIV Cohort.

Both DAGNAE and DAIG are involved in a multitude of continuing medical education (CME) activities, and HIV/AIDS-treating physicians in Germany routinely attend several educational events each month. Many also participate—often presenting their own scientific contributions—in the International AIDS Conference, the Conference on Retroviruses and Opportunistic Infections (CROI), the Interscience Conference on Antimicrobial Agents and Chemotherapy (ICAAC), or the International AIDS Society (IAS) conferences, in addition to other international, national and regional meetings.

Economics

In Germany, there are two different kinds of health insurance systems: statutory health insurance and private health insurance. Since health insurance is mandatory under federal law for all employees with an annual gross salary below €47,700 (US$74,310) (the limit for the year 2007), about 90% of Germans are covered by statutory health insurance. The monthly contribution to health insurance is about 15% of gross monthly income, with employees and employers each paying half of the contributions. Employees with an annual gross salary higher than the above-noted limit, as well as the self-employed, can choose between the two types of insurance. Less than 2% of the German population lacks health insurance coverage.

For most HIV-positive patients in Germany, healthcare costs (i.e. expenditures for antiretroviral therapy, diagnostics, or hospitalization) are covered by the state health insurance. There are scarcely any data on direct and indirect costs of care for HIV-infected patients living in Germany. In 2006, DAGNAE initiated an 18-month cohort study collecting pharmacoeconomic data on PLWHA nationwide. In order to obtain a good overview of the broad range of HIV care costs, private practices as well as hospitals and other outpatient care facilities are participating in this study.

In Germany, annual direct treatment costs are estimated to be as high as €20,000–30,000 (US$31,157–46,736) per case. Pharmacoeconomic and clinical data on 201 HIV-infected patients were collected in a single-centre study during the years 1997, 2000 and 2001 [45]. In this evaluation, the mean annual direct costs for antiretroviral drugs ranged between €17,746 (US$27,646) and €16,007 (US$24,937) per patient. Declining costs for additional drugs and hospitalization led to a decrease of about one third of the mean total direct cost, from €35,865 (US$55,873) in 1997 to €24,482 (US$38,140) in 2001. In 2001, two-thirds of all direct costs were attributed to HAART. Higher costs for patients in advanced stages of disease were common during the follow-up period.

Conclusion

By the end of 2006, 56,000 HIV-infected people were living in Germany, and the annual incidence of new HIV infections was approximately 2600. Almost half of the HIV-infected population of Germany is currently receiving HAART (as estimated by pharmaceutical companies based on their sales data). Most HIV-infected patients are treated and cared for in private practices and other outpatient care facilities. For about 90% of PLWHA, healthcare costs are covered by the state health insurance programme.

Most HIV/AIDS-treating physicians in Germany initiate antiretroviral treatment mainly based on clinical symptoms and/or a low CD4 count of 200–250 cells/mm^3. Viral load is only a secondary criterion for starting treatment. The proportion of patients in a deep salvage situation is ≤5%, and most of these patients had already started treatment in the pre-HAART era.

With the advent of the nationwide cohort study of the Competence Network for HIV/AIDS, it is hoped that a deeper collaboration with other European and international cohorts will be established.

References

1. UNAIDS/WHO. (2006). *AIDS epidemic update: December 2006*. Geneva: UNAIDS. Available at http://data.unaids.org/pub/EpiReport/2006/2006_EpiUpdate_en.pdf

2. Marcus U, Starker A. (2006). HIV und AIDS. In: Robert Koch Institut, ed. *Gesundheitsberichterstattung des Bundes*. Vol. 31. Berlin: Oktoberdruck.

3. Hamers FF, Batter V, Downs AM, Alix J, Cazein F, Brunet JB. (1997). The HIV epidemic associated with injecting drug use in Europe: geographic and time trends. *AIDS* 11:1365–74.

4. Deutsche AIDS-Stiftung. (2006). Ein trauriges Jubiläum – Rückblick auf 25 Jahre AIDS. *Stiftungkonkret* 2: 4–5.

5. *Der Spiegel*. (1982). Schreck von drüben. *Der Spiegel* 22: 187–188, May 31, 1982.

6. Jaeger H. (1983). Das Acquired Immune Deficiency Syndrome. Epidemiologie, Diagnose, Klinik, Therapie. *Deutsches Ärzteblatt* 26: 23–32.

7. Koegl C, Wolf E, Jessen H, *et al*. (2007). No Benefit from Early Treatment in Primary HIV-Infection? 14th Conference on Retroviruses and Opportunistic Infections, 25–28 February 2007, Los Angeles, USA. [Abstract 125 LB]

8. Mueck D, Balogh A-M, Wolf E, Koegl C, Jaegel-Guedes E, Jaeger H. (2007). Berufstätigkeit und Bildungsniveau bei HIV-infizierten Frauen und Männern in Deutschland. 3rd German-Austrian AIDS Conference, Frankfurt, Germany. [Abstract A.45]

9. Kuecherer C, Poggensee C, Korn K, *et al.* (2006). High level of resistant HIV-1 in newly diagnosed patients both with documented seroconversion and with unknown date of infection. 4th European HIV Drug resistance Workshop 2006, Monte Carlo, France. [Abstract 10]

10. Somogyi S, Poggensee G, Pauli G, *et al.* (2006). Occurrence of HIV-1 subtypes in Germany: results from the HIV-1 seroconverter study of the Robert Koch-Institut. 4th European HIV Drug resistance workshop, Monte Carlo, France. [Abstract P1.13]

11. Concorde Coordinating Committee. (1994). MRC/ANRS randomised double-blind controlled trial of immediate and deferred zidovudine in symptom-free HIV infection. *Lancet* 343:871–81.

12. Allen TM, Altfeld M, Yu XG, *et al.* (2003). HIV-1 Superinfection Despite Broad CD8+ T-cell Responses Containing Replication of the Primary Virus. 10th CROI, Boston, USA. [Abstract 307]

13. Cavert W, Notermans DW, Staskus K, *et al.* (1997). Kinetics of response in lymphoid tissues to antiretroviral therapy of HIV-1 infection. *Science* 276:960–4.

14. Arasteh K, Gölz J, Marcus U, Rockstroh J, Salzberger B, Vielhaber B. (2005). *Deutsch-österreichische Empfehlungen zur postexpositionellen Prophylaxe der HIV-Infektion. Teilaktualisierung Stand Juni 2005.* Available at http://www.daignet.de/media/PDF_D_A_antiretroviral_06_05.pdf

15. Vogel M, Wolf E, Ummard K, *et al.* (2006). Injection site reactions (ISR) and success of HAART influence continued use of enfuvirtide (T20). VIII International Congress on Drug Therapy in HIV Infection, Glasgow, Scotland. [Abstract 183]

16. Miller V, Sabin C, Hertogs K, *et al.* (2000). Virological and immunological effects of treatment interruptions in HIV-1 infected patients with treatment failure. *AIDS 2000* 14:2857–67.

17. Delaugerre C, Peytavin G, Dominguez S, *et al.* (2005). Virological and pharmacological factors associated with virological response to salvage therapy after an 8-week of treatment interruption in a context of very advanced HIV disease (GigHAART ANRS 097). *J Med Virol* 77:345–50.

18. Lisziewicz J, Rosenberg E, Lieberman J, *et al.* (1999). Control of HIV despite the discontinuation of antiretroviral therapy. *N Engl J Med* 340:1683–4.

19. El-Sadr WM, Lundgren JD, Neaton JD, *et al.* (2006). CD4+ count-guided interruption of antiretroviral treatment. *N Engl J Med* 355:2283–96.

20. Maggiolo F, Ripamonti D, Callegaro A, *et al.* (2006). CD4-guided STI: four-year follow-up of a controlled, prospective trial. XVI International AIDS Conference, Toronto, Canada. [Abstract WEAB0202]

21. Wolf E, Hoffmann C, Procaccianti M, *et al.* (2005). Long-term consequences of treatment interruptions in chronically HIV-1-infected patients. *Eur J Med Res* 10:1–7.

22. Arribas J, Pulido F, Delgado R, *et al.* (2006). Lopinavir/ritonavir as single-drug maintenance therapy in patients with HIV-1 viral suppression: forty-eight week results of a randomized, controlled, open label, clinical trial (OK04 Study). XVI International AIDS Conference, Toronto, Canada. [Abstract THLB0203]

23. Cameron W, da Silva B, Arribas J, *et al.* (2006). A two-year randomized controlled clinical trial in antiretroviral-naïve subjects using lopinavir/ritonavir (LPV/r) monotherapy after initial induction treatment compared to an efavirenz (EFV) 3-drug regimen (Study M03–613). XVI International AIDS Conference, Toronto, Canada. [Abstract THLB0201]

24. Delfraissy JF, Flandre P, Delaugerre C, *et al.* (2006). MONARK Trial (MONotherapy AntiRetroviral Kaletra): 48-Week analysis of lopinavir/ritonavir (LPV/r) monotherapy compared to LPV/r + zidovudine/lamivudine (AZT/3TC) in antiretroviral-naïve patients. XVI International AIDS Conference, Toronto, Canada. [Abstract THLB0202]

25. Goelz J, Wolf E, Moll A, Koegl C, Jaeger H. (2006). Single-agent HAART with lopinavir/r (LPV/r) in ART-naïve and pre-treated HIV-1-infected patients. XVI International AIDS Conference, Toronto, Canada. [Abstract THPE0134]

26. Castagna A, Danise A, Menzo S, *et al.* (2006). Lamivudine monotherapy in HIV-1-infected patients harbouring a lamivudine-resistant virus: a randomized pilot study (E-184V study). *AIDS* 20:795–803.

27. Salzberger B, Hartmann P, Hanses F, *et al.* (2005). Incidence and prognosis of CMV disease in HIV-infected patients before and after introduction of combination antiretroviral therapy. *Infection* **33**:345–9.

28. Hoffmann C, Wolf E, Fatkenheuer G, *et al.* (2003). Response to highly active antiretroviral therapy strongly predicts outcome in patients with AIDS-related lymphoma. *AIDS* **17**:1521–9.

29. Hoffmann C, Tabrizian S, Wolf E, *et al.* (2001). Survival of AIDS patients with primary central nervous system lymphoma is dramatically improved by HAART-induced immune recovery. *AIDS* **15**:2119–27.

30. Mauss S, Wolf E, Hans J. (1999). Changing incidence of mycobacterial diseases in German patients with HIV infection. *AIDS Read* **9**:391–2.

31. Oette M, Kaiser R, Daumer M, *et al.* (2006). Primary HIV drug resistance and efficacy of first-line antiretroviral therapy guided by resistance testing. *J Acquir Immune Defic Syndr* **41**:573–81.

32. Wolf E, Koegl C, Hoffmann C, *et al.* (2004). Low dose stavudine: as effective as standard dose but less side effects. XV International AIDS Conference, Bangkok, Thailand. [Abstract WePeB5861]

33. De Santis M, Carducci B, De Santis L, Cavaliere AF, Straface G. (2002). Periconceptional exposure to efavirenz and neural tube defects. *Arch Intern Med* **162**:355.

34. Fundaro C, Genovese O, Rendeli C, Tamburrini E, Selvaggio E. (2002). Myelomeningocele in a child with intrauterine exposure to efavirenz. *AIDS* **16**:299–300.

35. Riddler SA, Haubrich R, DiRienzo G, *et al.* (2006). A prospective, randomized, phase III trial of NRTI-, PI- and NNRTI-sparing regimens for initial treatment of HIV-1 infection – ACTG 5142. XVI International AIDS Conference, Toronto, Canada. [Abstract THLB0204]

36. Hughes S, Parry-Billings K, Givens N, *et al.* (2006). PREDICT1: a novel randomised prospective study design to determine the clinical utility of prognostic screening for HLA-B*5701 (Study CNA106030). VIII International Congress on Drug Therapy in HIV Infection, Glasgow, Scotland. [Abstract 118]

37. Dupke S, Berg T, Hintsche B, Mayr C, Schlote F. (2006). Impact of different TAMs on outcome of a HAART regimen with ABC+3TC+AZT (Trizivir) and TDF. VIII International Congress on Drug Therapy in HIV Infection, Glasgow, Scotland. [Abstract 226]

38. Mauss S, Wolf E, Jaeger H. (1999). Reversal of protease inhibitor-related visceral abdominal fat accumulation with recombinant human growth hormone. *Ann Intern Med* **131**:313–4.

39. Neumann T, Woiwoid T, Neumann A, *et al.* (2003). Cardiovascular risk factors and probability for cardiovascular events in HIV-infected patients: part I. Differences due to the acquisition of HIV-infection. *Eur J Med Res* **8**:229–35.

40. Klinker H. (2005). Therapy of Chronic Hepatitis C – How to Manage "Problem Patients"? *Klinikarzt* **34**:140–145.

41. Wasmuth J-C, Rockstroh JK. (2006). HIV and HBV/HCV Coinfections. In: Hoffman C, Rockstroh J, Kamps BS, eds. *HIV Medicine 2006, 14th Edition.* Flying Publisher. p541–553. Available at http//:www.hivmedicine.com (last accessed 26 April 2007).

42. Rockstroh JK. (2006). Management of hepatitis C/HIV coinfection. *Curr Opin Infect Dis* **19**:8–13.

43. Vogel M, Nattermann J, Baumgarten A, *et al.* (2006).Treatment of sexually transmitted acute HCV infection in HIV-positive individuals. 46th Interscience Conference on Antimicrobial Agents and Chemotherapy, San Francisco, USA. [Abstract H1060]

44. Vogel M, Voigt E, Schafer N, *et al.* (2005). Orthotopic liver transplantation in human immunodeficiency virus (HIV)-positive patients: outcome of 7 patients from the Bonn cohort. *Liver Transpl* **11**:1515–21.

45. Stoll M, Claes C, Schulte E, Graf von der Schulenburg JM, Schmidt RE. (2002). Direct costs for the treatment of HIV-infection in a German cohort after the introduction of HAART. *Eur J Med Res* **7**:463–71.

Chapter 9

Country review: Italy

Renato Maserati

Background

The HIV/AIDS situation in Italy in the 10 years since the highly active antiretroviral therapy (HAART) era began has been, and still is, shaped by two key factors. First, diagnosis, management and treatment for HIV-infected patients have been provided over these years by a network of clinical centres that are, in almost all cases, the infectious disease (ID) units in hospitals across the country. Some outpatient services for drug addiction (SERTs, an acronym that stands for *SERvizio di Tossicodipendenze*) and dermatology units may also prescribe, dispense and monitor the effects of antiretroviral drugs. There are currently 138 ID units operating in Italy, either in local, regional or teaching (university) hospitals, and all are working within the framework of the government-funded National Health System (NHS) (*Sistema Sanitario Nazionale*). This network is run by highly experienced clinical personnel and is supported by a number of laboratories (virology, immunology, pharmacology) that are unevenly distributed geographically, but available to most physicians. This, together with the relative youth of ID physicians as compared with those in other medical subspecialties, means that a shortage of human resources may affect the field of HIV medicine, although this is not predicted in other medical fields in the near future.

The second factor is the universal access policy implemented by the Italian NHS, which allows free evaluation and treatment for all HIV-infected residents of Italy. This entitles all people living with HIV/AIDS (PLWHA), whether or not they have entered the country legally, to receive the most appropriate care for their HIV infection from diagnosis to prescription of HAART, with follow-up at any ID centre. This has meant that all antiretroviral drugs licensed by the European Agency for the Evaluation of Medicinal Products (EMEA) in the last decade have been quickly made available to Italian PLWHA and their caregivers at no cost to the individual patient. However, the extensive coverage provided by the NHS is now under a great deal of pressure due to rising costs and an increased demand for responsible and efficient use of resources.

The growing perception of budgetary constraints on NHS activities, including drug coverage, has led to a burgeoning private health system based on insurance programmes and/or direct out-of-pocket spending by those who can afford it. In 2003, the government expenditure on health as a percentage of total health expenditure was 75.1%, while private expenditure on health was 24.9% [1]. The latter percentage has steadily grown in the last few years. It must be noted, however, that patients with infectious and/or transmissible diseases, particularly those living with HIV/AIDS, are still receiving complete medical care in public hospitals, where all ID wards are located. Furthermore, co-payment for diagnostic procedures, drugs and visits—a measure devised to increase the efficiency of the NHS—is not requested in the case of HIV-positive patients. This makes them exempt from any healthcare-related expenses in the same way that certain other groups of patients—for example, pregnant women, the disabled or individuals with chronic diseases—already are.

The HIV epidemic in Italy

Currently, there are an estimated 110,000–130,000 HIV-infected people living in Italy, meaning that the prevalence in a population of about 58.7 million is between 187 and 222 HIV infections per 100,000 residents. The surveillance system for HIV/AIDS is based on data flowing to the National AIDS Operations Centre (*Centro Operativo AIDS*, or COA) at the *Istituto Superiore di Sanità* (ISS) in Rome. AIDS cases have been consistently reported since the beginning of the epidemic. From 1982 to December 2005, 56,076 AIDS cases were reported to the COA (1577 cases in 2005). Of these, 34,757 (62%) were deceased at the end of 2005. Incidence rates for AIDS cases reported in 2005 ranged from 0.8 to 5.8 per 100,000 residents, depending on the region, with the highest incidence in Lombardy, where the Milan metropolitan area is located. A North–South split was also evident, with the more industrialized northern part of Italy still harbouring most of the cases [2].

While the absolute number of cases has been decreasing since 1995, some noteworthy changes have taken place in the demographics of the epidemic: AIDS is being diagnosed in an increasingly old age group: in 1985, median ages were 29 years for men and 24 years for women, but by 2005, median ages had risen to 41 for men and 38 for women (Figure 9.1). In the same period, the proportion of AIDS cases diagnosed in women remained basically stable at 23% and 25% of cases, respectively [2].

Analysis of the risk factors leading to AIDS (Figure 9.2) shows that the percentage of patients infected through injection drug use is now approximately 30%, after peaking in the late 1980s. Men who have sex with men (MSM) currently comprise around 20% of AIDS cases in Italy, a percentage that has remained quite stable over time, while there has been a steady increase in the rate of heterosexually transmitted HIV infection leading to AIDS. In 2005, around half of AIDS cases were diagnosed in heterosexuals who had either: had multiple sex partners, including sex workers (7440 cases); had contact with an active or former injection-drug-using (IDU) partner (2738 cases); or (most interestingly) had come from regions where HIV infection is endemic, or had sexual contact with someone coming from such areas of the world (1110 cases).

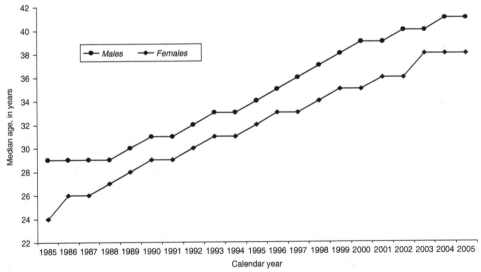

Fig. 9.1 Patients' age (median, in years) at time of diagnosis, subdivided by gender and year of diagnosis.

Source : [2]

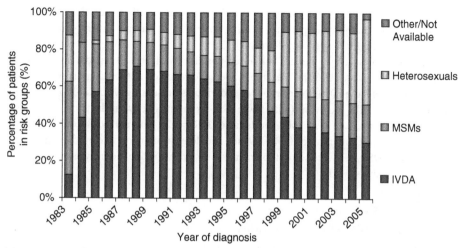

Fig. 9.2 Percentage of patients belonging to different risk groups, according to the year of AIDS diagnosis.

Source: [2]

Since 1996, the reporting system has also collected data on the time span between the first diagnosis of HIV infection and the clinical manifestations of full-blown AIDS according to the US Centers for Disease Control and Prevention (CDC) 1993 classification system. In the last decade (Figure 9.3) a growing proportion of patients—20.6% in 1996, 52.6% in 2005—have had an AIDS diagnosis within six months of their first HIV-positive test, indicating an increasing percentage of 'AIDS presenters', as was noted in a cohort study published a few years ago [3]. In that study of 3483 consecutive HIV-positive patients followed in Milan between January 1993 and December 2000, the proportion of AIDS presenters, strictly defined in that study as those developing AIDS within one month of receiving a positive HIV diagnosis, rose from 13.8% prior to 1997 to 32.5% after that year. Upon publication, the authors concluded that' In Italy, AIDS

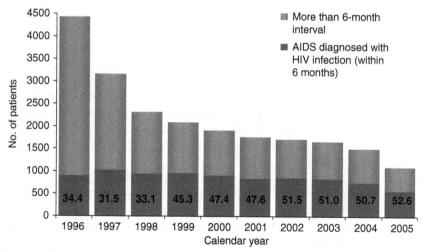

Fig. 9.3 Interval between the first diagnosis of HIV infection and AIDS diagnosis.

Notes: On the vertical axis, the absolute number of cases per calender year. Figures on the lower part of bars indicate the 'AIDS-presenter' percentage for that year (%).

Source: [2]

occurs mainly in subjects unaware of their HIV status (especially males, the elderly and those infected heterosexually) or in patients refusing antiretroviral therapy (mainly intravenous drug users who do not refer to specialized centres)' [3].

In another analysis of the Italian 'late tester' population [4], based on adults with AIDS diagnosed between January 1996 and December 2002 and reported to the Italian registry established by the COA as of June 2003, the number of individuals presenting with full-blown AIDS at the time of their first HIV diagnosis (with fewer than six months between the two events) rose from 19.95% in 1996 to 50.47% in 2002 (odds ratio (OR)=1.25 per year; 95% confidence interval (CI):1.23–1.27; test for trend p<0.001). When the determinants of a delayed diagnosis of HIV infection in AIDS cases were sought, being a late tester was independently associated (through multivariate analysis) with:

- male gender;
- age (under 32 years or over 39 years);
- acquisition of HIV infection by behaviours other than injection drug use;
- living in central or southern regions of Italy as opposed to northern regions; and
- having been diagnosed as HIV-infected after 1996–7.

The mean CD4 count in late testers was 83 cells/mm^3 versus 127 cells/mm^3 in non-late testers (p<0.001), and this difference was coupled with an increased proportion of *Pneumocystis jirovecii* pneumonia (PCP/ PJP), toxoplasmic encephalitis and Kaposi's sarcoma (KS) in late testers (OR=2.18, 1.24, and 2.14, respectively). By contrast, other AIDS-defining conditions such as oesophageal candidiasis and wasting syndrome were more common in non-late testers. AIDS presenters also had a significantly higher risk of presenting multiple AIDS-defining illnesses (OR=2.15 for the second illness, 3.03 for the third, and 2.44 for the fourth).

The lack of awareness of HIV status was associated, not unexpectedly, with a lower proportion of patients on HAART in late testers when compared with other patients with AIDS diagnosed in the same period (6.05% versus 61.71%, respectively, OR=25.05; 95% CI:21.40–29.33). What was more surprising was that people with a low level of education (fewer than six years of schooling) or a high one (more than eight years of schooling) were more likely to be late presenters than those who had attended school for six to eight years, corresponding to junior high school in the Italian school system. This association remained after adjusting for age, gender and risk category.

As of December 2005, there were 746 paediatric AIDS cases reported to the COA, or 1.3% of the total number of AIDS cases reported, most of them acquired perinatally in babies born to IDU mothers. The sharp decrease in the number of paediatric AIDS cases since 1997 (275 in 1994–5 versus 35 in 1996–7) is likely to be the result of both the increase in chemoprophylaxis given to pregnant women to avoid vertical transmission, and the effects of HAART in children. Since 1994–5, no cases of paediatric AIDS in haemophiliacs have been reported. Among the 693 cases of vertically acquired HIV infection leading to paediatric AIDS, more than half (357 cases) were born to mothers identified as IDUs, while 35.9% (249 cases) were born to heterosexually infected mothers. [2].

Time trends indicate that AIDS cases have become more frequent in foreign-born individuals over time (4.5% of cases in 1994–5, 17.9% in 2004–5). An increasing number of individuals, either legal immigrants or those classified as illegal migrants, have arrived in Italy from endemic areas such as sub-Saharan Africa in the last decade. This population may harbour a disproportionately high percentage of patients with sexually transmitted infections (STIs), including HIV, when compared to Italian-born citizens. In a study published in 2004 on 61,789 STI cases reported to the Italian National Registry for STIs between 1991 and 1999 [5], 6847 (11.2%) were found among foreigners, 47.1% of them Africans. The HIV prevalence among non-Italian patients with STIs was 5.5% (95% CI:4.9–6.2), with significant differences by continent of origin: the overall HIV prevalence in individuals with STIs from South America was 16.7% versus 9.4% found in Italians. In the same study, immigrants from sub-Saharan Africa had an HIV prevalence higher in MSM (28.6%) than in heterosexuals (8.9%), even though this rate is the highest found among non-Italian heterosexuals.

The data presented and discussed thus far refer to AIDS cases. While full-blown AIDS cases have been reported and analyzed since 1982, only five regions or provinces have been consistently reporting new HIV infections since 1985. Another four regions are currently reporting newly diagnosed HIV infections (Veneto since 1988, Piemonte since 1999, Puglia since 2000 and Liguria since 2004) [2]. The number of new infections, which peaked during the late 1980s and steadily decreased during the 1990s, seems to be increasing again in some areas (e.g. in 2004 it was reported to be 9.3 per 100,000 inhabitants in the province of Modena). This appears to be increasingly related to sexual exposure among both heterosexuals and MSM, and decreasingly to injection drug use. The percentage of new HIV diagnoses in non-nationals increased from 11.1% in 1992 to 31.7% in 2004.

Quite recently, a survey was carried out in five of eight surveillance areas (representing 24.1% of Italian residents) on HIV infections diagnosed in non-Italian nationals during the period 1992–2004 [6]. The number of new infections was compared with the number of residence permits issued by the Ministry of the Interior in the same time period and for the same geographical areas. The total number of new HIV infections was 17,040, of which19.2% were in non-nationals, with Africans representing the greatest proportion (53.8%). Over half (51%) of infections were diagnosed in heterosexuals, 56% of whom were men. Women seem to contract HIV at a younger age (25–29 years) than men (15.5% of whom were infected between 30 and 34 years of age).

Although the incidence of new HIV infections adjusted for age and gender was 5.5 times greater among legal immigrants than among native-born Italians (29.6 per 100,000 permits versus 5.4 per 100,000 population in 2004, respectively), the incidence in foreign-born residents decreased between 1992 and 2005 from 88.3 per 100,000 permits to 41.9 per 100,000 permits. This figure may underestimate the real impact that HIV infection in migrants from endemic areas is currently having on the Italian NHS, given that a large proportion of these individuals are not appearing in any statistical survey due to their status as illegal aliens.

The arrival of new migrants in Italy is not likely to decrease in the next few years. The HIV epidemic is far from being controlled in most of the areas they arrive from, particularly sub-Saharan Africa and Eastern Europe, with the latter representing a global 'hot spot' due to the ongoing spread of HIV among IDUs [7]. It is therefore unlikely that the burden of new HIV/AIDS cases in foreigners living in Italy will decrease in the near future. Two additional features associated with retroviral infection in this population are of note. First, migrants from endemic areas such as Africa or the former Soviet Union are a high risk for active or latent tuberculosis (TB) [8], with all the infection control and treatment problems that this implies. Second, the cultural, religious and linguistic barriers that exist between varying ethnic groups and Italians may seriously hinder attempts to properly diagnose and treat HIV/AIDS in these populations.

While immigrants may pose new challenges to caregivers and public health officials, other groups that have traditionally comprised a large proportion of PLWHA are showing a discernible and sustained decrease in HIV incidence. A study conducted by the COA and other governmental bodies based on data collected from across Italy [9] has evaluated the changes in the epidemiology of HIV infection in IDUs attending the national SERT network (the outpatient units for drug addiction where IDUs receive methadone or buprenorphine substitution therapy and where they may be diagnosed and treated for addiction-related conditions). HIV testing, while not mandatory, is offered to all SERT clients, particularly IDUs. If the patient is ELISA-negative (enzyme-linked immunosorbent assay), he or she is encouraged to repeat the testing every six months. Data from 510 of 555 SERTs (92%) for the period 1990–2000 and showed that the number of attendees, the percentage of heroin and cocaine users and the percentage of those tested for HIV in 1990 and 2000 were, respectively: 66,702 versus 145,897; 90.7% versus 82.7%; and 59.5% versus 46%.

While the overall prevalence of HIV infection in the same study period was 19.8%, and significantly higher in women than in men (26% versus 18.7%), the annual HIV prevalence from 1990 to 2000 decreased from 30.8% (95% CI:30.3–31.2) to 15.8% (95% CI:15.5–16.1) (chi-square for linear trend p<0.0001), with a sharp decrease between 1990 and 1996 followed by a levelling-off. This trend between 1990 and 2000 was maintained even when data were sorted by gender, with prevalence decreasing from 33.8% to 22.6% in females and from 30.2% to 14.7% in males. Once these data were disaggregated for region of residence, almost all regions of Italy showed the same trend, with the following exceptions: Emilia-Romagna in the north, with a stable, high prevalence among SERT attendees; Campania in the south, which remained at low levels throughout the survey period; and the Mediterranean island of Sardinia, which saw a 23% increase in HIV prevalence between 1990 and 2000.

HIV is also a major health problem in Italian prisons. The increasing number of IDUs incarcerated since the early 1980s, the possible connections between immigration from endemic areas and crime, injection drug use among prisoners, tattooing using makeshift, unsterilized equipment, and unprotected sexual activities all make the overcrowded Italian prisons a critical place for controlling the epidemic. One of the main issues is the decreasing percentage of inmates who undergo voluntary HIV testing. This dropped from 49.4% in 1991 to 37.7% in 2001 and to 17.5% in the first half of 2006, with significant differences among regions. In 2006, for example, inmates incarcerated in Piemonte, Liguria, Veneto or Emilia-Romagna were tested in 74.8%, 61.3%, 59.5% and 51.2% of cases, respectively, while in large southern regions like Campania, Calabria and Sicilia, these figures were 10.5%, 18.9%, and 17.4%. Data from 1991–2001 showed that prevalence in new inmates undergoing the test decreased from 9.7% to 2.6% (3.7% in the first half of 2006), probably thanks to a decrease in the proportion of IDUs jailed in that period (32.6% in 1991, 8.1% in 2001). These figures are largely incomplete and may also be misleading due to the voluntary nature of HIV testing in Italian prisons. Data would probably be more reliable if other screening policies, such as unlinked anonymous testing, could be implemented. Studies are needed to determine why so many inmates refuse to be tested, and every effort should be made to determine the seroprevalence in the inmate population that is not tested at the time of incarceration.

The implementation of HAART remains worrying in prisons: while it has been demonstrated that the availability of antiretroviral drugs has led to a sharp decrease in AIDS cases in many different countries, including Italy, it has also been repeatedly reported that inmates show a lower level of adherence than PLWHA in the outside community. This could be mitigated by using a substantially different approach relying more on directly observed therapy (DOT), which was shown in an Italian study [10] to be more effective than self-administered regimens.

Data on HIV-2 infection in Italy are relatively old and limited to certain parts of the national population. In a study carried out in a single, large ID centre where, at the time, more than 3,000 HIV-positive patients were being followed, only 19 patients were identified as HIV-2 [11], and this was considered the first report of HIV-2 in Italy. All patients were immigrants from West Africa and were probably infected through heterosexual contact. Twelve of them also had a positive HIV-1 RNA plasma viraemia (> 50 copies/mL).

In 2001, a study was carried out on 349 patients enrolled in the Italian Cohort Naïve for Antiretrovirals (ICONA) to search for non-clade B subtypes, which were detected in 19 cases (5.4%) [12]. It was also reported that the percentage of patients carrying non-clade B virus before and after 1997 was 1.9% and 8.4%, respectively (p=0.008). Among Caucasians, heterosexual infection and female gender were significantly associated with the presence of non-clade B subtypes (p=0.001 and 0.005, respectively). Non-clade B HIV-1 was present in 14.5% of the heterosexuals who were found to be HIV-1 positive after 1997, 60% of whom were women. Four strains turned out to be F, two were A, one was C, one was G, and 11 (57.9 %) were non-clade B recombinant subtypes. Another, more recent, study published in 2005 highlighted wide regional differences in non-clade B infection rate in Italy [13]. When 347 samples from Toscana and Puglia were analyzed, 18.1% and 10.8% respectively were non-clade B subtypes. Most interestingly, since 52 strains from non-Italian patients were included, it was shown that in both of these regions, the percentage of non-clade B viruses was 52.1% (Toscana) and 72.4% (Puglia) in immigrants versus 6.1% and 3% in native Italians. This study demonstrated that HIV-1 infection from non-B subtypes in Italy should no longer be considered restricted to immigrants from endemic areas.

Co-infection with hepatitis viruses is generally seen as a major problem in southern Europe, where the seroprevalence of hepatitis C virus (HCV) and hepatitis B virus (HBV) is generally higher than in the central and northern parts of the continent. In the EuroSIDA cohort including 3048 HIV-positive patients, the prevalence of HIV/HCV co-infection was 33%, but when only IDUs were analyzed, this figure rose to 75% [14]. The burden of rapidly progressing liver disease and increased risk of hepatotoxic reactions, as happens in co-infected patients, appears to be particularly significant in IDUs. In the 4656 patients of the ICONA cohort, the prevalence of HCV co-infection was reported to be 17% [15], similar to the figure derived from an epidemiological investigation in southern Italy [16]. Among 131 HIV-positive subjects living in Campania, 19.4% were also HCV-positive, but the largest group of HIV/HCVco-infected patients (84.6%) comprised IDUs. Genotypes 1a and 3a were more frequent in co-infected patients, while 1b and 2a/c were the leading subtypes in the control HCV-positive cohort. In the whole of Italy, the burden represented by HBV infection has steadily declined over the years as a consequence of marked improvements in public health measures and the implementation of a vaccination programme [17].

Since 1991, all infants and 12-year old adolescents have been immunized against HBV through a mandatory vaccination programme. Universal screening of pregnant women was also implemented in order to identify newborns at risk of acquiring HBV. These efforts notwithstanding, it is estimated that there are at least 1.2–1.5 million people, mostly over 50 years of age, who are chronic carriers of HBV in Italy, and that 1200 people per year are acutely infected by this virus.

The incidence of TB in Italy decreased in the general population from ten to seven cases per 100,000 inhabitants between 1995 and 2004. In a study of 1360 HIV-positive individuals initially evaluated in 28 ID units in Italy between May 1995 and April 1996 [18], 95 (7.0%) were tuberculin-positive. After a median follow-up of 104.3 weeks (range 4–154.6), TB was diagnosed in 18 patients (11 pulmonary; 3 extrapulmonary; 4 both sites). The overall incidence rate was 0.79 per 100 person-years (95% CI:0.51–1.31).

Managing PLWHA in Italy

National guidelines for diagnosing and managing PLWHA have been provided since the beginning of the epidemic by the Italian National Health Institute (*Istituto Superiore di Sanità*, or ISS) in Rome, which also hosts the COA. The ISS represents the main epidemiological observatory collecting and analyzing data about HIV/AIDS in Italy. As described earlier, antiretroviral drugs in Italy are widely available at no cost to the individual patient, and their use is supposed to be strictly monitored by caregivers working within the ID units. Recent data from market surveys obtained by the pharmaceutical industry showed that the nucleoside reverse transcriptase inhibitor (NRTI) most widely prescribed in Italy as of the summer of 2006 was lamivudine (3TC) (27% of all NRTIs), followed by: tenofovir (TDF) (21%); the fixed-dose combination (FDC) of 3TC plus zidovudine (ZDV), or Combivir® (18%); stavudine (d4T) (9%); didanosine (ddI) (8%); and the FDC of ZDV plus abacavir (ABC) plus 3TC, or Trizivir® (5.5%). The rest of the molecules (including the most recent FDCs such as Truvada® and Kivexa®) trail behind and below the 5% share cut-off.

A similar, quite conservative picture emerges from the protease inhibitor (PI) and non-nucleoside reverse transcriptase inhibitor (NNRTI) market figures. The leading PI remains lopinavir/ritonavir (LPV/r) (42%), followed by atazanavir (ATV) (26%), nelfinavir (NFV) (10%), fosamprenavir (fAPV) (9%), and others below the 5% cut-off.

What may be surprising is the large market share that NFV still holds and the fact that indinavir (IDV) is still prescribed to about 3% of patients on PIs. Antiretroviral drugs such as tipranavir (TPV) or darunavir (DRV) do not have a large impact on these numbers, either because of their particular niche or because they not yet available beyond an early access programme (EAP) programme.

As for NNRTIs, efavirenz (EFV) has the lion's share with 69% of the market in this class, but nevirapine (NVP) has a proportion far higher (31%) than in most other European countries. Delavirdine (DLV) has never been available in Italy. It remains unclear why so many patients are still treated with drugs or regimens such as PIs unboosted by ritonavir (RTV), tymidine analogue NRTIs, or sub-standard combinations like dual-NRTI regimens, which have largely been abandoned in other European countries. There may be several reasons for this, including a conservative approach to HIV/AIDS clinical management, the lack of universal availability of the same drugs (e.g. some regional governments or individual hospitals within the same region may show different attitudes in making new drugs available to physicians, including new and more costly FDCs), and a different interpretation of international guidelines.

Recently, a group of Italian experts from major HIV/AIDS centres around the country published the results of a consensus workshop on the clinical management of HIV-positive patients [19]. It reflected the current attitudes of leading HIV/AIDS-treating physicians in Italy, and it may be interesting to see how different their recommendations and guiding principles are when compared with those of physicians who work in smaller hospitals or are less experienced in this field.

The methodology used for the consensus workshop, which was held in Rome in June 2005, was to have a small group of experts prepare a series of statements addressing four key questions concerning HAART:

◆ When to start treatment
◆ How to start treatment
◆ When to switch treatment
◆ What treatment to switch to

Statements received a score from AI to CIII according to the widely used Infectious Diseases Society of America (IDSA) evidence-grading scale, which grades the strength of a recommendation using letters (A=good, B=moderate, C=poor) and the quality of this evidence using roman numerals (I=properly randomized, controlled trials; II=other published studies; III=expert opinion). Each statement was then reviewed by a panel of 10–15 other experienced HIV/AIDS-treating physicians and, if necessary, rewritten. On the second day of the workshop, the statements were discussed in a plenary session in which all participants had the opportunity to discuss and influence the final form that statements would take by using a tele-voting system. Only top-scoring statements were immediately transferred to the final document; otherwise, they were discussed again until a wider consensus was reached. Recommendations emerging from the workshop were, by and large, similar to those formulated by other scientific societies around the world. What emerged as somewhat more unusual may be summarized in the following points:

♦ There seems to be less emphasis on HIV RNA plasma viral load than on absolute CD4+ T-cell count for starting therapy. This translates in a B/II indication to initiate therapy in asymptomatic patients with less than 350 CD4 cells/mm^3. Initiation above this threshold may be reasonable in a rapidly deteriorating situation (CD4 count decay >100 cells/mm^3 or HIV RNA plasma viral load >100,000 copies/mL). The immediate treatment of any symptomatic patient or of anyone whose CD4 count is below the 200 cells/mm^3 cut-off received an A/I grade.

♦ The indications for choosing the most appropriate HAART combination in treatment-naïve patients rely on LPV/r but also on EFV or NVP—the latter NNRTI to a lesser degree (B/I versus A/I for EFV). It may be worth noting that in the summer of 2005, when the panel convened, fAPV/r and SQV/r received the same B/I score. ATV/RTV, although still not approved for treatment-naïve patient therapy in the European Union (EU) as of October 2007, was indicated as '… a good alternative to [LPV/r]' [19]. The use of unboosted PIs (including NFV and unboosted ATV) had a B/I recommendation for patients intolerant to RTV or with baseline conditions, such as elevated cardiovascular risk or advanced liver impairment, that strongly contraindicated the use of RTV. As far as the NRTI component of HAART is concerned, the following combinations for treatment-naïve subjects received an A/I score: ZDV plus 3TC; TDF plus 3TC or emtricitabine (FTC); ABC plus 3TC.

♦ In terms of switching therapy in cases of first-line treatment failures (see Table 9.1), a prompt modification of HAART was recommended even after a low level of viral rebound. Furthermore, a wider use of resistance testing was recommended to better identify the second-line regimen. These recommendations make the Italian guidelines the most proactive on therapy switch due to failure in comparison to contemporary indications recommended by the US Department of Health and Human Services (DHHS) [20], the British HIV Association

Table 9.1 Recommendations for interventions in case of first-line treatment failure.

Condition	Intervention	Strength and quality of evidence
<1 log copies/mL in HIV RNA pVL reduction from baseline after 4 weeks	Assess adherence Assess possible interactions Determine plasma drug levels	A/III A/III B/II
Confirmed HIV RNA pVL >50 copies/mL after 24 wks (never undetectable)	Switch drugs following adherence and resistance testing indications	A/II
Confirmed HIV RNA pVL >50 copies/mL (rebound after undetectability)	Switch drugs following adherence and resistance testing indications	A/II
Increase of <25 to 50	Assess causes of immune suppression	B/II
CD4+ cells/mm^3 after 24 weeks with successful HIV RNA pVL reduction <50 copies/mL	Consider immune-adjuvant drugs (e.g. IL-2)	C/II

Source: Modified from [18].

(BHIVA) [21], the International AIDS Society–USA (IAS) [22] and the French Ministry of Health [23]. A therapy change is also recommended in cases of toxicity, poor adherence, or even patient's choice. The use of drugs such as interleukin 2 (IL-2) is considered, even at low strength, in discordant patients with a successful viral control in plasma but without an appreciable increase in CD4 count.

♦ Even though any use of cyclic supervised (or structured) therapy interruption is discouraged due to both its dangers and its substantial inefficacy in boosting specific HIV immune responses, it was recognized that patients (and their doctors) tend to stop a successful regimen for a number of reasons, including treatment fatigue and the desire to limit drug-related toxicities. Therefore, specific indications for stopping and resuming HAART are pragmatically provided in the guidelines.

Italian advocacy and support groups

As in almost all industrialized countries, Italy has seen the growth of a number of advocacy groups that foster knowledge of HIV infection and AIDS, promote campaigns for prevention and against discrimination toward PLWHA, and interact with governmental agencies and regional health authorities on access to care, as well as pointing out the unmet needs that the PLWHA community has to face daily and publishing bulletins and journals on this topic. The role of these advocacy groups is so well recognized that it has been institutionalized in what is called the *Consulta delle Associazioni per la lotta contro l'AIDS* (the conference of associations for the fight against AIDS, also referred to as the Italian Community Advisory Board, or ICAB). The *Consulta* holds a regular meeting approximately every two months before the *Commissione Nazionale per la lotta contro l'AIDS* (the Italian Ministry of Health's advisory body on health policies associated with HIV/AIDS) formally convenes. The mandate of the *Commissione* is to acknowledge the proposals it receives from the *Consulta* and translate these into recommendations for the Ministry of Health. Lately, the *Consulta* has begun to interact more directly with the pharmaceutical industry and clinical researchers in an effort to obtain quicker answers for the therapeutic and strategic needs of PLWHA.

The groups comprising the *Consulta* represent a cross section of experience and backgrounds; some are devoted to the care of special patient groups such as children or haemophiliacs, others represent gay-bisexual issues, and some are based within the Catholic Church. Although they may differ in terms of membership, financial resources, and their impact on local, regional and national communities, all of them have active websites, most run telephone hotlines, and some regularly publish bulletins and newsletters.

HAART as patients see it: the LONGIS Study

Some data are available on patients' perceptions of the aims and perils of HAART in Italy, although none is comprehensive. A survey of 359 patients was carried out by the Nadir Foundation, a nationwide advocacy group based in Rome, during the first quarter of 2006. Patients were recruited either through the Internet, by phone, or were directly interviewed by a Nadir Foundation volunteer.

More than half the patients (53.2%) were first diagnosed as HIV-infected as early as 1995. Patients resided mainly in north-central Italy (18.1% in the north-east; 34.5% in the north-west; 37% in central Italy), with and 10.3% residing in the south. Most men (67.3%) were in their fifth decade (mean age: 42 years); 46.5% were MSM, 23.4% were heterosexual and 18.4% were IDUs [Nadir Foundation, unpublished data].

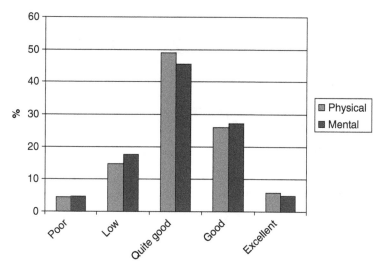

Fig. 9.4 Longis Study. Physical and mental status (359 patients).

Source: Nadir foundation, unpublished data.

When the interview took place, 53.8% of patients identified themselves as smokers (24.8% smoking ≥1 pack per day), while most (64%) did not drink any alcohol. As already widely reported in Southern Europe, co-infection with hepatitis viruses was quite common in this cohort: 45% of patients were co-infected with either HBV or HCV. Most of the patients (82.4%) were on HAART, while 12.3% had stopped their drugs for different reasons, and only 5.3% had never been treated. Among the treated group, 21.8% were on their first-line regimen, 16.3% on their second, 19.7% on their third and, notably, 42.2% were on fourth-line regimens or beyond. Despite previous exposure to antiretroviral drugs, 62.7% of them had an HIV RNA plasma viraemia <50 copies/mL, and this was well matched by the concomitant data on CD4 counts; a CD4 count above 200 cells/mm3 was declared by 86% of the individuals interviewed, with only 11.4% below this threshold (2.5% did not remember their most recent CD4 value).

When asked about their physical and mental well-being, most survey participants stated that they considered their health status to be 'average' (see Figure 9.4), independent of their immuno-virologic conditions. It is interesting to note that 49.3% reported no complaint about their current therapy, while 42.6% complained about side effects, 11.5% about dosing, and 7.1% about the number of pills per day (cumulatively, 18.6% complaining about pill burden). Since side effects were thought to be so relevant in determining a patient's acceptance of treatment, patients were also asked to identify and rate these as either 'mild–moderate' or 'severe–intolerable'. Abdominal bloating was most commonly reported in both categories (50% reporting it as mild–moderate, 16.7% as severe–intolerable), followed by diarrhoea and fatigue reported as mild–moderate (in 42% and 39.7% of patients, respectively) and by sleep disturbances and fatigue reported as severe–intolerable (15.1% and 11.1%, respectively). On the other hand, the 'pill burden' was reported to be quite low, since 52% of those interviewed stated they were taking four pills per day or fewer, mainly (66.8%) in two divided doses.

Self-reported adherence also appeared to be quite good, with 77% of patients considering themselves 'very good' or 'excellent' in their daily adherence to treatment; 85.3% claimed that they had either never missed or had missed only one dose within the month prior to the survey. However, most of these patients (83.1%), in an apparent contradiction to the adherence figures

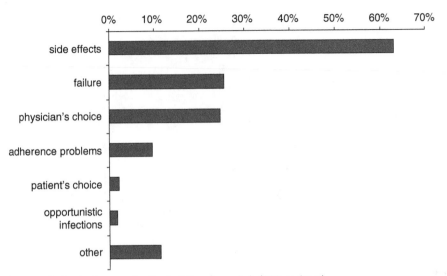

Fig. 9.5 Longis Study. Reasons for the last therapy switch (230 patients).

Source: Nadir foundation, unpublished data.

above, asked for a more 'friendly' regimen; 42.9% would have preferred fewer doses per day, and 54.4% a reduced number of pills per day. The survey data are summarized in Figure 9.5.

Finally, when patients were asked about the reasons for their last regimen switch, if any, more than 60% pointed to drug-related side effects, while virologic failure was identified by around 25%; 25% indicated 'physician's choice', while 'adherence' was the reason given by less than 10%.

Conclusions

Few, if any, success stories in the history of medicine can compare with what HAART has done for PLWHA in the industrialized world. It has turned a progressive, dreadful and lethal disease that was taking millions of lives into a chronic, manageable condition. Even if one could hardly describe it as one long honeymoon, the momentum still holds; most patients enjoy a full life, and current antiretroviral drug combinations are more compact, less toxic and easier to take than those available 10 years ago. The more advanced lines of treatment today may even try to achieve what was, until just a few years ago, only thought achievable in treatment-naïve patients: the complete suppression (below the limit of detection) of HIV RNA plasma viral load. This is being reported in most clinical centres, as seen in a recent cross-sectional evaluation of the *Policlinico San Matteo* Hospital cohort in Pavia in August 2006. Of 687 patients treated with HAART, 531 (77.3%) had an undetectable viral load, despite the fact that 55% of the patients with <50 copies/mL were on their third-line regimen or beyond.

While it is more difficult to report and analyze prevention or management of side effects compared with treatment efficacy, a recent multi-centre survey (the SIMONE Study) [24] may provide some reliable data in this regard. In this study, conducted between February and April 2005, data on 1243 individuals attending 12 HIV/AIDS clinics throughout north-central Italy were analyzed to determine the prevalence of metabolic syndrome (MS), defined as the presence of three or more of the following:

◆ a waist measurement >102 cm for men and >88 cm for women;

◆ high triglycerides (>150 mg/dL);

- low HDL cholesterol (<40 mg/dL for men and < 50 mg/dL for women);
- hypertension (=135/ =85 mm Hg);
- high blood glucose (=110 mg/dL).

The syndrome was found in 22% of the patients (95% CI:19.7–24.3), being present in 17.4% of women and 23.8% of men. The most frequent abnormality found was a high level of plasma triglycerides (in 52.2%), and at least one of the MS-defining alterations was found in 80.5% of all patients. In a multivariate analysis, the following were associated with MS:

- age (OR=1.71; 95% CI:1.46–2.00);
- body mass index (BMI) >25 (OR=3.00; 95% CI:2.37–3.76);
- lipodystrophy (OR=2.32; 95% CI:1.72–3.15);
- high plasma cholesterol (OR=1.56; 95% CI:1.08–2.25); and
- use of IDV (OR=4.3, 95% CI:1.7–11).

Despite the robust, continued success of HAART, which has translated into improved clinical outcomes for PLWHA living in Italy, there remain both new and ongoing challenges to be faced, and unmet needs to be answered. These include, among others: the pressure that new waves of immigrants (many of them illegal) from hyperendemic areas will place on Italy's health system in a time of shrinking budgets; a fading awareness within institutions, the media and amongst individuals of the ongoing HIV epidemic, coupled with the continued presence of stigma in some social milieux; and patients' call for simpler, more compact, less toxic antiretroviral drug regimens.

Acknowledgements

The author wishes to thank Anna Colucci, Barbara Suligoi (*Istituto Superiore di Sanità*) and Simone Marcotullio (Nadir Foundation) for providing data and friendly support.

References

1. World Health Organization. *WHO Statistical Information System (WHOSIS). Core Health Indicators.* Available at http://www3.who.int/whosis/core/core_select_process.cfm?country=ITA&indicator=NHA (accessed on 26 November 2006).

2. Suligoi B, Boros S, Camoni L, Lepore D, Ferri M, Roazzi P. (2006). Aggiornamenti dei casi di AIDS notificati in Italia e delle nuove infezioni da HIV al 31 dicembre 2005. *Not Ist Super Sanità* **19** (Suppl 1):3–23.

3. Castelnuovo B, Chiesa E, Rusconi S, *et al.* (2003). Declining incidence of AIDS and increasing prevalence of AIDS presenters among AIDS patients in Italy. *Eur J Clin Microbiol Infect Dis* **22**:663–9.

4. Longo B, Pezzotti P, Boros S, Urciuoli R, Rezza G. (2005). Increasing proportion of late testers among AIDS cases in Italy, 1996–2002. *AIDS Care* **17**:834–41.

5. Giuliani M, Suligoi B, and the Italian STI Surveillance Working Group. (2004). Differences between non-national and indigenous patients with sexually transmitted infections in Italy and insight into the control of sexually transmitted infections. *Sex Transm Dis* **31**:79–84.

6. Camoni L, Salfa MC, Regine V, *et al.* (2006). HIV incidence estimate among non-nationals in Italy. Abstracts of 5th International Conference on Urban Health (ICUH), 25–28 October 2006, Amsterdam, Netherlands. [Abstract 23]

7. Stvilia K, Tsertsvadze T, Sharvadze L, *et al.* (2006). Prevalence of hepatitis C, HIV, and risk behaviors for blood-borne infections: a population-based survey of the adult population of T'bilisi, Republic of Georgia. *J Urban Health* **83**:289–98.

8. Baussano I, Bugiani M, Gregori D, Pasqualini C, Demicheli V, Merletti F. (2006). Impact of immigration and HIV infection on tuberculosis incidence in an area of low tuberculosis prevalence. *Epidemiol Infect* **134**:1353–9.

9. Suligoi B, Magliocchetti N, Nicoletti G, Pezzotti P, Rezza G. (2004). Trends in HIV prevalence among drug-users attending public drug-treatment centres in Italy: 1990–2000. *J Med Virol* **73**:1–6.

10. Babudieri S, Aceti A, d'Offizi GP, Carbonara S, Starnini G. (2000). Directly observed therapy to treat HIV infection in prisoners. *JAMA* **284**:179–80.

11. Quiros Roldan E, Castelli F, Pan A, *et al.* (2001). Evidence of HIV-2 Infection in Northern Italy. *Infection* **29**: 362–363.

12. Balotta C, Facchi G, Violin M, *et al.* (2001). Increasing prevalence of non-clade B HIV-1 strains in heterosexual men and women, as monitored by analysis of reverse transcriptase and protease sequences. *J Acquir Immune Defic Syndr* **27**:499–505.

13. Monno L, Brindicci G, Lo Caputo S, *et al.* (2005). HIV-1 subtypes and circulating recombinant forms (CRFs) from HIV-infected patients residing in two regions of central and southern Italy. *J Med Virol* **75**:483–90.

14. Buffet-Janvresse C, Peigue-Lafeuille H, Benichou J, *et al.* (2003). HIV and HCV co-infection: Situation at six French university hospitals in the year 2000. *J Med Virol* **69**:7–17.

15. Becker S. (2004). Liver Toxicity in Epidemiological Cohorts. *Clin Infect Dis* **38**(Suppl 2):S49–55.

16. Rendina D, Vigorita E, Bonavolta R, *et al.* (2001). HCV and GBV-c/HGV infection in HIV positive patients in southern Italy. *Eur J Epidemiol* **17**:801–7.

17. Zanetti AR, Romanò L, Zappá A, Velati C. (2006). Changing patterns of hepatitis B infection in Italy and NAT testing for improving the safety of blood supply. *J Clin Virol* **36**(Suppl 1):S51–S55.

18. Girardi E, Antonucci G, Vanacore P, *et al.* (2000). Impact of combination antiretroviral therapy on the risk of tuberculosis among persons with HIV infection. *AIDS* **14**:1985–1991.

19. Carosi G, Torti C, Andreoni M, *et al.* (2006). Key questions in antiretroviral therapy: Italian Consensus Workshop (2005). *J Antimicrob Chemother* **57**:1055–64.

20. US National Institutes of Health. *Panel on Clinical Practice for Treatment of HIV Infection. Guidelines for the Use of Antiretroviral Agents in HIV-1-Infected Adults and Adolescents October 6, 2005.* Available at http://AIDSinfo.nih.gov (accessed 1 March 2006).

21. Gazzard B on behalf of the BHIVA Writing Committee. (2005). British HIV Association (BHIVA) guidelines for the treatment of HIV infected adults with antiretroviral therapy (2005). *HIV Med* **6**(Suppl 2):1–61.

22. Yeni PG, Hammer SM, Hirsch MS, *et al.* (2004). Treatment for adult HIV infection: 2004 recommendations of the International AIDS Society–USA Panel. *JAMA* **292**:251–65.

23. Delfrassy JF on behalf of the Direction Générale de la Santé's expert panel.(2004). *Prise en charge des personnes infectées par le VIH.* Paris: Editions Flammarion.

24. Bonfanti P, Ricci E, de Socio G, *et al.* (2006). Metabolic syndrome: a real threat for HIV-positive patients?: Results from the SIMONE study. *J Acquir Immune Defic Syndr* **42**:128–31.

Chapter 10

Country review: United States of America

Renslow Sherer

Introduction

In the United States in 1994, the HIV epidemic continued its relentless expansion: 80,691 people were diagnosed with AIDS and 112 people died from AIDS-related complications every day [1,2]. People living with HIV/AIDS (PLWHA), community activists and clinical care-givers were increasingly frustrated with inadequate prevention efforts and equally inadequate treatment options. Although regimens comprised of double nucleoside reverse transcriptase inhibitors (NRTIs) were shown to be superior to single drug therapy in 1994, the actual survival benefit was one or two additional years at best, drug toxicities and resistance were growing problems, and overall mortality from AIDS was undiminished.

Highly active antiretroviral therapy (HAART) began in the United States in 1995 with the first clinical trials of triple drug combination therapy. It is no exaggeration to say that the subsequent reversal of morbidity and mortality was unparalleled in the history of medicine and infectious disease control. People living with AIDS who had been wasted and bedridden rose from their beds when they started HAART, regained their lost weight, and returned to productive lives. In Chicago, for example, mortality rates fell by more than 61% between 1995 and 1997, and the daily census in the only public hospital fell from 75 to 25 in the same period [3,4]. A study of the impact of HAART on the United States in its first decade quantified the extent of the 'miracle' of HAART during this decade [5]: over 3 million life years were saved by HAART in the United States from 1996–2005, making the discovery of HAART the single most important therapeutic reversal of an infectious disease epidemic in the history of medicine.

In this chapter, we will consider selected aspects of the first decade of HAART in the United States. We begin with a review of the epidemiology and the scientific understanding of the pathogenesis of HIV disease in 1994. Then we will briefly consider the societal impact of AIDS and the role of community activists, and turn to the state of treatment in 1994 and the early HAART era that followed, with emphasis on rapid access to treatment and early lessons with treatment adherence and toxicity. To better describe the impact of HAART at the local level, we will consider this era in Chicago with an emphasis on the public sector. Thereafter, we will examine the issues that emerged in the early HAART era—particularly adherence, treatment toxicity, and drug resistance — that have greatly influenced trends in treatment outcomes, and will conclude with some observations for the coming decade of HIV/AIDS in the United States.

AIDS in the United States, 1994

By 1994, AIDS had become the leading cause of death in the United States among young adults aged 25–44, with 41,930 reported deaths in 1994 and an estimated total annual mortality of 55,000–60,000 [2]. As noted in Figure 10.1, the annual increase in AIDS cases was about 3%, and the US Centers for Disease Control and Prevention (CDC)- expanded case definition in 1993 to include people with CD4 counts below 200 cells/mm^3 and people with pulmonary tuberculosis (TB) more than doubled reported AIDS cases thereafter [6]. Two-thirds of cases were identified in the highest incidence states, including New York, California, Florida, Texas, New Jersey, Illinois, Maryland and Georgia. Half of all AIDS cases were in young adults aged 30–39, and 18% were in women. Seven thousand infants were born to HIV-infected women each year, and an estimated 2000 children were born HIV-positive per year [7]. The epidemic was moving into the second wave, with rising new infection rates occurring in African American and Latino men and women. Reported cases of AIDS in 1994 reflected transmissions from a decade earlier and showed the majority of cases to be in minority populations, with 39% in African Americans and 19% in Latinos [8]. Similarly, the proportion of risk behaviours was evolving, with increasing prevalence of reported AIDS cases among injection drug users (IDUs) (26%) and heterosexual transmission (12%), and a proportional decline in homosexually active men who, nonetheless, remained the highest percentage risk group with 44% of cases.

In 1994, data on the incidence of HIV infection were limited to states in which HIV was a reportable illness and to data from local surveillance and cohort studies. Available HIV data clearly indicated that a more rapid expansion of the epidemic into IDUs, women, young homosexually active men and people with sexually transmitted infections (STIs) was occurring, with disproportionately rising HIV incidence rates in communities of colour. For example, HIV seroprevalence among IDUs entering drug treatment centres from 1988–1993 was higher among African American and Latino IDUs than among white IDUs [9]. A higher prevalence of HIV

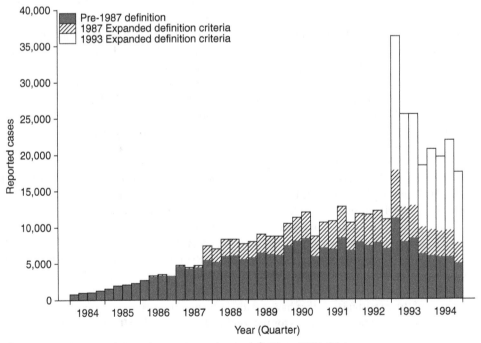

Fig. 10.1 AIDS reported cases, by quarter and case definition, 1984–94.*

* Includes Guam,Puarto Rico, the US Pacific Islands and the US Virgin Islands.
The expanded AIDS surveillance case definition implemented 1 January 1993 includes conditions that occur earlier in HIV disease. Persons diagnosed with these conditions before January 1993 were reported to CDC during 1993 and 1994, accounting for the substantial increase in the number of reported cases.
Source: [6]

among IDUs was found in the North-East (27%) compared to the South (12%), the Midwest (7%) and the West (3%). Also at this time, the annual incidence of AIDS among the sexual partners of IDUs, most of whom were women, was increasing, primarily among African American women [10].

The Pediatric ACTG 076 study results in 1993 showed a reduction in perinatal HIV transmission with from 25% to 8.8% with the use of zidovudine (ZDV), a stunning and unexpected finding [11]. HIV testing of pregnant women became a high priority in order to prevent perinatal transmission and raised the complex issues of the reproductive rights of the mother, as well as her right to treatment for her own health. In 1991, only 25% of pregnant women in the United States had been tested for HIV compared with 19% of the all women aged 18–44 years, but strategies to advise all pregnant women to undergo HIV testing were rapidly developing [12]. Although success was achieved with voluntary testing programmes of pregnant women in multidisciplinary settings, many legislatures took up mandatory testing initiatives for pregnant women.

Societal impact of AIDS, 1994

By 1994, most Americans knew someone living with AIDS, or they knew someone with a friend or family member living with AIDS. In spite of episodic media sensationalism about AIDS, there was more widespread public awareness about the disease, better knowledge of HIV prevention, and a more consistently compassionate response to the need for effective care and treatment for people living with AIDS than in the first decade of the epidemic. The visible and supportive role of public figures with HIV infection, such as Magic Johnson in 1991 and Arthur Ashe, Jr. in 1992, contributed to gradual acceptance and increasing tolerance in the United States. Other stories attracted national sympathy and revulsion at AIDS stigma; for example, the Ray family in Florida had three haemophiliac boys who were denied entrance to school when it became public that they were HIV-positive. Within weeks, the family was shunned in their community and their home was burned to the ground, forcing them to move.

The reality of AIDS was devastating in the homes and communities of people living with the disease. Funerals were commonplace, not only in gay communities in New York, Chicago and San Francisco, but in rural and suburban America, as many urban people living with AIDS chose to return to their home towns to die. For thousands of affected individuals, AIDS was an agonizing illness with a twofold burden. The pain, suffering and debilitation from the illness were often severe and prolonged for the individual and his or her family. The additional burdens of shame and stigma felt by people living with AIDS and their loved ones were often as painful, or more painful, to bear than the disease itself.

The gradual improvement in tolerance towards AIDS did not alter the occurrence of sporadic acts of intolerance and discrimination towards both PLWHA and people at risk of AIDS; indeed, the frequency of these episodes rose with the growing epidemic. Gay men and lesbians who had lived with homophobia and discrimination found that AIDS intensified the virulence and intensity of the attacks. Similarly, IDUs, who were used to discriminatory practices in healthcare and criminal justice settings, found that AIDS aggravated the frequency and the degree of animosity and stigma manifested towards them.

The unique issues of AIDS for women were gaining national recognition. Too often, women were treated as vessels for perinatal transmission prevention without regard to their own reproductive rights and health. Women were often identified as HIV-positive at the time of labour and delivery, and the complex issues of reproductive choices for women with HIV were not addressed. The majority of women living with HIV were African American and Latino, and half were IDUs. Those women infected with HIV or at high risk for infection and their advocates quickly realized that they would need to mobilize politically in order to gain care and prevention strategies that are most appropriate for women. Often lost in the heated and politicized debates on this issue was the tragedy of AIDS in two and even three generations in a single family.

Ryan White, a 10-year-old haemophiliac boy from Indiana who contracted HIV via blood transfusion, became a national symbol of intolerance and discrimination that evolved into a symbol of care and compassion. Due to exhaustive efforts by PLWHA and their advocates and caregivers to secure emergency relief for HIV/AIDS care and support services in the late 1980s, the Ryan White Comprehensive AIDS Resources Emergency (CARE) Act was enacted in 1990 [13]. The CARE Act was the first of its kind dedicated to a single disease entity. Although the CARE Act is beyond the scope of this case study, it was an admission of the weaknesses in the United States healthcare system, particularly for the poor and the working poor of the country. In the pre-HAART era, the CARE Act provided a strong measure of hope for healthcare and compassionate support for PLWHA and their families by providing US$200 million per year for the first five years. The CARE Act has been reauthorized twice since, in 1996 and 2000, and currently serves more than 500,000 Americans annually with appropriations in 2006 exceeding US$2 billion.

In parallel with the devastating societal impact of AIDS was the rise in political activism among the affected communities and their advocates, often joined by their families and health caregivers. Much of the progress against HIV/AIDS would not have occurred, and would not have occurred as quickly, without the political activism of the most seriously affected groups, starting with the gay community. The CARE Act's creation was activists' most visible success, for several reasons:

◆ It led to the most innovative and far-reaching health-related national legislation in the United States since the creation of Medicare (a health insurance programme administered by the US government that covers people who are either age 65 and over, or who meet other special criteria) and Medicaid (the largest source of funding for medical and health-related services for people with limited income in the United States);

◆ The CARE Act itself made an immediate and lasting impact on the care, treatment and support of PLWHA; and

◆ Perhaps more importantly, the CARE Act proved the ability of activists to work within the national political system to achieve their desired goals.

Other urgent objectives appeared achievable, such as: renewed attention to increased funding for prevention and risk reduction efforts; improvements in care systems at the state and local levels, including better care for women and children living with HIV, and for IDUs; continued work on stigma reduction and anti-discrimination; better prevention and clinical management of opportunistic infections (OIs); and basic science progress towards a vaccine. However, these objectives paled before the next greatest priority for all AIDS stakeholders: the search for the cure.

The pathogenesis and treatment of AIDS, 1994

Although the scientific understanding of the natural history and pathogenesis of AIDS in 1994 was relatively primitive by modern standards, considerable progress had been made. The isolation of HIV had enabled the development of the diagnostic HIV antibody test, the characterization of the natural history of HIV disease, the protection of the blood supply, and the development of antiviral therapy. However, HIV was understood to be a slow-moving infection with a prolonged latency period. Although additional HIV target cells and reservoirs such as the gonads and the central nervous system had been identified, AIDS pathogenesis was poorly understood. HIV disease progression was relentless and strongly associated with a CD4 cell decline of 100 cells/mm^3 per year, with more rapid progression in a quarter of those infected, and with rare individuals identified as 'long-term non-progressors' in whom the usual course of CD4 cell decline, disease progression and OIs was not seen.

The standard of care for antiretroviral therapy (ART) in 1994 was double NRTI therapy on the basis of the CPCRA FIRST study, the European Delta study and the ACTG 184 study, all of which compared double versus single NRTI therapy. The overall impact of the benefit was modest, with sustained CD4 cell increases for an additional one or two years, as compared with ZDV monotherapy, followed by treatment failure and CD4 count declines. At the same time, there was growing evidence of resistance to NRTIs with both single- and dual-drug ART.

Data from 1993's IX International AIDS Conference in Berlin on the optimal time to initiate ART were discouraging. Following the ACTG 016 and 019 studies of early ZDV monotherapy in 1990, treatment initiation was recommended when CD4 counts were below 500 cells/mm^3 [14]. However, these recommendations were modified when the Concorde study and the Veterans Administration (VA) collaborative study showed no benefit in starting ART treatment in patients with CD4 counts between 200 and 500 cells/mm^3, compared with patients who started treatment with CD4 counts below 200 cells/mm^3 or at the onset of significant clinical signs and symptoms. These variations were reflected in the short-lived HIV treatment guideline panels that were convened by the US National Institutes of Health (NIH).

Figure 10.2 illustrates the gradual improvement in life expectancy in people with AIDS in the United States since the beginning of the epidemic [15]. The period between 1985 and 1990 shows the impact of painstaking improvements in the diagnosis and prevention of OIs and the limited impact of early ART monotherapy, first with ZDV, and subsequently didanosine (ddI). The most important therapeutic advance during this period was *Pneumocystis carinii* pneumonia (PCP) prophylaxis; as shown in Figure 10.2, PCP prophylaxis reduced mortality by 50%. This observation provided an early lesson for the treatment of PLWHA, that ART was only one component

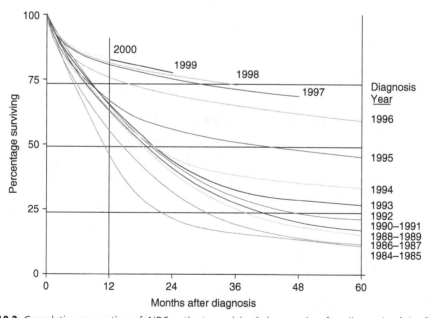

Fig. 10.2 Cumulative proportion of AIDS patients surviving*, by months after diagnosis of the first AIDS-defining opportunistic illness, for different years of diagnosis of the opportunistic illness.

* By product-limit method of survival analysis

of effective treatment, and that physician training and experience, OI treatment and prophylaxis, nutrition, and management of co-morbidities were also important. This lesson has presented additional challenges in present efforts to rapidly scale up care and treatment in the developing world.

New drug discovery and the NIH research agenda

The search for the cure in the United States was led by the pharmaceutical industry and the AIDS Clinical Trials Group (ACTG) of the NIH. The development of AZT (azidothymidine) by Burroughs-Wellcome in 1986 was followed by Bristol-Myers Squibb's ddI in 1992, and both were used as monotherapy until the landmark studies showing superior efficacy of double NRTIs in 1994, as noted above. During the period from 1988 to 1994, the NIH and the ACTG were increasingly criticized for conducting too many studies of AZT monotherapy to the exclusion of other new drug development.

Activist scrutiny shed light on the laborious process of new drug discovery and clinical trial design at the NIH, as well as the process of new drug approval and licensure by the Food and Drug Administration (FDA). An explicit objective of the activist agenda became the inclusion of PLWHA in the design, implementation and oversight of clinical trials. This notion, which is widely accepted today, was a radical departure from standard NIH procedure at the time. Treatment activist leaders from the Treatment Action Group (TAG) led the interaction with the FDA's AIDS Research Evaluation Working Group. Activists from the Lambda Legal Defense Fund, Project Inform, and ACT UP/New York (AIDS Coalition to Unleash Power) led advocacy efforts with the FDA to expedite the approval of new drugs. There were many other advocates for improved care and treatment at the national and local levels who were relentless in their activist interaction with the scientific and medical establishments. The leadership of Anthony Fauci, who was then and still is the Director of the NIH's National Institute of Allergy and Infectious Diseases (NIAID), was also central to these changes. He personally engaged with activists and succeeded in transforming a hostile and sometimes uninformed activist community into a well-informed, if often contentious, partner in the effort to expedite the process of new drug discovery, research and approval. From these often volatile interactions, the value of collaboration between researchers and PLWHA, without whom no clinical trials could be successfully conducted, was fully recognized for the design and conduct of the clinical trials.

Case study: AIDS in Chicago in 1994

In order to view the extraordinary impact of HAART, it is useful to consider a single city—Chicago—in the United States. In 1994, the HIV epidemic in Chicago passed two unfortunate milestones: the cumulative total cases of AIDS exceeded 10,000, and the total number of deaths in 1994 alone exceeded 1000 [16]. Important local trends included the fastest growth among women, adolescents, people of colour, IDUs and cases of heterosexual transmission. The fastest-growing areas of Chicago were the south and west sides of the city, in which the highest rates of infant mortality, TB, STIs and poverty were also located. More than 30,000 people were estimated to be living with HIV/AIDS in the greater Chicago Title I Eligible Metropolitan Area (EMA), defined as the City of Chicago, suburban Cook County and seven surrounding counties. However, only 11,000 PLWHA were identified and in care—around a third of those infected.

The major provider of public health services in Chicago was Cook County Hospital and its affiliated clinics in the Bureau of Health Services. In 1994, 1801 patients received primary care at the Cook County Hospital's HIV Primary Care Center, and together with patients from the network of county satellite clinics, 3351 patients were in care in the public sector, or 30% of those in care in the region. Hence, in Chicago, as in the rest of the United States, an increasing burden of HIV care was being shouldered by the public sector.

A closer look at the patients at Cook County Hospital in 1994 reveals the coming second wave of HIV in the United States [17]. Of 1801 patients, 530 (30%) were women, 71% were African American, 14% Latino (6% Mexican, 6% Puerto Rican and 2% other), 13% were white, and 1% were Asian. Thirty-three patients (1.6%) were teens aged 14–20. By risk behaviour, 35% were IDUs, 32% were gay/bisexual men, 24% had multiple heterosexual contacts, 1.4% were haemophiliac or transfused and 6% had HIV-infected parents. By stage of illness, 51% of patients had AIDS and 49% HIV infection with CD4 count above 200 cells/mm³. Thirty-two pregnant women living with HIV received care in 1994, as well as 128 patients with HIV/TB co-infection, three of whom had multi-drug resistant (MDR)-TB. By April 1994, 1181 PLWHA had died at Cook County Hospital since 1982. Finally, the enormous dependence of this population on the CARE Act and the services in the public sector is apparent in their payer mix data: 2% were privately insured, 39% were Medicaid enrolled, 3% were covered by Medicare/Social Security Administration (SSA) and 79% had no coverage. A typical clinic day in 1994 is described in Table 10.1.

Like other 'one stop' HIV caregivers in the United States, Cook County Hospital's HIV Primary Care Center became more sophisticated in providing a wide range of needed services to this diverse population. In addition to the 9121 primary medical care visits in 1994, the Center had 3355 mental health visits, 2362 chemical dependency counselling visits, 1620 clinical trial visits, and 12,819 case management visits, for a total of 29,829 distinct service visits in 1994 [17]. A third of this volume was located in a specialized clinic for women, children and families living with HIV, The Cook County Women and Children Program, which provided co-located paediatric, obstetrical and gynaecological care, medical care, reproductive counselling, early child development, on-site day care and other specialized services. This unique array of services culminated in the building of a specialized ambulatory facility, The CORE Center, in 1998 [18].

The rapidity of the rise in HIV cases in the public sector in Chicago in 1994 can be seen from the outcomes of HIV screening, case detection, and referral that were conducted in other sites at Cook County Hospital. One such site was the Ambulatory Screening Clinic, a walk-in public clinic that served 70,000 patients annually. A study of 1000 consecutive patients in 1992

Table 10.1 Patients from a single clinic day at Cook County Hospital, 1994

Patients
Acute withdrawal in a young African American heroin user
A pregnant HIV-positive Latina woman needing reproductive counselling
A young white gay man with new HIV, struggling with informing his partner
An African American family coping with a dying daughter
A young white woman seeking woman-centred contraception
An African American college professor recovering from PCP
A suicidal 55-year-old bisexual African American man with new HIV infection
A homeless white man with asymptomatic early infection needing busfare
An acutely ill Latino man with fever, chills, and altered mental status
An HIV-positive African American prisoner from the Cook County Jail

Source: Clinic record of Renslow Sherer, M.D.

demonstrated that, among the 515 (51%) patients with an STI, the HIV seroprevalence rate was 8% [19]. Another source of referrals was the HIV testing service at Cook County Hospital. Of the 4827 people tested in 1994, 395 (8.2%) were HIV-seropositive, of whom 250 were men and 145 were women. Of the 750 adolescents who agreed to HIV testing, eight (1.1%) were HIV-positive [20]. In sum, the rapidity of the rise in HIV cases in the Chicago area, and in particular in the public sector, was threatening to overwhelm the capacity for effective service delivery in 1994.

The early HAART era in the United States, 1995–2000

The HAART era began with critical advances in HIV pathogenesis. In 1995, *in vitro* studies defined HIV kinetics using one of the first FDA-approved protease inhibitors (PIs), ritonavir (RTV). A key element in this discovery was the extraordinary potency of PIs, which were shown to have the ability to reduce the viral load *in vitro* by 2–3 logs, far exceeding the potency of the existing classes of drugs. Ritonavir enabled the calculation of the HIV production rate of 10 billion virions per day and first- and second-order viral kinetics [21].

Of equal importance was the delineation of the plasma HIV viral RNA and its predictive value in the natural history of HIV disease. At Vancouver's groundbreaking XI International AIDS Conference in 1996, the Multicenter AIDS Cohort Study(MACS) researchers presented data showing that viral load strongly predicted HIV disease progression, leading to a dictum held dearly by HIV virologists to this day—'It's the virus, stupid' [22]. For the first time, researchers gave serious consideration to the possibility of viral eradication and a cure.

Two other breakthroughs set the stage for the HAART era in the United States. The first was the discovery of the composition and function of aspartyl protease enzyme by Dale Kempf and his colleagues in 1990, which led to Abbott Laboratories' development of RTV, saquinavir (SQV) by Roche Laboratories and indinavir (IDV) by Merck & Co., and which permanently linked PIs with the remarkable accomplishments of the early HAART era [23]. In addition, development of the first non-nucleoside reverse transcriptase inhibitor (NNRTI), nevirapine (NVP), by Boerhinger Ingelheim in 1995 was a key step, although its value was somewhat underappreciated at the time [24].

To the astonishment and excitement of everyone present, the XI International AIDS Conference ushered in the HAART era with a flourish. Two clinical trials permanently changed the course of HIV treatment history. Study 035 dramatically established the superiority of the combination of AZT, lamivudine (3TC) and IDV, over AZT and 3TC, or IDV monotherapy, in 93 treatment-naïve patients [25]. And Study 1090 showed the superiority of NVP in combination with 3TC and another NRTI over two NRTIs, in treatment-experienced but NVP-naïve patients [26]. The observation in Study 035 that the majority of drug-naïve patients achieved an undetectable viral load with average CD4 cell increases above 100 cells/mm^3 after 48 weeks was the finding that heralded the HAART era and provoked the greatest excitement. These outcomes far exceeded previous AIDS treatment trial outcomes and inspired hopes for long-term viral control and prevention of serious OIs, hopes that were to be realized in the early HAART era.

The impact of HAART in Chicago

The impact of HAART in Chicago was profound. Overall, from 1995 to 1997, there was a 61% decline in mortality. Figure 10.3 shows AIDS mortality from 1990–8 for the city of Chicago, and the impact of HAART. As shown, significant and comparable declines were observed in whites, African Americans and Latinos [3]. There were also comparable declines in the death rates in Chicago by gender, as shown in Figure 10.4. For both male and female African Americans, the total declines were the greatest, and the resulting case fatality rates in 1998 remained higher than for whites and Latinos.

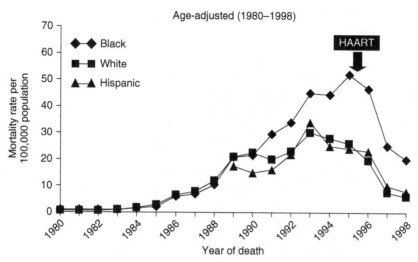

Fig. 10.3 HIV-associated mortality rates in Chicago by race and ethnicity, 1980–98.
Source: [3]

This study was the first in the United States on the impact of HAART in an entire urban population, and the outcomes were entirely consistent with reports from cohorts in clinical care in the private sector. For example, one report of 1255 patients in nine clinics in eight US cities found a mortality decline of 70%, from 29 deaths in 1995 to nine deaths in 1997 [27]. The data from the city of Chicago analyzed more than 30 times the number of fatalities and found a decline from 953 deaths in 1995 to 377 in 1997 [28].

In the pre-HAART era in the United States, it was found that declines in morbidity and mortality did not differ by sex, race or risk of HIV when access to care and treatment were ensured [29]. The Chicago mortality data suggest that the early HAART era had an equal impact on PLWHA in Chicago, regardless of race or gender. An analysis of mortality rates at Cook County Hospital found similar outcomes: mortality declined by 48% from 1995 to 1997, and by 62% from 1995 to 1998 [30]. Another study at Cook County Hospital demonstrated the value of

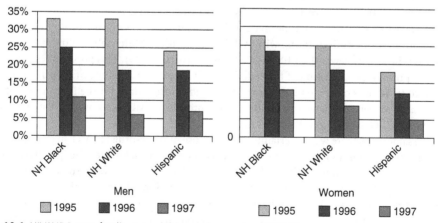

Fig. 10.4 HIV/AIDS case fatality rates (Chicago, by gender, 1995–7).
Source: [28]

HIV support services such as case management, drug counselling and mental health counselling in the retention of PLWHA; retention in primary care was 22% higher for patients who received these services compared with those in whom the need was unmet [17]. An invaluable lesson of the early HAART era was the need for comprehensive services to meet the diverse needs of PLWHA, which included access to HAART but went far beyond ART to include such support services as child care, reproductive counselling for women and families, co-location of paediatric and obstetric care with primary HIV care, primary and secondary HIV and STI prevention, and other specialty services—even transportation to the clinic.

Access to antiretroviral drugs varied in public and private treatment settings in the first year. For example, IDV was available only to private patients through a national pharmacy service for the first year following its approval by the FDA, but public patients, who were dependent on the public pharmacy, were unable to access IDV until 1998. RTV and SQV were available, but each had major limitations such as serious side effects and low bioavailability, respectively. When early reports of the combination of low-dose RTV and SQV first emerged, several advantages were apparent, including twice-daily dosing, reduced side effects and lack of dietary requirements [31]. A study at Cook County Hospital reported that 71% of patients had achieved viral loads <500 copies/mL after two years, and later studies confirmed the superiority of this twice-daily combination over indinavir-based regimens [32,33]. These early studies of the boosted PI combination of RTV and SQV anticipated two key features of the early HAART era in the United States: the urgent issue of treatment adherence and regimen simplification, and the preference for boosted PIs in international guidelines in the late HAART era.

The impact of HAART in the United States

As in Chicago, the impact of HAART across the United States was immediate and profound. People living with AIDS who had been wasted and bedridden regained their appetites, regained lost weight within weeks of starting HAART, and returned to productive lives. AIDS-related deaths declined precipitously by 61% from 1995 to 1997, which was an identical decline to that seen in Chicago, and AIDS dropped to the fifth most common cause of death among adults aged 25–44, as shown in Figure 10.5 [34]. Hospitalizations fell dramatically, as did the incidence of AIDS-associated OIs, and many private hospitals closed their AIDS wards. Figure 10.6 shows the decline in PCP, *Mycobacterium avium* complex (MAC), and cytomegalovirus (CMV) infection in PLWHA in the HIV Outpatient Study (HOPS) cohort from 1994 to 1999, from 7–20 events per 100 patient years to below five for each infection [27].

The impact of ART to prevent perinatal HIV transmission was equally profound. The estimated number of children living with AIDS in the United States fell by 90%, from nearly 1000 cases in 1992 to fewer than 100 in 2002 (Figure 10.7) [17, 35]. This progress resulted from the widespread implementation of the Pediatric ACTG protocol for the use of AZT in the second and third trimesters of pregnancy, intrapartum, and for the infant for the first month of life. These outcomes served as a beacon of hope for the promise of ART as a powerful tool to prevent mother-to-child transmission (PMTCT) of HIV.

At the same time, there was uncertainty about the use of triple-drug HAART in pregnancy due to the limited data on ART during pregnancy. This uncertainty highlighted the special reproductive issues for women living with HIV/AIDS and galvanized them (and their advocates) to demand adequate research into ART in pregnant women and equal consideration of the care and treatment of women for their own health, as well as for PMTCT and the health of the child. Similarly, the first HIV guidelines from the US Department of Health and Human Services (DHHS) in 1998 included the recommendation that women be treated with HAART according to recommended indications regardless of pregnancy status [36].

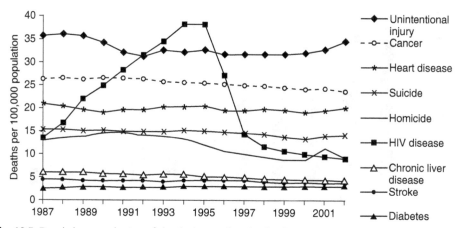

Fig. 10.5 Trends in annual rates of death due to the nine leading causes among persons 25–44 years of age, USA, 1987–2002.

Notes: For comparison with data for 1999 and later years, data for 1987–1988 were modified to account for ICD-10 rules instead of ICD-9 rules.

Source: [34].

Among the first consequences of the success of HAART was the formation of a permanent panel of experts to set national standards for its effective use. The NIH convened a panel of HIV experts in 1996 to articulate the principles of HIV treatment, and a second panel to create the first national guidelines for the use of ART in adults and adolescents based on those principles [37]. These panels promulgated a 'hit hard and hit early' strategy, recommending the initiation of HAART when CD4 counts were below 500 cells/mm^3 and/or the viral load exceeded 10–20,000 copies/mL. While these thresholds have been altered in subsequent versions, the overarching principles of treatment, i.e. to lower the viral load as much as possible—ideally, to below detection—and to raise the CD4 count as much as possible, remain unchanged to the present day.

The first guidelines summarized the current advances in the understanding of the pathogenesis of HIV, the critical roles and predictive values of the CD4 count and viral load, and the use of these tools to monitor therapeutic progress. Similarly, guidelines presented the current

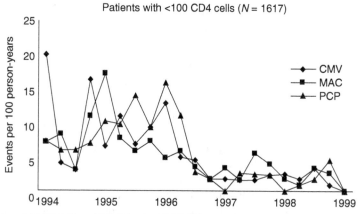

Fig. 10.6 Rates of CMV, PCP and MAC in the HOPS Cohort, 1994–9.

Source: [27] update: Palella, personal Communication, 1999.

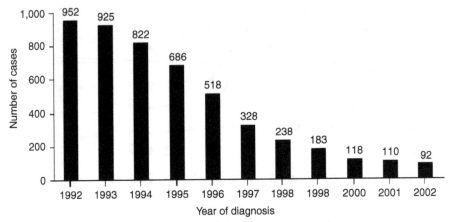

Fig. 10.7 Estimated numbers of AIDS diagnoses in children <13 years of age, by year of diagnosis, 1992–2002, United States.

Source: [35].

understanding of the variations in the natural history of untreated HIV disease, the relationship between the CD4 count and disease progression and the relationship between the slope of the CD4 count decline and the viral load.

The first treatment guidelines also addressed issues that continue to require the careful consideration of clinicians and patients today. These include:

- treatment toxicity and single-drug switches due to toxicity;
- issues related to treatment discontinuation;
- the need for optimal dosing of medications and the highest possible level of adherence to prescribed regimens and doses;
- the fact that changing regimens may constrain future treatment options, and therefore should be undertaken cautiously and according to specific virologic, immunologic and clinical criteria;
- that HAART in women, pregnant women, and children should be based on the same principles with the same goals of prolonging life, reducing morbidity and mortality, and improving the quality of life; and
- that, because HAART does not render patients non-infectious, even with better than adequate virologic control, the same principles of HIV prevention should be recommended to, and followed by, PLWHA who are taking HAART.

Adherence rapidly emerged as a critical threat to treatment success in the early HAART era. Initial studies suggested that taking more than 95% of doses was required for optimal treatment responses. These data came primarily from patients on unboosted PIs, for which the drug level necessary to maintain the antiviral effect is perilously close to the maximal plasma concentration, and thus unboosted PIs were particularly vulnerable to incomplete adherence. Although IDV had the fewest gastrointestinal side effects among the PIs, it quickly became a symbol of the complexity of HAART regimens because it required two pills to be taken on an empty stomach three times daily, and the ingestion of 40 ounces of water or more daily to prevent kidney stones. A standard regimen of IDV, AZT and 3TC would therefore require a total of 12 pills per day and a great deal of inconvenience, and many patients were unable to achieve or sustain adequate compliance. Subsequent versions of the DHHS Guidelines included a far more extensive section on treatment adherence.

By 1998, the need for better research and strategies on adherence led to two national initiatives, one regarding research convened by the Forum on Collaborative Research, and a second regarding practical implementation strategies by the Midwest AIDS Training and Education Center (MATEC). The pharmaceutical industry responded in several ways, including the investigation of simplified dosing strategies for existing drugs. Some of these were successful, such as the change from thrice-daily nelfinavir (NFV) to twice-daily dosing and the co-formulation of ZDV and 3TC as Combivir®, while others, such as boosted or twice-daily IDV, were unsuccessful. A second avenue of investigation was new drug discovery of once-daily compounds. This led to the development and approval of the NNRTI efavirenz (EFV), which is currently the most prescribed first-line antiretroviral drug in the United States, and once-daily second-generation PIs, including atazanavir (ATV), lopinavir (LPV) and the pro-drug fosamprenavir (fAPV).

The toxicity of antiretroviral drugs also emerged as a critical threat to the promise of HAART during its early era. Toxicity was found to be the most common reason for discontinuation, with gastrointestinal toxicity due to PIs leading to discontinuation in half of patients who stopped taking their medications. The DHHS Guidelines listed treatment toxicities and noted the importance of preparing patients for possible side effects, including overlapping side effects with other important medications for PLWHA, such as cotrimazole for PCP prophylaxis.

In the early HAART era, the first signs of serious long-term toxicities with antiretroviral regimens, and particularly with PI-containing regimens, were seen. Among these were lipid elevations and unexpected diabetes mellitus and insulin resistance in patients on PIs. Additionally, the NRTIs were seen to have several disparate side effects with common elements, such as AZT-associated myositis, which was clearly associated with mitochondrial toxicity in muscle cells. These observations anticipated the class effect of mitochondrial toxicity that has been linked to stavudine (d4T)-associated peripheral neuropathy, ddI-associated pancreatitis and neuropathy, and lactic acidosis, with all NRTIs.

In addition, the first signs of morphologic changes, particularly facial and limb lipoatrophy, were being reported in patients on HAART; this manifestation was found to be related to mitochondrial toxicity in adipocytes due to the NRTIs d4T and ddI and, to a lesser extent, ZDV. At the same time, the so-called protease paunch, with excess fat accumulation centrally as well as irregular fatty deposits elsewhere in the body, such as the dorso-cervical fat pad or 'buffalo hump', were associated with PIs at the end of the pre-HAART era in 1998–1999 [38].

These observations were devastating to the hopes of PLWHA for long-term health and normalcy, if not treatment eradication and cure, that characterized the early HAART era. Worst of all was the possibility that HAART itself could lead to the same kind of public exposure and recognition as AIDS itself had done in the past, due to the striking characteristics of the gaunt, lipoatrophic facies that results from the loss of facial subcutaneous fat. In the popular mind and the press, the same antiretroviral regimens that were heralded as the 'end of AIDS' and the promise of prolonged health were now viewed as potentially toxic and disfiguring. Renewed pressure was put on the research establishment to clarify the causes of this dreadful new set of side effects and to identify ways to treat them, as well as to find alternative treatments, a search that continues to the present.

Another threat to the enormous success and promise of HAART was the emergence of HIV drug resistance. The success of the first antiretroviral regimens in treatment-naïve patients contrasted with the outcomes of HAART in those PLWHA who had had prior treatment with single- and double-drug therapy. Treatment success was far more difficult to achieve in these patients, and resistance to the new PIs was more common. A second growing threat was the rise in transmitted drug resistance. This issue was also addressed thoroughly in the first HIV treatment guidelines, with the admonition that the best way to manage resistance is to prevent it through the use of maximally potent regimens in treatment-naïve patients.

HAART changed the natural history of HIV disease. Several cohort studies showed that fewer people were dying from AIDS-related complications, and the causes of morbidity and mortality shifted to a greater frequency of non HIV-associated causes. At Cook County Hospital, for example, non-HIV causes of death in PLWHA rose from 8% in 1995 to 32% in 2000 (Figure 10.8) [39]. Two-thirds of this mortality was due to chronic liver disease. Note also the sobering reality that, while the death rate from AIDS had fallen substantially, HAART had not removed all HIV-associated morbidity and mortality. At that time in the United States, as now, most patients presented with AIDS and CD4 counts below 200 cells/mm³, and many died from their first OI. Others failed to get the benefit from HAART due to adverse effects, drug resistance, poor adherence, lack of durable access to care and treatment, and other reasons.

An unexpected consequence of HAART that bears on these observations has recently been identified. Several cohort studies have shown that HAART has an impact on both HIV and non-HIV causes of mortality. The Data Collection on Adverse events of Anti-HIV Drugs (D:A:D) study is an observational study to determine the incidence of cardiovascular disease and other causes of morbidity and mortality. As shown in Figure 10.9 [40], the risk of mortality from all causes, including non-HIV causes such as cardiovascular disease, kidney disease and non-HIV cancers, increases as the CD4 count declines. These data suggest that HAART has a beneficial impact on both HIV and non-HIV causes of morbidity and mortality, and point towards a critical area for future research [41].

The final impediment to the success of HAART, an issue that is no less urgent in the present day, is the disparities in access to care and treatment of PLWHA. Access to HAART was immediate in 1996 for patients in the private sector. However, access to HAART among public sector patients varied widely among states. Patients at the lowest end of the economic spectrum were able to gain access to HAART over time under Title II of the CARE Act through the AIDS Drug Assistance Program (ADAP). However, the administration of ADAP was at the discretion of state governments, and thus wide disparities existed among the states and persist into the late HAART era, as described below.

The late HAART era, 2000–2006

The late HAART era in the United States has been characterized by new drugs and formulations with improved regimen simplification and lower toxicities, new treatment targets such as viral entry and integrase, better treatment options for the treatment-experienced patient,

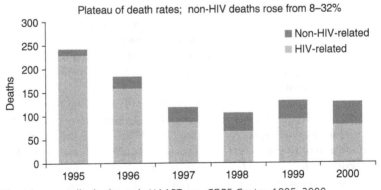

Fig. 10.8 Changing mortality in the early HAART era, CORE Center, 1995–2000.

Source: [39].

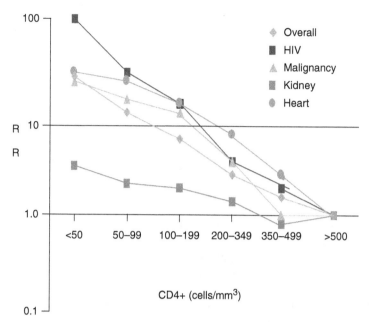

Fig. 10.9 Relative risk of HIV and non-HIV causes of death by CD4 strata in the D:A:D Study. *Source*: [40].

broader research into novel strategies and more progress on durable treatment outcomes. Several first-line regimen options of five or fewer pills administered once daily exist, including a single three-drug combination pill containing EFV, tenofovir (TDF) and emtricitabine (FTC) (Truvada®). The frequency of first-line regimen failures fell to below 10% in some clinical trials and cohorts, and long-term studies showed the leading regimens to have durable effects, with over two-thirds of patients achieving viral loads below detection, without symptoms or unacceptable side effects, for periods of three to seven years [42].

As another example of the remarkable progress in the late HAART era, the most recent version of the DHHS Guidelines revised its goals for heavily treatment-experienced patients. Recent trials of tipranavir (TPV), darunavir (DRV), maraviroc (MRV) and raltegravir (RAL) in heavily treatment-experienced patients have shown that 50% or more can achieve an undetectable viral load and significant CD4 cell increases with combinations of the newest drugs, as long as two or more active drugs and one new class of drugs are included in the regimen [43].

Unfortunately, access to care and treatment remains a growing threat in the late HAART era. By 2002, 80,035 PLWHA were on HAART with support from ADAP, which represented a 154% increase from 1996 to 2002, and 257,279 prescriptions were filled in June 2002. The costs associated with this programme increased 366% from 1996 to 2002, and the total budget was US$878 million, which was over four times its original cost in 1990 [44]. The programme participants largely reflected the demographics of AIDS at the time: 33% were African Americans, 37% were white, 25% were Latino and 1% were Asian and Pacific Islander; 22% of participants were women. Half of the participants had incomes below the federal poverty level, which at the time was an annual income of US$8,860, and 27% were uninsured at the time of the HIV/AIDS diagnosis. Three states—California, New York, and Florida—had participant levels from 10,000–15,000, with annual ADAP budgets of US$6–14 million. Illinois was the eighth highest state with 1500 enrollees and an annual budget of US$2.2 million. Thirteen states, including Texas and Georgia, had limited enrolment and/or prolonged waiting lists. At that time,

ADAP was experiencing a serious budget shortfall at the national and state levels, with a deficit of US$145 million at the end of 2002. Conservative estimates in 2002 were that 100,000 US residents with HIV/AIDS in need of treatment were unable to access HAART. In 2006, the ADAP spent US$790 million nationwide [45]. Because the CARE Act received level funding from 2004–6, while AIDS prevalence has increased significantly, ADAPs were further stretched by 2006, waiting lists were growing and drug formularies were increasingly restricted.

For those in the United States able to access HAART, the late HAART era has seen important additional advances in drug formulations and new drug development. The success of Combivir® led to co-formulations of second-line NRTIs and the nucleotide TDF in the form of Truvada® as well as Epzicom™ (co-formulated abacavir (ABC) and 3TC). Both of these co-formulations have the advantage of a single pill once daily, which, with EFV, provides a very simple regimen of two pills per day. The other important benefit of these drugs is the absence of mitochondrial toxicity and lipoatrophy, which has led to their widespread replacement of the thymidine analogue nucleosides as initial HAART agents. In 1996, Atripla™, which is co-formulated EFV, TDF and FTC, was approved as the first one-pill once-daily regimen, as noted above. Among the second-generation PIs, Kaletra® was approved in 2002 as the first co-formulated PI combining LPV and RTV. Along with ATV and fAPV, the new PIs were better tolerated and had higher potency, particularly when used boosted with RTV. The additional attribute of the boosted PIs was the remarkable infrequency of drug resistance associated with them, even in the presence of prolonged virologic failure, as best shown by the LPV developmental trials. By the end of the first decade of HAART, even more potent third-generation PIs—tipranavir (TPV) and darunavir (DRV)—had been developed that were active against viruses resistant to all other members of the class [46, 47]. As well, promising second-line NNRTIs such as the experimental drugs etravirine (formerly TMC 125) and rilpivirine (formerly TMC 278) were entering into phase III trials and expanded access [43].

The most remarkable therapeutic breakthroughs in the late HAART era have been the novel HIV targets, including a variety of viral entry targets, integrase, and viral maturation. Enfuvirtide (ENF), which blocks the fusion of entry proteins, both proved the concept of the therapeutic viral entry blockade and added an important ray of hope for the heavily resistant and treatment-experienced patient [48]. More recently, two CCR5 entry protein inhibitors—maraviroc (MRV) and vicriviroc—have shown promise in early clinical trials; maraviroc gained FDA approval in 2007 [43]. Two integrase inhibitor candidate drugs are in later stages of development, with the Merck & Co. compound RAL available by expanded access and showing remarkable potency and tolerability [43]. The pipeline for other novel targets, such as viral maturation, is robust.

Because of the emergence of serious long-term treatment toxicities, interest in treatment interruption arose in the late HAART era as a means to reduce toxicity and cost. Most of the interruption strategies in most stages of illness failed to show benefit while showing a cost of interruption, most commonly either HIV disease progression or drug resistance. Discontinuation of HAART in the advanced patient with a heavily resistant virus, treatment interruption in acute HIV infection, and so-called 'structured treatment interruption' strategies have all failed. There have been limited successes with CD4-guided treatment interruptions that call for withdrawal of HAART when CD4 cells exceed a given threshold, usually 350–500 cells/mm^3, but only when HAART is resumed at a threshold of 300–350 cells/mm^3 or more. The landmark Strategies for Management of Anti-Retroviral Therapy (SMART) study of 5472 enrolled patients showed conclusively that a lower threshold for resumption of HAART of 250 cells/mm^3 was too low, and the risk of HIV disease progression or death was 1.6 times greater in the treatment discontinuation group [49]. A surprising finding was the greater incidence of non-HIV morbidity and mortality due to cardiovascular and renal disease and other causes in the treatment discontinuation group compared with the group that stayed on treatment. As with the D:A:D mortality data above, HAART is clearly playing a beneficial role for both HIV and non HIV causes of mortality.

Summary and future considerations

Highly active antiretroviral therapy represents a stunning achievement. In the first decade of HAART in the United States, more than 3 million productive years of life were saved, and a relentlessly progressive and fatal illness was transformed into a manageable chronic illness. However, a challenging scientific agenda remains for the treatment of HIV disease. Addressing the diverse needs of PLWHA with comprehensive services has been shown to be optimal, but such systems are complex to develop, manage and replicate. Effective care requires both HAART and more than HAART, i.e. an experienced physician or clinician with a comprehensive system of care and support.

Adherence is a persistent problem for some patients in spite of the reduction of toxicities and the simplification of regimens. Alternate strategies, including directly observed therapy, are needed to address this issue in chronically non-adherent patients. Though diminished in severity and frequency, treatment toxicity remains a difficult problem, and a deeper understanding of the morphologic and metabolic complications of HAART, as well as better alternatives to the often disfiguring facial lipoatrophy, dorso-cervical fat pad and lipomata, remain important priorities. With more morbidity and mortality in this era due to non HIV-related conditions, further research and better treatment alternatives are needed for co-morbidities such as infection with hepatitis C virus (HCV) and the growing impact of cardiovascular disease. There are many manifestations of HIV that are less responsive to HAART, such as neurological consequences and some neoplasms, particularly non-Hodgkin's lymphoma. As PLWHA age, the overlapping issues of HIV disease and aging are becoming apparent. And with the stabilization of HIV disease, more couples with HIV are seeking the means to conceive children without the risk of HIV infection.

A challenging scientific agenda also remains for HIV prevention strategies. This should garner a greater portion of the attention and resources of the AIDS scientific establishment, given the maturity of HAART. Recent promising advances in circumcision, microbicides and HIV vaccine research suggest that real progress is coming in the near future. Moreover, HAART itself has made a substantial contribution to HIV prevention. Although HAART is an imperfect prevention tool that should always be accompanied by traditional methods of HIV prevention, it was invaluable to learn that with every log decline in plasma viral load due to HAART, the risk of HIV transmission declines 2.45 times [50].

Too often, the process of basic and clinical research itself, the infrastructure and personnel necessary to conduct it, the resources to support it, and the patients and subjects who participate in it, are overlooked in the consideration of the lessons of HAART. This is no small irony, as there would be no HAART era without these individuals and these systems. A critical lesson of the HAART era is the need to expand clinical and basic research on behalf of PLWHA. An important corollary, as the scientific establishment has increasingly engaged in trials and research in the developing world, is the absolute requirement for the thorough involvement of PLWHA in the design and implementation of these trials, and for the highest standards of conduct for research in these settings as can be found in the United States.

The final lessons learned from the first decade of HAART concern our responsibility to ensure access to HAART for all Americans and the need to nurture the political clout of the AIDS advocacy coalition and direct its energies to the proper priorities. The deficiencies in the US healthcare system that have continued to deny access to HAART to an estimated 100,000 Americans with HIV disease must be overcome. The same powerful coalition for AIDS advocacy that enabled the creation of the CARE Act, the integration of PLWHA into NIH research design and implementation, and the reform of outdated procedures at the FDA must maintain vigilance to overcome the obstacles to HIV/AIDS care and treatment delivery in the United States. At a moment in US history when national healthcare reform is being debated, and when so many advocates and researchers are engaged in the battle against AIDS in Africa and elsewhere in the developing world, the powerful AIDS advocacy coalition can use its strong voice on behalf of those PLWHA in the United States who do not have access to HAART.

The last lesson of the first decade of HAART concerns the responsibility of the United States to maintain and expand the global effort to achieve access to HIV care and treatment beyond the 2 million people in the world who are currently receiving HAART. The contributions to date through the US President's Emergency Program for AIDS Relief (PEPFAR), the Global Fund to Fight AIDS, Tuberculosis and Malaria, and private efforts are the largest in the world, but they still have fallen far short of the amount that could be given. As Harvard economist Jeffrey Sachs has argued, there are enough resources in the world to end poverty and achieve adequate healthcare, including HAART, for the people of the developing world, if the political will is present [51]. For those who have experienced the miracle of HAART in the United States and will reap its benefits in the decades to come, the lasting lesson of HAART is the urgency of the mission to share the miracle and provide durable HIV care and treatment throughout the world.

References

1. US Centers for Disease Control and Prevention (CDC). (1996). *AIDS/HIV Surveillance Report, 1995, (Vol 7: No 2)*. Atlanta: US Department of Health and Human Services, Public Health Service.

2. US Centers for Disease Control and Prevention (CDC). (1996). Update: Mortality Attributable to HIV Infection Among Persons Aged 25–44 – United States, 1994. *Morbidity and Mortality Weekly Report (MMWR)* **45**:121–125.

3. Whitman S, Murphy J, Cohen M, Sherer R. (2000). Marked declines in human immunodeficiency virus-related mortality in Chicago in women, African Americans, Hispanics, young adults, and injection drug users, from 1995 through 1997. *Arch Int Med* **160**:365–369.

4. Sherer R, Pulvirenti J, Cohen M, *et al.* (1998). Six-year improvement in HIV hospital outcomes at Cook County Hospital, Chicago: Impact of AIDS Care Units and HAART. Fifth International Conference on Retroviruses and Opportunistic Infections, 2 February 1998, Chicago, USA. [Abstract #206]

5. Wallensky RP, Paltiel AD, Losina E, *et al.* (2006). The survival benefits of AIDS treatment in the United States. *J Infect Dis* **194**:11–19.

6. US Centers for Disease Control and Prevention (CDC). (1996). Summary of Notifiable Diseases, United States, 1996. *MMWR* **45**:1–28.

7. US Centers for Disease Control and Prevention (CDC). (1996). HIV testing among women aged 18–44 years – United States, 1991 and 1993. *MMWR* **45**:733–737.

8. US Centers for Disease Control and Prevention (CDC). (1997). Update: Trends in AIDS Incidence, Deaths, and Prevalence – United States, 1996. *MMWR* **46**:166–173.

9. Prevots RD, Allen DM, Lehman JS, *et al.* (1996). Trends in HIV seroprevalence among injection drug users entering drug treatment centers, United States, 1988–1993. *Am J Epidemiol* **143**:733–42.

10. US Centers for Disease Control and Prevention (CDC). (1996). AIDS associated with injecting drug use – United States, 1995. *MMWR* **45**:392–398.

11. Connor EM, Sperling RS, Gelber R, *et al.* (1994). Reduction of maternal-infant transmission of human immunodeficiency virus type 1 with zidovudine treatment. *New Engl J Med* **331**:1173–80.

12. US Centers for Disease Control and Prevention (CDC). (1996). HIV testing among women aged 18–44 years – United States, 1991 and 1993. *MMWR* **45**:733–737.

13. Health Resources and Services Administration. *Reports and Studies: Ryan White HIV/AIDS Program Appropriations*. Available at http://hab/hrsa.gov/reports/funding.htm (accessed April 30, 2007).

14. Advisory Group on HIV Early Intervention, American Medical Association. (1994). Human Immunodeficiency Virus Early Intervention Guidelines, Second Edition. *Arch Fam Med* **3**:988–1002.

15. US Centers for Disease Control and Prevention (CDC). (1994). *HIV/AIDS Surveillance report, Vol 6:No 2,* Atlanta: US Department of Health and Human Services. p1–39.

16. Chicago Department of Public Health. (1994). *AIDS Report, 1994.* Chicago: Chicago Department of Public Health.

17. Sherer R, Stieglitz K, Narra J, *et al.* (2002). HIV Multidisciplinary Teams Work: Support Services Improve Access to and Retention in HIV Primary Care. *AIDS Care* **14**(S):S31–S44.

18. Sherer R and Cohen M. (1998). The CORE Center for Prevention, Care, and Research of Infectious Disease. *Chicago Medicine* **101**:12–17.

19. Ansell DA, Tzyy-Chyn H, Straus M, Cohen M, Sherer R. (1994). HIV and Syphilis Seroprevalence among clients with Sexually Transmitted Diseases Attending a Walk-In Clinic at Cook County Hospital. *Sex Trans Dis* **21**:93–96.

20. Cohen G, Sherer R, Cohen M, Williamson M, Albrecht G. (1994). The Change in Demand for HIV counseling and testing among 20,000 inner city minority patients at Cook County Hospital, Chicago, 1987–1993. X International AIDS Conference, 7–12 August 1994, Yokohama, Japan. [Abstract C512]

21. Perelson AS, Essinger P, Cao Y, *et al.* (1997). Decay of HIV-1 infected compartments during combination therapy. *Nature* **387**:188–91.

22. Mellors JW, Munoz A, Giorgi JV, *et al.* (1996). Plasma viral load and CD4+ lymphocytes from 200 to 500/mm3. *Ann Int Med* **335**:1081–90.

23. Kempf D, Norbeck DW, Codacovi L, *et al.* (1990). Structure-based, C2 symmetric inhibitors of HIV protease. *J Med Chem* **33**(10):2687–9.

24. Boehringer Ingelheim. (2006). *Viramune*® (nevirapine) package insert. Ingelheim, Germany: Boehringer Ingelheim.

25. Hammer S. Gulick R, Havlir D, *et al.* (1997). A controlled trial of two nucleoside analogues plus indinavir in persons with human immunodeficiency virus infection and CD4 counts of 200 per cubic millimeter or less. *New Engl J Med* **337**:725–33.

26. Lange JM. (2003). Efficacy and durability of nevirapine in ART naïve patients. *Jl Acquir Immune Defic Syndr* **34**(Suppl 1):S40–52.

27. Pallela FJ, Delaney KM, Moorman AC, *et al.* (1998). Declining morbidity and mortality among patients with advanced human immunodeficiency virus infection. *N Engl J Med* **338**:853–860.

28. Sherer R, Pulvirenti J, Cohen M, *et al.* (1998). Six-year improvement in HIV hospital outcomes at Cook County Hospital, Chicago: Impact of AIDS Care Units and HAART. Fifth International Conference on Retroviruses and Opportunistic Infections, 2 February 1998, Chicago, USA. [Abstract 206]

29. Chaisson RE, Keruly JC, Moore RD. (1995). Race, sex, drug use, and progression of HIV disease. *N Eng J Med* **333**:751–756.

30. Sherer R, Jasek J, Cohen M, *et al.* (1999). 48% decline in mortality from 1995–1997 in HIV patients at Cook County Hospital in Chicago. American Public Health Association Conference, 8 November 1999, Chicago, USA. [Abstract 4594]

31. Cameron DW, Japour AJ, Xu Y, *et al.* (1999). Ritonavir and saquinavir combination therapy for the treatment of HIV infection. *AIDS* **13**:213–244.

32. Sherer R, Rajaram V, Maclean M, Teter C. (1999). Two-year follow-up of therapy with Ritonavir and Saquinavir plus two NRTIs: Viral and CD4 outcomes, metabolic complications, and implications for salvage therapy. *Antiviral Therapy* **4**:21–23.

33. Kirk O, Katzenstein TL, Gerstoft J, *et al.* (1999). Combination Therapy containing ritonavir plus saquinavir has superior short-term antiretroviral efficacy: a randomized trial. *AIDS* **13**:9–16.

34. US Centers for Disease Control and Prevention (CDC). (1998). United States HIV and AIDS cases reported through June, 1998. *HIV/AIDS Surveillance Report* **10**:1–40.

35. US Centers for Disease Control and Prevention (CDC). (2002). *HIV/AIDS Surveillance Report* **14**:15. Atlanta: US Department of Health and Human Services

36. Connor EM, Sperling RS, Gelber R, *et al.* (1994). Reduction of maternal-infant transmission of human immunodeficiency virus type 1 with zidovudine treatment. *New Engl J Med* **331**:1173–80.

37. US Centers for Disease Control and Prevention (CDC). (1998). Report of the NIH Panel to Define Principles of Therapy of HIV Infection and Guidelines for the Use of Antiretroviral Therapy in Adults and Adolescents. *MMWR* **47**(RR-5):1–96.

38. Max B, Sherer R. (2000). Management of Adverse Effects of Antiretorviral Therapy and Medication Adherence. *Clin Inf Dis* **30**(Suppl 2):S96–116.

39. Green L, Cohen M, Sherer R, *et al.* (2002). Trends in causes of death by gender in Chicago since HAART, 1996 – 2000. XIX World AIDS Conference, 5 July 2002, Barcelona, Spain. [Abstract 337]

40. Weber R, Fris-Muller F, Sabin C, *et al.* (2005). HIV and non-HIV-related deaths and their relationship to immunodeficiency: The D:A:D Study. 12th Conference on Retroviruses and Opportunistic Infections (CROI), 22–25 February 2005, Boston, USA. [Abstract 595]

41. Weber R, Fris-Muller F, Sabin C, *et al.* (2005). HIV and non-HIV-related deaths and their relationship to immunodeficiency: The D:A:D Study. 12th Conference on Retroviruses and Opportunistic Infections (CROI), 22–25 February 2005, Boston, USA. [Abstract 595]

42. United States Department of Health and Human Services. (2007). *Guidelines for the Use of Antiviral Agents in HIV-1 Infected Adults and Adolescents, April 17, 2007*. Available at http://AIDSinfo.nih.gov (accessed April 30, 2007).

43. Kuritzkes D. (2007). New agents and new paradigms: The complexity of CCR5 inhibition. 14th Conference on Retroviruses and Opportunistic Infections (CROI), 27 February 2007, Los Angeles, USA. [Abstract 108]

44. Kaiser Family Foundation. (2003). *ADAP Summary, April, 2003*. Available at http://KFF.org (accessed May 12, 2003).

45. Health Resources and Services Administration. *Ryan White CARE Act Overview*. Available at http://hab/hrsa.gov/reports/funding.htm (accessed April 30, 2007).

46. Boehringer Ingelheim. (2006). *Aptivus*® (tipranavir) package insert. Ingelheim, Germany: Boehringer Ingelheim.

47. Ortho Biotech. (2007). *Prezista* ᵀᴹ *(darunavir) package insert*. Bridgewater NJ, USA: Ortho Biotech.

48. Roche Laboratories Inc. and Trimeris, Inc. (2006). *Fuzeon*® (enfuvirtide) package insert. Nutley, NJ, USA: Roche Laboratories Inc. and Trimeris, Inc.

49. The Strategies for the Management of Anti-Retroviral Therapy (SMART) Study Group.(2006). CD4 guided interruption of antiretroviral therapy. *New Engl J Med* **355**:2359–61.

50. Quinn TC, Wawer MJ, Sewankambo M, *et al.* (2000). Viral load and heterosexual transmission of HIV1: Rakai Cohort Study Group. *New Engl J Med* **342**:921–9.

51. Sachs JD. (2005). *The End of Poverty – Economic Possibilities for Our Time*. London, UK: Penguin Press. p43–47.

Chapter 11

US Cohorts review: The HIV Outpatient Study (HOPS) and the Multicenter AIDS Cohort Study (MACS)

Frank J. Palella, Jr*, Anne C. Moorman, and
John T. Brooks (HOPS); John Phair*, Lisa Jacobson,
Roger Detels, Joseph Margolick and
Charles Rinaldo (MACS)

Introduction

Knowledge about the basic mechanisms of disease has increased to a great extent over the past 20 years, as has medical science's ability to translate knowledge gained into innovations that can be applied to patients. This is largely due to clinical research, whose earliest recorded history traces as far back as the court of King Nebuchadnezzar II, as documented in the Old Testament [1]. However, the first widely known clinical study was conducted by James Lind, a Scottish physician who, while serving as surgeon on HMS Salisbury in the late 1770s, experimented on a parallel control group of 12 sailors—all afflicted with scurvy—to whom he administered six different treatments to ultimately demonstrate that citrus fruit cures scurvy [2]. Since this earliest of trial-and-error studies, the number of clinical trials conducted worldwide has risen exponentially. In the United States alone, for example, the number of clinical trials performed in 2005 was 8386 and, at an average annual growth rate of 5.8%, experts predict their number will reach more than 13,000 by 2011 [3].

In the field of HIV medicine, interventional and observational studies have been used to great effect in determining the safety and efficacy of anti-HIV medications as well as tracking health outcomes among HIV-positive patients treated with highly active antiretroviral therapy (HAART) [4]. Observational studies—in the form of cohort studies—have been a key tool for a spectrum of investigations, including the characterization of HIV natural history, identification of non-interventional factors influencing HIV disease progression, and the evaluation of therapies and interventions for adverse effects and intended (beneficial) effects [4]. Among the largest—and most cited—cohort studies in the United States are HOPS (HIV Outpatient Study) and MACS (Multicenter AIDS Cohort Study). An overview of both these studies is presented below.

1. The HIV Outpatient Study

The HIV Outpatient Study (HOPS) is a prospective observational cohort study that was initiated in 1993 by the US Centers for Disease Control and Prevention (CDC), and is currently expected

* Corresponding authors.

to continue collecting and analyzing longitudinal data on HIV-infected outpatients until mid-2011. It is the longest-running and only remaining US government-sponsored multi-site prospective cohort of a diverse spectrum of people living with HIV infection and receiving routine clinical care in the United States.

The objectives of the HOPS are:

♦ to describe and monitor trends in the demographics, symptoms, diagnoses and treatment of a dynamic population of HIV-infected outpatients seen in clinics across the United States;

♦ to describe factors associated with clinical, immunologic and virologic success, such as prolonged survival; and

♦ to describe emerging problems with long-term HIV infection and its treatment.

This continuously enrolling cohort includes HIV-infected individuals seen at up to 12 (currently eight) clinics specializing in the treatment of HIV infection in seven US cities: Chicago; Denver; Stony Brook, NY; Oakland/San Leandro, CA; Philadelphia; Tampa, FL; and Washington, DC. Earlier sites that are no longer active were also located in Atlanta and Portland, OR. The physicians at HOPS sites routinely care for hundreds of HIV-infected patients every year. From 1993–2007, longitudinal data were collected on more than 8000 HIV-infected ambulatory patients seen at over 300,000 outpatient visits during over 32,000 person-years of follow-up (median 2.6 years). Approximately 2500 patients actively participate in the HOPS annually.

At baseline, data collected include information on sociodemographics and risk behaviours such as smoking, alcohol consumption and drug use. During follow-up, clinical data from all visits are continuously collected through real-time chart abstraction by trained personnel at each participating site. These data include symptoms, probable and confirmed diagnoses, prescribed drug treatments (including dosages, formulations and frequencies), and results of all laboratory tests, including local laboratory normal limits. HIV-specific laboratory data include CD4 counts, HIV viral load determinations, and results of HIV genotypic and phenotypic resistance testing. These data are entered into an electronic data collection system and transmitted monthly to a contracted data management company.

The HOPS began in 1993 with enrolment of approximately 1800 patients. To maintain the open cohort, each study site continuously enrols new HOPS patients. A median 12.4% of patients are lost annually due to death (2.9%) or loss to follow-up (9.5%). At the three current private-practice HOPS clinics (Denver; Tampa, FL; Washington, DC), with approximately 1000 patients and comprising 40% of the existing HOPS population, all new and existing patients are offered enrolment in the HOPS, and clinic enrolment rates have been maintained at over 95% of the total clinic population. At the five participating university-based clinics (Chicago; Denver; Philadelphia; Stony Brook, NY; Washington, DC) with approximately 1500 patients, comprising 60% of the active HOPS patient population, new enrolment is limited in order to maintain the cohort at a stable size while capturing at least 25% of the participating investigators' active clinic population. The percentage of clinic patients enrolled in the HOPS ranges from 26% to 95%, or 169 to 444 active HOPS patients per clinic.

Table 11.1 summarizes sociodemographic characteristics of all HOPS patients seen since 1993, as well as those active in 2006. Of all those seen since 1993, 19.5% have been female, 30.6% African American, and 10.8% Latino. Fifty percent of participants have been men who have sex with men (MSM), 23.2% had an HIV risk of high-risk heterosexual activity, and 14.1% have used injection drugs. Payment for medical services was from public funding sources (Medicare, Medicaid, Ryan White or others) for 43.1%, and 46.1% were privately insured. Sixty-one percent

Table 11.1 Demographic characteristics of the HIV Outpatient Study (HOPS) cohort, 1993–2006

Demographics	n (%)	n (%)
Gender		
Male	6632 (80.5%)	2018 (77.5%)
Female	1610 (19.5%)	586 (22.5%)
HIV Risk		
Men who have sex with men (MSM)	4738 (57.5%)	1520 (58.4%)
Injection drug use (IDU)	1162 (14.1%)	254 (9.8%)
High risk heterosexual sex partners	1915 (23.2%)	694 (26.7%)
Other/unknown	427 (5.2%)	136 (5.2%)
Race		
White	4597 (55.8%)	1435 (55.1%)
Black	2518 (30.6%)	814 (31.3%)
Latino	894 (10.8%)	288 (11.1%)
Other	233 (2.9%)	67 (2.6%)
Method of payment for medical services		
Private health insurance	3800 (46.1%)	1410 (54.1%)
Public payer (Medicare, Medicaid, Ryan White, other)	3551 (43.1%)	961 (36.9%)
Other/unknown	897 (10.8%)	233 (8.9%)
AIDS case status at most recent follow-up		
AIDS	5027 (61.0%)	1535 (58.9%)
No AIDS	3215 (39.0%)	1069 (41.1%)
	Total cohort 1993-2006 (n=8242)	Patients active in 2006 (n=2604)

of patients had met the AIDS case definition by their last follow-up. Of the 2604 currently active patients, 22.5% are female, 31.3% African American and 11.1% Latino. Fifty-eight percent are MSM, 26.7% have had an HIV risk of high-risk heterosexual activity, and 9.8% have used injection drugs. Payment for medical services is from public sources for 36.9%, while 54.1% are privately insured. The AIDS case definition has been met by 58.9% of currently active patients.

Over the past decade, diverse and numerous analyses have been conducted using the HOPS data. Some of these are summarized below.

Survival and disease trends and responses to HAART

The HOPS was among the first cohorts to demonstrate the marked and sustained clinical efficacy of HAART use, reporting both a 10-fold decline in death rates associated with its widespread introduction and similarly dramatic declines in AIDS-related opportunistic infections (OIs), particularly among people with CD4 counts <100 cells/mm3 [5] (Figure 11.1). Subsequent HOPS work identified factors associated with achieving durable clinical responses to HAART, as measured by changes in CD4 counts and reductions in both plasma HIV RNA levels and OI rates, and profiled changes over time in antiretroviral therapies prescribed by HIV providers [6–10].

Analyses of HOPS data have also shown that AIDS-related death and OI rates have remained durably low among HAART recipients, while the causes of death among HAART recipients have shifted from AIDS-related to non AIDS-related illnesses, notably pulmonary, cardiovascular, renal and hepatic disorders, as well as non AIDS-associated malignancies [11] (Figure 11.2a).

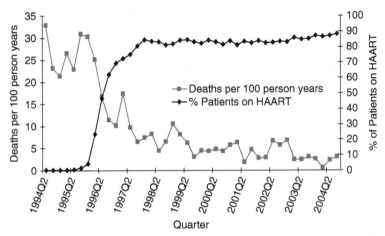

Fig. 11.1 Mortality and HAART use over time — HOPS patients with CD4 nadir <100 cells/mm³ as of 31 December 2004 (last quarter).

Similarly, while overall hospitalization rates have declined markedly among HOPS participants [12], non AIDS-related conditions have become as frequent causes of hospitalization as OIs (Figure 11.2 b,c) (K. Buchacz, unpublished data, 2007).

The HOPS has also monitored and published data on patterns and incidence rates of specific infections, both opportunistic and non-opportunistic, during both the pre-HAART and HAART eras [13,14]. These reports have included profiles of the safety of discontinuing drug prophylaxis for *Pneumocystis jiroveci* (formerly *P. carinii*) pneumonia among HAART-treated patients with stably increased CD4 counts (>200 cells/mm³) [15,16], as well as the potential value of novel antimicrobial prophylaxis interventions for the prevention of cryptosporidiosis in patients with AIDS [17,18]. HOPS data (in conjunction with data from the CDC Adult and Adolescent Spectrum of Disease project) have also been used more recently to monitor trends in cancer incidence among HIV-infected persons in care. While incidence rates of traditionally AIDS-defining malignancies such as non-Hodgkin's lymphoma (NHL) and Kaposi's sarcoma (KS) have declined, rates of cervical cancer and several non AIDS-defining malignancies (e.g. malignant melanoma, Hodgkin's lymphoma, colon cancer, prostate cancer) have remained largely unchanged [19,20]. When compared to incidence trends describing the same malignancies in the general population, NHL and KS have been the only cancers that declined differentially (although their incidence remains elevated compared with the general population), whereas only anal cancer increased differentially.

Analyses of HOPS data have contributed vital observations to the ongoing debate over the optimal timing of HAART initiation. HOPS data were among the first to suggest that initiating treatment at higher CD4 counts, not only above 200 cells/mm³, but also possibly above 350 cells/mm³, improves survival [21–23] without increasing the risk of developing peripheral neuropathy and anaemia [24,25]. Ongoing analyses are under way to assess the risk of developing HIV-associated body habitus abnormalities and HIV antiretroviral drug resistance among patients who initiated HAART at various CD4 counts. More recent HOPS data have demonstrated significant survival benefits associated with the use of HIV susceptibility testing (both genotypic and phenotypic) as typically used to guide HAART treatment selection, regardless of when treatment was initiated. Survival benefits associated with the use of HIV drug resistance testing were evident among HAART-experienced people, as well as among therapy-naïve individuals with CD4 counts below 200 cells/mm^3 [26].

Other HOPS data have shown that response to HAART is not attenuated among individuals with large body mass indices (BMI) [27]. The observation that 43% of current HOPS partici-pants meet clinical criteria for being overweight or obese (BMI >25) has led some pharmaceuti-cal manufacturers to consider actively including such patients in their pharmacokinetic evaluations of new antiretroviral drugs. Previously, such 'non-normals' who constituted a growing proportion of people living with HIV infection would have been excluded based on weight.

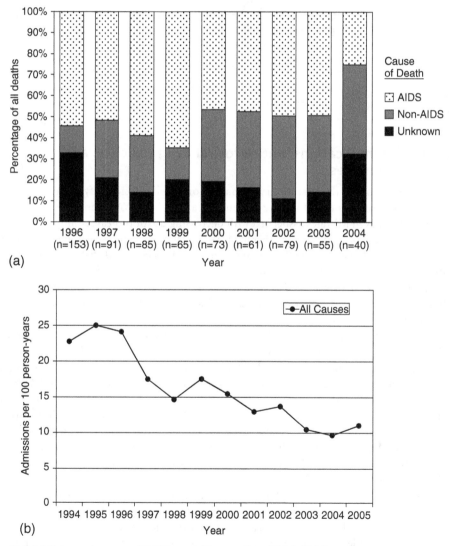

Fig. 11.2 (a) Rates and causes of HOPS mortality over time (1996–2004).
(b) Rates of HOPS hospitalizations (1994–2005).

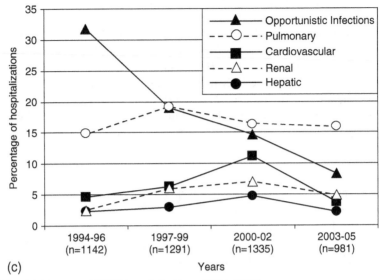

(c)

Fig. 11.2 (*Cont*) (c) Causes of HOPS hospitalizations (1994–2005).

Metabolic complications, antiretroviral drug toxicities and co-morbid illnesses

The HOPS was among the first observational cohort studies to identify increased rates of myocardial infarctions (MIs) among patients treated with HAART and to subsequently document declines in MI rates associated with decreasing use of protease inhibitors (PIs) and more aggressive use of lipid-lowering therapy [28–31]. HOPS patients have also participated in cross-sectional studies evaluating the prevalence of HIV-associated body habitus abnormalities (both lipoatrophy and lipoaccumulation) and the factors associated with their development [32–34]. This work demonstrated that, in addition to certain antiretroviral drugs, stage of HIV infection and patient age are associated with increased risks for body habitus abnormality development.

Reports from the HOPS have contributed to a better understanding of renal disease among HIV-infected individuals. Early analyses corroborated reports that kidney disease is among the leading causes of morbidity and mortality for African American HIV-infected patients [35]. When concern emerged over renal toxicity associated with tenofovir use, analyses of HOPS data provided a means of evaluating this issue in a large and diverse cohort of patients in routine clinical care. Findings revealed that while tenofovir (TDF) use is associated with statistically significant decreases in calculated creatinine clearance and serum phosphate, these changes are small and stable, rarely lead to drug discontinuation, and are unlikely to be associated with adverse clinical outcomes [36,37] or to be augmented by co-administration with ritonavir (RTV) [38].

HOPS work has also contributed to an improved understanding of clinical outcomes in persons chronically co-infected with HIV and viral hepatitis, a co-morbidity increasingly prevalent among HIV-infected individuals. HOPS analyses have described hepatitis A and B vaccination rates and have identified remediable barriers to vaccine receipt [39,40]. The long-term follow-up, large size and representative diversity of the HOPS cohort have also allowed estimation of chronic hepatitis C virus (HCV) co-infection prevalence among those infected with HIV. These data were among the few US data available to calculate anticipated needs for HCV-related morbidity in the 2007 reauthorization of the Ryan White CARE Act, which is the safety net programme that provides care and support to medically indigent HIV-positive patients in the United States.

Areas of ongoing investigative inquiry in the HOPS

The HOPS investigators plan to continue trend analyses in HIV-related morbidity and mortality, in antiretroviral drug use, in the spectrum of HIV- and treatment-related complications and co-morbid conditions, and in the rates and causes of hospitalization and death. Analyses to examine new trends in the utilization of HIV drug resistance testing, the prevalence of specific genotypic and phenotypic antiretroviral resistance determinants, and the impact of drug resistance on clinical outcomes are under way. Evaluations of the timing of HAART initiation, rates of survival, and associated adverse events and toxicities are ongoing. Monitoring of the evolving prevalence and incidence of chronic viral hepatitis B and C co-infections among HIV-infected individuals and the efficacy and toxicity of HAART for these individuals is also ongoing. Monitoring of the prevalence and incidence of cardiovascular disease-related morbidity and mortality, and risk factors for developing and preventing future illness, continues.

2. The Multicenter AIDS Cohort Study

The Multicenter AIDS Cohort Study (MACS) was funded in 1983 by the US National Institute of Allergy and Infectious Disease (NIAID), and recruitment of participants began in early 1984. In the more than 20 years since its initiation, more than 1000 papers have originated from investigators in the MACS detailing the results of the study. The initial rationale for funding this epidemiological investigation was to collect specimens that could potentially be of use in identifying an infectious agent as the cause of the acquired immunodeficiency syndrome (AIDS) and to delineate the natural history of pre-AIDS in men who have sex with men (MSM), the first epidemiologically identified group at high risk of developing the syndrome [41]. Coincident with initiation of recruitment, the Gallo and Levy laboratories confirmed the findings of Barre-Sinoussi *et al.* of a retroviral etiology of the syndrome [42–44], and within a year the immunoassay for antibodies to the virus became available [45].

With the availability of the antibody assay, it was determined that approximately 60% of the recruits into the MACS were, in fact, uninfected [46]. The study thus evolved into an investigation of the natural history of uninfected men developing incident HIV infection and of men with more advanced established infection. Recruitment was reopened to increase the number of African Americans in the cohort in 1987, and again in 2001 to augment the participation of younger African American and Latino men. The advent of HAART in the latter part of 1995 resulted in a third shift in the objectives of the study; the focus became the delineation of benefits and possible adverse effects of this revolutionary treatment.

Methodology

The four MACS clinical sites are located in Baltimore, Pittsburgh, Chicago and Los Angeles; the data coordinating centre, or Center for Analysis of the MACS (CAMACS), is at Johns Hopkins University's Bloomberg School of Public Health. The participants are seen at the clinics every six months. The protocol for data collection was agreed upon by the MACS investigators before recruitment was initiated. It is reviewed and updated semi-annually. At each visit, the partici-pants are interviewed regarding their health in the prior six months, their use of medications, and risk behaviours. They undergo a focused physical examination and are bled. Uninfected men are monitored for development of antibody to HIV. Both infected and uninfected participants are monitored for evidence of hepatitis B virus (HBV) and HCV; in addition, serum chemistries including blood glucose, haemoglobin A1c, hepatic function tests and serum lipids are measured. T-cell phenotyping is obtained on both infected and uninfected men, and HIV RNA copy number is determined in each infected man at each visit. Peripheral blood mononuclear cells, cell pellets, serum and plasma are banked in local and national repositories for use by MACS and non-MACS investigators. For participants with severe immunodeficiency, outcomes are continuously ascertained by phone calls review of participants' medical records and collection of death certificates. All data is sent to CAMACS following editing at local sites.

The study

The majority of incident HIV infections were recorded in the first three years of the study [47]. The average annual incidence of new infections in the years 1984 to 1987 was greater than four per 100 person-years. Since 1988, the average annual incidence has been one per 100 person-years or fewer. By late 1995, more than 60% of the men who entered the study with evidence of infection had developed clinical AIDS, as defined by the occurrence of an OI or neoplastic condition, and 90% of these participants with AIDS died before effective antiretroviral therapy became available. As of January 1996, a total of 2737 infected participants had been identified, including 542 men with incident infections. The infected cohort available in 1996 for evaluation of the impact of HAART totalled 1228, and 1094 have remained active in the ensuing 10 years. This subset of the 1094 participants included 206 with a previous diagnosis of clinical AIDS and 446 who were naïve to antiretroviral therapy. The median age was 42 years (Table 11.2).

The treatment-naïve participants had a median CD4 count of 499 cells/mm^3. In contrast, those who were treatment-experienced had a median CD4 count of 256 cells/mm^3. Median HIV RNA values were 23,334 and 37,629 copies/mL, respectively (Table 11.3).

The use of HAART increased rapidly during 1996 and 1997, and by the first half of 1998, 75% of the infected cohort was receiving HAART. Its initial users had low CD4 counts (<200 cells/mm^3), but with time, participants with higher CD4 counts began treatment with HAART [48]. In the first half of 1998, the median CD4 count of those initiating HAART was 441 cells/mm^3. The corresponding CD4 count of those remaining HAART-naïve consequently rose with time. Thus, by the second half of 1999, the median CD4 count was 523 cells/mm^3 in the

Table 11.2 Description of MACS seropositives[a] as of January 2006

Seroprevalent		Seroconverter	Total
Overall	2195	542	2737
Number alive 1/1/96	877 (40%)	351 (65%)	1228 (45%)
Active since 1/1/96	764 (87%)	330 (94%)	104 (89%)
Clinical AIDS by 1996	143 (19%)	63 (19%)	206 (19%)
ART-naïve[b]	297 (39%)	149 (45%)	446 (41%)
Median age (IQR) 1996	42 (38,46)	41 (36,46)	42 (37,46)
Range	25,68	24,63	24,68

[a] Includes seroprevalent and seroconverters whose first seropositive visit was ≤1/1/96

[b] ART-naïve is defined as no use of antiretrovirals prior to 1996 among participants continuing to be active from 1996 onwards

Table 11.3 HIV biomarkers[a] of active MACS participants according to treatment status, 1 January 2006

	Antiretroviral Therapy History		
	Naïve	**Experience**	**Overall**
CD4 cells/mm³			
Mean	529	279	371
Median	499	256	337
IQR	340; 688	92; 414	165; 515
Range	10; 1662	0; 1800	0; 1800
% ≤350	27	67	52
CD8 cells/mL			
Mean	1032	946	978
Median	952	859	899
IQR	693; 1224	554; 1218	604; 1221
Range	119; 4043	36; 2853	36; 4043
HIV RNA copies/mL			
Mean	75 607	141 721	117 617
Median	23 334	37 629	29 675
IQR	4,619; 81 015	7,060; 141 977	6,239; 115 300
Range	<50; 1 785 483	<50; 4 371 653	<50; 4 371 653

[a] Biomarkers assessed at last visit in period 1989–96

remaining 106 infected men who had not begun HAART. By the beginning of 2005, close to 80% of participants without clinical AIDS and 95% of those with clinical AIDS were on HAART.

HAART was extremely effective at a population level. The incidence of AIDS following enrolment in the MACS was approximately six per 100 person-years from 1984 to 1987. It rose to more than 10 in the period 1988 to 1994, and fell to five between 1995 and 2000. Since 2001, the average annual incidence has been two or less per 100 person-years. The relative hazard of progressing to AIDS was 1.52 in the years 1987 to 1990, in comparison with the referent period of 1990 to 1993, when nucleoside reverse transcriptase inhibitor (NRTI) combination therapy was beginning to be used by the infected cohort. There was little change in the hazard of progression in the calendar period 1993 to 1996, but post-1996 the relative hazard of progression decreased to 0.30 in the members of the cohort at equal duration of infection, and to 0.31 at equal CD4 counts and levels of HIV RNA [49].

In the first three years of effective therapy, suppression of HIV replication below 50 copies/mL was maintained by 50% of HAART users; 13% demonstrated rebound to greater than 400 copies/mL at least on one occasion, and 37% never suppressed below 400 copies/mL. Progression to AIDS was 2.5 times more prevalent among those who did not suppress and 50% more prevalent among those who rebounded in comparison with those who maintained CD4 counts >250 cells/mm3 and HIV RNA below 1000 copies/mL. The relative hazard for those with higher HIV RNA levels was 4.6 as compared with the group with the lower levels of viral replication. Far greater relative hazards were noted in men with lower CD4 counts. The greatest increases in CD4 counts were noted in men with the lowest counts at initiation of effective therapy; however, men with counts remaining below 100 cells/mm³ who were on HAART had a relative hazard of 33 for development of clinical AIDS. The incidence of KS [50,51] and dementia [52] decreased dramatically in parallel with the drop in the occurrence of OIs in the first years of the HAART era [53]. Decreases in the occurrence of lymphoma were less marked [50].

Progression to AIDS in the pre-HAART era was noted a median of 8.9 years after seroconversion; death occurred a median of 2.7 and 1.3 years after the CD4 count reached 200 cells/mm^3 and the development of clinical AIDS, respectively [54,55]. In contrast, progression to AIDS among men initiating HAART with CD4 counts above 200 cells/mm^3 was less than 10% in the ensuing three years and remained low in the ensuing years of the HAART era [56]. Effects on mortality were even more dramatic. From January 1990 to December 1994, 50% of participants with AIDS died within less than two years, and close to 90% were dead within four years. In contrast, during the 42 months from January 1995 to June 1998, less than 40% of men with AIDS died within three years. Less than 30% of the men who were diagnosed with clinical AIDS in the three years from July 1998 to June 2001 died in the next six years. The median survival in the participants developing AIDS in the calendar period July 2001 to December 2003, using Weibull models, has been estimated to be 16 years [57].

The costs or adverse effects of therapy unfortunately became apparent in the first years of HAART use. The men receiving HAART in the MACS were compared with those infected men not on therapy, and with uninfected participants. Clinically, the most obvious problems were the neuropathies due to the retroviral infection and therapy with didanosine (ddI) or stavudine (d4T), especially when used in combination as the NRTI backbone of a HAART regimen [58], and fat redistribution [59]. In addition, decreases in renal function [60] and serum lipid increases were documented in men receiving HAART. The lipid changes were documented in a subset of men with incident infection. The onset of HIV infection was followed by decreases in serum lipids during untreated infection and then increases with initiation of HAART [61]. Systolic hypertension was seen after two years of HAART, most frequently in African American participants over the age of 50 with an increased body mass index and who smoked or had used tobacco. Diastolic hypertension was not noted until men had received HAART for more than five years [62]. Diabetes, prediabetes and insulin resistance were significantly more common in recipients of PI-based regimens than in the uninfected cohort [63,64]. The metabolic syndrome was also diagnosed in both the infected and uninfected cohort, but was more frequent in men receiving HAART. Infected participants had significantly more hypertriglyceridaemia, lower high-density lipoprotein concentrations, and hyperglycaemia; however, they were less likely to have an elevated waist circumference than the uninfected men with the metabolic syndrome [65].

Conclusion

The MACS cohort as of mid-2006, 10 years after the widespread use of HAART, includes 178 men with clinical AIDS, 1059 AIDS-free infected men, and 1421 uninfected participants. The advent of widespread use of HAART has resulted in a major change in the focus of this ongoing study. Infected men are living much longer than in the pre-HAART era and are consequently at risk of diseases associated with aging in Western societies. The mean age of the HIV-infected survivors of the original cohort is 50; the mean age of the uninfected men who volunteered in 1984–5 is 54. Thus the investigation has the ability to evaluate the interaction of HIV infection, age and HAART in age-matched infected and uninfected men who have similar lifestyles. The current goals of the investigation are to delineate more clearly both the long-term benefits and adverse effects of prolonged but effective HAART in this older group of volunteers. Ongoing investigations include a longitudinal evaluation of carotid artery atherosclerosis and coronary artery calcification, the role of HBV and HCV in long-term outcomes of treated HIV infection, functional magnetic resonance imagery (MRI) evaluation of the central nervous system in infected men over the age of 50 receiving HAART, the impact of HAART upon risk-taking behaviour by infected and uninfected men, the impact of the concurrent epidemic of methamphetamine use upon the risk of acquiring infection, and progression of HIV infection and the interaction of HIV and advancing age in the surviving cohort. These investigations should provide insights into the impact of HIV infection and HAART in older individuals.

References

1. Twyman R. (2004). *A Brief History of Clinical Trials*. Available at http://genome.wellcome.ac.uk/doc_WTD020948.html(accessed August 31, 2007).

2. Rolleston HD. (1915). James Lind, pioneer of medical hygiene. *Journal of the Royal Naval Medical Service* 1:181–190.

3. BCC Research. (2006). *The Clinical Trials Business: Strategic Report*. Wellesley, Massachusetts: Business Communications Company.

4. Gange SJ, Kitahara MM, Saag MS, et al. (2004). Cohort profile: The North-American AIDS. Cohort collaboration on Research and Design. *Int J Epidemiology* 36:294–301

5. Palella F, Delaney K, Moorman A, *et al.*, the HIV Outpatient Study (HOPS) Investigators. (1998). Declining Morbidity and Mortality in an Ambulatory HIV-Infected Population. *New Engl J Med* >**338**:853–60.

6. Palella F, Chmiel J, Kirby K, the HOPS Investigators. (2005). Determinants of enhanced survival among triple class antiretroviral experienced, virologically non-suppressed patients in the HIV Outpatient Study (HOPS). 43rd Infectious Diseases Society of America Annual Meeting, 6–9 October 2005, San Francisco, USA.. [Abstract 780]

7. Palella F, Baker R, Chmiel J, Moorman A, Holmberg S, the HOPS Investigators. (2005). Comparative treatment outcomes among persons with advanced HIV infection receiving PI versus NNRTI-based first ever HAART in the HIV Outpatient Study (HOPS). 43rd Infectious Diseases Society of America Annual Meeting, 6–9 October 2005, San Francisco. [Abstract 788]

8. Holmberg S, Hamburger M, Moorman A, Wood K, Palella F, the HOPS Investigators.(2003). Factors associated with maintenance of long-term plasma human immunodeficiency virus RNA suppression. *Clin Infect Dis* **37**:702–707.

9. Palella F, Chmiel J, Moorman A, Chan C, Holmberg S, the HOPS Investigators. (2002). Durability and predictors of success of HAART for ambulatory HIV-infected patients. *AIDS* **16**:1617–1626.

10. Weidle PJ, Lichtenstein KA, Moorman AC, *et al.* (2000). Factors associated with the successful modification of antiretroviral therapy. *AIDS* **14**:491–497.

11. Palella F, Baker R, Moorman A, Chmiel J, Wood K, Holmberg S, the HOPS Investigators. Mortality and morbidity in the HAART era: changing causes of death and disease in the HIV Outpatient Study (HOPS). *JAIDS* **43**:27–34.

12. Buchacz K, Moorman A, Richardson J, *et al,*. the HOPS Investigators. (2006). Temporal trends in hospitalizations and hospitalization-associated diagnoses in the HIV Outpatient Study (HOPS) during 1994–2002. XVI International AIDS Conference, 13–18 August 13–18, 2006, Toronto, Canada..[Abstract MOPE0071]

13. Grubb J, Moorman A, Baker R, Masur H. (2006). The Changing Spectrum of Pulmonary Disease in Patients with HIV Infection on Anti-Retroviral Therapy. *AIDS* **20**:1095–1107.

14. Moorman A, Holmberg S, Marlowe S, *et al,*. the HIV Outpatient Study (HOPS) Investigators. (1999). Changing conditions and treatments in a dynamic cohort of ambulatory HIV patients: the HIV outpatient study (HOPS). *Ann Epidemiol* **9**: 349–357.

15. Yangco B, Von Bargen J, Moorman A, Holmberg S, the HIV Outpatient Study (HOPS) Investigators. (2000). Discontinuation of chemoprophylaxis against *Pneumocystis carinii* pneumonia in patients with HIV infection. *Ann Intern Med* **132**:201–205.

16. Moorman A, Von Bargen J, Palella F, Holmberg S, the HIV Outpatient Study(HOPS) Investigators. (1998). *Pneumocystis Carinii* pneumonia incidence and preventivechemoprophylaxis failure in an ambulatory HIV-infected population. *JAIDS* **19**:82–188.

17. Holmberg SD, Moorman AC, Von Bargen JC, *et al.*, the HIV Outpatient Study (HOPS) Investigators. (1998). Possible effectiveness of clarithromycin and rifabutin for cryptosporidium chemoprophylaxis in HIV disease. *JAMA* **279**:384–386.

18. Holmberg S, Moorman A. (2001). Possible bias of ascertainment in assessing chemoprophylaxis for cryptosporidiosis. (Letter). *AIDS* **15**:1589.

19. Patel P, Hanson D, Novak R, *et al.*, the HOPS and ASD Investigators. (2006). Incidence of AIDS defining and non-AIDS defining malignancies among HIV-infected persons. 13th Conference on Retroviruses and Opportunistic Infections, 5–9 February 2006, Denver, CO, USA. [Abstract 813]

20. Patel P, Novak R, Tony T, *et al.*, the HOPS Investigators.(2004). Incidence of non-AIDS defining malignancies in the HIV Outpatient Study (HOPS). 11th Conference on Retroviruses and Opportunistic Infections, 8–11 February 2004, San Francisco, USA. [Abstract 81]

21. Holmberg SD, Palella FJ, Lichtenstein KA, Havir DV. (2004). The case for earlier treatment of HIV infection. *Clin Inf Dis* **39**:1699–1704.

22. Palella FJ, Holmberg SD, Chmiel J. (2004). HIV Survival Benefit Associated with Earlier Antiretroviral Therapy (letter). *Ann Intern Med* **140**:579.

23. Palella F, Knoll M, Chmiel J, *et al.*, the HOPS Investigators. (2003). Survival benefit of initiating antiretroviral therapy in HIV-infected persons in different CD4+ cell strata. *Ann Intern Med* **138**:620–262.

24. Lichtenstein K, Armon C, Buchacz K, Moorman A, Wood K, Brooks J, the HOPS Investigators. (2006). Early, Uninterrupted Antiretroviral Therapy is Associated with Improved Outcomes and Less Toxicities in the HIV Outpatient Study (HOPS). 13th Conference on Retroviruses and Opportunistic Infections, 5–9 February 2006, Denver, CO, USA. [Abstract 769]

25. Lichtenstein K, Armon C, Baron A, Moorman A, Wood K, Holmberg S, the HOPS Investigators.(2005). Modification of the incidence of drug-associated symmetrical peripheral neuropathy by host and disease factors in the HIV Outpatient Study cohort. *Clin Infect Dis* **40**:148–157.

26. Palella F, Carmon C, Chmiel J, *et al.*, the HOPS Investigators. (2007). Enhanced survival associated with use of HIV susceptibility testing among HAART-experienced patients in the HIV Outpatient Study (HOPS)., 14th Conference on Retroviruses and Opportunistic Infections, 25–28 February, 2007, Los Angeles, CA, USA. [Abstract M-103]

27. Tedaldi E, Brooks JT, Weidle P, *et al.*, the HIV Outpatient Study (HOPS) Investigators.(2006). Increased body mass index does not alter response to initial highly active antiretroviral therapy (HAART) in HIV-1 infected patients. *JAIDS* **43**:35–41.

28. Holmberg S, Moorman A, Greenberg A. (2004). Trends in rates of myocardial infarction among patients with HIV (Letter). *New Engl J Med* **350**:730–732.

29. Holmberg S, Moorman A, Tong T, *et al.*, the HOPS Investigators. (2002). Protease inhibitor use and adverse cardiovascular outcomes in ambulatory HIV-infected persons. *Lancet* **360**:1747–1748.

30. Lichtenstein K, Armon C, Buchacz K, Moorman A, Wood K, Brooks J, HOPS Investigators. (2006). Analysis of Cardiovascular Risk Factors in the HIV Outpatient Study (HOPS) Cohort. 13th Conference on Retroviruses and Opportunistic Infections, 5–9 February 2006, Denver, USA. [Abstract 735]

31. Iloeje UH, Yuan Y, L'Italien G, *et al.* (2005). Protease inhibitor (PI) exposure may increase the risk of cardiovascular disease (CVD) in human immunodeficiency virus (HIV) infected patients. *HIV Med* **6**:1–8.

32. Lichtenstein K, Armon C, Moorman A, Wood K, Holmberg S, HOPS Investigators. (2004). A 7-year longitudinal analysis of IL-2 in patients treated with highly active antiretroviral therapy (Correspondence). *AIDS* **18**: 2346–8.

33. Lichtenstein K, Delaney K, Ward D, Moorman A, Wood K, Holmberg S, the HOPS Investigators. (2003). Development of and risk factors for lipoatrophy (abnormal fat loss) in ambulatory HIV-1 infected patients. *JAIDS* **32**:48–56.

34. Lichtenstein K, Ward D, Moorman A, *et al.*, the HOPS Investigators. (2001). Clinical assessment of HIV-associated lipodystrophy in an ambulatory population. *AIDS* **15**:1389–1398.

35. Krawczyk C, Holmberg S, Moorman A, Gardner L, McGwin G, the HOPS Investigators. (2004). Factors Associated With Chronic Renal Failure in HIV-Infected Ambulatory Population. *AIDS* **18**:1–8.

36. Buchacz K, Brooks JT, Tong T, *et al.*, the HIV Outpatient Study (HOPS) Investigators. (2006). Evaluation of hypophosphatemia in tenofovir disoproxil fumarate (TDF)-exposed and TDF-unexposed HIV-infected out-patients receiving highly active antiretroviral therapy. *HIV Medicine* **7**:451–456.

37. Young B, Buchacz K, Baker RK, *et al.*, (2007). Renal function in tenofovir-exposed and -unexposed patients receiving highly active antiretroviral therapy (HAART) in the HIV Outpatient Study (HOPS) cohort. *JIAPAC*.

38. Buchacz K, Young B, Baker RK, *et al.*, the HIV Outpatient Study (HOPS) Investigators. (2006). Renal function in patients receiving tenofovir with ritonavir/lopinavir or ritonavir/atazanavir in the HIV Outpatient Study (HOPS) cohort. *JAIDS* **43**:626–628.

39. Tedaldi E, Baker R, Moorman A, *et al.*, the HOPS Investigators. (2003). Influence of coinfection with hepatitis C virus on morbidity and mortality due to human immunodeficiency virus infection in the era of highly active antiretroviral therapy. *Clin Infect Dis* **36**:363–367.

40. Tedaldi E, Baker K, Moorman A, *et al.*, the HOPS Investigators. (2004). Hepatitis A and hepatitis B vaccination practices for ambulatory patients. *Clin Infect Dis* **38**:1483–1489.

41. Kaslow RA, Astrow DG, Detels R, Phair JP, Polk B., Renaldo Jr R. (1987). The Multicenter AIDS Cohort Study: rationale, organization and selected characteristics of the participants. *American Journal of Epidemiology* **126**:310–318.

42. Barre-Sinoussi F, Chermann JL, Rey F, *et al.* (1983). Isolation of a T-Lymphotropic retrovirus from a patient at risk for acquired immune deficiency syndrome (AIDS). *Science* **220**:868–871.

43. Gallo RC, Salahuddin SZ, Popvic M, *et al.* (1984). Frequent detection and isolation of cytopathic retroviruses (HTLV-III) from patients with AIDS and at risk for AIDS. *Science* **224**:500–503.

44. Levy J, Hoffman AD, Kramer SD, Landes JA, Shimabukuro JM, Oshiro LS. (1984). Isolation of lymphocytopathic retroviruses from San Francisco patients with AIDS. *Science* **225**:840–842.

45. Weiss SH, Goedert JJ, Sarngadhasan MG, Bodner AJ. (1985). The AIDS Seroepidemiology Collaborative Working Group, Gallo, R.C., Blattner, W.A.: screening test for HILV-III (AIDS Agent) Antibodies. *JAMA* **253**:221–225.

46. Kingsley LA, Detels R, Kaslow R, *et al.* (1987). Risk factors for seroconversion to human immuno-deficiency virus among male homosexuals. Results from the Multicenter AIDS Cohort Study. *Lancet* **1**:345–9.

47. Kingsley LA, Zhou SYJ, Bacellar H, *et al.* (1991). Temporal Trends in human immunodeficiency virus type 1 serocoversion, 1984–1989. A report from the Multicenter AIDS Cohort Study (MACS). *American Journal of Epidemiology* **134**:331–339.

48. Yamashita TE, Phair JP, Munoz A, *et al.* (2001). Immunologic and virologic response to highly active antiretroviral therapy in the Multicenter AIDS Cohort Study. *AIDS* **15**:735–746.

49. Detels R, Munoz A, McFarlane G, *et al.* (1998). Effectiveness of potent antiretroviral therapy on time to AIDS and death in men with known infection duration. *JAMA* **280**:1497–1503.

50. Jacobson LP, Yamashito TE, Detels R, *et al.* (1999). Impact of potent antiretroviral therapy on the incidence of Kaposi's Sarcoma and non-Hodgkin's lymphoma among HIV-1 infected individuals. *Journal of Acquired Immune Deficiency Syndrome* **111**:534–541.

51. Tam HK, Zhang ZF, Jacobson LP, *et al.* (2002). Effect of highly active antiretroviral therapy on survival among HIV-infected men with Kaposi's sarcoma and non-Hodgkin's lymphoma. *International Journal of Cancer* **98**:916–922.

52. Sacktor N. (2002). The Epidemiology of human immunodeficiency virus-associated neurological disease in the era of highly active antiretroviral therapy. *Journal of Neurovirol* **8**:115–121.

53. Detels R, Tarwater P, Phair JP, Margolick J, Riddles SA, Munoz A. (2001). Effectiveness of potent anti-retroviral therapies on the incidence of opportunistic infections before and after AIDS diagnosis. *AIDS* **15**:347–355.

54. Munoz A, Xu J. (1996). Models for the inoculation of AIDS and variation according to age and period. *Statistics in Medicine* **15**:2459–2473.

55. Enger C, Graham N, Peng Y, *et al.* (1996). Survival from early, intermediate and late stages of HIV infection. *JAMA* **275**:1329–1334.

56. Cole SR, Hernan MA, Robins JM, *et al.* (2003). Effect of highly active antiretroviral therapy on time to acquired immunodeficiency syndrome or death using marginal structural models. *American Journal of Epidemiology* **158**:687–694.

57. Schneider MF, Gange SJ, William CM, *et al.* (2005). Patterns of the hazard of death after AIDS through the evolution of antiretroviral therapy: 1984–2004. *AIDS* **19**:2009–2018.

58. Reisler R, Jacobson L, Gupta S, *et al.* (2005). Chronic kidney disease, and the use of HAART in the Multicenter AIDS Cohort Study. 12th Conference on Retroviruses and Opportunistic Infections, 2005, Boston, USA. [Abstract 818]

59. Brain T, Wang Z, Chu H, *et al.* (2006). Longitudinal anthropometric changes in HIV-infected and HIV-infected men. *Journal of Acquired Immune Deficiency Syndrome* **43**:356–362.

60. McArthur JC. (1995). Neurological diseases associated with HIV-1 infection. *Current Opinion of Infection Diseases* **8**:74–84.

61. Riddler SA, Smit E, Cole SR, *et al.* (2003). Impact on HIV infection and HAART on serum lipids in men. *JAMS* **289**:2978–2982.

62. Seaberg EC, Munoz A, Lu M, *et al.* (2005). Association between highly active antiretroviral therapy and hypertension in a large cohort of men followed from 1984 to 2003. *AIDS* **19**:953–960.

63. Brown T., Cole SR, Li X, *et al.* (2005). Antiretroviral therapy, and the prevalence and incidence of diabetes mellitus in the MACS. *Archives of Internal Medicine* **165**:1179–1884.

64. Brown TI, Cole SR, Kingsley LA, *et al.* (2005). Cumulative exposure to nucleoside analog reverse transcriptase inhibitors is associated with insulin resistance markers in the Multicenter AIDS Cohort Study. *AIDS* **19**:1375–1385.

65. Palella F, Wang Z, Chu H, *et al.* (2006). Correlates of the Metabolic Syndrome among HIV seropositive and seronegative men in the Multicenter AIDS Cohort Study., 13th Conference on Retroviruses and Opportunistic Infections, 2006, Denver, USA. [Abstract 747]

Chapter 12

The French Hospital Database on HIV (FHDH) ANRS CO 4

Dominique Costagliola

Introduction

In France, the prevalence of HIV infection at the end of 2005 was estimated at 134,000 based on the direct method, and at 106,000 based on back-calculation, with a plausible range of 88,000 to 185,000. It is currently increasing by approximately 3500 cases a year. While the first known case of AIDS occurred in 1978, and diagnostic surveillance was initiated in 1982, new diagnoses of HIV infection have only been systematically reported since March 2003. In 2005, notification of seropositivity covered only around 66% of cases, and it was estimated that about 7000 new diagnoses of seropositivity were made that year. Heterosexual intercourse was the main route of infection among people who discovered they were seropositive in 2005, half of whom were from sub-Saharan Africa. HIV continues to spread among men who have sex with men (MSM), while the incidence of HIV infection among injection drug users (IDUs) continues to fall.

Since 1987, when zidovudine (ZDV) was registered in France, antiretroviral therapy (ART) has been initiated or modified in hospitals, with general practitioners only permitted to renew prescriptions. The coverage of healthcare expenses linked to HIV infection is 100% for all HIV-positive patients who are enrolled in the ALD 30 programme, the chronic and/or severe disease programme within the national social security plan that covers health expenses in France. Antiretroviral therapy became available in March 1996 through expanded access programmes.

Data from the French Hospital Database on HIV (FHDH), which included 50–60% of HIV-infected patients in hospital care, were used to describe HIV patients, the use of ART and its impact on clinical progression (CD4 counts and plasma HIV RNA), and morbidity in the last 10 years. Mortality was assessed using the *Mortalité* 2000 [1] and *Mortalité* 2005 [2] studies.

The French Hospital Database on HIV

The FHDH was created in 1992 in order to collect clinical information on HIV-infected patients managed in HIV/AIDS centres (CISIH). It is managed by the UMR S 720 (Clinical and Therapeutic Epidemiology of HIV Infection) team at the *Institut National de la Santé et de la Recherche Médicale* (INSERM), on which the author serves as Principal Investigator.

Patients are eligible for inclusion if they are infected by HIV-1 or HIV-2, are managed in a CISIH, and give their written informed consent. At the first CISIH visit, a patient dossier is created to record basic information such as transmission group, date of first seropositive diagnosis, date of infection (if available) and clinical history of HIV infection. Information on clinical parameters (e.g. AIDS-defining events, other diagnoses), biological variables (e.g. viral load, CD4 count) and treatment characteristics (e.g., antiretroviral drugs, primary and secondary prophylaxis, treatment of clinical events) are collected at each hospitalization (inpatient or outpatient) and at each visit to the CISIH if a clinical and/or therapeutic event has occurred, or at least every six months in all cases.

The project was approved by the *Commission nationale de l'informatique et des libertés person-elles* (CNIL), France's watchdog organization for electronic information, on 27 November 1991 (*Journal Officiel,* 17 January 1992). Because of the need to return to patient files to validate data for specific research projects, CNIL's approval for a local access list was obtained in 1999. The U720 team performed regular data audits in local centres to compare data in the medical records and in the local database.

In 1995, the CISIH Clinical Epidemiology Group (CEG), based on the FHDH, was created. The aim of this group is to ensure that analyses can be initiated by the centres that produce the data—more than 100 hospital units nationwide. Since its inception in November 1995, CEG has led to the creation of several clinician- or U720 team member-initiated task forces. All data-generating units and U720 team members involved in the studies are members of CEG, which is coordinated by U720. A scientific committee with a maximum of 40 members debates CEG research themes and selects projects according to their feasibility and scientific pertinence. The committee undergoes renewal of a third of its members every two years.

The FHDH is drawn from 62 hospitals distributed among 29 of the 30 CISIH centres and includes data on 101,000 patients aged 13 years or over who were seen at least once between 1 January 1992 and 30 June 2005 with a mean follow-up of 60 months. Since 2000, the database has participated in the ART Cohort Collaboration and, since 2006, in the Concerted Action on SeroConversion to AIDS and Death in Europe (CASCADE), as well as Collaboration of Observational HIV Epidemiological Research in Europe (COHERE), studies. The database is supported within the framework of the *Agence Nationale de Recherche sur le SIDA* (ANRS) coordinated cohort action.

One of the main advantages of the database is its large size at a time when the incidence of all opportunistic diseases has markedly diminished, allowing the continuous study of the clinical course of HIV disease, the comparison of biological and clinical outcomes, and the occurrence of rare complications that may be either HIV- or treatment-related.

Besides research projects, the database facilitates the study and description of the epidemiology of HIV infection in patients in hospital care in France, since ART in France is initiated or modi-fied only in hospitals. By 31 October 2004, 77,449 patients were enrolled in the ALD 30 programme (described above) for HIV infection. With 44,080 patients being followed in 2004, the database is estimated to be 57% complete, and comparison with data from the VESPA study [3] indicates that it is representative of those in care in France (Tables 12.1 and 12.2).

An aging population

In 2004, women represented 31% of HIV-positive patients, a slight increase from 1996 (27%). Among the 44,080 patients who had at least one recorded follow-up visit in 2004, one in four men and one in eight women were over 50 years of age, which partially explains the wide diversity in patient morbidity. One in four women, but only one in 17 men, were of sub-Saharan African origin. HIV seropositivity had been diagnosed a median of 7.5 years previously in women and 9.7 years previously in men.

Frequent prescription of antiretroviral drugs

In 2004, 81% of patients were receiving ART, compared with 69% in 1996 and 85% in 2000. The figures are slightly lower in 2004 than in 2000, reflecting the evolution of the recommenda-tions of treatment over time. Twelve per cent of patients were treatment-naïve, while 7% had interrupted treatment (5% in 2000). Among the patients receiving treatment, 6% were still

Table 12.1 Characteristics of patients followed in 1996, 2000 and 2004

	1996 n=36,521	2000 n=44,016	2004 n=44,080
Demographic data			
Age (years)[a]	36 (31–42)	39 (34–45)	42 (36–48)
Sex (male)	73%	71%	69%
Transmission group			
Men who have sex with men (MSM)	37%	35%	34%
Injection drug users (IDUs)	24%	19%	14%
Heterosexual	29%	36%	41%
Others or unknown	10%	10%	11%
Origin			
Sub-Saharan Africa	4%	8%	12%
Clinical data			
Time since HIV diagnosis (years)[a]	5.5 (2.5–8.8)	7.5 (3.5–11.5)	9.2 (3.8–14.3)
AIDS (category C disease)	27%	23%	23%
Biological data			
CD4 cell count (/mm³)[a]	271 (130–439)	426 (265–616)	430 (284–609)
HIV RNA copies per mL[a]	-	<500 (<500–6,800)	<500 (<500–4,560)
ARV treatment			
Never	25%	10%	12%
Not treated in the given year but previously treated	6%	5%	7%
One NRTI	5%	1%	1%
Two NRTI	37%	10%	5%
HAART	27%	74%	75%
Inpatient hospitalization			
At least once in the given year	23%	15%	11%

[a] Numbers are median (Q1-Q3)

taking a dual nucleoside reverse transcriptase inhibitor (NRTI) regimen (53% in 1996), while 93% were receiving multi-drug therapy (39% in 1996).

Relatively satisfactory immunologic and virologic status but frequent hospitalizations

In 2004, the distribution of CD4 counts and viral loads was similar in men and women, with a median CD4 count of 430 cells/mm³ (interquartile range (IQR): 284–609) and viral loads below 500 copies/mL in 65% of patients. One in four men and one in five women had developed AIDS. In the same year, 11% of monitored patients had been hospitalized at least once, compared to 23% in 1996.

Patients first managed in 2004

Women represented 37% of newly managed patients in the FHDH in 2004. The patients' median age was 37 years. Heterosexual intercourse was the source of infection in 81% of female cases and 34% of male cases, while homosexual intercourse was the source of infection in 45% of male cases. Thirteen per cent of newly managed patients had AIDS, compared to 16% in 1996.

The median duration of known seropositivity was seven months when management started, but one in four patients had known they were seropositive for more than 17 months. The median

Table 12.2 Demographics of patients enrolled in 1996, 2000 and 2004

	1996 n=8882	2000 n=4808	2004 n=3839
Demographic data			
Age (years)[a]	35 (30–41)	36 (30–43)	37 (30–44)
Sex (male)	73%	65%	63%
Transmission group			
Men who have sex with men (MSM)	37%	26%	28%
Injection drug users (IDUs)	19%	9%	4%
Heterosexual	32%	50%	52%
Others or unknown origin	12%	15%	16%
Sub-Saharan Africa	6%	18%	23%
Clinical data			
Time since HIV diagnosis (years)[a]	2.3 (0.5–7.1)	0.6 (0.2–2.8)	0.5 (0.2–1.4)
AIDS (category C disease)	16%	15%	13%
Biological data			
CD4 cell count (/mm³)[a]	284 (130–466)	322 (148–512)	324 (160–509)
HIV RNA copies per mL[a]	-	24,500 (1932–12,900)	25,300 (1960–121,000)
ARV treatment in the given year			
Never	40%	36%	46%
One NRTI	7%	3%	2%
Two NRTI	41%	5%	2%
HAART	12%	56%	50%
Inpatient hospitalization			
at least once in the given year	22%	25%	22%

[a] Numbers are median (Q1-Q3)

CD4 count was 324 cells/mm³ (IQR: 160–509) and the median viral load was 25,300 copies/mL (IQR: 1,960–121,000).

Patients starting their first treatment in the first half of 2005: Impact of late presentation

The characteristics of patients starting their first antiretroviral regimen in the first half of 2005 were studied after excluding pregnant women and patients with primary infection under six months old, as these two categories require specific management. In 2005, 51% of patients beginning first-line ART had AIDS or a CD4 count below 200 cells/mm³, 37% had a count between 200–350 cells/mm³, and 12% had a count above 350 cells/mm³. Treatment was started late in more than half the patients, owing to late presentation.

It should be noted that about 36% of patients enrolled in the FHDH between 1997 and 2004 with CD4 counts below 200 cells/mm3 or with an AIDS-defining illness, which is the definition of late presentation in the database; this situation has not improved since 1996 (Figure 12.1) [4]. Factors associated with late management were older age, gender and geographic origin (odds ratio (OR)=1.5 for women from sub-Saharan Africa, 1.6 for men not from sub-Saharan Africa, and 1.9 for men from sub-Saharan Africa, compared with women not from sub-Saharan Africa (p<0.001 for the three ORs)). MSM were managed earlier than patients belonging to all other transmission groups (OR=1.6; p<0.001). The relative risk of death associated with late management

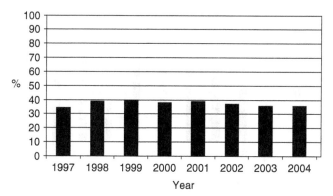

Fig. 12.1 Percentage of patients with late access to care per year of enrolment.

was 13.9 during the first six months after enrolment in the FHDH and remained significantly higher during the first four years, relative to subjects whose management started earlier. Efforts must be made to encourage patients who know they are infected to come forward for treatment and to encourage earlier screening, especially of heterosexual men, immigrants from sub-Saharan Africa and people over 50 years of age.

Multi-drug antiretroviral regimens comprised two NRTIs and one protease inhibitor (PI) for 62% of patients, two NRTIs and a non-nucleoside reverse transcriptase inhibitor (NNRTI) for 26%, and three NRTIs for 8%. Among the 10 most frequently prescribed combinations (59% of all prescribed combinations), nine corresponded to the 'preferred options' recommended in 2004 guidelines, and only one was defined as 'other choices' (ZDV + lamivudine (3TC) + abacavir (ABC) represented 5% of first-line regimens). Seven per cent of patients received a combination including atazanavir (ATV), which is not authorized for this purpose in either Europe or the United States. Trials assessing this product in treatment-naïve patients are still ongoing at the time of writing.

Evolution of the biological status of patients treated between 1996 and 2005

Figure 12.2 shows the percentage of patients receiving ART per year of follow-up. This percentage rose from 27% in 1996 to 74.5% in 2001 and has remained stable at around 75% since then.

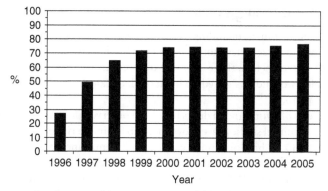

Fig. 12.2 Percentage of patients receiving ART per year of follow-up.

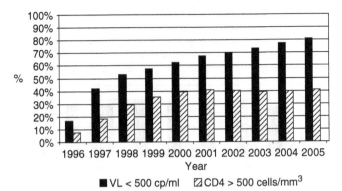

Fig. 12.3 Evolution of the percentage of patients receiving antiretroviral treatment for at least six months with viral load <500 copies/mL and with CD4 >500 cells/mm³.

Among patients who have been on ART for at least six months, the percentage of those with a viral load <500 copies/mL has increased every year since 1996, from 17% in 1996 to 63% in 2000, to 78% in 2004, and to 81% in the first half of 2005 (Figure 12.3). Over the same period, the percentage of patients with CD4 counts within the normal range (>500 cells/mm³) increased from 8% in 1996 to 39% in 2000 and has remained around 40% since then. Therefore, although the virologic effectiveness of treatment has constantly improved since 1996, the same is not true for the immunologic effectiveness, as only 40% of treated patients reached a normal value.

Morbidity and mortality in the HAART era

AIDS and survival after AIDS diagnosis

The incidence of AIDS among patients being followed has decreased from eight per 100 patient-years of follow-up in 1996 to two per 100 patient-years since 2001. An analysis of survival after AIDS focusing on cases diagnosed between 1993–5 and between 1998– 2000 shows that 47% of patients died, 63% of these from AIDS-defining disorders. The five-year probability of AIDS-related death fell from 40% (95% confidence interval (CI):38–41) in the period 1993–5 to 11% (95% CI:10–12) (p<0.001) in 1998–2000, while the five-year probability of death from causes unrelated to AIDS fell from 20% (95% CI:19–21) to 12% (95% CI:10–13) (p<0.001) in the same periods, respectively [5].

Non AIDS-defining malignancies

Recent epidemiological studies, including one from the FHDH, show that non AIDS-defining malignancies are two to three times more frequent in HIV-infected patients than in the general population [6–8]. Nevertheless, there are large differences according to gender and type of cancer: for example, two studies showed no higher risk of cancer in HIV-infected women than in uninfected women [6,9].

Carcinogenic effects of antiretroviral drugs have been observed *in vitro*, but, with the exception of Hodgkin's disease, clinical studies have shown no increase in the risk of cancer since the advent of multi-drug ART [6,7]. The global improvement in the immune status of the HIV-infected population that has resulted from widespread use of ART has not been accompanied by a reduction in the incidence of non AIDS-defining malignancies. Thus, while immunosuppression is a known risk factor for cancer, other factors also appear to be at work in HIV-infected patients.

Co-infection by oncogenic viruses (Epstein-Barr, human herpes virus type 8, human papilloma virus, and hepatitis B and C viruses) and increased exposure of HIV-infected subjects to known risk factors such as tobacco smoke, alcohol and malnutrition, could be complicating factors. Currently, the most frequent and/or most serious cancers in terms of mortality among HIV-infected patients are Hodgkin's disease, lung cancer and, to a lesser extent, anal cancer and hepatocellular carcinoma [10].

Vascular disorders

Cardiovascular and cerebrovascular disorders are emerging causes of illness and death among HIV-infected subjects [1,11–13]. Epidemiological studies show a high frequency of cardiovascular risk factors (especially smoking) in HIV-infected patients [14–16]. Moreover, they point to an association between the risk of cardiovascular and cerebrovascular disease and the metabolic complications of multi-drug ART, including lipid disorders, insulin resistance and Type 2 diabetes [13,17]. The negative impact of multi-drug ART on cardiovascular status has been demonstrated for PI-containing combinations [11,12] but not for NNRTI-containing combinations [17].

Primary pulmonary hypertension [18], although rare, has a far higher incidence in HIV-infected patients (76 cases per 100,000 patient-years) than in the general population (0.17 per 100,000 patient-years). As in the general population, incidence is higher among women and IDUs. The risk of primary pulmonary hypertension is associated with immunosuppression, but it is also higher in patients with CD4 counts above 350 cells/mm^3 (33 per 100,000 patient-years) than in the general population. In a 2004–5 study of 10,547 patients in 15 French clinical units, the estimated prevalence of primary pulmonary hypertension was 0.21% [19].

Thromboembolic disorders have rarely been studied in HIV-infected patients, but data from the ANRS CO3 Aquitaine cohort suggest that further research is necessary [20].

More varied causes of death

The *Mortalité* 2005 survey (ANRS EN19) was designed to document causes of death among HIV-infected adults in France in 2005. A total of 335 centres participated. Among the 912 reported deaths (median age 46 years, 76% men), the main causes were AIDS-defining illnesses (37%), cancers unrelated to AIDS or hepatitis (17%), viral or non-viral hepatitis (15%), cardiovascular disorders (9%), non AIDS-defining infections (5%) and suicide (5%) [2].

The increasing diversity of causes of death observed in the *Mortalité* 2000 survey, which analyzed 964 deaths [1], thus seems to have expanded further in 2005. AIDS accounted for fewer deaths than before (47% in 2000), while cancer, hepatitis B and C infection, cardiovascular disease and suicide remained frequent causes of death. In 2000, malignancies unrelated to AIDS and to hepatitis accounted for 11% of deaths, hepatitis B and C for 11%, cardiovascular disorders for 7% and suicide for 4%.

Conclusion

The face of the HIV epidemic in France has changed over the last 10 years, now affecting more women, and women from sub-Saharan Africa in particular. It is therefore a challenge to adapt the management of HIV infection to these new patients in a context of budgetary restriction in the public hospital system.

In a country where 100% of health expenses are covered, 75% of patients in care were being treated with ART in 2005. The treatment is virologically effective (viral load <500 copies/mL) in about 80% of treated patients, but a third of newly enrolled patients are not seen for the first time until they are at an advanced stage of HIV infection (AIDS or CD4 count <200 cells/mm^3).

The risk of death remains higher in these patients for about four years after the beginning of care. One needs to encourage earlier diagnosis, especially among heterosexual men, immigrants from sub-Saharan Africa and people over the age of 50, as well as to avoid late management of patients who are aware of their infection, notably by counselling patients at risk of being lost to follow-up and by issuing reminders when visits are irregular or missed altogether.

Causes of death and illness are becoming more diverse, largely because of the aging of the HIV-infected population, the high frequency of risk factors for cardiovascular disease and cancer, and the effects of HIV and ART. Besides HIV infection itself, risk factors such as smoking, cardiovascular disease and cancer should be taken into account during long-term management.

References

1. Lewden C, Salmon D, Morlat P, et al. (2005). Causes of death among HIV-infected adults in the era of potent antiretroviral therapy: emerging role of hepatitis and cancers, persistent role of AIDS. Int J Epidemiol 34:121–130.

2. Lewden C, May T, Rosenthal E, et al., le groupe Mortalité 2005 en collaboration avec Mortavic. (2006). Causes de décès en France en 2005 des adultes infectés par le VIH et évolution par rapport à 2000. Bulletin Hebdomadaire Epidémiologique (BEH) 48:379–382.

3. Lert F, Obadia Y, Equipe de l'étude Vespa. (2004). Comment vit-on en France avec le VIH/sida? Population et sociétés 406:1–4.

4. Lanoy E, Mary-Krause M, Tattevin P, et al., ANRS CO04 French Hospital Database on HIV, Clinical Epidemiological Group. (2007). Frequency, determinants and consequences of delayed access to care for HIV infection in France. Antivir Ther 12:89–96.

5. Grabar S, Lanoy E, Allavena C, et al. (2007). Survival after the first AIDS defining illness and causes of death before and after potent antiretroviral therapy. Results from the French Hospital Database on HIV. 14th Conference on Retroviruses and Opportunistic Infections, 25–28 February 2007, Los Angeles, USA. [Abstract K-130]

6. International Collaboration on HIV and Cancer. (2000). HAART and incidence of cancer in HIV-infected adults. J Nat Cancer Inst 92:1823–1830.

7. Herida M, Mary-Krause M, Kaphan R, et al. (2003). Incidence of non-AIDS-defining cancers before and during the highly active antiretroviral therapy era in a cohort of human immunodeficiency virus-infected patients. J Clin Oncol 21:3447–3453.

8. Clifford GM, Polesel J, Rickenbach M, et al. (2005). Cancer risk in the Swiss HIV Cohort study: associations with immunodeficiency, smoking, and highly active antiretroviral therapy. J Nat Cancer Inst 97:425–432.

9. Hessol NA, Seaberg EC, Preston-Martin S, et al. (2004). Cancer risk among participants in the women interagency HIV study. J Acquir Immune Defic Syndr 36:978–985.

10. Bonnet F, Lewden C, May T, et al. (2004). Malignancy-related causes of death in human immunodeficiency virus-infected patients in the era of highly active antiretroviral therapy. Cancer 101:317–324.

11. Friis-Moller N, Sabin CA, Weber R, et al. (2003). Combination antiretroviral therapy and the risk of myocardial infarction. N Engl J Med 349:1993–2003.

12. Mary-Krause M, Cotte L, Simon A, et al. (2003). Increased risk of myocardial infarction with duration of protease inhibitor therapy in HIV-infected men. AIDS 17:2479–2486.

13. D'Arminio Monforte A, Sabin CA, Phillips AN, et al. (2004). Cardio- and cerebrovascular events in HIV-infected persons. AIDS 18:1811–1817.

14. Friis-Moller N, Weber R, Reiss P, et al. (2003). Cardiovascular disease risk factors in HIV patients – association with antiretroviral therapy. Results from the D:A:D study. AIDS 17:1179–1193.

15. Saves M, Chene G, Ducimetière P, *et al.* (2003). Risk factors for coronary heart disease in patients treated for human immunodeficiency virus infection compared with the general population. *Clin Infect Dis* **37**:292–298.

16. Benard A, Tessier JF, Rambeloarisoa J, *et al.* (2006). HIV infection and tobacco smoking behaviour: prospects for prevention? ANRS CO3 Aquitaine Cohort, 2002. *Int J tuberc Lung Dis* **10**:378–383.

17. D:A:D Study group, Friis-Møller N, Reiss P, Sabin CA, *et al.* (2007). Class of antiretroviral drugs and the risk of myocardial infarction. *N Engl J Med* **356**:1723–1735.

18. Mary-Krause M, Costagliola D, the Clinical Epidemiology Group of the Centre d'Information et de Soins de l'Immunodéficience Humaine.(2001). Primary pulmonary hypertension and HIV infection. 21ème Réunion Interdisciplinaire de Chimiothérapie anti-infectieuse, 2001, Paris, France. [Abstract 10/C2]

19. Sereni D, Sitbon O, Lascoux-Combe C, *et al.* (2006). Prevalence of pulmonary arterial hypertension in HIV positive outpatients in the HAART era. Conference on Retroviruses and Opportunistic Infections, 5–8 February, 2006, Denver, USA. [Abstract 744]

20. Bonnet F, Chêne G, Lawson-Ayayi S, *et al.*, Groupe d'Epidemiologie Clinique du SIDA en Aquitaine. (2006). Causes of severe morbidity in HIV-infected patients. Aquitaine cohort 2000–2004: the importance of bacterial infections, cardio-vascular, digestive, and psychiatric morbidity. XVI International AIDS Conference, 13–18 August 2006, Toronto, Canada. [Abstract MoPDB02]

Chapter 13

EuroSIDA: a prospective observational study of chronic HIV infection across the European continent

Jens D. Lundgren*, Ole Kirk and Amanda Mocroft

Introduction

There are currently over 1.5 million people across Europe infected with HIV (Figure 13.1). In the last decade, the HIV epidemic in Europe has intensified in the eastern region, especially in the Baltic countries, notably the Russian Federation and Ukraine (Figure 13.2). In Western Europe, new infections are now mostly imported from highlyendemic areas of the world, although active transmission—especially among high-risk subpopulations of society—still occurs. Thus, the prevalence of HIV has increased dramatically on the European continent in the last decade.

There are significant problems with the management of patients affected by this public health crisis. Available antiretroviral therapy (ART), although extremely effective, does not cure HIV and hence has to be continued for life. Other limitations are the development of resistance, adverse effects of treatment, and the requirement for strict adherence. ART is expensive and access to care varies tremendously across the European continent; access remains limited in many countries in Eastern Europe. Furthermore, a significant proportion of the infected people are also infected with other chronic viral infections (e.g. hepatitis B virus (HBV) and hepatitis C virus (HCV)), which may adversely affect their prognosis. As the course of chronic infection continues, and if access to care is not dramatically improved, tuberculosis (TB) will become a major public health issue. Of particular concern is multi-drug resistant (MDR)-TB, which is prevalent in the general population in Eastern Europe. In addition, whereas most clinical research has studied people infected with the B subtype of HIV, the non-B subtype is increasing in prevalence across the continent.

The EuroSIDA study was initiated in 1994 to study the clinical implications of the issues outlined above and provide a continued surveillance mechanism for detection of emerging problems at a European level. The study's primary objective remains to prospectively study demographic, clinical, therapeutic, virologic and laboratory data from those infected with HIV across Europe in order to determine the long-term virologic, immunologic, and clinical outcomes.

Collaborators and funders

EuroSIDA is based on a unique collaboration among clinicians in 94 clinical centres in 33 European countries, plus Israel and Argentina. A list of participants in the study appears at the

---

* Corresponding author.

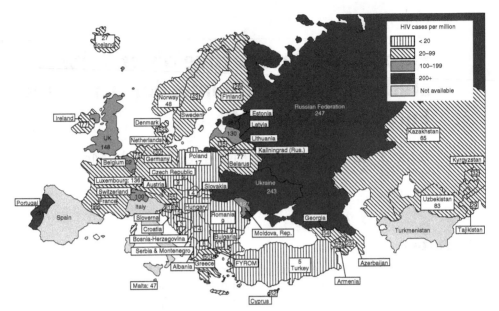

Fig. 13.1 New infection in 2005 across Europe, by country.

Source: [1]

end of the chapter. Sites contribute long-term follow-up data on a fraction of their patients to the study's coordinating centre, where the central database is located. Additional data are added to the central database from four central laboratories analyzing the central plasma repository located at the coordinating centre. The database analysis is centralized at the statistical centre.

Since its inception, EuroSIDA has been sponsored by the European Commission and, most recently, via the Sixth Framework Programme. The study has also received financial support from a large number of pharmaceutical companies manufacturing antiretroviral drugs.

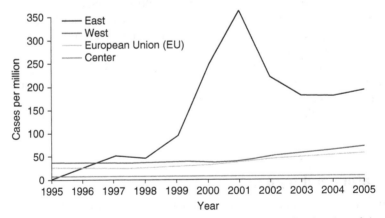

Fig. 13.2 New HIV infections in Europe according to year and WHO-defined region of the continent.

Source: [2]

Finally, the study group members and their institutions contribute indirectly by dedicating their time and effort pro bono.

Purpose of the cohort study

The specific objectives of EuroSIDA, falling into three main categories, follow.

1. To examine the efficacy of ART and its limiting factors

(a) *Durability of virologic efficacy of first-line ART.* We study factors associated with short- and long-term viral load outcomes (virologic failure/detection of resistance). For example, the influence of gender, ethnicity, HIV subtype, co-infection with HBV and/or HCV (and HCV subtype), age, geographical location and time frame.

(b) *Virologic outcomes of second-line and subsequent antiretroviral regimens, including those inpatients with multiple class failure.* In studying outcomes of second-line (i.e. after initial viral load failure) and subsequent regimens, we again examine the above-mentioned factors, but the baseline treatment history and resistance pattern become crucial additional factors to consider.

(c) *Viral rebound after achieving viral suppression.* It is vital to increase our understanding of the reasons for loss of viral load responses (viral rebound). We study the presence of resistance and assess evidence of inadequate drug exposure and/or of superinfection by analyzing stored plasma samples from the time of viral rebound.

(d) *Resistance accumulation in people with viraemia remaining on the same regimen.* Little is known about how rapidly resistance develops in people remaining on the same antiretroviral regimen. This is likely to depend on the resistance already present, the specific drugs used, and possibly other factors. Increased understanding of this issue is important for clinical judgements concerning which strategies to adopt in patients with virologic failure and few remaining drug options.

(e) *CD4 count and clinical outcomes.* At each treatment phase we also study CD4 count and clinical outcomes, including death. Generally, CD4 count and clinical outcomes are a consequence of poor virologic outcomes. However, in patients with multi-drug resistance and ongoing viraemia, the surrogacy of viral load outcomes for clinical outcomes starts to break down. i.e. CD4 counts remain stable and clinical progression does not occur despite relatively high viral load. CD4 count outcomes then become the main focus.

(f) Detailed analysis of specific resistance patterns emerging under various regimens in people infected with different viral subtypes. Each drug regimen and viral subtype is potentially associated with a different pattern of emerging resistance mutations, and this is likely to affect responses to subsequent regimens.

2. To detect current or emerging late-onset adverse events among patients on ART

(a) *Long-term study of incidence of potential adverse effects of ART.* Longer-term exposure to ART may result in dysfunction within a variety of organ systems, including the peripheral nervous system, the cardiovascular system, the liver, pancreas, kidneys, adipose tissue and bones. Also, endocrine complications may emerge, such as insulin resistance and type 2 diabetes mellitus. Lactic acidosis may develop due to impaired mitochondrial function. The frequency, causal relationship with specific antiretroviral drugs, and possible consequences (e.g. whether dyslipidaemia, lipodystrophy and/or impaired glucose tolerance induced by ART accelerate the atherosclerotic process and thus enhance risk of cardiovascular disease) are studied. EuroSIDA collects data on incidence of specific potential adverse effects and on treatment-limiting toxicities. In addition, information on new potential toxicities is collected by revising the data collection form at regular intervals (most recently to include questions regarding lactic acidosis, pancreatitis, renal failure and bone fractures).

(b) *The impact of adverse events on mortality risk.* We aim to assess whether patients with ART toxicities have an increased risk of death as compared with patients who do not experience such toxicities.

(c) *Influence of co-infection with HBV and HCV.* The immunodeficiency induced by HIV may accelerate the process of liver fibrosis progression due to HBV/HCV, and this is expected to be an increasing clinical problem as patients live longer with HIV. Patients co-infected with HBV and/or HCV are excluded from most trials of new antiretroviral drugs, and information on how these drugs function in co-infected patients is therefore limited. Most antiretroviral drugs are metabolized via hepatic enzyme systems, and there is some evidence to suggest that such drugs are more poorly tolerated in hepatitis co-infected patients, due either to added liver toxicity and/or decreased drug metabolism leading to additional hepatic toxicity. We are assessing whether the outcomes mentioned in 2(a) differ according to the presence of hepatitis co-infection. The pharmaco-epidemiology of HCV and HBV treatment will be examined.

(d) *Relationship between levels of specific drugs and toxicity.* The relationship between toxicity and drug levels for: raised lipids, with several drugs; cessation of efavirenz (EFV) due to central nervous system (CNS) toxicity with levels of the drug; and hepatotoxicity with nevirapine, is assessed.

3. To continue surveillance of HIV in clinics around Europe to describe temporal changes and regional differences

The study provides a large and quality-assured surveillance system to monitor the following key parameters of overall health status. New patients are added to the study regularly to ensure up to date and regional representation of the European HIV clinic population.

(a) *The overall pattern of HIV-related diseases and death, and the possible emergence of new drug-related morbidities.* Cause of death is becoming increasingly important as fewer patients die from HIV-related immunodeficiency, and there is an increasing need to classify deaths according to whether or not they are due to HIV-induced immunodeficiency and to study specific causes, such as liver-related deaths. For example, the influence of HBV and HCV infection on the mortality risk is examined, and incidences of death due to any newly identified adverse events is tracked.

(b) *The overall prevalence of patients with advanced immunodeficiency.* Although this group of patients has declined steadily since 1994, it is unclear whether this will continue as an increasing proportion of patients experience triple-class failure, or to what extent future treatment developments will improve their advanced immunodeficiency.

(c) *Prevalence of resistance in treatment-naïve patients.* The prevalence of resistance mutations detected in treatment-naïve patients is monitored.

(d) *HIV subtype diversity.* This may be important if differences in response to ART are identified.

(e) *Genotypic resistance pattern in drug-experienced patients.* It is important to study models of transmission of HIV in order to understand what patterns of resistant virus are circulating in patients with viraemia.

(f) *Virologic response to initial ART.* Monitoring of virologic response to initial ART is important in assessing the efficacy of therapy in practice. Any improvement in drug tolerability, adherence or efficacy might be expected to lead to increasingly favorable responses, while any significant increase in the transmission of drug-resistant virus could lead to a deterioration in response over time. Such monitoring of response to ART could provide an indication of both increased transmission of resistant virus and of its practical impact.

(g) *The overall prevalence of MDR-TB.* The prevalence of MDR-TB in the general population in Eastern Europe, where the treatment of TB and HIV can occur in separate clinics, may be as high as 15–25%. Only a fraction of HIV-infected patients receive ART, and the population with severe immunodeficiency is expected to increase markedly over the next five years. As a consequence, a large-scale epidemic of MDR-TB may emerge that may subsequently spread to other areas of Europe, with crucial public health implications. EuroSIDA, in collaboration with other cohorts and TB clinics in Eastern Europe, has initiated a study to directly assess this.

(h) *The overall prevalence of HBV and HCV co-infection (including HCV subtype) and of treatment for these infections.* Currently, approximately 30% of patients seen in clinics across Europe are co-infected with HCV and 10% with HBV. HCV exists in four subtypes, with distinct differences in terms of virulence and susceptibility to specific anti-HCV therapy and possibly to ART. Furthermore, HBV replication is inhibited by drugs used to treat HIV (e.g. lamivudine (3TC) and tenofovir (TDF)), although there is some evidence to suggest that the virus may develop resistance from continued selective pressure from these therapies. In addition to the epidemiology of HCV subtypes, the extent of treatment across Europe, or its outcome, for HBV or HCV co-infection with HIV is being studied.

(i) *The introduction of and utilization of newly developed ART.* Antiretroviral therapy, and especially newly licensed antiretroviral drugs, is costly. It is generally unknown how rapidly new drugs or regimens are taken up in different regions of Europe, what proportion of eligible patients start on newly available regimens, or, indeed, how these new drugs or regimens are incorporated into currently available regimens. The epidemiology of how new drugs are introduced across Europe will be studied.

Methodology

EuroSIDA is a prospective, multi-centre, multi-national study of patients with HIV-1 infection [3]. At recruitment, in addition to demographic and clinical information, a patient's complete ART history is collected, together with the eight most recent CD4 counts and viral load measurements. Data are extracted from patient notes onto follow-up forms at six-month intervals. Most of the data are collected from the clinics as part of routine care and are extracted from patient records by trained study personnel; a low but increasing percentage of data is transferred from local or national ongoing cohort studies. A case record form is sent to the sites with pre-printed patient-specific data from previous rounds of data capture in order for the site to cross-check the data in the central database. Intensive control programmes are implemented to ensure optimal quality of all aspects of the conduct of the study.

Additionally, a central plasma repository has been created to study the viral epidemiology of HIV (resistance and subtypes (9255 resistance tests, more than 5000 patient subtyped)), to embark on measuring levels of drugs used in ART, to further virologically characterize HBV and HCV from patients in the study and to perform population-based drug level determinations.

Enrolment

Seven cohorts have been recruited to date, the first in May 1994 (3116 patients) and the latest in January 2006 (2337 patients) (Table 13.1). A total of 16,100 consecutive patients will be enrolled by 2009 by adding an eighth cohort of 2500 patients in 2008 to ensure that all regions of Europe in which the HIV epidemic is prevalent are represented. This is to allow the study to provide timely information on the clinical presentation and outcome of European patients infected with HIV as well as long-term follow-up. By early 2010, it is projected that a total of 83,000 prospective person-years of follow-up will have been collected within EuroSIDA (with prospective follow-up of up to 15 years).

Participant demographics

As of April 2007, 14,262 HIV-1 infected patients in 94 centres across 33 European countries, Israel and Argentina were included in the study (Table 13.1 and Figure 13.3). Table 13.2, which is divided into four regions according to clinic location, illustrates the demographic characteristics of the patients from each region at the time that they were enrolled into EuroSIDA. Patients are recruited from all regions of Europe, and the study aims to include patients into the study in approximately the same proportion as the whole HIV-infected population across Europe. For example, Southern and Eastern Europe have a predominance of injecting drug users (IDUs), and proportionally more women, infected with HIV and hence there are proportionally more of these groups of patients included in the study. As has been generally observed, HIV infection through heterosexual contact has increased in all regions over time, reflecting not only an increase in this mode of transmission but also of immigration from regions where HIV is endemic.

Review and analysis of cohort study data

As of April 2007, a total of 66,445 person-years of prospective follow-up data had been collected from the participating patients (Figure 13.4); of which 18,312 were collected from patients

Table 13.1 Actual and estimated number of patients recruited into the EuroSIDA study

Date	Cohort	Number patients enrolled per cohort	Number patients enrolled (%) per cohort Eastern Europe	Cumulative number	Cumulative number (%) Eastern Europe
May-94	I	3116	0	3116	0
Dec-95	II	1365	0	4481	0
Apr-97	III	2841	0	7322	0
Apr-99	IV	1225	303 (24.7)	8547	303 (3.5)
Sep-01	V	1257	709 (56.4)	9804	1012 (10.3)
Nov-03	VI	2121	553 (26.1)	11,161	1565 (13.1)
Nov-05	VII	2337 [2,500]	999 [1,250] (42.8)	14,229 [13,661]	2564 [2.736] (18.0)
Apr-08	VIII	[2500]	[1250] (50.0)	[16,161]	[3986] (24.7)

Source: EuroSIDA, private communication

* Note: The numbers in brackets refer to the estimated number of patients expected to be recruited.

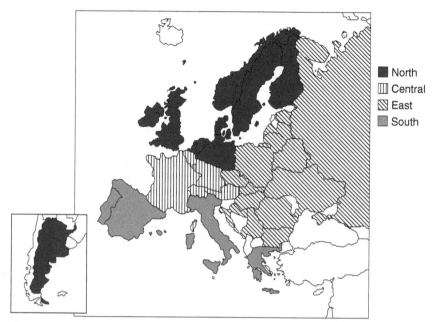

Fig. 13.3 Countries participating in Europe and regions identified for the purpose of subdivision of the continent. Of note are two countries outside the European continent: Israel and Argentina.

enrolled in cohort I, 9291 from cohort II, 19,675 from cohort III, 7062 from cohort IV, 4694 from cohort V, 6926 from cohort VI and 485 from cohort VII (Table 13.1).

The number of patients under active follow-up in EuroSIDA has steadily increased over the last decade (Figure 13.5), with a marked 'bump' in 1997 when the large cohort III was enrolled. At present, more than 8000 patients are under active follow-up. Of 14,262 patients, 2582 are known to have died. The rate of loss to follow-up is 37 patients lost per 100 person-years of follow-up, with relatively higher rates in clinics that have recently joined the study and that

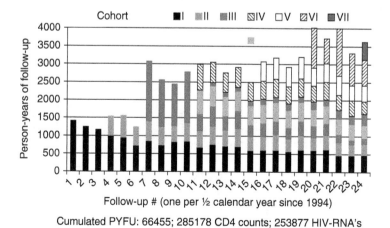

Cumulated PYFU: 66455; 285178 CD4 counts; 253877 HIV-RNA's

Fig. 13.4 Number of person-years collected within each of the seven sub-cohorts of EuroSIDA (see Table 13.1 for details) since inception of cohort I in 1994.

Table 13.2 Characteristics of patients at entry into EuroSIDA, sorted by clinic location.

		North	West	South	Central East and East combined	Total
All		3708	3428	4562	2564	14,262
Gender	Females % (n)	16.6 (617)	22.4 (769)	26.6 (1212)	34.4 (882)	24.4 (3480)
Race	Non-white % (n)	13.9 (517)	27.9 (957)	7.2 (327)	2.3 (60)	13.1 (1861)
Exposure group	Homosexual % (n)	60.3 (2237)	47.0 (1612)	30.5 (1390)	22.2 (568)	40.7 (5807)
	IDU % (n)	13.6 (505)	15.8 (540)	33.5 (1528)	40.6 (1042)	3615 (25.4)
	Heterosexual % (n)	20.1 (747)	27.1 (929)	30.4 (1387)	31.5 (808)	27.1 (3871)
ART-experienced	% (n)	74.5 (2761)	84.9 (2910)	80.4 (3666)	54.5 (1398)	75.3 (10,735)
CD4 count	Cells/µL median (IQR)	230 (104-370)	285 (141-428)	280 (129-438)	390 (251-561)	286 (141-440)
Age	Median (IQR)	38.5 (33.0-45.7)	38.6 (33.0-45.7)	35.6 (31.1-41.8)	31.5 (26.1-38.9)	36.4 (31.1-43.6)
HIV RNA level[a]	Copies/mL median (IQR)	3.08 (1.91-4.56)	2.70 (1.70-4.08)	2.72 (1.90-4.22)	2.91 (2.00-4.35)	2.85 (1.90-4.28)
Viral suppression[a]	% <500 copies/mL (n)	42.0 (867)	49.1 (1099)	46.4 (1227)	46.7 (815)	46.1 (4009)
Prior AIDS	% (n)	32.4 (1203)	29.5 (1012)	26.9 (1225)	20.7 (530)	27.8 (3970)
Hepatitis C status	Negative % (n)	38.3 (1420)	39.4 (1351)	31.0 (1416)	43.4 (1113)	37.2 (5300)
	Positive % (n)	10.5 (390)	9.4 (323)	17.9 (816)	38.8 (994)	17.7 (2523)
	Unknown % (n)	51.2 (1898)	51.2 (1754)	51.1 (2330)	17.8 (457)	45.2 (6439)
Hepatitis B status	Negative % (n)	61.9 (2295)	49.0 (1678)	46.2 (2106)	79.8 (2045)	57.0 (8124)
	Positive % (n)	4.9 (181)	3.9 (133)	3.8 (171)	4.8 (122)	4.3 (607)
	Unknown % (n)	33.2 (1232)	47.2 (1617)	50.1 (2285)	15.5 (397)	38.8 (5531)

[a] Data available at entry for % (n) in North 55.6 (2063); West 65.3 (2239); South 58.0 (2645) and Central East 68.1 (1745).

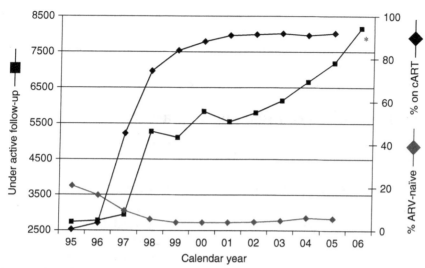

Fig. 13.5 Number of patients under active follow-up in EuroSIDA in the last decade, with indication of the proportion of these patients that are on combination antiretroviral therapy (cART) and that are antiretroviral (ARV)-naïve.

follow patients with variable adherence to regular appointments. However, due to rigorous data quality checks, many patients assumed to be lost later re-enter the study after some time away from their clinic.

For an idea of the size of the database, note that it contains, for example, a total of 285,178 CD4 counts and 253,877 HIV RNA level determinations with a median interval between determinations for both variables of three months (interquartile range: 2–4).

EuroSIDA has contributed data to inter-cohort collaborations on issues for which the size of EuroSIDA was not sufficiently large to properly address the scientific question posed. Some of these collaborations have been 'one-offs' in which data were merged for a specific project, and others have been of longer standing, where the protocol stipulates repeated merging of data. Additionally, data from EuroSIDA were used to estimate sample sizes for the two ongoing phase III interleukin (IL)-2 trials—ESPRIT and SILCAAT. These collaborations included (in chronological order):

◆ Estimation of sample size in ESPRIT (1998–2006) [4];
◆ Safety of discontinuation of disease-specific chemoprophylaxis collaboration (2001) [5,6];
◆ Collection of data for the Data on Adverse Effects of anti-HIV Drugs (D:A:D study) collaboration (1999–ongoing) [7–15];
◆ ART cohort collaboration (2001–ongoing) [16–19].
◆ Pre-HAART nucleoside reverse transcriptase inhibitor (NRTI) exposure and viral rebound collaboration (2003) [20];
◆ The Pursuing Later Treatment Options (PLATO) Collaboration (2004) [21];
◆ CoDe (2004–ongoing; <http://www.cphiv.dk/CoDe/tabid/55/Deafualt.aspx>);
◆ 3TC and liver-related death in HBV collaboration (2006) [22];

- COHERE (Collaboration of Observational HIV Epidemiological Research Europe (2006 – ongoing; <http://www.cohere.org>);
- Co-infection with Mycobacterium tuberculosis among HIV-infected patients in Europe; a prospective European multi-cohort study (2006–ongoing); <http://www.cphiv.dk/HIVTB/tabid/284/Default.aspx>)

Lessons learned and contributions to practice

EuroSIDA has provided insight into various aspects of the management of patients who are chronically infected with HIV, as summarized below.

Variations in disease presentation and outcome across Europe

Regional variation across Europe in terms of the time taken to approve access to new drugs between 1995 and 1998 is likely to have resulted in regional differences in survival in that period [23]. At the same time, there were regional differences in the proportion of patients with a poor virologic response to combination antiretroviral therapy [24]. However, these regional variations in survival have since been reduced, reflecting reduced dependence on the availability of novel single agents to maintain health and suppress viral replication, and a more streamlined process for making drugs available to those in need [25].

ART and outcomes across Europe in the last decade

Over the last decade, the prognosis for patients living with HIV across the European continent has improved dramatically (Figure 13.6). Not only have survival rates improved [3,26,27], but risk of non-fatal AIDS-related malignant [28–30] and opportunistic complications [29,31–35], as well as rates of hospital admissions [36], have been reduced dramatically. Similarly, improved prognoses were observed in individuals infected with HIV through injection drug use [37,38], in immigrants to Europe from other continents [39], and in women [40]. The benefits have been maintained up to the present time.

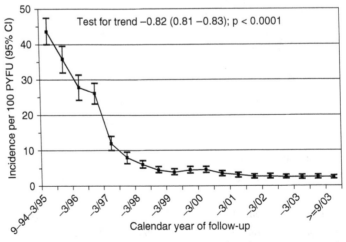

Fig. 13.6 Incidence of AIDS or death in EuroSIDA in the last decade.

Note: update of: Mocroft at al, Lancet 1998, 2000 & 2003.

The ability of ART to reverse immunodeficiency

When combination ART became available, there were widespread concerns that patients with profound levels of immunodeficiency would remain immunodeficient despite increased CD4 counts when HIV replication was reduced by the therapy—i.e. holes would remain in the immune system that could not be filled. However, several observations have somewhat eased these concerns. First, the risk of disease progression was reduced markedly once the CD4 counts were increased [41]. Second, once the CD4 count increased and the disease-specific chemoprophylaxis was discontinued, these opportunistic diseases only developed very infrequently. This was initially shown for the most frequent opportunistic disease—*Pneumocystis carinii* pneumonia (PCP) [5,35], and subsequently for other, less common infections as well [6]. Consequently, it became the standard of care to discontinue disease-specific chemoprophylaxis once the chronic HIV disease was well managed and the CD4 counts had increased on combination ART.

Determinants of response to combination ART

Much of the research effort in EuroSIDA has focused on this topic, ranging from the role of HIV subtypes [42] and how drug-related mutations evolve under various types of antiretroviral drugs [43], to determinations of factors other than HIV that predict the slope of CD4 counts in completely suppressed patients [44] and the finding that the risk of HIV-specific disease progression was comparable for a given set of CD4 counts and HIV RNA levels [45]. This finding supports using these two laboratory markers as surrogates of disease progression. A surrogate marker for clinical progression is characterized by the fact that changes in the marker reliably predict changes in clinical outcome.

Benefits of incompletely suppressive ART

Although most patients initiating combination ART achieve complete suppression of viral replication, this is not true for all [46,47]. The extent to which treatment remains of benefit in this situation remains undefined. However, the rate of disease progression in patients with advanced immunodeficiency (CD4 counts <50 cells/mm^3) has gradually declined as the number of drugs the patients receive has increased [48]. In patients on incompletely suppressive combination antiretroviral therapy, the HIV RNA levels have increased only slightly over extended periods of exposure to a single regimen, and this has been associated with slightly *increased* CD4 counts [49], contrary to what might be expected based on the natural history of chronic HIV infection. This finding was refined further to show that the CD4 count slope remains positive as long as the HIV RNA levels are below 10,000 copies/mL or below 1.5 log$_{10}$ copies/mL from pre-ART levels [21] (see Figure 13.7). However, use of incompletely suppressive combination ART leads to accumulation of drug-related mutations as long as the virus remains partly susceptible to the drugs used [50]. Hence, a strategy of using non-suppressive ART should only be used in situations where the number of remaining active drugs is too low to completely suppress viral replication and where the lack of therapy would leave the patient with high absolute risks of developing opportunistic disease.

Adverse effects of combination ART

Exposure to combination ART for five years is associated with a doubling of the risk for cardiovascular disease [9,10,15], an adverse effect likely to be exclusively linked to exposure to one of the three main drug classes—the protease inhibitors (PIs) [15]. Prediction of risk based on the

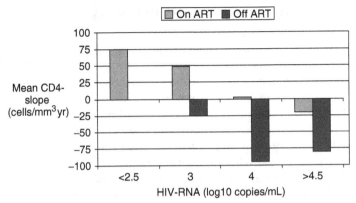

Fig. 13.7 CD4 slopes in patients with stable HIV RNA levels either on or off antiretroviral therapy. Of note: for a given HIV RNA level, the CD4 slope tends to be more positive in patients on versus those not on ART.

Note: Modified from: PLATO: Ledergerber *et al*, Lancet, 2004.

Framingham equation (developed in the general population) predicted this risk [7,13], suggesting that at least part of the drug effect is mediated via conventional cardiovascular risk factors [10]. EuroSIDA has studied factors associated with treatment-limiting side effects [51,52] and liver failure (see below).

Hepatitis virus co-infection

In EuroSIDA, 8% of the cohort has shown evidence of chronic infection with HBV [53] and 33% with HCV [52]. Although co-infection increases the risk of liver-related deaths, these patients have responded equally well to combination ART compared with HIV mono-infected individuals [53,54]. While treatment-limiting adverse effects are, as a rule, seen more frequently in patients with evidence of HIV-HCV co-infection, no particular antiretroviral drug has been shown to be more poorly tolerated than another [52]. With the introduction of combination ART, the risk of liver-related deaths has gradually declined over time [15,55], probably as a consequence of improved immune function, and resulting in a reduced rate of progression of the underlying liver disease (see Figure 13.8). However, once the improvement in number of CD4 counts in the statistical models was taken into account, there remained a residual excess risk of liver-related deaths for longer periods of exposure to combination ART [15,55]. This relatively weak—but reproducible—safety signal is being investigated further.

Treatment of HIV-HBV co-infection was associated with a reduced risk of liver-related deaths [22]. Whereas specific treatment is available to treat HCV infection, relatively few patients in EuroSIDA have initiated treatment for HIV-HCV infection yet, although the proportion of patients with HCV and HIV who are receiving appropriate treatment is increasing over time [56].

Future research using the EuroSIDA cohort

EuroSIDA is currently funded to assess the clinical outcomes of the patients already enrolled as well as an additional cohort of patients scheduled to be enrolled in 2008–10 by the European Commission. The size of the study, with clinical sites in over 30 countries, makes EuroSIDA the largest ongoing multi-national cohort in the world, and ideally suited to evaluate regional

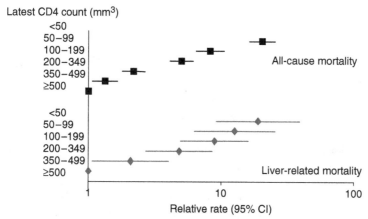

Figure 13.8 Multivariable relationships with death rate (all-cause and liver-related) and according to the latest CD4 count.

Note : Modified from: D:A:D: study: Weber *et al*, Arch Intern Med 2006

differences in care and outcomes. A future focus area will be possible differences within Eastern European countries.

Efforts related to further virologic characterization of HIV and the two dominant hepatitis viruses will be intensified. Since the central plasma repository contains samples spanning the last decade, important new information on longer-term changes will be generated. Of particular interest are the selective effects on HIV from using various incompletely suppressive antiretroviral regimens and the rate at which the cohort acquires HIV with drug-related mutations.

The study of possible adverse effects of ART will continue to be a focus area. The outcomes to be evaluated will expand as new potential adverse events arise, but will include renal failure, pancreatitis, bone fractures and non AIDS-defining malignancies in addition to liver failure and cardiovascular disease. Possible changes in the profile of causes of death will be studied as a potential generator of emerging signals of change in the health of HIV-infected populations over time.

While antiretroviral drugs cause adverse effects, their clinical benefits are also well documented. Many such adverse effects are organ-specific pathologies for which ART, by its ability to reduce viral replication and improve immune function, may also be of benefit. Hence, analysis to further understand the risk/benefit ratio of using antiretroviral drugs over extended periods of time in various subgroups will be another important focus area in the future.

In Europe, more than half of the 1.5 million HIV-infected patients are co-infected with HCV. EuroSIDA will continue to expand the understanding of how this viral infection interacts with the host and how it can best be managed.

Acknowledgements

Sponsorship

The European Commission BIOMED 1 (CT94–1637), BIOMED 2 (CT97–2713), the Fifth Framework (QLK2–2000–00773) and the Sixth Framework (LSHP-CT-2006–018632) programmes have been the primary sponsors of the study. Unrestricted grants were also provided by Boehringer-Ingelheim, Bristol-Myers Squibb, Gilead, GlaxoSmithKline, Merck and Co., Pfizer, Roche and Tibotec. The participation of centres from Switzerland was supported by a grant from the Swiss Federal Office for Education and Science.

The multi-centre study group on EuroSIDA (national coordinators in parenthesis)

Argentina: (M Losso), A Duran, Hospital JM Ramos Mejia, Buenos Aires. **Austria:** (N Vetter), Pulmologisches Zentrum der Stadt Wien, Vienna. **Belarus:** (I Karpov), A Vassilenko, Belarus State Medical University, Minsk; VM Mitsura, Gomel State Medical University, Gomel; O Suetnov, Regional AIDS Centre, Svetlogorsk. **Belgium:** (N Clumeck), S De Wit, B Poll, Saint-Pierre Hospital, Brussels; R Colebunders, Institute of Tropical Medicine, Antwerp. **Bulgaria:** K Kostov, Infectious Diseases Hospital, Sofia. **Croatia:** J Begovac, University Hospital of Infectious Diseases, Zagreb. **Czech Republic:** (L Machala), H Rozsypal, Faculty Hospital Bulovka, Prague; D Sedlacek, Charles University Hospital, Plzen. **Denmark:** (J Nielsen), J Lundgren, T Benfield, O Kirk, Hvidovre Hospital, Copenhagen; J Gerstoft, T Katzenstein, A-B E Hansen, P Skinhøj, Rigshospitalet, Copenhagen; C Pedersen, Odense University Hospital, Odense, L Oestergaard, Skejby Hospital, Aarhus. **Estonia:** (K Zilmer), West-Tallinn Central Hospital, Tallinn; Jelena Smidt, Nakkusosakond Siseklinik, Kohtla-Jörve. **Finland:** (M Ristola), Helsinki University Central Hospital, Helsinki. **France:** (C Katlama), Hôpital de la Pitié-Salpétière, Paris; J-P Viard, Hôpital Necker-Enfants Malades, Paris; P-M Girard, Hospital Saint-Antoine, Paris; JM Livrozet, Hôpital Edouard Herriot, Lyon; P Vanhems, Université Claude Bernard, Lyon; C Pradier, Hôpital de l'Archet, Nice; F Dabis, Unité INSERM, Bordeaux. **Germany:** (J Rockstroh), Universitöts Klinik, Bonn; R Schmidt, Medizinische Hochschule, Hannover; J van Lunzen, O Degen, University Medical Center Hamburg-Eppendorf, Infectious Diseases Unit, Hamburg; HJ Stellbrink, IPM Study Center, Hamburg; S Staszewski, JW Goethe University Hospital, Frankfurt; J Bogner, Medizinische Poliklinik, Munich; G. Fätkenheuer, Universität Köln, Cologne. **Greece:** (J Kosmidis), P Gargalianos, G Xylomenos, J Perdios, Athens General Hospital; G Panos, A Filandras, E Karabatsaki, First IKA Hospital; H Sambattakou, Ippokration Genereal Hospital, Athens. **Hungary:** (D Banhegyi), Szent Lásló Hospital, Budapest. **Ireland:** (F Mulcahy), St. James's Hospital, Dublin. **Israel:** (I Yust), D Turner, M Burke, Ichilov Hospital, Tel Aviv; S Pollack, G Hassoun, Rambam Medical Center, Haifa; S Maayan, Hadassah University Hospital, Jerusalem. **Italy:** (A Chiesi), Istituto Superiore di Sanità, Rome; R Esposito, I Mazeu, C Mussini, Università Modena, Modena; C Arici, Ospedale Riuniti, Bergamo; R Pristera, Ospedale Generale Regionale, Bolzano; F Mazzotta, A Gabbuti, Ospedale S Maria Annunziata, Firenze; V Vullo, M Lichtner, Università di Roma la Sapienza, Rome; A Chirianni, E Montesarchio, M Gargiulo, Presidio Ospedaliero AD Cotugno, Monaldi Hospital, Napoli; G Antonucci, F Iacomi, P Narciso, C Vlassi, M Zaccarelli, Istituto Nazionale Malattie Infettive Lazzaro Spallanzani, Rome; A Lazzarin, R Finazzi, Ospedale San Raffaele, Milan; M Galli, A Ridolfo, Ospedale L. Sacco, Milan; A d'Arminio Monforte, Istituto Di Clinica Malattie Infettive e Tropicale, Milan. **Latvia:** (B Rozentale), P Aldins, Infectology Centre of Latvia, Riga. **Lithuania:** (S Chaplinskas), Lithuanian AIDS Centre, Vilnius. **Luxembourg:** (R Hemmer), T Staub, Centre Hospitalier, Luxembourg. **Netherlands:** (P Reiss), Academisch Medisch Centrum bij de Universiteit van Amsterdam, Amsterdam. **Norway:** (J Bruun), A Maeland, V Ormaasen, Ullevål Hospital, Oslo. **Poland:** (B Knysz), J Gasiorowski, Medical University, Wroclaw; A Horban, Centrum Diagnostyki i Terapii AIDS, Warsaw; D Prokopowicz, A Wiercinska-Drapalo, Medical University, Bialystok; A Boron-Kaczmarska, M Pynka, Medical Univesity, Szczecin; M Beniowski, E Mularska, Osrodek Diagnostyki i Terapii AIDS, Chorzow; H Trocha, Medical University, Gdansk. **Portugal:** (F Antunes), E Valadas, Hospital Santa Maria, Lisbon; K Mansinho, Hospital de Egas Moniz,

Lisbon; F Maltez, Hospital Curry Cabral, Lisbon. **Romania**: (D Duiculescu), Spitalul de Boli Infectioase si Tropicale 'Dr. Victor Babes', Bucharest. **Russia**: (A Rakhmanova), Medical Academy Botkin Hospital, St Petersburg; E Vinogradova, St Petersburg AIDS Centre, St Peterburg; S Buzunova, Novgorod Centre for AIDS, Novgorod. **Serbia**: (D Jevtovic), The Institute for Infectious and Tropical Diseases, Belgrade. **Slovakia**: (M Mokráš), D Staneková, Dérer Hospital, Bratislava. **Spain**: (J González-Lahoz), V Soriano, L Martin-Carbonero, P Labarga, Hospital Carlos III, Madrid; B Clotet, A Jou, J Conejero, C Tural, Hospital Germans Trias i Pujol, Badalona; JM Gatell, JM Miró, Hospital Clinic i Provincial, Barcelona; P Domingo, M Gutierrez, G Mateo, MA Sambeat, Hospital Sant Pau, Barcelona. **Sweden**: (A Karlsson), Karolinska University Hospital, Stockholm; PO Persson, Karolinska University Hospital, Huddinge; L Flamholc, Malmö University Hospital, Malmö. **Switzerland**: (B Ledergerber), R Weber, University Hospital, Zürich; P Francioli, M Cavassini, Centre Hospitalier Universitaire Vaudois, Lausanne; B Hirschel, E Boffi, Hôpital Cantonal Universitaire de Genève, Genève; H Furrer, Inselspital Bern, Bern; M Battegay, L Elzi, University Hospital, Basel. **Ukraine**: (E Kravchenko), N Chentsova, Kiev Centre for AIDS, Kiev. **United Kingdom**: (S Barton), St. Stephen's Clinic, Chelsea and Westminster Hospital, London; AM Johnson, D Mercey, Royal Free and University College London Medical School, London (University College Campus); A Phillips, MA Johnson, A Mocroft, Royal Free and University College Medical School, London (Royal Free Campus); M Murphy, Medical College of Saint Bartholomew's Hospital, London; J Weber, G Scullard, Imperial College School of Medicine at St. Mary's, London; M Fisher, Royal Sussex County Hospital, Brighton; R Brettle, Western General Hospital, Edinburgh. **Virology group:** B Clotet (Central Coordinator) plus ad hoc virologists from participating sites in the EuroSIDA Study.
Steering Committee: F Antunes, B Clotet, D Duiculescu, J Gatell, B Gazzard, A Horban, A Karlsson, C Katlama, B Ledergerber (Chair), A D'Arminio Montforte, A Phillips, A Rakhmanova, P Reiss (Vice-Chair), J Rockstroh.
Coordinating Centre Staff: J Lundgren (project leader), O Kirk, A Mocroft, N Friis-Møller, A Cozzi-Lepri, W Bannister, M Ellefson, A Borch, D Podlekareva, C Holkmann Olsen, J Kjær, L Peters, J Reekie.

References

1. Hamers FF, Devaux I, Alix J and Nardone A. (2006) HIV/AIDS in Europe: trends and EU-wide priorties. Eurosurveillance 2006 **11:** 06123.
2. EuroHIV. (2006). HIV/AIDS surveillance in Europe. End year report 2005, No. 73.
3. Mocroft A, Ledergerber B, Katlama C, *et al.* (2003). Decline in the AIDS and death rates in the EuroSIDA study: an observational study. *Lancet* **362:**22–29.
4. Mocroft A, Neaton J, Bebchuk J, *et al.* (2006).The feasibility of clinical endpoint trials in HIV infection in the highly active antiretroviral treatment (HAART) era. *Clin Trials* **3:**119–132.
5. Ledergerber B, Mocroft A, Reiss P, *et al.* (2001). Discontinuation of secondary prophylaxis against Pneumocystis carinii pneumonia in patients with HIV infection who have a response to antiretroviral therapy. Eight European Study Groups. *N Engl J Med* **344:**168–174.
6. Kirk O, Reiss P, Uberti-Foppa C, *et al.* (2002). Safe interruption of maintenance therapy against previous infection with four common HIV-associated opportunistic pathogens during potent antiretroviral therapy. *Ann Intern Med* **137:**239–250.
7. Law M, Friis-Moller N, Weber R, *et al.* (2003). Modelling the 3-year risk of myocardial infarction among participants in the Data Collection on Adverse Events of Anti-HIV Drugs (DAD) study. *HIV Med* **4:**1–10.
8. Friis-Moller N, Weber R, Reiss P, *et al.* (2003). Cardiovascular disease risk factors in HIV patients–association with antiretroviral therapy. Results from the DAD study. *AIDS* **17:**1179–1193.

9. Friis-Moller N, Sabin CA, Weber R, *et al.* (2003). Combination antiretroviral therapy and the risk of myocardial infarction. *N Engl J Med* **349**:1993–2003.

10. d'Arminio A, Sabin CA, Phillips AN, *et al.* (2004). Cardio- and cerebrovascular events in HIV-infected persons. *AIDS* **18**:1811–1817.

11. Fontas E, van LF, Sabin CA, Friis-Moller N, *et al.* (2004). Lipid profiles in HIV-infected patients receiving combination antiretroviral therapy: are different antiretroviral drugs associated with different lipid profiles? *J Infect Dis* **189**:1056–1074.

12. Thiebaut R, El-Sadr WM, Friis-Moller N, *et al.* (2005). Predictors of hypertension and changes of blood pressure in HIV-infected patients. *Antivir Ther* **10**:811–823.

13. Law MG, Friis-Moller N, El-Sadr WM, *et al.* (2006). The use of the Framingham equation to predict myocardial infarctions in HIV-infected patients: comparison with observed events in the D:A:D Study. *HIV Med* **7**:218–230.

14. Weber R, Sabin CA, Friis-Moller N, *et al.*(2006). Liver-related deaths in persons infected with the human immunodeficiency virus: the D:A:D study. *Arch Intern Med* **166**:1632–1641.

15. Friis-Moller N, Reiss P, Sabin CA, *et al.* (2007). Class of antiretroviral drugs and the risk of myocardial infarction. *N Engl J Med* **356**(17):1723–1735.

16. Chene G, Sterne JA, May M, *et al.* (2003). Prognostic importance of initial response in HIV-1 infected patients starting potent antiretroviral therapy: analysis of prospective studies. *Lancet* **362**:679–686.

17. d'Arminio MA, Sabin CA, Phillips A, *et al.* (2005).The changing incidence of AIDS events in patients receiving highly active antiretroviral therapy. *Arch Intern Med* **165**:416–423.

18. Egger M, May M, Chene G, *et al.* (2002). Prognosis of HIV-1-infected patients starting highly active antiretroviral therapy: a collaborative analysis of prospective studies. *Lancet* **360**:119–129.

19. May MT, Sterne JA, Costagliola D, *et al.* (2006). HIV treatment response and prognosis in Europe and North America in the first decade of highly active antiretroviral therapy: a collaborative analysis. *Lancet* **368**:451–458.

20. No named authors. (2004). Nucleoside analogue use before and during highly active antiretroviral therapy and virus load rebound. *J Infect Dis* **190**:675–687.

21. Ledergerber B, Lundgren JD, Walker AS, *et al.* (2004). Predictors of trend in CD4-positive T-cell count and mortality among HIV-1-infected individuals with virological failure to all three antiretroviral-drug classes. *Lancet* **364**:51–62.

22. Puoti M, Cozzi-Lepri A, Arici C, *et al.* (2006). Impact of lamivudine on the risk of liver-related death in 2,041 HBsAg- and HIV-positive individuals: results from an inter-cohort analysis. *Antivir Ther* **11**:567–574.

23. Chiesi A, Mocroft A, Dally LG, *et al.* (1999). Regional survival differences across Europe in HIV-positive people: the EuroSIDA study. *AIDS* **13**(16):2281–2288.

24. Mocroft A, Miller V, Chiesi A, *et al.* (2000). Virological failure among patients on HAART from across Europe: results from the EuroSIDA study. *Antivir Ther* **5**:107–112.

25. Bannister WP, Kirk O, Gatell JM, *et al.* (2006). Regional changes over time in initial virologic response rates to combination antiretroviral therapy across Europe. *J Acquir Immune Defic Syndr* **42**:229–237.

26. Mocroft A, Vella S, Benfield TL, *et al.* (1998). Changing patterns of mortality across Europe in patients infected with HIV-1. EuroSIDA Study Group. *Lancet* **352**:1725–1730.

27. Mocroft A, Katlama C, Johnson AM, *et al.* (2000). AIDS across Europe, 1994–98: the EuroSIDA study. *Lancet* **356**:291–296.

28. Kirk O, Pedersen C, Cozzi-Lepri A, *et al.*(2001). Non-Hodgkin lymphoma in HIV-infected patients in the era of highly active antiretroviral therapy. *Blood* **98**:3406–3412.

29. d'Arminio MA, Cinque P, Mocroft A, *et al.* (2004). Changing incidence of central nervous system diseases in the EuroSIDA cohort. *Ann Neurol* **55**:320–328.

30. Mocroft A, Kirk O, Clumeck N, *et al.* (2004). The changing pattern of Kaposi sarcoma in patients with HIV, 1994–2003: the EuroSIDA Study. *Cancer* **100**:2644–2654.

31. Kirk O, Gatell JM, Mocroft A, *et al.* (2000). Infections with Mycobacterium tuberculosis and Mycobacterium avium among HIV-infected patients after the introduction of highly active antiretroviral therapy. EuroSIDA Study Group JD. *Am J Respir Crit Care Med* **162**(3 Pt 1):865–872.

32. Mocroft A, Oancea C, van Lunzen J, *et al.* (2005). Decline in esophageal candidiasis and use of antimycotics in European patients with HIV. *Am J Gastroenterol* **100**:1446–1454.

33. Podlekareva D, Mocroft A, Dragsted UB, *et al.* (2006). Factors associated with the development of opportunistic infections in HIV-1-infected adults with high CD4+ cell counts: a EuroSIDA study. *J Infect Dis* **194**:633–641.

34. Weverling GJ, Mocroft A, Ledergerber B, *et al.* (1999). Discontinuation of Pneumocystis carinii pneumonia prophylaxis after start of highly active antiretroviral therapy in HIV-1 infection. EuroSIDA Study Group. *Lancet* **353**:1293–1298.

35. Yust I, Fox Z, Burke M, *et al.* (2004). Retinal and extraocular cytomegalovirus end-organ disease in HIV-infected patients in Europe: a EuroSIDA study, 1994–2001. *Eur J Clin Microbiol Infect Dis* **23**:550–559.

36. Mocroft A, Monforte A, Kirk O, *et al.* (2004). Changes in hospital admissions across Europe: 1995–2003. Results from the EuroSIDA study. *HIV Med* **5**:437–447.

37. Mocroft A, Gatell J, Reiss P, *et al.* (2004). Causes of death in HIV infection: the key determinant to define the clinical response to anti-HIV therapy. *AIDS* **18**:2333–2337.

38. Mocroft A, Madge S, Johnson AM, *et al.* (1999). A comparison of exposure groups in the EuroSIDA study: starting highly active antiretroviral therapy (HAART), response to HAART, and survival. *J Acquir Immune Defic Syndr* **22**:369–378.

39. Blaxhult A, Kirk O, Pedersen C, *et al.* (2000). Regional differences in presentation of AIDS in Europe. *Epidemiol Infect* **125**:143–151.

40. Moore AL, Kirk O, Johnson AM, *et al.* (2003). Virologic, immunologic, and clinical response to highly active antiretroviral therapy: the gender issue revisited. *J Acquir Immune Defic Syndr* **32**:452–461.

41. Miller V, Mocroft A, Reiss P, *et al.* (1999). Relations among CD4 lymphocyte count nadir, antiretroviral therapy, and HIV-1 disease progression: results from the EuroSIDA study. *Ann Intern Med* **130**:570–577.

42. Bannister WP, Ruiz L, Loveday C, *et al.* (2006). HIV-1 subtypes and response to combination antiretroviral therapy in Europe. *Antivir Ther* **11**:707–715.

43. Cozzi-Lepri A, Ruiz L, Loveday C, *et al.* (2005). Thymidine analogue mutation profiles: factors associated with acquiring specific profiles and their impact on the virological response to therapy. *Antivir Ther* **10**:791–802.

44. Mocroft A, Phillips AN, Ledergerber B, *et al.* (2006). Relationship between antiretrovirals used as part of a cART regimen and CD4 cell count increases in patients with suppressed viremia. *AIDS* **20**:1141–1150.

45. Olsen CH, Gatell J, Ledergerber B, *et al.* (2005). Risk of AIDS and death at given HIV-RNA and CD4 cell count, in relation to specific antiretroviral drugs in the regimen. *AIDS* **19**:319–330.

46. Phillips AN, Ledergerber B, Horban A, *et al.* (2004). Rate of viral rebound according to specific drugs in the regimen in 2120 patients with HIV suppression. *AIDS* **18**:1795–1804.

47. Mocroft A, Ledergerber B, Viard JP, *et al.* (2004). Time to virological failure of 3 classes of antiretrovirals after initiation of highly active antiretroviral therapy: results from the EuroSIDA study group. *J Infect Dis* **190**:1947–1956.

48. Miller V, Phillips AN, Clotet B, *et al.* (2002). Association of virus load, CD4 cell count, and treatment with clinical progression in human immunodeficiency virus-infected patients with very low CD4 cell counts. *J Infect Dis* **186**:189–197.

49. Cozzi-Lepri A, Phillips AN, Miller V, *et al.* (2003). Changes in viral load in people with virological failure who remain on the same HAART regimen. *Antivir Ther* **8**:127–136.

50. Cozzi-Lepri A, Phillips AN, Ruiz L, *et al.* (2007). Evolution of drug resistance in HIV-infected patients remaining on a virologically failing combination antiretroviral therapy regimen. *AIDS* **21**:721–732.

51. Mocroft A, Staszewski S, Weber R, *et al.* (2007). Risk of discontinuation of nevirapine due to toxicities in antiretroviral-naive and -experienced HIV-infected patients with high and low CD4+ T-cell counts. *Antivir Ther* **12**:325–333.

52. Mocroft A, Rockstroh J, Soriano V, *et al.* (2005). Are specific antiretrovirals associated with an increased risk of discontinuation due to toxicities or patient/physician choice in patients with hepatitis C virus coinfection? *Antivir Ther* **10**:779–790.

53. Konopnicki D, Mocroft A, de Wit S, *et al.* (2005). Hepatitis B and HIV: prevalence, AIDS progression, response to highly active antiretroviral therapy and increased mortality in the EuroSIDA cohort. *AIDS* **19**:593–601.

54. Rockstroh JK, Mocroft A, Soriano V, *et al.* (2005). Influence of hepatitis C virus infection on HIV-1 disease progression and response to highly active antiretroviral therapy. *J Infect Dis* **192**:992–1002.

55. Mocroft A, Soriano V, Rockstroh J, *et al.* (2005). Is there evidence for an increase in the death rate from liver-related disease in patients with HIV? *AIDS* **19**:2117–2125.

56. Mocroft A, Rockstroh J, Soriano V, *et al.* (2006). Limited but increasing use of treatment for hepatitis C across Europe in patients coinfected with HIV and hepatitis C. *Scand J Infect Dis* **38**:1092–1097.

Chapter 14

The Swiss HIV Cohort Study (SHCS)

Huldrych F. Günthard and Bernard Hirschel*

Introduction

Switzerland is unique in that 50% of HIV-infected patients and 68% of AIDS patients are followed as part of the Swiss HIV Cohort Study (SHCS). The SHCS is an ongoing multi-centre research project dealing with HIV-infected adults aged 16 years or older. Established in 1988, the SHCS adopted its present structure and mode of operation in 1995: separation between infrastructure and research budgets; performance-based remuneration towards infrastructure allocated to each centre; implementation of a quality control programme; and research targeting specific focus areas. In 2000, the budget was transferred from the Federal Office of Public Health (FOPH) to the Swiss National Science Foundation (SNSF), and the SHCS grant was placed under the latter agency. Patients undergo standard clinical and laboratory examinations every six months. Thus, a high standard of care is provided, and quality control of treatment is guaranteed. Regular data mining, complemented by targeted research projects, provides insights into epidemiology, clinical care, development of HIV drug resistance, and many other aspects of the HIV epidemic.

In 2003, the SHCS combined two studies on HIV in pregnant women and HIV-infected children, both of which had been ongoing since the late 1980s, into the Swiss Mother+Child HIV Cohort Study (MoCHiV). Another important subproject concerns genetics and focuses on the genetic variants that are associated with differences in disease progression and toxicity of antiretroviral drugs. Since 2006, consent for participation in the SHCS has also included consent for genetic analyses. Currently, the DNA of more than 4000 individuals is available for studies such as:

- whole genome association studies in patients who can provide data on viral setpoint and who have a known date of HIV seroconversion. This is a collaborative European project supported by the Center for HIV-AIDS Vaccine Immunology (CHAVI), which is itself a consortium of universities and academic research centres worldwide supported by the US National Institutes of Health (NIH);

- evolutionary genetic assessment of proteins involved in antiretroviral defence. This includes the reconstruction of ancestral proteins and structural analysis of protein differences among humans and non-human primates; and

- pharmacogenetics of antiretroviral agents, with analysis of genes involved in cytochrome P450, drug transport genes, lipid metabolism and mitochondria.

Within the SHCS, expenses for procedures that are necessary for routine management (e.g. viral load measurements, CD4 counts, blood chemistries and counts) are paid for by the Swiss medical

* Corresponding author.

insurance programme; Switzerland has universal medical insurance, with medical insurance companies functioning roughly like public utilities. A grant from the SNSF totalled 3–4 million Swiss Francs (about US$2.4–3.2 million) per year from 2000 to 2006, and pays for data entry, databases, quality control and coordination, with approximately 1 million Swiss Francs (US$ 823,000) per year for self-administered research projects. These are approved and supervised by a scientific board comprising representatives from each study centre. This system fosters cooperation and is quite nimble—projects have been approved and funded in as little as one month, although a delay of two to four months is more typical—but has been harshly criticized for its lack of outside peer review.

The SHCS has stimulated the creation of other cohort projects in Switzerland, including a hepatitis C cohort constituted in 2002 and cohorts pertaining to transplantation and inflammatory bowel disease in 2007.

Epidemiology

The first AIDS case in Switzerland was diagnosed in 1981 [1]. The number of cases peaked at almost 800 in 1994, with 700 people dying from AIDS-related complications. After 1995 these figures dropped sharply to reach 217 newly diagnosed AIDS cases and 65 deaths caused by AIDS in 2005, when approximately 15,000 people infected with HIV-1 were living in Switzerland. There were more than 2000 new HIV diagnoses per year when HIV antibody tests were first introduced; this has since declined to fewer than 1000 [2] (see Figure 14.1).

New developments

Since 2001, approximately 700–800 new HIV infections have been reported each year. Primarily due to extensive needle exchange and methadone and heroin substitution programmes, few infections still occur among injecting drug users (IDUs). Among heterosexuals, some new HIV infections have been seen in Swiss residents infected in sub-Saharan Africa or South-East Asia, whereas others occur in immigrants. However, there is no evidence of increasing infection among heterosexuals in Switzerland. In contrast, the number of new infections among Swiss men who have sex with men (MSM) has increased since 1998 and represents a priority target for prevention (see Figure 14.1).

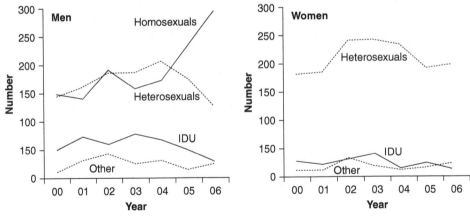

Fig. 14.1 Number of newly diagnosed HIV infections in Switzerland per year, 2000–2006.

Source: Bull.OFSP 2006; No 46/06, pages 953–962.

The prevalence of HIV drug resistance in primary and recently infected HIV patients remained stable at approximately 10% between 1996 and 2005. In particular, there was no increase in transmitted multi-drug resistant HIV-1 strains seen over this period. The prevalence of resistance in the whole HIV population is estimated at 19% and was approximately 25% in patients on HAART (highly active antiretroviral therapy) in 2005 [3]. Patients who have started HAART are less likely to harbour drug resistant virus, as compared with those who began with relatively ineffectual monotherapy or dual therapy in the 1990s. We therefore expect drug resistance to decrease over the next decade.

Treatment strategies

In the early years of the epidemic, opportunistic infections (OIs) dominated patient care. Theoretically, most of these could be treated effectively, but in reality, a series of half-won battles predicted ultimate defeat. Significant gains in survival necessitated prevention, first through the use of antibiotics against the most common OIs, then using antiretroviral drugs to prevent or reverse immune suppression.

The history of OI prevention is neatly bracketed by two publications from the SHCS, both of which appeared in the *New England Journal of Medicine*. In 1991 [5], we established the efficacy of pentamidine for the prevention of *Pneumocystis carinii* pneumonia, and in 2001 [6], we showed that prophylaxis could safely be withdrawn in patients who, thanks to HAART, had raised their CD4 count to more than 200 cells/mm^3.

Antiretroviral therapy (ART) was introduced in 1987 with azidothymidine (AZT)-monotherapy, followed by a short period of dual drug therapy. In 1996, triple combination therapy—or HAART—became the standard of care [7]. Estimates for HAART use in 2005 are available from the SHCS, where 22.3% of the study participants were not on treatment, 56% were on triple drug regimens, 19.2% were on more than three drugs (not counting the protease inihibitor (PI) ritonavir (RTV) at sub-therapeutic dosing for pharmacokinetic boosting), and 2.5% were on single or dual drug therapy. Today, first-line treatment consists of either RTV-boosted PI- or non-nucleoside reverse transcriptase inhibitor (NNRTI)-based regimens combined with two nucleoside or nucleotide analogues. The SHCS has pioneered several structured treatment interruption (STI) trials. While no benefit in terms of lower viral setpoint was observed after repeated STIs, CD4-guided therapy interruption using 350 cells/mm^3 as a cut-off to reintroduce treatment seemed to be safe over a two-year period [8]. At present, STIs are only recommended within study protocols or when serious drug toxicity occurs.

The effect of HAART

HAART has been successful in slowing disease progression and lowering mortality from HIV infection in Switzerland. The incidence of OIs and HIV-related cancers such as Kaposi's sarcoma and non-Hodgkin's lymphoma has dramatically fallen since 1996, and mortality from AIDS decreased from 700 in 1994 to 65 in 2005, a reduction of 91%. Full suppression of viral replication (<50 HIV RNA copies/mL) is key to long-term treatment success because persistent low-level replication leads to the emergence of drug resistance with subsequently higher risk of treatment failure.

In Switzerland, access to HAART was early and rapid. Figure 14.2 shows uptake of therapy in the SHCS from 1991 to 2006.

Patients who continue to die from AIDS-related complications fall into two categories:

◆ those who either refuse treatment or are unaware that they are infected and present with advanced AIDS symptoms that prove fatal despite treatment; and

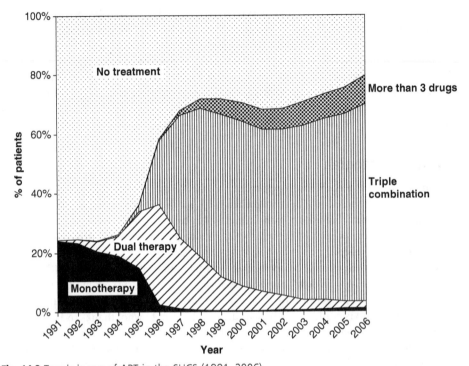

Fig. 14.2 Trends in use of ART in the SHCS (1991–2006)

Source: HIV cohort study database, 2006; Dr Alain Nguyen, infectious discase unit, Geneva Hospital, Switzerland.

- those who cannot be treated because of viral resistance or intolerance. Many of these patients have other medical conditions that make treatment difficult, such as advanced liver disease due to hepatitis C.

Figure 14.3 illustrates survival rates for patients with CD4 counts below 200 cells/mm³ for the period 1988–2000.

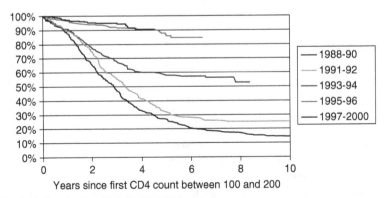

Fig. 14.3 Survival of patients with 100–200 CD4 counts.

Source: Swins HIV cohort-study, update November 2005.

Monitoring

CD4 counts were available when the first AIDS cases occurred in the 1980s, viral load measurements were introduced in 1994, and resistance testing became routine in 2000. Studies from the SHCS have shown that genotyping as a guide to treatment decisions leads to more strategic use of drug regimens compared with reliance on treatment history alone, and that genotype-optimized HAART has the potential to lower healthcare costs. Therapeutic drug monitoring (TDM), which monitors a patient's plasma drug concentration, has been used routinely since 2003 [9]. It is particularly helpful to assess adherence, reduce toxicity and identify insufficient drug levels.

Side effects

In an extensive standardized survey within the SHCS, 47% of patients on HAART presented with clinical and 27% with laboratory adverse events plausibly attributed to treatment. Among the latter, 25% were graded serious or life-threatening (grades 3 or 4) [10]. Hyperlactataemia was a common finding, but severe symptomatic hyperlactataemia and lactic acidosis were rare, mainly occurring with stavudine (d4T) and didanosine (ddI), two antiretroviral drugs that are no longer used in Switzerland. No association was found between osteonecrosis and HAART, but there was an association with the CD4 nadir before treatment. Severe toxicities have become less frequent with newer drugs.

Hepatitis C and B (HCV/HBV) co-infection

In the SHCS, 31% of patients are HCV co-infected. The SHCS has demonstrated that treatment with pegylated interferon and ribavirin in a real-life clinical setting achieves sustained virologic response rates similar to those in randomized clinical trials, namely 28.4% for genotype 1/4 and 51.8% for genotype 2/3 [11]. However, only 12.5% of HCV RNA-positive individuals underwent HCV treatment, which is consistent with other studies. This relatively low number is due to the complexity of therapy in conjunction with ART, problems of adherence, and psychiatric co-morbidity, particularly in substance abusers. Liver-related death was the most frequent cause of non AIDS-related death. Improving HCV treatment will be of great importance for the future. Compared with HCV, the prevalence of HBV co-infection in Switzerland is low.

Conclusion

Intensive and frequently adjusted prevention programmes targeting different transmission groups, including needle exchange and substitution programmes, have controlled the spread of HIV infection in Switzerland, but high rates of infection among MSM continue to be a challenge. Morbidity and mortality have dropped spectacularly over the last decade due to HAART. Many HIV-related deaths now occur due to HCV co-infection, which remains difficult to treat.

References

1. Swiss HIV Cohort Study. (2006). *Swiss HIV Cohort Study*. Available at www.shcs.ch (accessed 7 February 2007).

2. Francioli P, Vogt M, Schadelin J, *et al.* (1982). Acquired immunologic deficiency syndrome, opportunistic infections and homosexualty. Presentation of three cases studied in Switzerland. *Schweiz Med Wochenschr* **112**:1682–1687.

3. Anonymous. (2006). L'épidémie de VIH en Suisse à l'automne 2006. *Bulletin de l'Office fédéral de la santé publique* **2006**:953–961.

4. Yerly S, Jost S, Telenti A, *et al.* (2004). Infrequent Transmission of HIV-1 Drug-resistant Variants. *Antivir Ther* **9**:375–384.

5. Hirschel B, Lazzarin A, Chopard P, *et al.* (1991). A controlled study of inhaled pentamidine for primary prevention of Pneumocystis carinii pneumonia. *N Engl J Med* **384**:1079–1083.

6. Ledergerber B, Mocroft A, Reiss P. (2001). Discontinuation of secondary prophylaxis against *Pneumocystis carinii* pneumonia in patients with HIV infection who have a response to antiretroviral therapy. Eight European Study Groups. *N Engl J Med* **344**:168–174.

7. Egger M, Hirschel B, Francioli P, *et al.* (1997). Impact of new antiretroviral combination therapies in HIV-infected patients in Switzerland: prospective multicentre study. *BMJ* **315**:1194–5.

8. Ananworanich J, Gayet-Ageron A, Le Braz M, *et al.* (2006). CD4-guided scheduled treatment interruptions compared with continuous therapy for patients infected with HIV-1: results of the Staccato randomized trial. *Lancet* **368**:459–465.

9. Marzolini C, Telenti A, Decosterd L, Biollaz J, Buclin T. (2001). Efavirenz plasma levels can predict treatment failure and central nervous system side effects in HIV-1-infected patients. *AIDS* **15**:1193–4.

10. Fellay J, Boubaker K, Ledergerber B, *et al.* (2001). Prevalence of Clinical and laboratory adverse events associated with potent antiretroviral therapy – The Swiss HIV Cohort Study. *Lancet* **358**:1322–7.

11. Egger M, Junghans C, Friis-Moller N, Lundgren JD. (2001). Highly active antiretroviral therapy and coronary heart disease: the need for perspective. *AIDS* **15**:S193-S201.

Chapter 15

The OPTIMA Cohort

Mark Holodniy

The Options in Management with Antiretrovirals (OPTIMA) study is the first tri-national collaboration between the US Department of Veterans Affairs (VA), Canadian Institutes for Health Research, and the UK Medical Research Council. The study cohort represents 368 very advanced HIV-1-infected patients with significant exposure to antiretroviral therapy (ART), multi-drug resistant virus and limited treatment options. OPTIMA is a prospective, randomized, 2-factorial design study looking at the clinical utility of a three-month antiretroviral drug-free period (ARDFP), and whether there is a difference in effectiveness between standard and 'mega-regimens' (five or more active antiretroviral drugs). At the time of writing the study is in its final year of follow-up. Although still blinded to treatment strategy, an ARDFP in the OPTIMA study has not resulted in safety concerns. Thus, the question of whether or not there is a favourable clinical response to standard or mega-ART preceded by an ARDFP will be answered in 2008. This chapter reviews the development of the cohort, the baseline characteristics and blinded analyses performed to date.

Introduction

Combination antiretroviral drug treatment regimens, commonly referred to as highly active antiretroviral therapy (HAART), have resulted in a substantial decrease in the incidence of AIDS and death in people with the human immunodeficiency virus (HIV) infection [1–3].

The duration of response to these regimens is limited in many patients by either the emergence of viral resistance or the development of toxicity. Over the last several years, there has been increasing evidence from clinical practice that standard ART fails in a significant proportion of patients [4]. Furthermore, subsequent treatment options are narrowed by the problem of accumulating HIV drug resistance, which culminates in variable levels of cross-resistance within each of the three main classes of antiretroviral drugs [5–7]. Resistance to increasing numbers of individual and classes of antiretroviral drugs is associated with increased risk of AIDS-associated events and death [8].

An effective virologic and immunologic response in ART re-treatment may be elicited by changing as many drugs of the combination as possible, particularly if a new class of drug is used and if the virologic breakthrough is of lower degree or shorter duration. In clinical practice, the virologic and immunologic response to switching therapy to three or four new drugs after antiretroviral regimen failure is often transient. Once a prolonged and significant virologic failure occurs on two different HAART regimens that have included all three classes of drugs, fewer treatment options are available. Although second-generation protease inhibitors (PIs) and new classes of antiretroviral drugs, such as entry and integrase inhibitors, could mitigate against this problem in the future, the optimal management of such patients currently remains unclear. The clinical dilemma posed in selecting treatments for patients facing this situation is the focus of the OPTIMA trial.

Effective options in multi-drug experienced HIV treatment failure are limited and include: continuing the current or similar regimen; waiting for new drugs to appear, recognizing that drugs may be ineffective after all three classes have been used in two regimens; employing a 'mega-regimen' (comprising five or more drugs), whereby more drugs are added than a standard three-drug HAART regimen; and, finally, stopping all or some of the drugs in a regimen for some period of time, known variously as 'drug-free period', 'drug holiday' or 'structured treatment interruption'.

The first question addressed by the OPTIMA trial is whether there is a difference in effectiveness between mega and standard antiretroviral regimens. Mega-ART is an experimental treatment strategy that has resulted in some success, defined by short-term virologic response. Essentially, the strategy is to treat with as many antiretroviral drugs as possible—defined in the OPTIMA study as five or more, although other studies have used up to nine antiretroviral (ARV) medications simultaneously—and maintain them for as long as possible. In previous studies, associated toxicity, though frequent, was manageable in many patients by supportive medication or drug substitution [9–11]. As clinical efficacy is related to clinical outcome as well as anti-HIV activity and toxicity of treatment, past validation of only surrogate marker responses of mega-HAART activity is of limited value. There are no randomized controlled trials with clinical endpoints (AIDS events or death) that compare mega-ART to standard HAART regimens.

The second question addressed by the OPTIMA trial is the clinical utility of an ARFDP. Its potential value in the presence of multi-drug resistance lies not only in a respite from pill-taking, some improved drug-related toxicity and improved quality of life (QOL), but also in the possibility that the activity and efficacy of a subsequent HAART regimen may be improved relative to such a regimen initiated without an interruption. In earlier small, uncontrolled studies, in the absence of pressure from antiretroviral drugs, most of the resistant blood plasma virus population returned to wild-type within two weeks to two months of discontinuation of ART [12], and was thus sensitive to drugs re-introduced after the ARDFP. Virologic response to subsequent regimens was correlated with the amount of resistance burden present after an ARDFP [13,14]. Although population sequencing of plasma HIV RNA indicated that wild-type virus re-emerged after treatment discontinuation, clonal analysis of viral variants indicated that antiretroviral drug-resistant HIV strains remained in the circulating quasi-species pool of viruses [15]. It was also observed that treatment interruption resulted in transient reduction in CD4 counts, probably as a result of increased replication and cytopathogenicity of wild-type virus [16]. Whether reduction in CD4 counts and subsequent rebound viraemia—with resultant partial reversion to wild-type, drug-susceptible HIV—resulted in increased clinical events, but was offset by relief of drug toxicity and subsequent response to re-treatment, was not known at the time of inception of the OPTIMA trial.

Several studies addressing this question in a variety of patient populations with multi-drug resistant virus have now been completed; they are reviewed elsewhere [17] and discussed briefly below. Enhanced virologic response to mega-ART was observed in patients with at least two months of ARDFP when compared to those patients who did not have an ARDFP in the French ANRS 097 GIGHAART study, despite an expected fall in CD4 counts during the ARDFP [18]. However, some studies have shown no virologic advantage (Spanish Retrogene study, AIDS Clinical Trials Group (ACTG) 5086 studies, CPCRA 064 study) and increased clinical endpoints (CPCRA 064 study), but no difference in survival rates after an ARDFP (CPCRA 064 study) [19–22]. It is possible that a temporary ARDFP may provide patients with an improved QOL without seriously affecting long-term survival, or possibly even improve survival, even with a standard antiretroviral regimen, because the patients are better able to tolerate the new therapy.

The concept of treatment interruptions had been supported previously by the US Department of Health and Human Services (DHHS) therapeutic guidelines panel, which stated in 1998 that, 'For patients with no rational alternative options who have virologic failure with return of viral load to baseline (pre-treatment levels) and declining CD4 T cell count, there should be consideration for discontinuation of antiretroviral therapy' [23]. However, based on studies completed to date, current DHHS guideline recommendations from 10 October 2006 now state, 'Discontinuing or briefly interrupting therapy (even with ongoing viraemia) may lead to a rapid increase in HIV RNA, a decrease in CD4 count, and increases the risk for clinical progression and is therefore not recommended' [23].

Despite recent clinical trial results and current guideline recommendations, controversy still exists as to whether there is any clinical benefit from treatment interruption. Most of the trials published to date have used different lengths of treatment interruption (two to four months), patients with different degrees of immunologic impairment, different post-interruption treatment regimens (standard versus mega-HAART) and study endpoints (virologic versus AIDS event and death rates). Many patients with multi-drug resistant and unsuppressed HIV viral load have pill fatigue or cumulative toxicities and have opted for self-imposed treatment interruptions of varying duration. However, the optimal duration of an ARDFP and treatment strategy, or whether any specific group of patients would benefit from this strategy, is not known.

There are important differences between the design of OPTIMA and the recently closed Strategies for Management of Antiretroviral Therapy (SMART) study that should also be mentioned. First, the two studies are testing different hypotheses regarding treatment. OPTIMA is studying whether a brief treatment interruption may improve response rates and tolerance to resumption of ART in patients with advanced disease and few or no HIV treatment options. SMART studied whether CD4 count could be used as a guide to starting and stopping treatment in less advanced patients with the objective of conserveing drug options and minimizing adverse effects of treatment. Second, the OPTIMA trial is studying patients who have failed standard therapies because of high-level HIV drug resistance. Study patients in SMART had mild to moderate HIV disease and a broad range of treatment options. Thirdly, treatment interruptions in OPTIMA are intended to last for 12 weeks, whereas patients in SMART could be off of antiretroviral drugs for many months. Results from the SMART trial were recently presented and found that continuous treatment was far superior compared with discontinuation based on a CD4 count threshold [24].

OPTIMA trial study design

OPTIMA is a prospective, multi-centre trial to study the optimal management of HIV-1–infected patients who have failed at least two conventional HAART regimens including all three classes of anti-HIV drugs [25,26]. The study is a 2 x 2 factorial, open, randomized multi-centre trial in which subjects were randomized to undergo an ARDFP for three months or not (no ARDFP), followed by either standard (four or fewer drugs) or mega- (five or more drugs) ART (Figure 15.1).

The primary outcome measure is the time to new or recurrent AIDS event or death from any cause (effectiveness) and time to development of a new non HIV-related serious adverse event (toxicity, non HIV morbidity). The secondary outcome measure is the time to development of a new non HIV-related serious adverse event and time to either of the primary endpoints. Quality of life is being assessed using computer-based instruments such as: time trade-offs (TTO) and standard gamble (SG) (both in VA patients only); visual analogue scale (VAS); EuroQol (EQ-5D); Health Utilities Index Mark 2 and Mark 3 (HUI3, HUI2); and the Medical

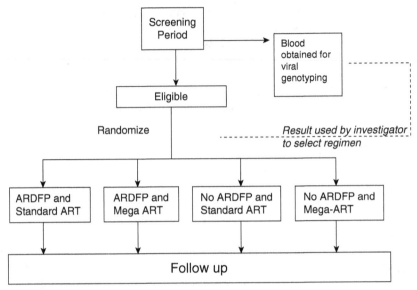

Fig. 15.1 OPTIMA study schema.
ARDFP = Antiretroviral drug-free period

Outcomes Study HIV (MOS-HIV). Additional analyses include incidence of grades 3 or 4 clinical or laboratory adverse events, changes in CD4 counts, HIV-1 viral load, resistance patterns and health economics (cost-effectiveness and cost-utility analyses from societal and payor perspectives).

The OPTIMA trial included male and female patients with advanced HIV disease and in whom regimens that included all three classes of antiretroviral drugs had failed. Patients were included if they have been on their current HIV regimen for at least three months and had a CD4 count of ≤300 cells/mm³ (or ≤15%) and a viral load ≥5000 copies/mL by the HIV-1 Amplicor Monitor polymerase chain reaction (PCR) assay (Roche), or ≥2500 by the Versant branched DNA (bDNA) assay (Bayer), while on that regimen. At the screening visit, a genotype and virtual phenotype were obtained to guide subsequent regimen decisions. Patients were seen at the baseline visit at which randomization to ARDFP or no ARDFP was determined. A second randomization was then performed to determine whether patients would receive a standard or mega-HAART regimen. Patients on ARDFP were seen at six weeks for a safety visit, and all patients were seen at 12 weeks and every three months during the first year, and every six months thereafter. Patients were to be seen for at least one year of follow-up. Quality of life assessments were performed, and blood samples (for T cell subsets, viral load and sample repository) were obtained at each visit.

Several factors contributed to slow recruitment in the study. Results from the CPCRA 064 study were published, and concerns were raised as to the merits of treatment interruption in patients living with AIDS [21]. Preliminary results from the SMART study further affected investigators' decisions in Canada and the United Kingdom in terms of enrolling patients. Finally, with the advent of more effective antiretroviral drug combinations and ritonavir (RTV)-boosted PI regimens, fewer subjects appeared to be available at the sites. The study was recalibrated from a sample size of 504 and 292 primary events based on ongoing event rates, and it was determined that a target accrual of 390 subjects and 232 primary events would provide sufficient power to answer the primary study question.

Baseline characteristics of the OPTIMA Cohort

At present, a total of 60 sites (25 VA sites, 17 in the United Kingdom and 18 in Canada) are participating in the OPTIMA trial. The final subject was recruited on 30 June 2006. A total of 425 subjects were screened, and 368 subjects were randomized. The VA recruited 288 (78%), Canada 41 (11%), and the UK 39 (11%) of the subjects. Baseline patient characteristics are presented in Table 15.1. The cohort is 98% male with a mean age of 47 years. Risk factors for HIV infection included men who have sex with men (MSM) (50%), injection drug use (IDU) (10%), and 25% heterosexual contact. Fifty percent were Caucasian, 30% black and 10% Latino. The mean and median CD4 counts were 127 cells/mm^3 and 109 cells/mm^3, respectively. The mean HIV-1 viral load was 4.82 log$_{10}$ copies/mL.

Prior ART history for the OPTIMA Cohort is listed in Table 15.2. Over 96% of patients have used more than three nucleoside reverse transcriptase inhibitors (NRTIs) (median five); at least one non-nucleoside reverse transcriptase inhibitor (NNRTI) (97%, median one), more than three PIs (63%, median three), and 2.5% were enfuvirtide (ENF)-experienced.

The first regimen on study is presented in Table 15.3. Because the study is still blinded, we are unable to break out the specific regimens by randomized study arm. Seventy percent of patients were placed on combination antiretroviral regimens that included two classes and between three and five drugs. Many of these regimens included ENF, various boosted PIs, and antiretroviral drugs available through expanded access programmes.

Baseline genotypic and virtual phenotypic resistance from the first 309 patients is presented in Tables 15.4a,b and Table 15.5, respectively. In this clinically advanced population, the prevalence of HIV drug resistance is significant. Over half the patients had evidence of significant thymidine-associated mutations (TAMs, T215Y and M41L) and NNRTI class resistance (K103N), and 50% had lamivudine (3TC)/emtricitabine (FTC) resistance (M184V). More than 40% had one or more HIV-1 protease gene primary PI mutations. Resistance was highly correlated with prior antiretroviral exposure.

In terms of baseline QOL scores, the OPTIMA Cohort has substantially reduced QOL scores compared to a comparable HIV-uninfected population. TTO and SG scores were generally higher than community-based preferences (HUI2/3, EQ-5D, VAS). When CD4 count and HIV viral load were separated, there was a trend towards lower scores in those patients with CD4 counts <129 cells/mm^3. Only EQ-5D scores were significantly lower in those OPTIMA patients with viral loads >59,000 copies/mL. The SG and TTO instruments were moderately correlated with each other (r=0.42) and poorly correlated with the VAS, EQ-5D and HUI3 (r≤0.29). The VAS, EQ-5D and HUI3 were moderately to strongly correlated with each other (r=0.57–0.86) [27]. The OPTIMA trial is the first study to compare this many QOL instruments using the same cohort and demonstrate significantly different findings among the instruments.

Primary outcome data to date

The mean follow-up per patient so far has been 1.8 years, accounting for 795 person-years of study. Subjects have spent 88% of the time on their allocated strategy. As of 1 September 2006, there were 84 deaths (59 HIV- or ART-related) and 123 AIDS-defining illnesses (77 new and 46 recurrent) in 77 patients. Thus, a total of 161 (43%) subjects have had a primary outcome for a calculated rate of 17.5 events per 100 person-years (total includes all adjudicated and unadjudicated endpoints at this time). The causes of AIDS events are listed in Table 15.6.

Table 15.1 OPTIMA subject baseline characteristics and demographics

	N
Total	**364**
Mean Age (SD)	**48.0 (8.56)**
Age Categories (%):	
31–40	68 (19)
41–50	153 (42)
51–60	119 (33)
>60	24 (7)
Gender (%):	
Male	355 (98)
Female	9 (2)
Race (%):	
White	179 (49)
Black	141 (39)
Asian	2 (1)
Latino	36 (10)
Native American/Aboriginal	2 (1)
Other	4 (1)
Mode of Infection (%):	
Blood	34 (9)
IV drug use	52 (14)
Heterosexual	84 (23)
MSM	174 (48)
Other	18 (5)
Pending	1 (<1)
AIDS at entry (%):	363 (>99)
HIV RNA copies/ml (%):	
<5k	30 (8)
5–50k	128 (35)
50–100k	62 (17)
>100k	143 (39)
Unknown	1 (<1)
Mean log (SD)	4.75 (0.7)
CD4 cells/mm^3:	
mean (SD)	127 (108)
min	1
max	594
median	108

Presumptive oesophageal candidiasis (EC) (41 events, 19.8%) and *Pneumocystis carinii* pneumonia (PCP, now *Pneumocystis jiroveci*) (20 events, 9.7%) have been the most common AIDS events.

As of 15 May 2006, there were 645 grade 3 or 4 adverse events in 178 patients. One hundred and seventy-four of these events in 82 patients led to a change in antiretroviral regimens. As of the same date, there were 559 serious adverse events (SAE) in 183 patients (including 60 deaths) (Table 15.7). A total of 154 unique patients experienced 490 non-AIDS SAEs, and 37 unique patients experienced 69 AIDS events. Some patients may have experienced AIDS and non-AIDS events as well as multiple events in different system organ classes (SOCs). The most common

Table 15.2 OPTIMA Cohort prior antiretroviral history

Class	Number	Patients
PIs	0	2
	1	54
	2	76
	3	58
	4	76
	5	64
	6	31
	>6	1
Total	-	362
Median	3	-
NRTIs	0	0
	1	1
	2	13
	3	36
	4	87
	5	103
	6	91
	7	26
	8	5
Total	-	362
Median	5	-
NNRTIs	0	13
	1	215
	2	112
	>2	22
Total	-	362
Median	1	-
Fusion inhibitors (FIs)	0	353
	1	9
Total	-	362
Median	0	-

non-AIDS SAEs were associated with infections (35%) and gastrointestinal disorders (10%). Only 28 events were thought to be related to ART.

Analyses conducted to date

Both AIDS and non-AIDS events can adversely affect clinical outcome and QOL for HIV-infected patients. The OPTIMA study team compared the type, frequency and QOL consequences of AIDS versus non-AIDS events in patients having advanced AIDS in the OPTIMA Cohort. Patients with AIDS-related events, non-AIDS SAEs or no serious clinical event were identified. Scores from the MOS-HIV QOL instrument [28], and both physical health status (PHS) and mental health status (MHS), were calculated at baseline, pre-event and post-event. Concurrent SAEs and AIDS events and those with missing MOS-HIV data were excluded. When this analysis was performed, 289 patients were enrolled, with a median CD4 count of 111 cells/mm^3. Of 37 deaths, 14 were HIV-related, seven unrelated and 13 yet to be adjudicated. There were 185 non-AIDS SAEs in 81 patients and 89 AIDS events in 53 patients. Mean baseline QOL scores for PHS and MHS using the MOS-HIV were low. There were no differences in pre-event

Table 15.3 Antiretroviral regimen after randomization in the OPTIMA study

Number of classes	Number of drugs	Total
1	1	1
	2	1
	3	8
	4	6
	5	2
	Total	18
2	2	1
	3	80
	4	61
	5	92
	6	11
	Total	245
3	3	10
	4	31
	5	42
	6	7
	Total	90
4	4	1
	Total	1

scores between groups. Compared to patients without events, the decrease in PHS scores was greater for SAEs (p=0.006) and the decrease in MHS scores was greater for both SAEs (p=0.013) and AIDS events (p<0.003). PHS and MHS score declines from pre- to post-event status did not differ between AIDS events and non-AIDS SAEs. However, significant decreases in pre-event to post-event scores occurred in PHS following SAEs (p=0.002) and in MHS following AIDS events (p=0.033). The conclusion from this analysis was that:

◆ non-AIDS SAEs are more common than AIDS-related events in OPTIMA patients and are associated with similar declines in QOL as AIDS events;

◆ the adverse effects of AIDS events and non-AIDS SAEs on physical and mental health status are similar;

◆ significant and similar declines in physical health status are associated with both non-AIDS SAEs and with AIDS events;

◆ significant declines in mental health status are associated with AIDS events but not with non-AIDS SAEs; and

◆ non-AIDS and AIDS events have comparable serious adverse effects on quality of life in this population [29].

Further analyses looked at this question using the HUI3, HUI2 and EQ-5D utility measures if an AIDS event occurred within one month of QOL assessment and if an SAE was ongoing within the instrument recall period. Mean utility scores did not change significantly from baseline to pre-event. Both AIDS-related and non-AIDS SAEs were associated with declines in health-related QOL when compared to those patients who did not have an event. HUI3 scores decreased significantly (pre- to post-event) for patients with AIDS (p=0.04) and non-AIDS SAEs (p=0.05), whereas ED-5D scores fell significantly only in patients with non-AIDS SAEs (p=0.02) [30]. Score declines related to SAEs were significantly greater in all three instruments compared to AIDS events [31]. Mixed-effect models were assessed. Time from baseline to the event was modelled as

Table 15.4a Frequency of HIV-1 reverse transcriptase (RT) gene mutations[a] in the OPTIMA Cohort (n=309)

RT MUTATIONS	N	Percent (%)
41L	161	52.1
103N	157	50.8
215Y	155	50.2
184V	156	50.5
62V	136	44.0
67N	119	38.5
210W	99	32.0
118I	95	30.7
74V	73	23.6
181C/I	72	23.1
70R	71	23.0
219Q/E	70	22.5
190S/A	67	21.7
190A	47	15.2
44D	47	15.2
215F	45	14.6
69D	43	13.9
188L/H	34	11.0
333E	42	13.6
108I	38	12.3
100I	34	11.0
115F	17	5.5
151M	10	3.2
225H	9	2.9
69INS	9	2.9
65R	9	2.9
116Y	8	2.6
106A/M	6	2.0

[a] Based on IAS-USA guidelines

a random effect, while all other covariates were modelled as fixed effects. Four models were fitted with independent variables including baseline score, time from baseline, event and change in CD4 count, HIV viral load, or both. Both non-AIDS SAEs and AIDS had a negative impact on QOL score.

The significance of SAE impact did not vary by adding the changes of CD4 count or viral load. After adjusting for all independent variables, non-AIDS SAEs had a stronger negative impact than AIDS on all QOL measures [32]. Thus, in different analyses, we continue to show that non-AIDS events dominate the overall burden of disease in this advanced HIV-infected population.

Table 15.4b Frequency of HIV-1 protease gene mutations[a] in the OPTIMA Cohort (n=309)

PR MUTATIONS	N	Percent (%)
63P	252	81.5
10F/I/V	201	65.0
71V/T	181	58.4
90M	151	48.9
54V/L/M	129	47.6
46I/L	140	44.3
62V	136	44.0
36I	127	41.1
82A/F/S/T	121	39.1
13V	103	33.3
84V	70	22.7
77I	100	32.4
64L/M/V	67	22.5
20M/R	63	20.3
33F	55	17.8
71T	46	14.9
60E	43	14.0
73S/A	34	11.0
58E	24	7.7
43T	23	7.1
32I	21	6.8
88D/S	21	6.8
24I	20	6.5
47V	19	6.1
53L	19	6.1
76V	17	5.5
69K	15	4.9
50V	12	3.9
30N	13	4.9
74P	11	4.6
11I	13	4.2
16E	10	3.2
48V	10	3.2
35G	6	1.9
50L	3	1.0

[a] Based on IAS-USA guidelines

Table 15.5 Baseline fold change for antiretrovirals using virtual phenotype in the OPTIMA Cohort

Drug Name	N	Mean fold change	SD	Cut-Off 1[a]	Cut-Off 2[a]
Abacavir	354	2.9	2.0	0.8	1.9
Amprenavir	354	5.4	9.4	0.9	2.0
Amprenavir/r	11	7.5	14.0	1.3	11.4
Atazanavir	103	25.3	32.5	2.7	32.9
Delavirdine	354	69.1	60.8	10[b]	
Didanosine	354	1.9	2.3	0.9	2.6
Efavirenz	354	133.3	152.0	3.4[c]	
Emtricitabine	103	27.3	24.8	3.5[c]	
Fosamprenavir	11	7.5	14.0	2.2[c]	
Indinavir	354	10.3	10.2	0.9	4.5
Indinavir/r	11	11.9	13.0	10.6	40.1
Lamivudine	354	26.1	22.1	1.0	3.4
Lopinavir	343	19.6	24.7	2.5[b]	
Lopinavir/r	11	18.0	29.5	9.7	56.1
Nelfinavir	354	17.7	15.1	1.3	7.3
Nevirapine	354	45.2	24.0	5.5[c]	
Ritonavir	354	50.0	61.0	3.5[b]	
Saquinavir	354	9.0	12.3	2.5[b]	
Saquinavir/r	11	8.7	14.3	7.1	26.5
Stavudine	354	1.6	1.4	0.9	2.0
Tenofovir	328	1.6	1.3	0.9	2.1
Tipranavir	11	1.3	0.8	1.2	5.4
Zalcitabine	354	1.7	1.5	2.0[b]	
Zidovudine	354	9.9	11.3	1.2	9.6

[a] Cut-off values for maximal (CCO1) and minimal (CCO2) clinical response.

[b] Historical cut-off values for antiretrovirals no longer in use, or no longer reported on the current virtual phenotype report.

[c] Biological cut-offs. No CCO established yet for these antiretrovirals.

Based on the significant impact that non-AIDS SAEs have on QOL, our group believes that non-AIDS SAEs should be considered as a component of primary outcome measures in future management trials of HIV treatment.

Finally, the relative burden of oesophageal candidiasis on QOL was examined in comparison with other AIDS-defining illnesses. Although it is an AIDS-defining illness, some have suggested that the degree of morbidity is lower with oesophageal candidiasis than other, more serious opportunistic infections (OIs). Since the clinical endpoints in the CPCRA 064 study were dominated by oesophageal candidiasis events, we felt it was important to determine whether the impact of OIs on QOL was similar. Of 300 subjects enrolled at the time of this analysis, 35 AIDS events occurred as a single isolated event and were included in the analysis.

Table 15.6 Primary endpoints in the OPTIMA trial as of 1 October 2006

	Total	
	N	%
Total number of events	**207**	**100**
Aspergillosis, invasive pulmonary	1	0.5
B-cell, non-Hodgkin's lymphoma	3	1.4
CMV retinitis	7	3.4
Cerebral toxoplasmosis	1	0.5
Chronic herpes simplex virus (HSV) mucocutaneous ulceration	6	2.9
Cryptococcosis, meningitis or extrapulmonary	3	1.4
Cryptosporidiosis	2	1
Oesophageal candidiasis	41	19.8
HIV wasting syndrome	9	4.3
HIV encephalopathy/ dementia	2	1
Herpes zoster virus (HZV), multidermatomal	1	0.5
Histoplasmosis, disseminated or extrapulmonary	1	0.5
KS	5	2.4
MAC, disseminated	6	2.9
Other CMV end-organ disease	5	2.4
Other indeterminate intracerebral lesion(s)	1	0.5
PCP	20	9.7
Progressive multifocal leukoencephalopathy (PML)	1	0.5
Primary cerebral lymphoma	1	0.5
Recurrent bacterial pneumonia	6	2.9
Rhodococcus equi disease	1	0.5
Death	84	40.6

Patients with oesophageal candidiasis (n=12) had better baseline PHS scores than those with other AIDS events (n=23) (mean score 41.7 versus 36.4, p=0.04). PHS score declined by a mean of 3.8 after other AIDS events, and increased by 1.2 after EC diagnosis (-3.8 versus +1.2, p=0.10 between groups), while MHS score did not appear to change (-2.9 versus -2.8, p=0.87). Compared with other AIDS events in the OPTIMA trial, oesophageal candidiasis was associated with higher physical health score at baseline, similar subsequent impact on mental health and lesser subsequent impact on physical health [33]. Thus, to better evaluate the impact of antiretroviral salvage strategies on clinical event rates, AIDS events may need to be weighted when used as outcomes in clinical trials.

The impact of hepatitis C virus (HCV) co-infection on survival and the onset of new AIDS events were also studied in the OPTIMA Cohort. Of the 311 patients for whom HCV status and follow-up data were available, 72 (23%) were HCV antibody-positive. Twenty-five per cent of HCV-positive patients died compared with 16% of HCV-negative patients. There was evidence

Table 15.7 Serious adverse events and causes of death in the OPTIMA Cohort

Deaths Reported as SAEs by System Organ Class (SOC)	Total
Cardiac disorders: total	4
Gastrointestinal disorders: total	1
Infections and infestations: total	25
Nervous system disorders: total	5
Renal and urinary disorders: total	5
General disorders and administration site conditions	7
Neoplasms benign, malignant, and unspecified	5
Respiratory, thoracic and mediastinal disorders	5
Metabolism and nutrition disorders	1
Surgical and medical procedures	1
Hepatobiliary disorders	1
Grand Total	60

Summary of non-AIDS Serious Adverse Events by System Organ Class (SOC)	Number	% of Total
Blood and lymphatic system disorders	30	5%
Cardiac disorders	26	5%
Ear and labyrinth disorders	1	<1%
Endocrine disorders	1	<1%
Eye disorders	2	<1%
Gastrointestinal disorders	55	11%
Hepatobiliary disorders	4	<1%
Immune system disorders	6	1%
Infections and infestations	135	28%
Investigations	13	3%
Metabolism and nutrition disorders	23	5%
Nervous system disorders	28	6%
Psychiatric disorders	9	2%
Renal and urinary disorders	33	7%
Skin and subcutaneous tissue disorders	5	1%
Social circumstances	4	<1%
Surgical and medical procedures	8	2%
Vascular disorders	16	3%
General disorders and administration site conditions	41	8%
Injury, poisoning, and procedural complications	8	2%
Musculoskeletal and connective tissue disorders	8	2%
Neoplasms benign, malignant, and unspecified	19	4%
Reproductive system and breast disorders	1	<1%
Respiratory, thoracic, and mediastinal disorders	14	3%
Grand Total	490	100%

Summary of AIDS Serious Adverse Events by System Organ Class (SOC)	Number	% of Total
Infections and infestations	60	87%
Neoplasms benign, malignant	6	9%
Nervous system disorders	3	4%
Grand Total	69	100%

to suggest that HCV is associated with impaired survival (hazard ratio (HR)=1.79; 95% confidence interval (CI):1.01–3.16, p=0.045). The effect size was similar after adjusting for mode of transmission (HR=1.70; CI:0.86–3.36, p=0.13), but after further controlling for (time dependent) number of antiretroviral drugs, the effect was attenuated (HR=1.37; CI:0.67–2.80, p=0.39). The median time to first switch/stop of on-study ART was 3.8 (0.03, 36) and 6.5 (0.03, 46) months in HCV-positive and HCV-negative patients, respectively. HCV-positive patients were no more likely than HCV-negative patients to experience an AIDS event during follow-up (23% versus 25%). We also found no statistically significant effect of HCV on time to a new AIDS event or death (HR=1.32; 0.84, 2.08, p=0.23). HCV co-infection in OPTIMA appears to increase the risk of mortality, but this effect might be partly explained by a shorter time to switching/stopping ART [34]. One possible reason may be that HCV-positive patients in OPTIMA are less able to tolerate ART.

The relationship between viral load and CD4 count response, and the subsequent development of primary endpoints in OPTIMA was recently analyzed [35]. A one log/mL decline in HIV-1 viral load at 24 weeks after starting an antiretroviral salvage regimen after randomization was considered successful. A Cox hazards model was used to examine the association between virologic response and time to a clinical event. For this analysis, 307 subjects were included, 167 (54.4%) of whom had a successful viral load response. Patients who had a one log or greater viral load reduction were significantly less likely to have an AIDS event or death compared with those who had no viral load response (13.2% versus 37.9%). Thus, a one log reduction in viral load was a significant predictor of AIDS or death (RH=0.71 per log decrease; 95% CI:0.55–0.92, p<0.001) and death alone, 12 of 167 (7.2%) versus 38/140 (27.1%) (RH=0.76 per log decrease; 95% CI:0.55–1.05, p<0.001).

When baseline CD4 count was divided into tertiles (<50, 51–200, and >200/mm^3), lower CD4 counts were significantly associated with AIDS or death (RH per cell=0.992; 95% CI:0.988–0.996, p<0.001) and with death only (RH per cell=0.989; 95% CI:0.984–0.94, p<0.001). When CD4 change was divided according to those subjects who had a less than or greater than 90/mm3 CD4 cell change, there was a trend towards having fewer clinical events in those patients who had a greater than 90 cells/mm3 CD4 cell increase. Thus, even in late salvage, regardless of the specific regimen or treatment strategy, baseline CD4 count and a significant reduction in viral load remain strong predictors of clinical outcome.

An extension of this analysis attempted to determine whether baseline level of resistance as measured by virtual phenotype (VircoType®, Virco) correlated with clinical outcome [36]. A Cox hazards model was used to assess both the univariate and multivariate contribution of baseline predictors (CD4 count, log viral load, resistance) to time to AIDS event or death. This analysis included 228 subjects. Baseline drug exposure and resistance are presented in Figures 15.2a and 15.2b. When PI, NRTI, and all class resistance were considered, only NRTI resistance in the univariate analysis was a significant predictor of time to AIDS event or death (RH=1.139; 95% CI:1.004–1.291, p=0.043). No aspect of resistance was significant in the multivariate analysis. When categorical definitions for resistance (number of antiretroviral drugs per class) were considered in a multivariate analysis, resistance to higher numbers of NRTIs, PIs, and to all antiretroviral drugs were significantly associated with an AIDS event or death (Table 15.8a). In the multivariate analysis, only resistance to five or more PIs was a significant predictor of clinical outcome (Table 15.8b). As before, CD4 count remained a significant predictor of time to AIDS or death. Baseline viral load level was not a significant predictor. Thus, there is some evidence to suggest that in the OPTIMA Cohort, a significant level of drug resistance burden is associated with clinical events.

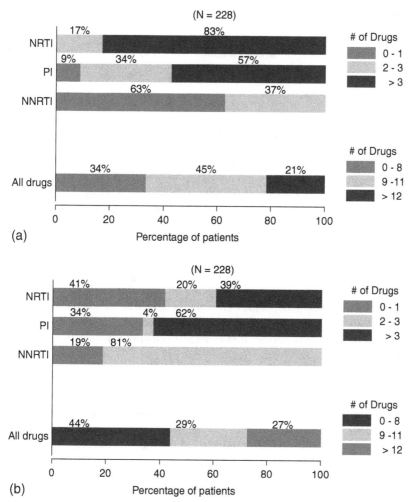

Fig. 15.2 (a) Drug exposure as measured by virtual phenotype in the OPTIMA Cohort; (b) Resistance as measured by virtual phenotype in the OPTIMA Cohort.

Table 15.8a ARV resistance-associated predictors of AIDS and death in the OPTIMA Cohort: univariate analysis

Predictor	Relative Hazard	95% CI	p value
NRTIs resistant (0–5 versus 6–7)	2.11	1.20–3.73	0.01
PIs resistant (0–5 versus 6)	1.56	0.90–2.71	0.11
All resistant (≤12 versus 13–16)	1.83	1.06–3.13	0.03

Table 15.8b ARV resistance-associated predictors of AIDS and death in the OPTIMA Cohort: multivariate analysis

Predictor	Relative Hazard	95% CI	p value
CD4 (per cell)	0.993	0.989–0.997	<0.001
Log pVL	1.23	0.70–2.15	0.46
PI resistance (≤5 versus 6)	1.85	1.03–3.32	0.04

Preliminary economic analyses from the VA OPTIMA population have yielded some interesting findings [Wei Yu, personal communication, 2006]. When compared to all HIV-infected veteran patients in care within the VA system, the mean cost for VA OPTIMA patients (n=273) in the year prior to randomization (1999) was 34% higher (in 2006 US dollars). Comparing pharmacy, inpatient and outpatient costs from the year prior to randomization to the first year on study, the average cost increased from US$20,280 to US$27,210. Pharmacy costs accounted for approximately 47% of the total cost. There was a trend toward increased inpatient costs after one year on the study, which correlated with a mean increase in days of inpatient care. Total pharmacy and antiretroviral drug costs increased 31% and 35%, respectively, after one year. Since this analysis is only looking at blinded data, some of the trends may be related to increased use of ENF, costs for mega-HAART, additional prescriptions to manage side effects, or inpatient hospitalization as a result of toxicity management. Further studies are planned once the study is unblinded to compare costs across treatment arms and across countries.

Discussion

The OPTIMA study will be unblinded in mid-2008. Results from the OPTIMA trial could become irrelevant if effective HIV treatment for multi-drug resistant infection became available, treatment regimens were developed that had a low likelihood of failure, or if sufficient numbers of tolerable treatment alternatives were available so that effective options would not become exhausted. Newer treatment regimens are becoming available that encourage adherence because of fewer side effects, lower pill burden and more convenient dosing schedules. Newer classes of drugs are being introduced, such as entry and integrase inhibitors, whose effectiveness is even less likely to be compromised by cross-resistance to regimens that have previously failed with conventional classes of antiretroviral drugs, but the long-term complications of these drugs and their propensity for developing resistance remains untested.

Despite these welcome trends, the problem of salvage treatment for patients with multi-drug resistant infection is unlikely to become trivial for several reasons. All antiretroviral regimens are known to lead to resistance if not rigorously adhered to or if used as part of an inadequately constructed combination. Concerns were expressed during OPTIMA protocol development that the introduction of antiretroviral drugs such as lopinavir (LPV) or other PI-boosted regimens, tenofovir (TDF), and ENF would make OPTIMA irrelevant. However, patients randomized in OPTIMA have failed regimens that include these drugs. Emerging trends in ARV drug resistance are likely to increase with time so that the problem of patients harbouring multi-drug resistant virus permitting few therapeutic options is likely to grow in parallel with the growth of the global HIV pandemic. The underlying rationale for OPTIMA, which seeks to find the best approach to salvage, should therefore continue to be of relevance.

The rationale for OPTIMA would also be compromised if other studies convincingly answered the questions posed by the study. The GIGHAART study provided important support for the concept that mega-HAART treatment and short-term treatment interruption could enhance virologic response, although it did not appear to provide benefit for clinical endpoints [18]. The CPCRA 064 study was terminated because of undesirable declines in CD4 count, increased AIDS events in the treatment interruption arm and the unlikelihood that further recruitment would show that treatment interruption offered any clinical benefit [21]. Although death rates were equal in both arms, the majority of clinical events were presumptive oesphageal candidiasis, which might have been avoided with more aggressive vigilance and oral candidiasis treatment. No randomized trials compare the risk and benefits of standard versus mega-HAART. Thus, the continuing question of how to manage multi-drug resistance, in the absence of studies to answer the clinical questions posed by OPTIMA, and emerging evidence supporting one of the study's more controversial hypotheses, serve to reinforce the ongoing relevance of the trial.

Although current HIV treatment guidelines recommend against complete treatment interruptions in patients on salvage treatment, the studies to date, summarized elsewhere [17], represent several different strategies. Varying lengths of treatment interruption (two to four months or longer), baseline CD4 count (and hence degree of immunologic impairment), type of follow-up antiretroviral regimen (standard versus mega-HAART), and investigator chosen or study required all make comparisons between trials difficult. In general, CD4 counts have decreased and HIV-1 viral load has increased during the treatment interruption period. Although an increase in AIDS-defining illnesses, driven primarily by presumptive oesophageal candidiasis, has been seen in some studies, no clinical benefit after complete treatment interruption has been seen to date.

Oesophageal candidiasis is a common infection and one of the earliest AIDS-defining events, occurring at a relatively early stage of immunosuppression. Approximately 10% of patients with AIDS will experience this infection during their lifetime. Unless the underlying immunodeficiency is corrected, approximately 60% will experience a relapse within six months of initial infection [37]. Thus, it is not surprising to see the increased number of cases in the CPCRA 064 and OPTIMA studies. Because it has a much diminished impact on mortality when compared with other opportunistic infections [38] and, in the absence of azole resistance, is easily treated in most patients, primary and secondary prophylaxis are rarely used as part of routine therapy. This has led some investigators to propose weighting OIs in terms of severity when designing and analyzing clinical trials when AIDS events are being considered as primary endpoints [39].

More recent data from several groups have shown that partial treatment interruption may offer a virologic and toxicity advantage over complete interruption or maintenance of a regimen to which a patient's HIV strain is completely resistant. In general, discontinuing NNRTIs and PIs has not resulted in any CD4 cell decline or viral load increases, whereas despite the presence of genotypic and phenotypic resistance, NRTIs appear to have some residual antiretroviral activity. Discontinuing NRTIs with maintenance of NNRTI- or PI-containing regimens has resulted in significant CD4 declines and viral load increases [40]. Larger studies will need to be performed to determine whether clinical outcome is affected by partial treatment interruptions.

A surprising finding in the OPTIMA trial is the impact of SAEs on the physical and mental health QOL among study subjects. Currently, non-AIDS SAEs outnumber and dominate primary clinical endpoints by four to one and are primarily manifested by infections and gastrointestinal events. In a recent meta-analysis from five randomized clinical trials, SAEs occurred significantly more often than AIDS events and were associated with similar risk of death [41]. Because of the importance of this finding and our ongoing findings on the impact of SAEs on QOL, non-AIDS SAEs are an important secondary endpoint and may be included in a composite endpoint together with AIDS events and death in the OPTIMA trial. Although a minority of SAEs appear to be related to antiretroviral drugs, we will not know what the contribution of treatment interruption or mega-HAART is to the prevalence of non-AIDS SAEs until the study is unblinded.

References

1. Hogg RS, Yip B, Kully C, *et al.* (1999). Improved survival among HIV-infected patients after initiation of triple-drug antiretroviral regimens. *CMAJ* **160**:659–65.

2. Palella FJ Jr, Delaney KM, Moorman AC, *et al.* (1998). Declining morbidity and mortality among patients with advanced human immunodeficiency virus infection. HIV Outpatient Study Investigators. *N Engl J Med* **338**:853–60.

3. Mocroft A, Vella S, Benfield TL, *et al.* (1998). Changing patterns of mortality across Europe in patients infected with HIV-1. EuroSIDA Study Group. *Lancet* **352**:1725–30.

4. Ledergerber B, Egger M, Opravil M, *et al.* (1999). Clinical progression and virological failure on highly active antiretroviral therapy in HIV-1 patients: a prospective cohort study. Swiss HIV Cohort Study. *Lancet* **353**:863–8.

5. Antinori A, Zaccarelli M, Cingolani A, *et al.* (2002). Cross-resistance among nonnucleoside reverse transcriptase inhibitors limits recycling efavirenz after nevirapine failure. *AIDS Res Hum Retroviruses* **18**:835–8.

6. Miller V, Larder BA.(2001). Mutational patterns in the HIV genome and cross-resistance following nucleoside and nucleotide analogue drug exposure. *Antivir Ther* **6**(Suppl 3):25–44.

7. Race E, Dam E, Obry V, Paulous S, Clavel F. (1999). Analysis of HIV cross-resistance to protease inhibitors using a rapid single-cycle recombinant virus assay for patients failing on combination therapies. *AIDS* **113**:2061–8.

8. Zaccarelli M, Tozzi V, Lorenzini P, *et al.* (2005). Multiple drug class-wide resistance associated with poorer survival after treatment failure in a cohort of HIV-infected patients. *AIDS* **19**:1081–9.

9. Montaner JS, Harrigan PR, Jahnke N, *et al.* (2001). Multiple drug rescue therapy for HIV-infected individuals with prior virologic failure to multiple regimens. *AIDS* **15**:61–9.

10. Miller V, Cozzi-Lepri A, Hertogs K, *et al.* (2000). HIV drug susceptibility and treatment response to mega-HAART regimen in patients from the Frankfurt HIV cohort. *Antivir Ther* **5**:49–55.

11. Rottmann C, Miller V, Staszewski S. (1999). Mega-HAART: preliminary results and correlation with baseline resistance. *Antivir Ther* **4** (Suppl 3):93–4.

12. Verhofstede C, Wanzeele FV, Van Der Gucht B, De Cabooter N, Plum J. (1999). Interruption of reverse transcriptase inhibitors or a switch from reverse transcriptase to protease inhibitors resulted in a fast reappearance of virus strains with a reverse transcriptase inhibitor-sensitive genotype. *AIDS* **13**:2541–6.

13. Miller V, Sabin C, Hertogs K, *et al.* (2000). Virological and immunological effects of treatment interruptions in HIV-1 infected patients with treatment failure. *AIDS* **14**:2857–67.

14. Izopet J, Massip P, Souyris C, *et al.* (2000). Shift in HIV resistance genotype after treatment interruption and short-term antiviral effect following a new salvage regimen. *AIDS* **14**:2247–55.

15. Hance AJ, Lemiale V, Izopet J, *et al.* (2001). Changes in human immunodeficiency virus type 1 populations after treatment interruption in patients failing antiretroviral therapy. *J Virol* **75**:6410–7.

16. Youle M, Janossy G, Turnbull W, *et al.* (2000). Changes in CD4 lymphocyte counts after interruption of therapy in patients with viral failure on protease inhibitor-containing regimens. Royal Free Centre for HIV Medicine. *AIDS* **14**:1717–20.

17. Pai NP, Lawrence J, Reingold AL, Tulsky JP. (2006). Structured treatment interruptions (STI) in chronic unsuppressed HIV infection in adults. *Cochrane Database Syst Rev* **3**:CD006148.

18. Katlama C, Dominguez S, Gourlain K, *et al.* (2004). Benefit of treatment interruption in HIV-infected patients with multiple therapeutic failures: a randomized controlled trial (ANRS 097). *AIDS* **18**:217–26.

19. Benson CA, Vaida F, Havlir DV, *et al.* (2006). A Randomized Trial of Treatment Interruption before Optimized Antiretroviral Therapy for Persons with Drug-Resistant HIV: 48-Week Virologic Results of ACTG A5086. *J Infect Dis* **194**:1309–18.

20. Ruiz L, Ribera E, Bonjoch A, *et al.* (2003). Role of structured treatment interruption before a 5-drug salvage antiretroviral regimen: the Retrogene Study. *J Infect Dis* **188**:977–85.

21. Lawrence J, Mayers DL, Hullsiek KH, *et al.* (2003). Structured treatment interruption in patients with multidrug-resistant human immunodeficiency virus. *N Engl J Med* **349**:837–46.

22. Lawrence J, Hullsiek KH, Thackeray LM, *et al.* (2006). Disadvantages of structured treatment interruption persist in patients with multidrug-resistant HIV-1: final results of the CPCRA 064 study. *J Acquir Immune Defic Syndr* **43**:169–78.

23. Panel on Antiretroviral Guidelines for Adult and Adolescents. (2006). *Guidelines for the use of antiretroviral agents in HIV-infected adults and adolescents.* Washington, DC: US Department of Health and Human Services. p1–113. Available at http://www.aidsinfo.nih.gov/ContentFiles/AdultandAdolescentsGL.pdf (accessed May 16, 2007).

24. El-Sadr WM, Lundgren JD, Neaton JD, *et al.* (2006). CD4+ count-guided interruption of antiretroviral treatment. *N Engl J Med* **355**:2283–96.

25. Kyriakides TC, Babiker A, Singer J, *et al.* (2003). An open-label randomized clinical trial of novel therapeutic strategies for HIV-infected patients in whom antiretroviral therapy has failed: rationale and design of the OPTIMA Trial. *Control Clin Trials* **24**:481–500.

26. Kyriakides TC, Babiker A, Singer J, Piaseczny M, Russo J. (2004). Study conduct, monitoring and data management in a trinational trial: the OPTIMA model. *Clin Trials* **1**:277–81.

27. Joyce V Araki SS, Sundaram V, *et al.*(2004). Utility-Based Assessments of Quality of Life in a Randomized Trial of Antiretroviral Therapy in Advance HIV Disease. Oral presentation, Society for Medical Decision Making Annual Meeting, 2004, Atlanta, GA, USA.

28. Wu AW, Rubin HR, Mathews WC, *et al.* (1991). A health status questionnaire using 30 items from the Medical Outcomes Study. Preliminary validation in persons with early HIV infection. *Med Care* **29**:786–98.

29. Brown ST, Singer J, Anis A, *et al.* (2004). Non-AIDS Serious Adverse Events are as Important as AIDS Events in Patients with Advanced Multi-Drug Resistance HIV Disease. XV International AIDS Conference, 2004, Bangkok, Thailand. [Abstract MoPeD3841]

30. Araki SS, Guh D, Singer J, *et al.* (2004).The Impact of AIDS-related Events and Non-AIDS Serious Adverse Events on Health-Related Quality of Life in a Multinational Trial of Antiretroviral Therapy. Society for Medical Decision Making, 2004, Atlanta, GA. [Abstract 5]

31. Anis AH, Sun H, Singer J, *et al.* (2005). AIDS-defining Events and Serious Adverse Events (SAE) in Patients with Advanced HIV Disease in the OPTIMA Trial: What affects patients Quality of Life most? 3rd International AIDS Society Conference on HIV Pathogenesis and Treatment, 2005, Rio de Janeiro, Brazil. [Abstract WePe12.9C04]

32. Anis AH, Sun H, Singer J, *et al.* (2005). The Longitudinal Pattern of Health Utility and its Determinants among Patients on Salvage Regimens with or without a Prior Treatment Interruption. 3rd International AIDS Society Conference on HIV Pathogenesis and Treatment, 2005, Rio de Janeiro, Brazil. [Abstract WePe12.9C18]

33. Cameron DW, Brown S, Youle M, *et al.* (2005). Relative Impact of Esophageal Candidiasis (EC) versus other AIDS events in the OPTIMA trial. 14th Annual Canadian Conference on HIV/AIDS Research, 2005, Vancouver, Canada. [Abstract 285P]

34. Ewings F, Angus B, Brown S, *et al.* (2006). The Effect of Hepatitis C virus on HIV progression in a late salvage population: Results from the OPTIMA study. 12th Annual Conference of the British HIV Association, 2006, Brighton, UK. [Abstract O15]

35. Singer J, Ayers D, Cameron W, *et al.* (2006). Predictors of Clinical Response to Salvage Therapy in a Late Salvage Population with Multi-drug resistant HIV in the OPTIMA Trial. 13th Conference on Retroviruses and Opportunistic Infections, 5–8 February 2006, Denver, CO, USA. [Abstract 526]

36. Singer J, Wu K, Cameron W, *et al.* (2005). Early HIV-RNA Response predicts clinical outcomes in a late salvage population. 3rd International AIDS Society Conference on HIV Pathogenesis and Treatment, 2005, Rio de Janeiro, Brazil. [Abstract WePe12.9C02]

37. Vazquez JA. (2003). Invasive esophageal candidiasis: current and developing treatment options. *Drugs* **63:**971–89.

38. Mocroft A, Youle M, Morcinek J, *et al.* (1997). Survival after diagnosis of AIDS: a prospective observational study of 2625 patients. Royal Free/Chelsea and Westminster Hospitals Collaborative Group. *BMJ* **314:**409–13.

39. Neaton JD, Wentworth DN, Rhame F, Hogan C, Abrams DI, Deyton L. (1994). Considerations in choice of a clinical endpoint for AIDS clinical trials. Terry Beirn Community Programs for Clinical Research on AIDS (CPCRA). *Stat Med* **13:**2107–25.

40. Deeks SG, Hoh R, Neilands TB, *et al.* (2005). Interruption of treatment with individual therapeutic drug classes in adults with multidrug-resistant HIV-1 infection. *J Infect Dis* **192:**1537–44.

41. Reisler RB, Han C, Burman WJ, Tedaldi EM, Neaton JD. (2003). Grade 4 events are as important as AIDS events in the era of HAART. *J Acquir Immune Defic Syndr* **34:**379–86.

Part 3

HAART in medium human development countries

Chapter 16

Country review: Brazil

Celso Ferreira Ramos-Filho* and
Cledy Eliana dos Santos

Introduction

Brazil is a medium-income developing country situated on the Atlantic coast of South America. It is the only Portuguese-speaking country in the Americas. With a land area of 8.5 million square kilometres, divided into 27 states, Brazil is the fifth-largest country in the world by geographical area, and with a population of 183.8 million (2007 estimate), it is the fifth most populous country in the world [1]. In the same year, Brazil's gross domestic product (GDP) reached US$799.4 million, for a per capita GDP of US$4,289 [2]. It is a medium human development country, placing 63rd among world nations in 2003 [3].

In 2002, public expenditure on education and health represented 4.2% and 3.6% of GDP, respectively, while national expenditure on research and development reached only 1% (1997–2002). From a socio-economic point of view, it is a country of inequalities, with a Gini coefficient of 59.3 [4].

There are also many disparities within the country, both within and between its five geographical regions, the states within each region, and different municipalities. For instance, in 2000, infant mortality in the North-East region was estimated at 53.13 per 1000, while in the South it was estimated at 22.20 per 1000, less than half the former. Similarly, as recently as 1996, more than 17% of births in the country's North-East region occurred outside a health unit or hospital, while in the South-East, this figure drops to less than 3% [5].

Brazil has a comprehensive public health system in which every citizen has a right to free medical care, although not necessarily to free medication in outpatient settings. However, there are regional disparities here too, with health professionals, facilities and equipment tending, in general, to be less abundant in the North and the North-East, the two least-developed regions [6]. Therefore, although in principle everyone has the same access to healthcare, in practice this may not be the case.

To understand the AIDS situation in Brazil it is important to be aware that Brazil is a huge, partially industrialized country with a large, unevenly distributed population, not well developed from a social point of view, with stark economic disparities between its component states and with an ambitious (and underfinanced), free healthcare system.

Epidemiology

The first case of AIDS in Brazil occurred in 1980 and was diagnosed retrospectively. As of June 2006, 433,067 cases had been reported to the national surveillance centre. From 1980 to 2005, there were 183,074 AIDS-related deaths; including the 11,026 deaths in 2006, the crude mortality rate comes to 6 per 100,000 population [7].

---

* Corresponding author.

Until the mid-1990s, the national incidence rate of AIDS kept growing, peaking at 19 cases per 100,000 people. Eighty per cent of these cases were concentrated in the South-East and the South. Notwithstanding the high incidence rates in these two regions, where the epidemic started early, incidence seems to have stabilized since 1998, although somewhat slowly. In the remaining three regions, this trend is not apparent, and the incidence is rising, especially in the North and West Central regions.

The epidemic has hit certain population groups hard, such as injection drug users (IDUs), men who have sex with men (MSM) and, in the early 1980s, individuals with a history of blood and blood product transfusion. Incidence has declined in children and in the 13– 29 year-old age group, while it has increased in older populations, particularly in individuals over 40 years of age. Of late, there has been a persistent increase in incidence among women, although a trend toward stabilization has appeared exclusively in females between 13 and 24 years of age. In men, there has been a marked and constant decrease among IDUs, and stabilization among MSM, but an increase among heterosexuals.

Since 1998, the annual number of AIDS-related deaths has kept fairly constant at around 11,000 cases, no doubt as the result of a policy of free access to antiretroviral treatment. The stable mortality rate is strongly influenced by results in the state of São Paulo and in the Federal District (corresponding to the country's capital, Brasília, and neighbouring cities) [8]. The male-to-female ratio for reported AIDS cases reached 26.5:1 in 1985 and has been steadily decreasing since, down to 1.4:1 in 2006.

A recent study (2004), estimated an overall HIV prevalence of 0.61% among individuals aged 15 to 49 years. Prevalence among males is estimated at 0.80%, and at 0.42% for females. The total number of infected individuals is thus 593,787, with the upper limit of the estimate set at 644,511 [9]. A previous study carried out in 2000 found a prevalence of 0.65%, for a point estimate of 597,443 individuals infected with HIV. This study did not find any significant differences with the results from a previous study in 1998 [10].

Thus, Brazil has faced differing 'sub-epidemics' since the early 1980s, with stabilization in some groups and geographical regions, but with dissimilar features in other places and groups. There are four important trends in the Brazilian epidemic, namely, that it is growing among heterosexuals, women, the poor and the inhabitants of smaller, more marginalized communities (due to migration into smaller communities).

HIV in Brazil

Subtypes

In all probability, HIV-1 came to Brazil from the United States, Europe, or both; therefore, subtype B predominates in most of the country, as would be expected, followed in frequency by subtypes F and C; occasionally, subtypes D and A are also present. In addition, two circulating recombinant forms (CRF), including CRF12_BF, a recombinant form that seems to be unique to South America, also occur [11–14].

As previously mentioned, the epidemic has differing dynamics and characteristics in the various regions of the country. For instance, a small study (31 samples) in Manaus, in the North, found almost equal prevalence of subtypes B and F [15]. In the South, subtype C has been on the increase, with a corresponding decrease in subtype B, the former being the predominant strain at present [16, 17].

HIV-2 was detected in Rio de Janeiro in the late 1980s, by polymerase chain reaction (PCR) analysis [18], but the finding has not been further confirmed.

HIV drug resistance

A countrywide study showed that resistance to antiretroviral drugs in treatment-naïve individuals was low (6.7% overall) in the early 2000s [19], as did a study in the city of São Paulo (6.3% for samples collected between 1998 and 2002). However, resistance among recently infected individuals was found to be 12.7%, compared with only 5% among individuals with long-standing infections, although these findings were not considered statistically significant [20]. Furthermore, a study in Santos, a port city in the state of São Paulo, showed a disturbing resistance prevalence of 25% for long-standing infections, and 36.8% for recent infections, in samples collected between 1999 and 2001 [21].

Since 2001, genotyping tests have been available and free of charge through the public health system throughout the country, in a special network of laboratories involving specially trained physicians, the *Rede Nacional de Genotipagem* (RENAGENO), or national network for genotyping. Patients are eligible if, after undergoing antiretroviral therapy (ART) for at least six months, virologic failure is suspected; in the case of pregnant women, the necessary minimum period of treatment is reduced to three months. Patients for whom the introduction of enfuvirtide (ENF) in the treatment regimen is being considered must have genotype testing. Patients are not eligible if their viral load is under 5000 copies/mL, or if they are considered to be non-adherent to treatment, or if they have had a previous genotyping test showing resistance to all available drugs. Treatment-naïve patients are not eligible.

There are an estimated 180,000 patients receiving ART in Brazil. The Brazilian National STD and AIDS Program (NATAP) began providing treatment for HIV and opportunistic infections in 1991 (not in 1996, as is widely and mistakenly believed). In November 1996, national legislation specifically made it mandatory for all levels of government to provide such treatment [22].

The new Brazilian Constitution issued in October 1988 stated in Article 196 that 'health is a right of all citizens and a duty of the State, guaranteed through social and economic policies aimed at reducing the risk of disease and other health hazards and through universal and equal access to actions and services destined to its promotion, protection and recovery' [*translation*] [23]. This is the constitutional basis of the Unified Health System (*Sistema Único de Saúde*, or SUS), with its three pillars: decentralization of management; comprehensive care, with priority given to preventive measures without adversely affecting care; and community involvement.

While the 1988 Constitution, when establishing the basis for the SUS, made it obligatory for the Brazilian State to provide medical care for any disease or medical condition to all Brazilian citizens, regardless of age, working status, socio-economic level, contribution, or payment to any specific fund or tax, HIV is the only disease for which a specific legal guarantee was created. As a result, HIV-infected patients are able to obtain antiretroviral and other drugs they need free of charge. This does not necessarily include the treatment of other outpatient conditions—viral hepatitis being a case in point—even for HIV-infected patients. Drugs for other important diseases, such as tuberculosis (TB), are available, but are not as easy to obtain.

The health system's structure

Treatment for HIV in Brazil is dispensed in more than 1000 public facilities throughout the country. A laboratory network has also been under development since 1997, with 96 units doing CD4 counts, 88 performing viral load tests and 20 involved in genotyping. This network has been built gradually over a period of about 20 years and is not a recent achievement, nor is it solely the result of the programme for free access to antiretroviral drugs. Since the availability of drugs does not in itself necessarily imply either a sufficient amount or adequate level of care, the Brazilian Ministry of Health (MOH) has also, in parallel with developing a policy of universal distribution of antiretroviral drugs, made efforts to ensure that people living with HIV/AIDS (PLWHA) receive comprehensive care.

At the end of 1987, the (pre-existing) national surveillance system had been notified of 2750 AIDS cases. Of these, roughly 77% had occurred in the two states of São Paulo (57.89%) and Rio de Janeiro (18.62%), with the majority of cases in the two state capital cities (44.26% and 15.9% of the country's total, respectively). Notwithstanding these small numbers and a relatively localized epidemic, training of physicians from all regions started in mid-1987; moreover, the March 1988 *Boletim Epidemiológico AIDS*, published monthly by the National STD/AIDS Program established in 1986, was already issuing the first 'Recommendations for the Implementation of Medical Care for AIDS in Brazil' [24]. Therefore, it can be confidently stated that an organized response to the HIV epidemic began early in Brazil.

It should be noted that at that time, and until 1990, the MOH was not actually in charge of medical care, but only of epidemiological surveillance, prevention, control of endemic diseases, and drug regulation.

Over the last decade, the SUS has gradually strengthened and supported the promotion of universal access to regional, decentralized healthcare, innovations in basic care and greater regulation of the private sector. The federal government is responsible for national policies, financing a large portion of the care services provided by states and municipalities and, in the specific case of AIDS care, the procurement of antiretroviral drugs [25]. States and municipalities are responsible for providing the actual medical care, including outpatient and inpatient facilities, clinical laboratory services, and surveillance data collection and analysis. However, a central computing facility in the MOH—the DATASUS—collects and stores this information. Therefore, in principle, a very complex system exists in which the federal government issues recommendations and finances most activities, the state governments coordinate the action, and the municipal administrations implement and execute the policies that have been developed. HIV and AIDS services are part of this healthcare structure.

The spread of the HIV epidemic in the country led the National STD/AIDS Program to establish specialized AIDS care services, but always with a view to integrating HIV treatment, care and prevention services into existing healthcare units. A number of different types of service provision were proposed and promoted, including outpatient clinics, day hospitals, homecare services and general hospitals. After the initial training of physicians, multidisciplinary teams were created, which called for further training of physicians, nurses, pharmacists, social workers, psychologists and other health professionals. Steps were taken to standardize laboratory procedures, procure diagnostic kits and guarantee their quality control, and, gradually, to develop facilities for viral load and CD4 count tests, including—since 2000—viral genotype testing.

Azidothymidine (AZT) became available on the private market in Brazil in 1988, and became available free of charge in 1991, but only through a restricted number of health units. At the same time, drugs for treatment and prevention of opportunistic infections (OIs), such as ganciclovir, pentamidine, fluconazole and others, were procured. Drugs for the treatment of Kaposi's sarcoma (KS), a very common condition at the time, were also made available free of charge. Instructions and guidelines on the use of these drugs were issued.

Since 1994, the MOH has promoted HIV prevention in all health and medical procedures. The ministry's other stated priorities are:

◆ to promote and facilitate access to services, and to guarantee the quality of care;

◆ to guarantee continuity of care within states and municipal districts;

◆ to guarantee training and ensure that the knowledge and skills of the multidisciplinary teams providing HIV care are kept up to date; and

◆ to guarantee the standardization of procedures and guidelines [26].

Today, the network of specialized HIV health services comprises 700 specialized outpatient clinics, 94 day care units, 53 homecare services and 432 accredited hospitals.

Changes in the profile of the epidemic have called for expanding the range of HIV services to include the management of IDUs, the reduction of vertical transmission of HIV and syphilis, dealing with issues related to ART adherence and administering directly observed therapy (DOT) for TB. As both the number of cases and their geographical distribution increase, the HIV care network is in a permanent state of expansion. Interestingly, medical care for PLWHA in Brazil is mainly given by specialist physicians trained in infectious diseases.

An analysis of HIV care and developing trends in Brazil for the period 1995–2006 was carried out based on types of procedure or care and using data from the MOH's central registry (DATA-SUS). A total of 11,139,690 HIV or AIDS events were found in that period. Of 9,206,870 consultations, 53.4% were carried out by physicians (41.1% by specialists, 17.4% by general practitioners), 17.5% by nurses, and 29.1% by other health professionals [27]. From 2000 on, a wider array of services was offered to the public.

Treatment

Guidelines—or rather, mandatory conditional instructions—were available as of 1991 for the treatment of HIV with AZT monotherapy and subsequently for treatment with didanosine (ddI). However, in March 1996, before the aforementioned congressional legislation had been enacted, a set of comprehensive guidelines was formulated by a large group of AIDS specialists brought together for this purpose by NATAP. Since then, three sets of national guidelines have been periodically reviewed and disseminated by NATAP for adults and adolescents, children, and pregnant women, respectively [28]. These guidelines are developed and reviewed by three different committees of physicians who are not necessarily affiliated with the MOH's central administration. This means that these committees have a fair degree of freedom and independence from government injunction.

At the time of writing, all drugs registered in the country are available through Brazil's health system, with the exception of delavirdine (DLV) and zalcitabine (ddC), which were withdrawn from the market by their producers, and the co-formulation of abacavir (ABC), lamivudine (3TC) and AZT (marketed as Trizivir®). Certain drugs marketed elsewhere are not currently available in Brazil, such as the protease inhibitors (PIs) tipranavir (TPV) and darunavir (DRV), the nucleoside reverse transcriptase inhibitor (NRTI) emtricitabine (FTC), and the co-formulations of ABC and 3TC (marketed as Kivexa®), of FTC and tenofovir (TDF) (marketed as Truvada®), and of efavirenz (EFV), FTC and TDF (marketed as Atripla™) [28].

Under Brazil's guidelines for adults and adolescents, treatment is not recommended for individuals with CD4 counts above 350 cells/mm^3, or without a CD4 count determination having been done. For patients with CD4 counts between 350 and 200 cells/mm^3, treatment should be considered. Symptomatic patients, and those with a CD4 count under 200 cells/mm^3 should be treated.

Preferred treatment is two NRTIs plus a non-nucleoside reverse transcriptase inhibitor (NNRTI); alternatively, a PI may be used instead of the latter. The combination regimen of AZT/3TC/EFV is the recommended first-line regimen. Patients with intolerance to AZT may be treated with ddI, ABC, or TDF (with some restrictions for the latter two). Stavudine (d4T) is no longer recommended as an NRTI backbone for the first-line antiretroviral regimen. The PIs of choice are lopinavir (LPV) and ritonavir (RTV)-boosted atazanavir (ATV). Alternatives to these are unboosted ATV, boosted saquinavir (SQV) and, in restricted cases, nelfinavir (NFV).

Treatment failure is characterized as a detectable viral load after 48 weeks of treatment, or a repeatedly detectable viral load after viral suppression had been obtained. When this occurs, a sample must be submitted for viral genotyping, as noted above, or empiric therapy may be initiated (according to recommendations established in the guidelines and taking into consideration the drugs previously used). ENF is available for patients with multi-drug resistant strains, provided that a recent genotype test has indicated at least one (other) drug to which the virus is presumptively sensitive.

Treatment of acute infection is not recommended, nor is the use of structured treatment interruption (STI). Therapeutic drug monitoring is not generally available, even outside the SUS.

Brazilian physicians seem, in the main, to follow these guidelines. A pilot study in Nova Iguaçu, a city on the outskirts of Rio de Janeiro, targeting an underprivileged population seen at a primary care centre, showed that no patient was prescribed a regimen contraindicated in the guidelines, and that 57 of 59 initial therapeutic regimens conformed entirely to the national guidelines [29]. Another study involving three sites in Rio de Janeiro gave comparable results, since only 2% of 984 patient records reported use of inappropriate regimens as defined by Brazil's national ART guidelines issued in 2000 [30].

Response to treatment has been the object of various studies. As a cautionary note, it should be kept in mind that Brazilian guidelines allowed for dual antiretroviral therapy until 2000. A cross-sectional study of adults taking ART for 6–24 months in five public clinics in Rio de Janeiro found that 82% of patients were 'responders' to treatment, with 69% achieving a decrease in their viral load of >1 log at 6 months of treatment; these results were comparable to those reported from more developed countries at the time of the study [31]. Another study of 454 patients whose treatment was started between 1996 and 2004 found a rate of viral failure (defined as a viral load >400 copies/mL after 6 months of treatment) of 28% [32]. Similar results were obtained in a retrospective cohort study of 485 drug-naïve, HIV-infected subjects from different care settings who started highly active retroviral therapy (HAART) between 1996 and 2004 in Rio de Janeiro. In this cohort, virologic failure was observed in 119 (25%) of the subjects [33].

A retrospective study examined the duration of benefit of ART in a group of patients seen at one hospital in São Paulo in the period 1996–2000. Treatment failure/cessation of therapy benefit was defined as:

♦ viral load higher than 1000 copies/mL after six months of therapy;

♦ increase in CD4 count of less than 10% of baseline values after the same period of time;

♦ treatment interruption due to drug intolerance;

♦ therapy abandonment, or death; and

♦ need for treatment intensification.

The mean estimated duration of benefit was 14.1 months [34].

There are few data on adverse reactions to antiretroviral drugs in Brazil. A recent prospective study in the state of Minas Gerais found a rate of 34.5% for adverse reactions among patients initiating their first treatment. The gastrointestinal (GI) tract was the area most affected (nausea 14.5%, vomiting 13.1%, diarrhoea 8.9%). Overall, 12% of patients changed their drug regimen because of adverse reactions, even though most of these reactions were considered 'light to moderate' in severity [35].

Results of free access to antiretroviral drugs

The results of providing wide access to ART have been studied in various publications. The frequency of hospital admissions due to AIDS in the public health system has not varied, standing at around 0.3%, despite increases in the number of AIDS cases and number of individuals on treatment. In 1998, 63% of all patients using antiretroviral drugs underwent hospitalization, while only 30% were hospitalized in 2003. At the same time, the number of individuals receiving drug treatment for HIV increased by a factor of 2.7 between 1997 and 2003 [36].

The implementation of free ART in Brazil coincides with a marked decrease in the expected numbers of AIDS-related hospital admissions, with a probable causal relationship. As part of an ongoing study, HIV/AIDS-related hospital admissions in Brazil during the first decade of ART were recently analyzed, with a focus on the expected and actual numbers, numbers of admissions averted, and corresponding impact on costs. For 2004, an estimated 206,353 HIV-infected patients were in care, 147,395 of whom were on HAART. Of these, 27,844 were admitted to public hospitals. When compared to the pre-ART (1996) hospitalization rates, approximately 167,211 admissions were averted in 2004 [37]. For the period 1996–2006, more than one million (1,200,609) hospital admissions were averted, for an estimated gross saving of US$434.1 million [38].

There is a paucity of data with regard to the impact of HAART on the occurrence of OIs. One study in Rio de Janeiro found a reduction of 81% in the risk of developing TB for patients on ART [39].

AIDS mortality is decreasing. In Brazil, median survival times for patients diagnosed with AIDS is increasing over time, from five months in the 1980s, to 18 months in 1995, to 58 months for those diagnosed in 1996 [40].

In the city of Rio de Janeiro, a gradual drop in AIDS-related mortality was observed from 1995 (26.75 per 100,000) to 2003 (13.62 per 100,000), a total decrease of 47.5%. This trend was reflected in the country as a whole, which saw a 27.1% decline in AIDS-related mortality between 1995 and 2002 [41]. Another study, also from Rio de Janeiro, found that the probability of survival after five years was 21% for patients diagnosed with AIDS before 1991, 50% for those diagnosed between 1991 and 1995, and 86% from 1996 onward. When compared with post-1996 figures, risk of death was nine times higher prior to 1991, and four times higher between 1991 and 1995 [42].

Notwithstanding the availability of free ART in the country, one of the mortality studies in Rio de Janeiro found that over 50% of the subjects who died had never received ART [41]. Similar results were observed in a hospital in São Paulo city, where the death rate in adults with AIDS decreased significantly between 1995 and 1999, from 29% to 19.8%. Lack of ART before hospitalization was associated with death during hospitalization (odds ratio (OR)=3.8), and survival was associated with previous use of three or more antiretroviral drugs (OR=0.15) [43]. Both studies seem to indicate that late diagnosis is associated with an increased risk of death. In the city of Rio de Janeiro, at least, there is evidence that physicians' lack of knowledge and expertise is linked to unfavourable outcomes [41]. A previously mentioned study from the city of Nova Iguaçu pointed to occasional, temporary shortages of antiretrovirals, difficulties in obtaining CD4 counts and viral load results in a timely fashion, and late presentation of patients with advanced symptomatic disease as causes for treatment failure [29].

Adherence to treatment is clearly an issue. However, in a nationwide study involving a random sample of 60 healthcare facilities in which 1,972 patients receiving ART were interviewed, the rate of adherence (defined as having taken more than 95% of prescribed pills in the three days prior to the interview) was 75%, considered to be adequate compared to adherence rates currently seen in industrialized countries. Predictors of non-adherence included facilities with smaller numbers of patients, missed appointments, complexity of regimens and number of pills required, and fewer than two years of formal education [44].

A study from the South-Eastern region state of Minas Gerais evaluated self-reported non-adherence to treatment (defined as the intake of less than 95% of prescribed doses in the three days preceding the interviews). Among 306 patients, the cumulative incidence of non-adherence was 36.9%, giving an incidence rate of 0.21 per 100 person-days. Multivariate analysis showed unemployment, use of alcohol, three or more adverse reactions, number of pills per day, changes in the antiretroviral regimen, and a longer period of time between the HIV test results and the initiation of treatment to be associated with non-adherence [45].

Co-infection

Tuberculosis

As expected, there is a high prevalence of TB among HIV-positive patients in Brazil. Until 1999, TB was the third most frequently seen OI in HIV-infected patients, reported in 18% of AIDS cases. It is now estimated that 17.7% of all reported TB cases in Brazil are in individuals infected with HIV. Prevalence studies among HIV-infected patients under follow-up have shown TB infection rates of up to 20.7%; TB is also frequently implicated as an associated cause of death for PLWHA [46]. Recently, a study in a reference centre in the South region found a TB infection rate of 27% in a sample of 204 HIV-infected patients [47].

Data regarding antituberculous drug resistance are scarce in Brazil. A study in the mid-1990s showed an overall resistance rate of 8.5% in treatment-naive patients; simultaneous resistance to isoniazide and rifampin was 1.1%. In a study of multi-drug resistant (MDR) cases of TB carried out with a systematic survey of HIV serology status, 8% of patients were found to be HIV-positive. In another, hospital-based study, prevalence of MDR bacilli isolated from HIV-infected patients was found to be 15%, while in uninfected patients the rate fell to 3% [48].

Another study, also hospital-based, and also from Rio de Janeiro, showed an MDR-TB rate of 28.85% in HIV-infected patients; this, however, was not significantly different from the results for uninfected patients [49]. Therefore, although TB is undoubtedly a very serious problem in HIV-infected individuals, multi-drug resistance does not seem to be particularly troublesome.

Hepatitis

HIV co-infection with hepatitis C virus (HCV) is undoubtedly important; however, given the varying importance of injection drug use in the epidemiology of HIV in the various parts of the country, an overall estimate is difficult. Published studies have reported HIV/HCV co-infection prevalence rates as diverse as 18%, 33%, and even 95% [50]. One study found a reduced survival for patients with both infections, but the reasons for this were not clear [51]. Although, theoretically, all Brazilian citizens are entitled to free and comprehensive medical care—in which treatment for hepatitis is certainly included—there is far less access to anti-hepatitis drugs (with the exception of 3TC) than to antiretroviral drugs.

Prevention

An overview of all preventive measures against HIV implemented in Brazil would be out of place in this treatment-specific chapter. Suffice it to say that, in 1992, when it was considering its first large-scale loan to Brazil for AIDS control, the World Bank predicted that, by 2000, Brazil would have 2 million HIV-infected people. In contrast, a recent study estimated the number of HIV-infected individuals between the ages of 15 and 49 in Brazil in 2004 to be, at most, 644,511—significantly below the World Bank's prediction [9].

Prevention and treatment are mutually reinforcing and must be considered in an integrated approach. As far as prevention is concerned, a wide range of measures have proved successful, including: universal access to condoms; women's empowerment; adoption of programmes relating to mother-to-child transmission; implementation of strategies targeting the most vulnerable groups and those populations at highest risk of infection; and the inclusion of issues related to HIV/AIDS in school curricula.

An effort is being made to incorporate educational and preventive activities into outpatient care in Brazil's SUS network. In an effort to characterize existing prevention and education activities within public health units that provide HIV/AIDS outpatient care, data from a central registry in the MOH for the period 1995–2006 were analyzed. A total of 387,345 educational activities in the context of medical care were registered; 76.3% took place inside healthcare units and 23.7% in the community. Of these, 76% were conducted by health professionals with a university-level education, and 24% by professionals with lower qualifications [Brazil: National STD/AIDS Program, unpublished data, 2007]. As the majority of these activities are, by and large, already being conducted by professionals with post-secondary education, this may preclude further expansion of such activities.

Conclusion

The HIV/AIDS epidemic in Brazil was detected early in the 1980s. Its progress seems to have been at least partially curbed by early and integrated response, including the establishment of an inclusive epidemiological surveillance system. The epidemic is characterized as concentrated since the prevalence among certain vulnerable groups is higher than 5%, but it is below 1% in the general population. The estimated overall prevalence has not varied greatly, standing at 0.65% and 0.61% in 2000 and 2004, respectively. There is a trend toward stabilization in the South and South-eastern regions, with evidence of an increase in the other three regions of the country.

An early response is also noted with regard to medical assistance and care for affected people. This has entailed training of health professionals, the establishment of a national network of specialized services, including laboratory facilities, and the provision of drugs for OI treatment as well as HIV and AIDS themselves. It should be emphasized that all HIV services and drugs are provided to patients entirely free of charge, as is the case for any other disease or condition in Brazil's health system (SUS).

Direct benefits obtained for the population include a major improvement in the quality of care and treatment services for HIV-infected patients, which in turn has resulted in increased life expectancy and a markedly better quality of life for them. Other benefits are the notable reduction, both in number and complexity, of hospitalizations, an increase in outpatient care, with related cost-savings, and the optimization of both human and financial resources.

References

1. Population Reference Bureau, Washington, DC. (2007). *2007 World Population Data Sheet*. Available at http://www.prb.org/Publications/Datasheets/2007/2007WorldPopulationDataSheet.aspx
2. United Nations, Statistics Division. (2007). *National Accounts Main Aggregates Database, Basic Data Selection*. New York: United Nations. Available at http://unstats.un.org/unsd/snaama/resultsGDP.asp?Series=1&CCode=76&Year=2005&SLevel=0&Selection=basic
3. Watkins K (Director). (2006). *Human Development Report 2005*. p 214–222. New York: United Nations Development Program. Available at http://hdr.undp.org/en/reports/global/hdr2005/
4. Ibid. (2005). p 270–273.
5. Simões CCS, Sabóia AL, Oliveira LAP, Belchior JR. (1999). *Evolution and perspective of childhood mortality in Brazil (1999)*. Rio de Janeiro: IBGE, Departamento de População e Indicadores Sociais (in Portuguese). p 45.
6. Diretoria de Pesquisas. (2006). *Health Statistics. Medico-sanitary Assistance 2005*. Rio de Janeiro: IBGE, Departamento de População e Indicadores Sociais (in Portuguese). p 162.

7. Simão M. (2006). Apresentaçao [Introduction] (in Portuguese). *Boletim Epidemiológico Aids DST* **III**:3. Available at http://www.aids.gov.br/data/documents/storedDocuments/%7BB8EF5DAF-23AE-4891-AD36-1903553A3174%7D/%7B6B12D137-92DF-4CF5-A35A-482AED64CBC0%7D/BOLETIM2006internet.pdf

8. Pascom AR, Fonseca MGP, Dhalia CBC. (2005). *Trends in the AIDS epidemic in Brazil and HIV/AIDS-related behavior, and response. July 2005. p12-18.* Available at http://www.aids.gov.br/main.asp?View={E62A8511-7150-4615-9BFA-10FDC4F4E642}

9. Szwarcwald CL, Souza PRB Jr. (2006). An estimate of the HIV prevalence in the Brazilian population 15 to 48 years of age, 2004 (in Portuguese). *Boletim Epidemiológico STD/AIDS* **III**,11-15.

10. Szwarcwald CL, Carvalho MF. (2001). An estimate of the number of individuals from 15 to 49 years of age infected by HIV, Brazil 2000 (in Portuguese). *Boletim Epidemiológico STD/AIDS* **XIV**:51-55.

11. Morgado MG, Guimaraes ML, Gripp CB, *et al.* (1998). Molecular epidemiology of HIV-1 in Brazil: high prevalence of HIV-1 subtype B and identification of an HIV-1 subtype D infection in the city of Rio de Janeiro, Brazil. *J Acquir Immune Defic Syndr Hum Retrovirol* **18**:488-94.

12. Bongertz V, Bou-Habib DC, Brigido LFM, *et al.* (2000). HIV-1 diversity in Brazil: genetic, biologic, and immunologic characterization of HIV-1 strains in three potential HIV vaccine evaluation sites. *J Acquir Immune Defic Syndr* **23**:184-93.

13. Guimaraes ML, dos Santos Moreira A, Loureiro R, Galvao-Castro B, Morgado MG. (2000). High frequency of recombinant genomes in HIV type 1 samples from Brazilian southeastern and southern regions. *AIDS Res Hum Retroviruses* **18**:1261-9.

14. Carr JK, Avila M, Gomez Carrillo M, *et al.* (2001). Diverse BF recombinants have spread widely since the introduction of HIV-1 into South America. *AIDS* **15**:F41-7.

15. Vicente ACP, Otsuki K, Silva NB, *et al.* (2000). The HIV epidemic in the Amazon Basin is driven by prototypic and recombinant HIV-1 subtypes B and F. *J Acquir Immune Defic Syndr* **23**:327-31.

16. Soares EAJM, Santos RP, Pellegrini JA, Sprinz E, Tanuri A, Soares MA. (2003). Epidemiologic and Molecular Characterization of Human Immunodeficiency Virus Type 1 in Southern Brazil. *J Acquir Immune Defic Syndr* **34**:520-6.

17. Soares EAJM, Martínez AMB, Souza TM, *et al.* (2005). HIV-1 subtype C dissemination in southern Brazil. *AIDS* **19**(suppl 4):S8-6).

18. Pieniazek D, Peralta JM, Ferreira JA, *et al.* (1991). Identification of mixed HIV-1/HIV-2 infections in Brazil by polymerase chain reaction. *AIDS* **5**:1293-9.

19. Brindeiro RM, Diaz RS, Sabino EC, *et al.* (2003). Brazilian network for HIV drug resistance surveillance (HIV-BResNet): a survey of chronically infected individuals. *AIDS* **17**:1063-9.

20. Barreto CC, Nishyia A, Araújo LV, Ferreira JE, Busch MP, Sabino EC (2006). Trends in antiretroviral drug resistance and clade distributions among HIV-1 infected blood donors in São Paulo, Brazil. *J Acquir Immune Defic Syndr* **41**:338-341.

21. Sucupira MCA, Caseiro MM, Alves K, *et al.* (2007). High levels of primary antiretroviral resistance genotypic mutations and B/F recombinants in Santos, Brazil. *Aids Patient Care* **21**:116-28.

22. Galvão J. (2002). Access to antiretroviral drugs in Brazil. *Lancet* **360**:1862-5.

23. República Federativa do Brasil. (1988). *Constituição da República Federativa do Brasil de 1988 (Brazilian Constitution, in Portuguese)*. Available at http://www.planalto.gov.br/CCIVIL_03/Constituicao/Constitui%C3%A7ao.htm

24. Loures LAM, Chequer PJN, de Sá CAM, Ramos Filho CF, Ayrosa Galvão PA, Marzochi KBF. (1988). Recommendations for the implementation of Medical Care for AIDS in Brazil (in Portuguese). *Boletim Epidemiológico AIDS* **I**:1-5.

25. Ministry of Health of Brazil. (2000).*The Brazilian Response to HIV/AIDS: Best Practices. Decentralized management model adopted in Brazil by the National Co-ordination for STD and AIDS. National Coordination for STD and AIDS.* Brasília: Ministry of Health. p91-93.

26. Santos CE, Vitoria MA, Lima JN. (2002). Building up an AIDS care services network In Brazil. The XIV International AIDS Conference, 2002, Barcelona, Spain. [Abstract ThOrF1514]

27. dos Santos C, Serafim JA, Okamura M, *et al.* (2007). Comprehensive Health Care for PLWHA in Brazil (1995–2006). 47th Annual Interscience Conference on Antimicrobial Agents and Chomotherapy, Chicago, 2007. [Presentation no. H–1729]

28. Government of Brazil. (2006). *National STD/AIDS Program, Recommendations for Therapy of Adults and Adolescents Infected with HIV.* Available at http://www.aids.gov.br/data/Pages/LUMISFB7D5720PTBRIE.htm

29. Carmody ER, Diaz T, Starling P, dos Santos APRB, Sacks HS. (2003). An evaluation of antiretroviral HIV/AIDS treatment in a Rio de Janeiro public clinic. *Trop Med Int Health* **8**:378–85.

30. Loo VS, Diaz T, Gadelha AM, *et al.* (2004). Managing HIV-infected patients on antiretroviral therapy in Rio de Janeiro, Brazil: do providers follow national guidelines? *AIDS Care* **16**:834–40.

31. Hofer CB, Schechter M, Harrison LH. (2004). Effectiveness of antiretroviral therapy among patients who attend public HIV clinics in Rio de Janeiro, Brazil. *J Acquir Imune Defic Syndr* **36**:96–71.

32. Tuboi SH, Harrison LH, Sprinz E, Schechter M, Albernaz RK, Schechter M. (2005). Predictors of virologic failure in HIV-1-infected patients starting highly active antiretroviral therapy in Porto Alegre, Brazil. *J Acquir Immune Defic Syndr* **40**:324–8.

33. May SB, Barroso PF, Nunes EP, *et al.* (2007). Effectiveness of highly active antiretroviral therapy using non-brand name drugs in Brazil. *Braz J Med Biol Res* **40**:551–5.

34. Medeiros R, Diaz RS, Castelo Filho A. (2002). Estimating the length of the first antiretroviral therapy regiment durability in São Paulo, Brazil. *Braz J Infect Dis* **6**:298–304.

35. Menezes de Pádua CA, César CC, Bonolo PF, Acurcio FA, Guimarães MDC. (2006). High incidence of adverse reactions to initial antiretroviral therapy in Brazil. *Braz J Med Biol Res* **39**:495–505.

36. Dourado I, Veras MASM, Barreira D, Brito AM. (2006). AIDS epidemic trends after the introduction of antiretroviral therapy in Brazil. *Rev. Saúde Pública* **40**(suppl):9–17.

37. dos Santos C, Silveiro O, Scapini R, *et al.* (2007). A Decade of HAART: effect on hospital admissions for HIV and AIDS in Brazil. 4th IAS conference on HIV Pathagenisis, Treatment and Prevention. Sydney, 2007. [Abstract TUPE B095]

38. dos Santos CE, Silveira O, Scapini R, *et al.* (2007). A Decade of HAART; effect on hospital admissions for HIV/AIDS in Brazil. 4th IAS Conference on HIV Pathogenesis, Treatment and Prevention, 2007, Sydney, Australia. [Abstract A-042–0127–04420]

39. Santoro-Lopes G, Pinho AMF, Harrison LH, Schechter M. (2002). Reduced Risk of Tuberculosis among Brazilian Patients with Advanced Human Immunodeficiency Virus Infection Treated with Highly Active Antiretroviral Therapy. *Clin Infec Dis* **34**:543–546.

40. Marins JRP, Jamal LF, Chen SY, *et al.* (2003). Dramatic improvement in survival among adult Brazilian AIDS patients. *AIDS* **17**:1675–82.

41. Saraceni V, Cruz MM, Lauria LM, Durovni B. (2005). Trends and characteristics of AIDS mortality in the Rio de Janeiro city after the introduction of highly active antiretroviral therapy. *Braz J Infect Dis* **9**:209–215.

42. Campos DP, Ribeiro SR, Grinsztejn B, *et al.* (2005). Survival of AIDS patients using two case definitions, Rio de Janeiro, Brazil, 1986–2003. *AIDS* **19**(suppl 4):S22–S26.

43. Casseb J, Orrico GS, Feijó RD, Guaracy L, Medeiros LA. (2001). Lack of prior antiretroviral therapy is associated with increased mortality among hospitalized patients with AIDS in Sao Paulo, Brazil. *AIDS Patient Care STDS* **15**:271–5.

44. Nemes MIB, Carvalho HB, Souza MFM. (2004). Antiretroviral therapy adherence in Brazil. *AIDS* **18**(suppl 3):S15–S20.

45. Bonolo PF, César CC, Acúrcio FA, *et al.* (2005). Non-adherence among patients initiating antiretroviral therapy: a challenge for health professionals in Brazil. *AIDS* **19**(suppl 4):S5–S13.

46. Laguardia J, Merchán-Hamann E. (2003). Risk factors for tuberculous disease in reported AIDS cases in Brazil, 1980 to 2000 (in Spanish). *Rev. Esp. Salud Publica* **77**:553–565.

47. Silveira JM, Sassi RAM, Oliveira Netto IC, Hetzel JL. (2006). Prevalence of and factors related to tuberculosis in seropositive human immunodeficiency virus patients at a reference center for treatment

of human immunodeficiency virus in the southern region of the state of Rio Grande do Sul, Brazil (in Portuguese). *J. bras. Pneumol* **32**:48–55.

48. Fandinho F, Kritski A, Hofer C, *et al.* (1999). Drug resistance patterns among hospitalized tuberculous patients in Rio de Janeiro, Brazil, 1993–1994. *Mem Inst Oswaldo Cruz* **94**:543–7.

49. Brito RC, Gounder C, Lima DB, *et al.* (2004). Drug-resistant Mycobacterium tuberculosis strains isolated at an AIDS reference center general hospital in Rio de Janeiro (in Portuguese). *J. bras. pneumol* **30**:335–342.

50. Mendes-Corrêa MCJ, Barone AA. (2005). Hepatitis C in patients co-infected with human immunodeficiency virus. A review and experience of a Brazilian ambulatory. *Rev Inst Med trop S Paulo* **47**:59–64.

51. Marins JRP, Barros MBA, Machado H, Chen S, Jamal LF, Hearst N. (2005). Characteristics and survival of AIDS patients with hepatitis C: the Brazilian National Cohort of 1995–1996. *AIDS* **19** (suppl 4):S27–S30.

Chapter 17

Country review: China

Zhang Fu-Jie,* Ray Y. Chen, Selina N. Lo and Ma Ye

Introduction

China is currently undergoing vast and unparalleled social and economic reform as part of the world's largest 'social experiment' to transform its centralized economy towards a market-oriented system [1]. Like any major reform, there are gaps and challenges in its implementation. Nowhere is this more evident and well illustrated than in the case of HIV/AIDS treatment and access to healthcare. This chapter will outline: first, the epidemiology of HIV/AIDS in China; second, the history and evolution of the Chinese government's response; third, the achievements of the national HIV/AIDS programme; and finally, its challenges as it moves towards a comprehensive integrated response to HIV/AIDS in China.

Overall epidemiology

The HIV epidemic in China has in some respects been typical of the course of HIV infection in other countries but, in other respects, has had its own unique characteristics. The first reported case of HIV in China occurred in 1985, in a foreign-born person living in China [2]. Rather than viewing that as a sentinel case, and in common with the views of many other countries at that time, the Chinese government considered AIDS to be a foreign problem and not an issue in China. Since then, the HIV epidemic in China has spread primarily among injection drug users (IDUs) and female sex workers (FSWs), and has begun to enter the general population in certain high-risk areas.

Unique to the Chinese HIV epidemic was the spread of the virus among former plasma donors (FPDs), predominantly in the early to mid-1990s. This was a cohort of mostly poor, rural farmers who sold blood plasma to illegal vendors collecting plasma under unsanitary conditions. There are no clear estimates of how many were infected via this route. Much less is known about the other high-risk groups in China, including FSWs and men who have sex with men (MSM). Overall, it is estimated that there are about 650,000 people currently living with HIV in China (Table 17.1), about 75,000 of whom have developed AIDS. Overall national HIV prevalence is 0.05%. In 2005 alone, there were an estimated 70,000 new HIV infections in China, with about 25,000 AIDS deaths [3]. Comprehensive reviews of this epidemiology have been published [4,5].

Transmission through injecting drugs

Injection drug use is a significant and growing problem, primarily in southern and western China. Yunnan province in southern China abuts the illicit drug trade's 'Golden Triangle', comprising Myanmar, Laos and Thailand. Drugs enter southern China and travel up through

* Corresponding author.

Table 17.1 Estimated numbers and percentages of HIV infection in China by risk group.

Risk Group	Estimated number of infections	Percentage of total HIV population
Injection drug users	288,000	44.3%
Female sex workers and their clients	127,000	19.6%
Partners of high-risk groups and general population	110,000	16.7%
Former plasma donors	69,000	10.7%
Men who have sex with men	47,000	7.3%
Mother-to-child transmission	9000	1.4%
Total	650,000	100%

Source: [3].

western China to central Asia. While the reported number of drug users in China was 1.05 million in 2003, the actual number is thought to be many times higher [4]. An estimated 45% of these are IDUs [5].

HIV infection was first recognized in 1989 among IDUs in Yunnan province. China currently estimates that approximately 288,000 drug users live with HIV/AIDS, accounting for 44.3% of total cases and making this the largest reported cohort of HIV-infected people, just ahead of those infected through sexual transmission. The provinces of Yunnan, Xinjiang, Guangxi, Guangdong, Guizhou, Sichuan and Hunan together account for 89.5% of HIV/AIDS cases among IDUs. HIV prevalence among drug users rose from 1.95% in 1996 to 6.48% in 2004. Among estimated new HIV cases in 2005, 48.6% were due to injection drug use, just behind sexual transmission (49.8%) [3]. China initiated pilot methadone and needle exchange programmes in 2002 and scaled up these programmes to all areas of China with high rates of injection drug use in 2005. Despite these efforts, however, national surveillance data reveal that 45.5% of IDUs share needles. Furthermore, 11% engage in high-risk sexual activities [3].

Transmission through heterosexual sex

Sexual practices in China swung like a pendulum during the twentieth century. Data from before 1950 showed extremely high rates of sexually transmitted diseases (STDs), but by the 1960s and 1970s China had essentially eliminated all STDs through a combination of public health and societal control measures [6]. However, with the 'opening up' of China in the 1980s, STDs came back with a vengeance [7]. Current estimates show that about 127,000 sex workers and their clients are infected with HIV, comprising 19.6% of total HIV cases, with about 109,000 partners of HIV-positive individuals and members of the general population infected, adding 16.7% to the estimated total [3].

With the sexual revolution currently taking place in China as shown by recent STD trends [8,9], sexual transmission is overtaking injection drug use as the primary means of HIV transmission. In fact, sexual transmission rates of HIV have risen steadily over the last several years to become the primary cause of new infections in 2005 at 49.8% [3]. In surveillance among the FSW population, overall HIV prevalence has now reached over 1%, with some areas reporting prevalence as high as 10% in this population [10]. Even higher are the HIV prevalence rates among sex workers who are also IDUs. Compounding this problem are the high rates of STDs in this population and the concurrent increased risk of HIV transmission [10–12]. The infected clients of these FSWs then serve as a bridge for HIV from the high-risk sex worker population to the clients' spouses and the general population. Evidence of this trend has been borne out in certain areas where rates of HIV in pregnant women exceed 1% (see perinatal transmission section, below). Reported rates of condom use in FSWs vary significantly [5] and are difficult to estimate due to the variation in usage rates between one-time partners and regular partners, the amount the client is willing to pay, and whether or not the sex worker feels the man 'looks clean' (and vice versa) [13].

Transmission through plasma donations

The most unique aspect of China's HIV epidemic has been infection among those who have sold blood plasma. Many commercial blood collection companies established blood plasma collection stations throughout rural central China between the late 1980s and the mid-1990s. The local populations, mostly poor farmers, were paid to provide blood plasma. To increase the frequency with which an individual could donate, the collection centre operators would return pooled red blood cells to the donating individuals to prevent anaemia [5]. As a result of these practices, official estimates at that time were that as many as 600,000 people were infected with HIV in this way, 100,000 of whom developed AIDS [14]. Studies of the prevalence of infection in this population have ranged up to 56% for HIV and 73% for hepatitis C virus (HCV), with high rates of co-infection [15]. Since plasma collection centres were closed in 1995, the incidence of HIV infection in this cohort has decreased dramatically. There is little injection drug use in these areas, and with China's one-child policy, the children who would have been exposed to HIV infection perinatally have generally already been infected. The incidence of HIV in these FPD areas is thus currently relatively low. Current estimates are that 69,000 FPD and blood product recipients are living with HIV/AIDS, accounting for 10.7% of total cases. Henan, Hubei, Anhui, Hebei and Shanxi provinces account for 80.4% of all cases in this cohort [3]. With relatively few incident cases now, and with prevalent cases gradually dying (despite treatment) from HIV-related and other causes, this cohort is slowly diminishing.

Transmission among MSM

Representative estimates of HIV infection in MSM in China are difficult to obtain, due to the strong cultural bias to be married and have male children to continue the family name. Traditionally, to be homosexual has not been culturally acceptable, and thus this cohort generally remains hidden. What is clear is that Chinese MSM often engage in high-risk sexual practices with both men and women and have poor knowledge about HIV/AIDS and what constitutes risky behaviour [16,17]. Published surveys of MSM demonstrate high rates of STDs, with an HIV prevalence ranging from 0–5% [18,19]. An estimated 47,000 MSM are currently infected with HIV, representing 7.3% of total HIV cases [3]. Compounding this problem is that, given the societal pressures they face, many MSM marry and do not tell their wives about their sexual practices. This group thus serves as another bridging population, albeit smaller than male clients of FSWs, through which HIV gains entry into the general populace.

Transmission through perinatal infection and paediatric infections

Overall prevalence estimates of HIV in pregnant women are low, at about 0.4% based on national surveillance data. In certain high-risk areas, however, sentinel surveillance sites have identified rates of HIV among pregnant women as high as 1.4% [20]. Although such high rates may be confined to certain localities, the extent to which the HIV epidemic has become generalized beyond those areas is not clear and is very worrying. An estimated 9000 cases of mother-to-child transmission (MTCT) occurred in 2005, accounting for 1.4% of total estimated HIV cases [3]. Actual transmission rates are much higher than reported rates, as paediatric HIV diagnosis in

China still relies on HIV antibody testing and thus cannot definitively diagnose HIV infection before the age of 18 months. HIV RNA and DNA testing is not done routinely due to a scarcity of laboratories that are able to process such sophisticated tests, and to the expense involved, which would have to be borne by the child's parents. Thus, about half of HIV-infected infants die before the age of 2 years [21], many of them before being definitively diagnosed.

Between 1985 and 2004, a total of 1820 HIV-infected children (0–17 years old) were reported through the national surveillance system. In October 2004, a national survey was conducted to update this figure. A total of 1259 children aged 17 or under were identified as still alive at the time of the survey. The six provinces with the highest prevalence (Henan, Yunnan, Anhui, Hubei, Guangxi and Shanxi) represented 88% of the total cases. Mother-to-child transmission of HIV accounted for 76% of cases, with 16% related to use of blood products. Despite the known benefits of antiretroviral therapy (ART) to prevent mother-to-child transmission (PMTCT) of HIV, only one mother of these infected children reported any use of ART during pregnancy [22]. Although PMTCT services are currently being scaled up in China with the goal of covering 90% of pregnant women by 2010, this programme, too, faces many challenges in terms of coverage, the late presentation of most pregnant women to health services, and lack of linkage at the local level to ART treatment services.

Migrant labourers and surplus men

One of the effects of China's booming economy is the growing economic divide between urban and rural areas. Large cities grow, develop and modernize at breakneck speed, while the farming countryside remains little changed from 20 years ago. The inequality of this economic divide is further emphasized by the fact that 80% of China's population lives in the countryside. As a result, an estimated 120 million migrant labourers have gone to the cities in search of better jobs and a better lifestyle. These migrant labourers, both men and women, are generally either single or separated from families, have limited education and lack good job skills. Women find jobs in the service industry—in hotels, restaurants, and hair salons or as household maids. Some end up selling sex, finding that they can make a better income this way. Men work in construction, mines, as long-distance truck drivers, or in other physically demanding occupations, and are often housed together in makeshift dormitories. These men, relatively young, separated from families for long periods, and working and living in an almost exclusively male environment, are at high risk for seeking the services of FSWs. Multiple studies have shown this cohort to practise high-risk sexual behaviours [23, 24] and to have varying rates of STDs [25, 26]. Although currently not known to be a high-prevalence HIV population, this group is certainly at high risk and has the potential to serve as another bridging population to their low-risk families, whom they generally see only once a year.

Many of these men—young, poor, and single—are known as 'surplus men', a phenomenon in China resulting from the societal preference for male children to carry on the family name. Much research and speculation has gone into this social consequence of China's one-child policy and the resulting imbalance in the gender ratio at birth [27,28]. In terms of HIV, there is a hypothetical concern that this cohort of single, sexually active men will serve as a nexus of HIV transmission between sex workers and the general population [29]. To know whether this concern is valid requires continued surveillance and monitoring of this cohort.

Molecular epidemiology

The molecular epidemiology of HIV-1 in China has, in general terms, followed the various transmission routes detailed above. Although the first HIV-1 infection was identified in Beijing in 1985, it is believed that HIV-1 first entered China through injecting drug users in Yunnan in the late 1980s, as separate subtypes B and B'. Subtype B, initially the predominant strain, was gradually replaced by subtype B'. HIV-1 subtype C strains were also identified among IDUs in the early 1990s, possibly from Indian IDUs, and spread rapidly through southern, central and north-western China via drug trafficking [30]. As a result of co-circulation with subtype B', two circulating recombinant forms (CRFs)—CRF07_BC and CRF08_BC—evolved [31] and subsequently spread along different drug trafficking routes across southern and north-western China [30, 32]. Recent data show that subtypes C and B'C make up about half of the total HIV-1 subtypes in Yunnan [33], with new recombinant strains continuing to arise among IDUs [34]. Subtype B', after entering Yunnan, somehow jumped to Henan and is the primary subtype among the FPD population throughout central China [35].

Sexual transmission of HIV, in contrast to the IDU and FPD cohorts, predominantly involves the CRF01_AE strain, although there have also been reports of the AE subtype in IDUs [36,37]. About 40% of HIV-1 infection in Yunnan is due to the AE subtype, which is cause for concern regarding a possible shift in transmission of HIV from the IDU cohort to the general population in Yunnan through sexual transmission [33]. Overall, subtypes B and B' comprise 38% of cases in China, CRF07_BC and CRF08_BC 45%, and CRF01_AE 15%. The remaining proportion is a combination of subtypes A and C, as well as CRF02_AG. Subtypes D and F, and HIV-2 have also been identified in China in small numbers.

Antiretroviral drug resistance

A small number of published studies have examined antiretroviral drug resistance in treatment-naïve and -experienced patients in China. Studies of treatment-naïve subjects have generally found low rates of drug resistance. One study sequenced 138 reverse transcriptase genes and 164 protease genes from about 400 subjects from across China and found at least one nucleoside reverse transcriptase inhibitor (NRTI) resistance mutation in 5.8%, a non-nucleoside reverse transcriptase inhibitor (NNRTI) resistance mutation in 1.5%, and a primary protease inhibitor (PI) resistance mutation in 0.6%. Secondary protease mutations, however, were found in 99% [38]. Other studies also identified low rates of primary resistance mutations in treatment-naïve patients [39,40]. In contrast, a small study of 45 treatment-naïve patients from Henan province found primary drug resistance mutations in 13.9% overall, including 8.3% in NRTI, 13.9% in NNRTI, and 11.1% in PI [41]. This study also examined 138 and 112 patients treated for three and six months, respectively, and found markedly increasing rates of drug resistance over time. Overall resistance mutations were identified in 45.4% of patients at three months and in 62.7% at six months. This increase was due primarily to changes in NNRTI mutations, which increased from 13.9% at baseline to 39.5% at three months and to 47.9% at six months. The NRTI mutations also increased somewhat over the same time periods, from 8.3% at baseline to 11.9% and then to 14.8%. Because PIs are used only minimally in China, resistance rates for PIs decreased over this period, from 11.1% to 2.0% to 0%, respectively. Why there was any PI resistance in the first place was not clear.

Other studies of treatment-experienced patients demonstrate similarly high rates of antiretroviral drug resistance, particularly to NNRTIs [42]. One study of 126 patients from four provinces in central China showed low rates of NRTI resistance (<5%) but high rates of NNRTI resistance (K103N 34.1%, Y181C 23.8%, G190A 15.1%) [39]. The development of these high rates of resistance shortly after treatment initiation is a concern for the long-term success of ART in China, particularly with the limited numbers of drugs currently available. Poor adherence certainly played a significant role in this resistance, particularly early in the roll-out of the national ART programme.

In some provinces, patients have been enrolled in treatment preparedness programmes through non-governmental organizations (NGOs) or local groups of people living with HIV/AIDS (PLWHA), with good results, even in groups that are traditionally thought to be poor adherents to treatment [43].

Spectrum of opportunistic infections and co-infections

Because only about 20% of the estimated 650,000 HIV-infected individuals have currently been identified, efforts to scale up surveillance are critically important. Outside of the large-scale screenings among the FPD cohort, the majority of patients are not diagnosed until they present with an opportunistic infection (OI). The spectrum of OIs seen in HIV-positive patients in China is similar to those seen elsewhere. *Pneumocystis carinii* pneumonia (PCP) is the most commonly seen OI, with tuberculosis (TB), both pulmonary and extra-pulmonary, oropharyn-geal candidiasis, cytomegalovirus (encephalitis, retinitis and gastrointestinal-tract infections), toxoplasmosis and cryptococcal meningitis also seen. Penicilliosis has been reported in southern China. Malignancies such as central nervous system (CNS) lymphoma, Hodgkin's and non-Hodgkin's lymphomas and Kaposi's sarcoma (KS) are also seen but are difficult to diagnose definitively. The Chinese HIV/AIDS treatment guidelines [44] recommend the use of OI prophy-laxis, similar to other international treatment guidelines (Table 17.2). In addition, the Chinese Free ART Manual recommends that all infants born to HIV-positive mothers be given cotrimox-azole prophylaxis from the age of 6 weeks up to 18 months, at which point HIV can be ruled out with an ELISA (enzyme-linked immunosorbant assay) test [45]. However, the national pro-gramme does not provide OI prophylaxis or cover the costs of OI treatments, which patients must purchase for themselves. Even though cotrimoxazole is relatively inexpensive, PCP prophy-laxis is prescribed and taken by patients inconsistently at best. Prophylaxis for other OIs is essen-tially non-existent due to the high cost of those medications.

China has the second highest TB burden in the world [46], and TB/HIV co-infection causes a significant proportion of the morbidity associated with AIDS, and vice versa. Among the chal-lenges to managing TB/HIV co-infection are: diagnosis of sputum smear negative for TB among AIDS patients; poor clinical recognition and management of TB and HIV amongst health staff in the different departments; difficult follow-up and adherence management, particularly in the rural areas of China; and cost to the patient of medication and treatment outside of that

Table 17.2 Chinese primary prophylaxis recommendations to prevent opportunistic infections

Opportunistic infection/pathogen	CD4+ cell count below which prophylaxis should begin	Prophylactic medicine	CD4+ cell count above which prophylaxis may be discontinued
Pneumocystis pneumonia	200 cells/mm^3	Cotrimoxazole 2 tablets/day if ≥60 kg; 1 tablet/day if <60 kg	>200 cells/mm^3 for ≥6 months
Mycobacterium avium complex	<50 cells/mm^3	Clarithromycin 500 mg twice each day or azithromycin 1200 mg/week	>100 cells/mm^3 for ≥ 6 months
Cytomegalovirus retinitis	<50 cells/mm^3	Ganciclovir, dosage not specified	100 cells/mm^3 for > ≥6 months
Toxoplasmosis	<100 cells/mm^3 and Toxo IgG+	Cotrimoxazole 2 tablets/day	>200 cells/mm^3 for >3–6 months

Source: [44].

delivered free of charge in the national programme. The Chinese government recognizes these problems and has developed several strategies to reduce the burden.

In early 2006, the Chinese Ministry of Health (MOH) issued a document outlining a TB/HIV co-infection pilot programme with four major objectives: the establishment of mechanisms for collaboration between TB and HIV departments; detection of TB cases among the TB/HIV population; screening for HIV among TB patients; and treatment and management of co-infected patients. Four provinces were selected for this pilot project: Guangxi Autonomous Region, Yunnan, Sichuan and Henan. Tuberculosis patients are screened for HIV infection using the 'opt out' method. Individuals who screen positive are referred to an HIV voluntary counselling and testing (VCT) centre for validation testing and further counselling. Confirmed HIV cases are followed at HIV treatment centres. Tuberculosis diagnosis among HIV/AIDS patients is performed in the HIV clinics. Patients are first screened for symptoms suggestive of TB, and further TB evaluation with chest X-ray and sputum smear and culture are conducted based on the outcome of the screening and the CD4 count. Once a diagnosis of TB/HIV co-infection is confirmed, patients are provided cotrimoxazole prophylaxis and anti-tubercular treatment. Initiation of ART is determined at the physician's discretion.

This pilot project is contributing to the scale-up of TB/HIV management, with the assistance of a significant contribution from the Global Fund to Fight HIV, Tuberculosis and Malaria (Global Fund). This programme, similar to the national Free ART Programme, faces problems of follow-up and referral, particularly with the changing face of migration within China, where *hukou* (registered hometown) residency often determines access to free national health services. Multi-drug resistant (MDR) TB in China reportedly contributes to a third of the world's cases of MDR TB [47], and although there are new national initiatives addressing this directly, they have not yet been linked to HIV programmes. As such, much work to address and link the jointly burdened arenas of TB and HIV treatment remains.

HCV/HIV co-infection is a major problem worldwide among IDUs. In China, this co-infection is highly prevalent not only in IDUs [48, 49] but also in FPDs [15, 50]. Although hepatitis B virus (HBV) infection is much more endemic in China than HCV, HBV/HIV co-infection seems to be far less of a problem in both FPD and IDU cohorts [50, 51]. These rates of hepatitis co-infection have implications for the treatment of these patients because HIV accelerates both HBV and HCV disease progression, and HCV increases the risk of adverse effects to HIV treatment [52,53]. In addition, HBV can be treated concurrently with HIV, depending on the drugs used. However, although some (but not all) of the drugs to treat HBV and HCV are available in China, most are priced far beyond the reach of the average person with the disease.

The history and evolution of the Chinese government's response to the AIDS crisis

The following section will outline, chronologically, the evolution of the national HIV/AIDS response, from the exigencies of delivering ART in sites lacking both comprehensive systems and trained personnel, to the development of a long-term strategy and dialogue whose goal is to provide good quality treatment to all who need it.

Although the first reported AIDS case in China was recognized in the mid-1980s, ART was not available through a government programme until 2002. Before then, individual drugs were available only to those who could afford to bring them into the country themselves or had contacts who could do so. This meant that HIV treatment was unavailable to the vast majority of those who needed it at that time—poor, rural farmers and IDUs. There were many reasons for this lack of availability, including the high cost of branded drugs, the lack of trained clinicians, particularly in the rural areas where most patients were located, and the lack of central government leadership at that time. Furthermore, stigma and discrimination among both medical staff and the community at large were high [54,55]. However, by the end of 2001, the central government's policies began changing for the better. In December 2001, the Division of Treatment and Care was established within the National Center for AIDS/STD Prevention and Control (NCAIDS) of the Chinese Center for Disease Control and Prevention (China CDC).

First pilot sites providing comprehensive treatment and care

In 2002, the Division of Treatment and Care initiated a pilot programme to provide free ART in Shangcai County, Henan Province, one of the areas hardest hit by HIV among the former plasma donating regions. The programme initially treated 100 patients using generic zidovudine (ZDV) with branded didanosine (ddI) and efavirenz (EFV). In addition, some of the first China CDC sites to start providing comprehensive, free HIV/AIDS treatment and care were those supported by the World Health Organization (WHO) in Suizhou County, Hubei Province, and by Médecins Sans Frontières (MSF) in Hubei and Guangxi Provinces, both in 2003.

Free antiretroviral drugs

In 2002, the government increased access to antiretroviral drugs by waiving tariffs and value-added taxes for imported drugs and by creating a fast-track process by which the State Food and Drug Administration (SFDA) could approve drugs manufactured in China [56]. By the end of 2002, Chinese pharmaceutical companies had received approval from the SFDA to produce generic versions of antiretroviral drugs not under patent protection in China: ZDV, ddI, stavudine (d4T) and nevirapine (NVP) [14]. The availability of these generic drugs at much-reduced prices compared to the branded versions enabled the government to scale up its free treatment programme, despite the limitations on regimen options due to cost and lack of access to certain branded drugs.

Initial efforts to scale up

In early 2003, the government began the scale-up of the free treatment programme through the China Comprehensive AIDS Response (China CARES) programme. This programme was designed to be an emergency response to the vast numbers of HIV-infected FPDs who were infected predominantly in the early to mid-1990s and who were, eight to ten years later, developing AIDS [57]. China CARES was initially launched in 51 counties across China and later scaled up to 127 counties in a total of 29 provinces. The central government dramatically increased HIV/AIDS-related budget allocation, from very little in 2000 to 800 million Chinese Yuan (about US$104.6 million) in 2004 and 2005 [58]; however, this budget has not covered all aspects of treatment. China CARES' beneficiary counties also received US$37,000–74,000 in matching funds from the central and local governments. Through China CARES, rural HIV-infected farmers who met the national treatment criteria were eligible for free treatment. The first-line regimen initially used was ZDV or d4T combined with ddI and NVP, all Chinese generic products. These drugs were distributed free through the national China CDC network. It was an ambitious plan implemented within a short time that resulted in, by the end of 2003, a cumulative total of 7000 people receiving free medicines [56].

Supportive national policy

National policy has existed since 2001 in the form of medium- and long-term plans [59] for HIV prevention and control. This was the beginning of a new era of government commitment to

HIV/AIDS efforts as a whole, and although not fully implemented, it set the stage for the treatment programmes that would follow soon after.

To highlight the central government's commitment to fight HIV, on World AIDS Day, 2003, Premier Wen Jiabao appeared on Chinese television publicly shaking hands with PLWHA at Beijing's Ditan Hospital. In conjunction with this visit, Wen also announced the new policy of 'Four Frees and One Care', which committed the government to providing the following:

- Free antiretroviral drugs to AIDS patients who are rural residents or people with financial difficulties living in urban areas;
- Free voluntary counselling and HIV screening tests;
- Free drugs to HIV-infected pregnant women for PMTCT, and HIV testing of newborn babies;
- Free schooling for children orphaned by AIDS; and
- Care and economic assistance for the households of PLWHA [60].

This policy formed the basis of the national Free ART Programme and broadened the scope of treatment from the China CARES counties to the entire country. While treatment did not become immediately available everywhere, scale-up moved outward from the original China CARES counties.

Although 'Four Frees and One Care' provided many benefits for those infected with HIV, many basic costs such as routine laboratory monitoring, OI treatment and hospitalizations were not included and continued to pose an effective barrier to treatment [61]. Two other policies were subsequently announced in 2004 to assist with this scale-up: 'Measures for Management of Drug Treatment of HIV/AIDS and Common OIs at No/Reduced Charge' ('Measures'), and 'Opinions Concerning the Management of HIV Antiviral Treatment' ('Opinions') [56]. 'Measures' extended the treatment responsibility from the China CDC system to the hospital system. It also clarified that the central government would be responsible for the costs of antiretroviral drugs, PMTCT drugs, and reagents for infant HIV diagnosis. The local governments would bear the costs of OI drugs and other barriers to accessing treatment. 'Opinions' defined management and implementation responsibilities for the Free ART Programme at the national, provincial, prefectural and county levels. Although these policies have helped considerably, implementation around the country is still inconsistent. Furthermore, this treatment is only accessible at one's registered hometown (*hukou*), which, as mentioned earlier, can pose a significant difficulty for migrant workers (discussed in more detail under 'Challenges', below).

In January 2006, the State Council decreed and promulgated a new regulation (No. 457) on AIDS prevention and treatment. This law protects the legal rights of PLWHA and obliges medical staff and institutions not to reject them. County-level governments and above are required to provide free antiretroviral drugs and low-cost medicines according to the patient's degree of economic difficulty.

In addition, the State Council China Action Plan for Reducing and Preventing the Spread of HIV/AIDS (2006–10) outlined several objectives for treatment in the country. Along with treatment coverage rates, the action plan also calls for the treatment of not less than 90% of patients for OIs by 2010.

China Free ART Manual

Guidelines about when to initiate treatment and what drugs to use are based on the China Free ART Manual [45]. This manual was developed by the MOH's HIV/AIDS Clinical Taskforce, a group composed of 25 of China's leading HIV/AIDS clinicians, virologists and public health personnel in conjunction with various international partners.

Eligibility for HIV treatment is based on meeting either clinical (WHO stage 3 or 4 disease) or laboratory (CD4 count <200 cells/mm^3) criteria. A total lymphocyte count of <1200 cells/mL may be used as a surrogate if a CD4 count is not available. The initial drug regimens used in the national Free ART Programme—ZDV or d4T in combination with ddI and NVP—formed the backbone of therapy until branded lamivudine (3TC) became available in 2005 as a result of Chinese government price negotiations. 3TC replaced generic ddI in the first-line regimen, and this combination remains the standard treatment regimen today.

The aforementioned changes in policy and programming created an environment of positive change in the arena of HIV/AIDS treatment. A number of achievements by the national programme have contributed to furthering this positive climate despite existing challenges.

Achievements of the national HIV/AIDS response

This section will briefly describe the results of the national adult and paediatric treatment programme as well as the use of, and access to, both traditional and western medicines. It will then describe some ongoing efforts to integrate programmes for training, laboratory and data systems.

Brief description of the national treatment programme at the end of 2006

The care model in China is described as community-based. There are several levels of healthcare provision; ART is provided at the county level, with routine follow-up, monitoring and care carried out at the village and township levels. Depending on the province, this may vary in terms of the treatment site and degree of coverage. In each province there is a referral mechanism to provincial and national clinicians if required by physicians at the county-level or below. Due to China's vast geographical size and population, some sites may treat relatively few patients, and hence further supervision may be needed to address more serious complications. By the same token, some county- and township-level clinicians in areas of higher prevalence have a wealth of experience with a high patient load. China CDC offices at each level collect patient data and are responsible for both stock management and distribution of drugs. Historically, it is important to note that although the China CDC system was established to manage the national treatment programme, the hospitals, administered by the Bureau of Health, began treating patients and collaborating with the China CDC long before any formal programme was envisaged. The MOH oversees all treatment and care activities, including training, development of technical guidelines, and technical assistance. The provincial health bureaus oversee the treatment programme by designating specific hospitals for infectious diseases and clinical training.

The cumulative number of individuals treated through the national treatment programme increased from 7000 at the end of 2003 to 30,640 by the end of 2006. According to the national treatment database (described in more detail below), 5497 of these patients have discontinued treatment (primarily because of side effects, adherence problems, and disease progression), 3381 have died, and 254 were lost to follow-up (Table 17.3). These data reflect the actual data received from local clinics, but are limited by reporting errors and biases inherent to observational databases.

Approximately 40% of patients initially remained on d4T/ddI/NVP due to the clinical success of this treatment. This has slowly been changing with the introduction of 3TC as a first-line drug. By the end of 2006, about 20% of patients were initiated on ZDV/3TC/NVP, with the remaining 80% receiving d4T/3TC/NVP. d4T was preferred over ZDV because of a relatively high rate of anaemia associated with ZDV in China; anecdotal evidence indicates that up to 20% of Chinese

Table 17.3 Status of antiretroviral treatment (ART) through the national Free ART Programme in China as of the end of 2006

	Number
Cumulative number on ART	30,640
Patients still on ART	25,143
Died	3381
Discontinued treatment	1489
Lost to follow-up	254
History of treatment with traditional Chinese medicine	2031

Source: National Centre for AIDS/STD Control and Prevention.

develop anaemia on ZDV. During pregnancy, however, ZDV is the preferred first-line drug. Other side effects observed on these two regimens include gastrointestinal disturbance (46%), rash (21%), peripheral neuropathy (13%), elevated liver enzymes (8%) and others (12%). For those unable to tolerate NVP or those with TB co-infection, a limited amount of branded EFV was negotiated by the government in 2004 for use in first-line regimens. Protease inhibitors (PIs) were not available through the national treatment programme until China produced a generic version of indinavir (IDV), which came on the market in 2005. Its use, however, has been limited by the necessity for thrice-daily dosing and the fact that there is no ritonavir (RTV) available for pharmacologic boosting of PIs.

Once patients begin ART, the effectiveness of long-term therapy is limited by the number and scope of antiretroviral drugs available. As of the end of 2006, the drugs available at no cost to the user through the national treatment programme were generic ZDV, d4T, ddI, NVP, and IDV, as well as branded 3TC and EFV. Thus, once treatment resistance develops, second-line options are very limited and third-line options non-existent. The MOH is negotiating with pharmaceutical companies for reduced pricing of the additional drugs needed.

Tenofovir (TDF) and lopinavir/ritonavir (LPV/r) have been targeted by national authorities for use in a second-line regimen under the national Free ART Programme, but these drugs are not currently obtainable. If negotiations are successful, these drugs will considerably improve the second-line treatment options available. To date, China has not taken advantage of compulsory licensing, which has been used by countries such as Brazil and Thailand, to secure additional antiretroviral drugs at lower prices.

Traditional Chinese medicine (TCM) is an integral part of Chinese society and is widely used by patients for a variety of general illnesses. Although TCM does not historically include rigorous research, clinical trials and evidence-based medicine, research is being done to evaluate the efficacy of such treatment. Results have been mixed, however, with one review concluding that TCM shows some promise for the treatment of HIV [62] and another finding a lack of sufficient evidence [63]. Although most practitioners in China would not advocate TCM as an alternative to ART, many believe that there is a role for TCM as an adjunct to ART to:

♦ boost the immune system to delay the need for ART;

♦ help alleviate symptoms related to AIDS; and

♦ help alleviate the adverse effects of western HIV medicines.

However, few studies have been conducted to determine the effects of drug interactions, and the national programme strongly advises caution if using TCM in conjunction with ART until further study is done. Despite this, there are anecdotal reports of patients being encouraged to use TCM in conjunction with, or even instead of, ART.

Monitoring and evaluation of the National ART Programme

Data on all patients receiving free ART through the national programme, estimated to be more than 95% of those being treated with ART in China, are captured in an ongoing observational database maintained at the NCAIDS, and the national treatment programme plans to improve HIV treatment in China through evidence-based research. Case report forms (CRFs) are completed for each patient at treatment initiation and at each follow-up visit. Information captured includes demographics, treatment regimen changes, laboratory values, clinical signs and symptoms, and self-reported adherence. These forms also serve as a standardized national medical record for all HIV patients on government-provided treatment. The CRFs are sent to the China CDC data management centre via DataFax, a data collection system that inputs data from a faxed image into an electronic database. As of the end of 2006, information from 30,640 patients had been entered into this database.

Several research projects using this database are under way to determine the impact of ART in China. Initial analyses, for example, show that mortality in high HIV prevalence areas decreased from 9.6% to 4.1% after the treatment programme was initiated (unpublished data). CD4 data from a small number of those on treatment show an initial CD4 count increase, which seems to taper off after 18 months (Table 17.4). The reasons for this trend are not clear, and the Division of Treatment and Care of NCAIDS of the China CDC is actively analyzing these data to improve national treatment standards and, eventually, to publish such analyses in peer-reviewed journals.

In addition, data quality control checks are being developed in order to understand the level of quality of the data. One brief quality control check of data from several provinces demonstrated an overall error rate of 10–20%. Efforts to improve the quality of these data are ongoing.

In a country as large as China, and with the rate of growth of the national treatment programme, monitoring and evaluation (M&E) of the programme is essential to long-term success. Over the course of 2007, in addition to improvements in the observational database being maintained, and with the help of national and international experts and funding, the Division of Treatment and Care plans to pilot M&E programmes in several provinces using outcome indicators that include CD4 count, viral load, quality of life, and clinical proficiency of physicians.

Paediatric HIV/AIDS programme

Children were part of the implementation of the national programme from its outset. However, treatment of children was limited by infant diagnostic methods and lack of paediatric formulations.

Table 17.4 Median CD4 cell counts for patients receiving treatment through the national Free ART Programme as of the end of 2006.

Months of treatment	Number of patients tested	Median CD4 count (cells/μl)	Interquartile range
0 (baseline)	21,531	159	60–270
6	2454	220	135–339
12	1884	251	163–375
18	1198	284	181–423
24	1122	283	172–410

Source: National Centre for AIDS/STD Control and Prevention.

Paediatric HIV treatment in China used split-dose adult formulation tablets until June 2005, when the Clinton HIV/AIDS Initiative (CHAI) donated paediatric formulations of antiretroviral drugs to China. Eighty-three children in Henan Province were initially started on paediatric formulation treatment at that time [22]. Since then, of the approximately 1800 known paediatric infections, approximately 600 children in 16 provinces have received paediatric treatment, 70% of whom are using paediatric formulation not yet available for purchase in China, thus relying on donation. Paediatric formulation drugs are currently procured through the new UNITAID initiative, and future procurement will include WHO-recommended fixed-dose combinations not yet available in China for either adults or children.

Although the paediatric programme has had much national political leadership support, the challenges of identifying HIV-positive pregnant women early, and linking them with maternal and child health PMTCT programmes, remain. Current efforts include scaling up PMTCT sites, expanding early infant diagnostic capacity and determining second-line therapy options for children in need. These efforts have been initiated with the collaboration of the maternal and child health service in a new pilot initiative of 'Family Care' in Guangxi Province, which has provided triple-drug therapy to pregnant women and early diagnosis of infants within a comprehensive, linked service. It is hoped that this will be expanded in the near future.

National training programmes and international support

Although treatment has been the Chinese government's most visible response to the HIV/AIDS crisis in China, the national programme has now moved far beyond its 'emergency response' beginnings to include training, laboratory infrastructure, M&E, and database management and research, with international partners providing assistance at each step. Training has been a critical component of the government scale-up because the vast majority of PLWHA are located in rural areas, where the medical infrastructure is weakest. China does have HIV specialists, but these experts are all based at universities or government institutions in major cities. Rural healthcare workers are often under-equipped for routine medical care, much less AIDS care. Training more rural clinicians to provide basic HIV/AIDS treatment and care has been a major activity of the Division of Treatment and Care of the China CDC. HIV/AIDS clinical training in China is essentially centralized training initiated to achieve two goals: to train existing infectious diseases physicians in HIV/AIDS management and care, and to ensure that at least 80% of all medical staff countrywide have knowledge of HIV/AIDS care and treatment.

Based on recommendations from the HIV/AIDS Clinical Taskforce, two types of training have been conducted so far. The first is a five-day course targeting provincial-level physicians who already have some HIV treatment experience. Over 2959 physicians have been trained through this course since 2003. The second is a two-month mini-residency held at nine urban hospitals throughout China. Over 1100 city- and county-level physicians have been trained in this way.

There have also been a number of collaborative projects with international organizations. The NCAIDS Division of Treatment and Care, the US CDC Global AIDS Program, CHAI, and the Anhui Provincial Health Bureau jointly established a rural training centre in a high HIV prevalence county in Anhui Province in 2004. An international HIV/AIDS clinician is based there to provide comprehensive, on-the-ground, hands-on training and support to county-level clinicians from across the country who rotate through the centre. Since its inception, a total of 80 physicians have received three-month training there.

In Yunnan Province, a clinical support model of mentorship has enabled the province to scale up ART treatment over a short period of time. Four sites were established in 2005 with support from foreign trainer-clinicians and a locally based project team.

Finally, some provinces have developed specialized training centres by integrating with existing medical and community care programmes and workshops run by NGOs and international organizations such as Family Health International (FHI), MSF, WHO, CHAI and various local Chinese organizations. Provincial authorities have also conducted their own training workshops, and international NGOs organize numerous small-scale training sessions as well. The Global Fund (Rounds 3 and 4 for China) has integrated health staff training into its core activities in the provinces.

All of these training methods and projects require ongoing funding, scale-up and qualified personnel. Given the size of the country and sheer numbers of health staff involved, this is a daunting exercise. Moreover, although the general objective of training is to increase clinical expertise, within these training programmes there is often little control over the motivation of those chosen to be trained, or any guarantee that they will resume HIV/AIDS treatment work after training. Many physicians who leave their posts for a period of weeks or months to attend training may even lose the income they normally would have earned during that time away. Thus, the success of the training programmes relies on good coordination among the different trainers, avoiding any duplication of efforts, and the ability to translate lessons learned on a wider scale.

Laboratories

The HIV/AIDS laboratory infrastructure in China has improved significantly in recent years. China currently has more than 5000 laboratories approved to perform HIV antibody testing. These approvals are provided at the provincial level and are based on a laboratory's ability to perform ELISA testing. There are also 102 laboratories across the country authorized to do Western blot validation testing. Approvals for these come from the China CDC for the laboratories in the CDC system, and from provincial authorities for laboratories outside the CDC system. In addition to scaling up the number of HIV testing locations, the China CDC has taken major steps over the last several years to improve the HIV laboratory infrastructure throughout China, with assistance from the WHO and the US National Institutes of Health (NIH).

Through the National AIDS Reference Laboratory (NARL) at the NCAIDS, a national external quality assurance proficiency testing (PT) network has been established that sends out PT panels to various laboratories across the country. The PT programme for HIV ELISA and Western blot testing began in 1998, and participating laboratories must pass this PT to maintain their approved status. The CD4/CD8 PT programme began in 2004 and sends panels to 67 laboratories twice a year. The HIV viral load PT programme, using NASBA (nucleic acid sequence based amplification) and RT-PCR, began in 2005 and sends panels to 21 laboratories once a year. Proficiency panels are also sent out for HBV surface antigen, HCV antibody, rapid plasma regain (RPR) for syphilis, HIV subtyping, the BED assay for early HIV infection diagnosis, and HIV drug resistance testing. More and more laboratories are participating in these PT programmes each year. Interpretation is done following international standards, with laboratories receiving passing or failing scores. The NARL also conducts practical and didactic training sessions on good laboratory practices and quality management for local laboratories.

A national HIV drug resistance surveillance network was established in 2004 by the NCAIDS of the China CDC. This network consists of four core laboratories located at the NCAIDS, the Academy of Military Medical Sciences in Beijing, the Shanghai CDC and the China Medical University in Shenyang, Liaoning Province. In 2004, this network performed a cross-sectional survey of HIV drug resistance among 14 provinces and established five sentinel surveillance sites in Henan, Anhui and Hubei Provinces. Surveillance was expanded to 29 provinces and autonomous regions in 2005, and to all 31 provinces and autonomous regions in 2006, with ongoing sentinel surveillance expanded from three provinces to 10. All four core laboratories participate in international genotype PT testing through the Virology Quality Assessment programme and have applied to join the WHO Global HIV Drug Resistance Surveillance Network.

Challenges

China needs to control its HIV epidemic and find, treat and care for those already living with HIV/AIDS. In a country of 1.3 billion people and multiple layers of health bureaucracy, this is a considerable challenge with no easy solution. Although the national HIV programme has accomplished much in a few short years, the scale-up has not been without its difficulties. Outlined below are the main challenges facing the scaling up of the national programme and the lessons learned thus far. Although it does not do justice to the complexity of the issues at hand, it is an attempt to describe the main obstacles and barriers China still faces regarding universal access. These are broadly divided into problems involving changes within China, particularly the healthcare system, and problems within the national treatment programme itself.

China's health system

China has embarked on a remarkable economic transformation over the past 30 years that has had tremendous benefits for its society but also some notable downsides, one of which is in the area of public healthcare. The economic reform plan of 'get rich first,' pioneered in 1978, has had widespread effects on investment in health, health worker financial security, insurance coverage, standards of care and the cost of care itself. This has occurred simultaneously with changes in the social fabric of China, whereby over 120 million rural poor have migrated to urban areas to seek work but are bereft of certain legal entitlements or access to health insurance [64]. During the period of economic reform, government expenditure on health as a percentage of gross domestic product (GDP) declined. In particular, funding for public health services such as surveillance and immunization is low. Fiscal decentralization, part of the social-economic reform, has left gaps between richer areas, whose governments have increased investments in health, and poorer regions, where hospitals have been forced to become increasingly self-reliant by raising patient fees. Healthcare workers have largely privatized their practices and charge high fees for service (FFS) to offset low wages and hospital and clinic financing. Simple care tends to be priced cheaply, while high technologies are priced considerably above cost [65]. This has led to an overuse of high-tech investigations, intravenous medications and more expensive drugs by clinicians in order to augment their meagre salaries.

This trend is accentuated by the general distrust of health providers by the poor Chinese population. Coupled with high costs of care, this can result in low utilization of hospitals by the rural poor and low medical insurance coverage of the population [1]. Pre-reform rural and government workers were covered by the nearly universal Labour Insurance and Government Insurance Schemes. After the reform, however, approximately 80% (640 million people in 2003) of the rural population and 50% of the urban population were no longer covered by health insurance [66]. There have been efforts in recent years to improve insurance coverage through a series of pilot schemes, but these mainly target catastrophic illnesses rather than basic services [1].

Problems with implementation of HIV/AIDS treatment through the public health system

One of the main difficulties with implementing a standard healthcare system is the large size of the country and the relative autonomy of each province. Although national mandates such as 'Measures' and 'Opinions' exist, how to implement and fund these mandates is often left up to each province to decide. Consequently, different provinces provide very different levels of service, depending on what they feel they can afford. For example, although HIV ELISA tests are provided free of charge, some provinces charge for Western blot confirmation; this results in many infections remaining 'undiagnosed' because Western blots are not performed to confirm the positive ELISA if the patient cannot afford the test.

CD4 counts are starting to be provided free of charge by some provinces. The central government recently purchased CD4 count and viral load technologies, but in general, coverage, particularly of the latter, is poor. Costs for routine laboratory monitoring, such as haematologies and chemistries, are borne by the patients themselves. Provincial policies on coverage of OI hospitalization fees also vary. Some provinces are developing coverage plans for AIDS-related hospitalizations, but with these plans generally based on reimbursement of expenses, hospitalizations are still unaffordable to many. Finally, indirect costs such as transportation, nutrition and infant feeding all depend on a person's ability to pay.

Compounding the issue is the national residence permit system in China, or *hukou*. All Chinese citizens have a registered place of residence, usually the place where they grew up. Changing this residence is difficult and generally requires a good job to sponsor you in the new location. The national Free ART Programme largely provides free treatment based on a person's *hukou*, so in effect, each person can only obtain free treatment from their registered place of residence. This causes significant difficulties for IDUs and sex workers, who are often quite mobile, as well as for the estimated 120 million migrant labourers in China, predominantly male and single. If diagnosed HIV-positive, sex workers must return to their home towns to obtain the free national medical treatment, even if they have good jobs where they are and no employment prospects back home.

The problem of ART scale-up amongst the populations of sex workers, migrants and IDUs is compounded by the *hukou* system and the illegality of their status. As these groups often do not have a fixed residence, are sometimes subject to arrest and are doubly stigmatized by having HIV, the challenge to provide good treatment and prevent further transmission is a difficult and urgent one. With regard to the IDU population, the government has significantly scaled up the number of methadone clinics and needle exchange programmes and is starting to integrate ART and methadone maintenance treatment. However, as a large proportion of the IDU population remains in detoxification centres and re-education camps, much more integration work needs to be done, as treatment is not yet available in these locations.

In regard to healthcare training, although a national training system is in place, there is little or no ongoing support for the majority of healthcare providers. Clinicians generally lack treatment experience and, especially in earlier times, did not know how to counsel patients well on antiretroviral drug side effects and the importance of treatment adherence, often resulting in poor adherence by the patient and the development of HIV drug resistance. Once resistance develops, very limited second-line treatment options remain through the national programme, as described above. When these options are exhausted, patients must either purchase expensive, branded second-line drugs themselves or remain on ineffective treatment. This is somewhat ironic in a country that possesses one of the world's largest manufacturing capacities for generic drugs. China is currently one of the major producers of active pharmaceutical ingredients (API) for antiretroviral drugs and has the capacity to produce nearly all first- and second-line drugs (Table 17.5) [67]. Certain Chinese pharmaceutical companies have also applied for WHO pre-qualification. Yet, due to patent barriers, China only produces five finished generic products for use in the country. All other APIs are exported and finished elsewhere and are not accessible to the majority of Chinese patients who need them but cannot afford them.

Because China is classified by the World Bank as a lower middle-income country, it does not qualify for some of the price reductions for medicines that have been obtained through the efforts of governments or international pharmaceutical companies for the least-developed countries. The SFDA is also undergoing major reform, which has resulted in delays in the registration of certain antiretroviral drug regimens. The central government is working towards a viable and sustainable second-line regimen for the national treatment programme, but when this will be realized is dependent on all the factors above.

Stigma against PLWHA continues to be widespread and has affected scale-up by discouraging many people from being tested and diagnosed. Moreover, although at national level the government has shown a commitment to tackle the HIV/AIDS crisis through the enactment of multiple new policies and work plans, at provincial and county levels there is often resistance. This results in a situation where the implementation of national policy at the local level is often limited by poor commitment [68]. The national government recently enacted legislation to protect the rights of PLWHA, but many provinces have yet to implement them. Moreover, the court system is also undergoing major reform, so few cases are brought to court.

Hospitals may not want to provide HIV care because they fear the impact it might have on their overall business by scaring away other patients, business they need in order to remain solvent. HIV screening of patients before any clinical procedure is common, with results not always provided to the patient. Those found to be HIV-positive may be turned away with other excuses. Within Chinese society, discrimination against HIV-infected individuals manifests as exclusion, isolation, loss of services, and gossip. This discrimination also extends to the infected person's uninfected family members.

The Chinese government is aware of these challenges, and the Treatment and Care Division of the NCAIDS at the China CDC has responded by increasing training through collaboration with international and national partners, working with adherence specialists, promoting community

Table 17.5 Active pharmaceutical ingredients for HIV drugs produced by major Chinese manufacturers

Drug	Pharmaceutical Manufacturers			
	Desano	Huahai	Mchem	Northeast
Zidovudine [a]	X		X	X
Stavudine [a]	X		X	X
Didanosine [a]	X	X		X
Lamivudine			X	
Nevirapine [a]	X	X	X	
Efavirenz			X	
Indinavir [a]	X	X	X	
Ritonavir	X		X	
Stavudine/Lamivudine/Nevirapine fixed-dose combination	X			

[a] Available as finished generic product in China.

Source: National Centre for AIDS/STD Control and Prevention.

care in conjunction with PLWHA groups and collaborating with the large-scale Global Fund effort to extend coverage. However, much more work remains to be done.

Conclusion

China is a country of stark contrasts. On the one hand, there is skyrocketing economic and technological capacity and growth, yet, on the other hand, there is also severe poverty and inequitable financing creating barriers to basic healthcare for PLWHA. Unlike other countries that were sensitized to AIDS long before antiretroviral drugs became available, China started ART training for management of HIV-positive patients concurrently with the start of health system reforms, without all the regimens in place and without a core group of physicians trained in OI management or ART. Despite this, the government has, in a relatively short period of time, trained and managed health staff and programmes that have had a significant and positive impact on both quantity and quality of HIV/AIDS treatment in China.

The commitment of the Chinese government to begin the national Free ART Programme was an encouraging step towards future healthcare equity. A formidable task remains, however, to scale up and equalize coverage around the country and maintain those already in treatment through the years ahead. Specific next steps have been described above and include obtaining a viable second-line treatment regimen, improving the quality of the national treatment programme through M&E and analysis of its observational database, improving treatment adherence rates and continuing to scale up laboratory assay quality and availability. The goals for treatment by the end of 2007 were:

- to have a cumulative total of at least 36,000 patients on ART;
- to provide treatment to 85% of identified paediatric HIV patients who require treatment;
- for new patients entering treatment, to maintain =80% on ART after one year; and
- to complete an ART monitoring and evaluation report in several pilot sites, including former plasma donor and IDU populations.

Successful treatment of PLWHA in China will require not only these specific steps, but also national policy work on financing and health systems, increased involvement of health workers and patients in programmes, capacity building at all levels, and ongoing education. China must find a way, through its own unique capacity, to not only strengthen and sustain its own programme, but also to share lessons learned, resources and experiences with other countries as its role in the global arena grows and evolves.

References

1. Wang H. (2005). China's fragmented health-system reforms. *Lancet* **366**:1257–8.
2. Zheng YY. (1988). First case of AIDS diagnosed in China. *Zhonghua Yi Xue Za Zhi* **68**:5–6.
3. PRC MoH, UNAIDS, WHO. (2006). *2005 Update on the HIV/AIDS Epidemic and Response in China.* Beijing: NCAIDS, China CDC.
4. He N, Detels R. (2005). The HIV epidemic in China: history, response, and challenge. *Cell Res* **15**:825–32.
5. Qian HZ, Vermund SH, Wang N. (2005). Risk of HIV/AIDS in China: subpopulations of special importance. *Sex Transm Infect* **81**:442–7.
6. Cohen MS, Henderson GE, Aiello P, Zheng H. (1996). Successful eradication of sexually transmitted diseases in the People's Republic of China: implications for the 21st century. *J Infect Dis* **174**(Suppl 2):S223–9.
7. Chen XS, Gong XD, Liang GJ, Zhang GC. (2000). Epidemiologic trends of sexually transmitted diseases in China. *Sex Transm Dis* **27**:138–42.

8. Parish WL, Laumann EO, Cohen MS, *et al.* (2003). Population-based study of chlamydial infection in China: a hidden epidemic. *JAMA* **289**:1265–73.

9. Chen ZQ, Zhang GC, Gong XD, *et al.* (2007). Syphilis in China: results of a national surveillance programme. *Lancet* **369**:132–8.

10. Chen XS, Yin YP, Liang GJ, *et al.* (2005). Sexually transmitted infections among female sex workers in Yunnan, China. *AIDS Patient Care STDS* **19**:853–60.

11. Chen XS, Yin YP, Liang GJ, *et al.* (2006). Co-infection with genital gonorrhoea and genital chlamydia in female sex workers in Yunnan, China. *Int J STD AIDS* **17**:329–32.

12. Galvin SR, Cohen MS. (2004). The role of sexually transmitted diseases in HIV transmission. *Nat Rev Microbiol* **2**:33–42.

13. Huang Y, Henderson GE, Pan S, Cohen MS. (2004). HIV/AIDS risk among brothel-based female sex workers in China: assessing the terms, content, and knowledge of sex work. *Sex Transm Dis* **31**:695–700.

14. Ma SJ, Hillier S, Zhang KL, *et al.* (2006). People's Republic of China. In: Beck EJ, Mays N, Whiteside A, Zuniga JM, eds. *The HIV pandemic: local and global implications*. Oxford: Oxford University Press. p282–99.

15. Qian HZ, Vermund SH, Kaslow RA, *et al.* (2006). Co-infection with HIV and hepatitis C virus in former plasma/blood donors: challenge for patient care in rural China. *AIDS* **20**:1429–35.

16. Zhang B, Liu D, Li X, Hu T. (2000). A survey of men who have sex with men: mainland China. *Am J Public Health* **90**:1949–50.

17. Liu H, Yang H, Li X, *et al.* (2006). Men who have sex with men and human immunodeficiency virus/sexually transmitted disease control in China. *Sex Transm Dis* **33**:68–76.

18. Zhang BC, Chu QS. (2005). MSM and HIV/AIDS in China. *Cell Res* **15**:858–64.

19. Choi KH, Liu H, Guo Y, Han L, Mandel JS, Rutherford GW. (2003). Emerging HIV-1 epidemic in China in men who have sex with men. *Lancet* **361**:2125–6.

20. Chen KT, Qian HZ. (2005). Mother to child transmission of HIV in China. *BMJ* **330**:1282–3.

21. Newell ML, Brahmbhatt H, Ghys PD. (2004). Child mortality and HIV infection in Africa: a review. *AIDS* **18**(Suppl 2):S27–34.

22. Zhang F, Au MC, Bouey PD, *et al.* (2007). The Diagnosis and Treatment of HIV-Infected Children in China: Challenges and Opportunities. *J Acquir Immune Defic Syndr* **44**:429–34.

23. He N, Detels R, Chen Z, *et al.* (2006). Sexual behavior among employed male rural migrants in Shanghai, China. *AIDS Educ Prev* **18**:176–86.

24. Wang B, Li X, Stanton B, Fang X, Lin D, Mao R. (2007). HIV-related risk behaviors and history of sexually transmitted diseases among male migrants who patronize commercial sex in China. *Sex Transm Dis* **34**:1–8.

25. He N, Detels R, Zhu J, *et al.* (2005). Characteristics and sexually transmitted diseases of male rural migrants in a metropolitan area of Eastern China. *Sex Transm Dis* **32**:286–92.

26. Hesketh T, Li L, Ye X, Wang H, Jiang M, Tomkins A. (2006). HIV and syphilis in migrant workers in eastern China. *Sex Transm Infect* **82**:11–4.

27. Ding QJ, Hesketh T. (2006). Family size, fertility preferences, and sex ratio in China in the era of the one child family policy: results from national family planning and reproductive health survey. *BMJ* **333**:371–3.

28. Hesketh T, Lu L, Xing ZW. (2005). The effect of China's one-child family policy after 25 years. *N Engl J Med* **353**:1171–6.

29. Tucker JD, Henderson GE, Wang TF, *et al.* (2005). Surplus men, sex work, and the spread of HIV in China. *AIDS* **19**:539–47.

30. Su L, Graf M, Zhang Y, *et al.* (2000). Characterization of a virtually full-length human immunodeficiency virus type 1 genome of a prevalent intersubtype (C/B') recombinant strain in China. *J Virol* **74**:11367–76.

31. Saksena NK, Wang B, Steain M, Yang RG, Zhang LQ. (2005). Snapshot of HIV pathogenesis in China. *Cell Res* **15**:953–61.

32. Beyrer C, Razak MH, Lisam K, Chen J, Lui W, Yu XF. (2000). Overland heroin trafficking routes and HIV-1 spread in south and south-east Asia. *AIDS* **14**:75–83.

33. Zhang Y, Lu L, Ba L, *et al.* (2006). Dominance of HIV-1 Subtype CRF01_AE in Sexually Acquired Cases Leads to a New Epidemic in Yunnan Province of China. *PLoS Med* **3**:e443.

34. Yang R, Xia X, Kusagawa S, Zhang C, Ben K, Takebe Y. (2002). On-going generation of multiple forms of HIV-1 intersubtype recombinants in the Yunnan Province of China. *AIDS* **16**:1401–7.

35. Su B, Liu L, Wang F, *et al.* (2003). HIV-1 subtype B' dictates the AIDS epidemic among paid blood donors in the Henan and Hubei provinces of China. *AIDS* **17**:2515–20.

36. Yu XF, Chen J, Shao Y, Beyrer C, Lai S. (1998). Two subtypes of HIV-1 among injection-drug users in southern China. *Lancet* **351**:1250.

37. Laeyendecker O, Zhang GW, Quinn TC, *et al.* (2005). Molecular epidemiology of HIV-1 subtypes in southern China. *J Acquir Immune Defic Syndr* **38**:356–62.

38. Si XF, Huang HL, Wei M, *et al.* (2004). Prevalence of drug resistance mutations among antiretroviral drug-naive HIV-1-infected patients in China. *Zhonghua Shi Yan He Lin Chuang Bing Du Xue Za Zhi* **18**:308–11.

39. Jiang S, Xing H, Si X, Wang Y, Shao Y. (2006). Polymorphism of the protease and reverse transcriptase and drug resistance mutation patterns of HIV-1 subtype B prevailing in China. *J Acquir Immune Defic Syndr* **42**:512–4.

40. Zhong P, Kang L, Pan Q, *et al.* (2003). Identification and distribution of HIV type 1 genetic diversity and protease inhibitor resistance-associated mutations in Shanghai, P. R. China. *J Acquir Immune Defic Syndr* **34**:91–101.

41. Li JY, Li HP, Li L, *et al.* (2005). Prevalence and evolution of drug resistance HIV-1 variants in Henan, China. *Cell Res* **15**:843–9.

42. Ma L, Sun J, Xing H, *et al.* (2007). Genotype and Phenotype Patterns of Drug-Resistant Human Immunodeficiency Virus 1 Subtype B' (Thai B) Isolated From Antiretroviral Therapy Failure Patients in China. *J Acquir Immune Defic Syndr* **44**:14–19.

43. Durier N, Loke C, Yang YN, Tang ZR, Sauvageot D. (2006). Antiretroviral therapy in intravenous drug users: results from a comprehensive routine HIV care project in Nanning, southern China Guangxi Zhuang autonomous region. XVI International AIDS Conference, August 2006; Toronto, Canada. [Abstract THPE0155]

44. Chinese CDC. (2005). *Guidelines for Diagnosis and Treatment of HIV/AIDS in China*. Beijing: Chinese Medical Association, Chinese Center for Disease Control and Prevention.

45. Zhang FJ, ed. (2005). *China Free ART Manual*. Beijing: Chinese Center for Disease Control and Prevention.

46. Wang L, Liu J, Chin DP. (2007). Progress in tuberculosis control and the evolving public-health system in China. *Lancet* **369**:691–6.

47. Zignol M, Hosseini MS, Wright A, *et al.*(2006). Global incidence of multidrug-resistant tuberculosis. *J Infect Dis* **194**:479–85.

48. Zhang C, Yang R, Xia X, *et al.* (2002). High prevalence of HIV-1 and hepatitis C virus coinfection among injection drug users in the southeastern region of Yunnan, China. *J Acquir Immune Defic Syndr* **29**:191–6.

49. Garten RJ, Zhang J, Lai S, Liu W, Chen J, Yu XF. (2005). Coinfection with HIV and hepatitis C virus among injection drug users in southern China. *Clin Infect Dis* **41**(Suppl 1):S18–24.

50. Xu JQ, Wang JJ, Han LF, *et al.* (2006). Epidemiology, clinical and laboratory characteristics of currently alive HIV-1 infected former blood donors naïve to antiretroviral therapy in Anhui Province, China. *Chin Med J* (Engl) **119**:1941–8.

51. Zhao M, Wang QY, Lu GH, Xu P, Xu H, McCoy CB. (2005). Risk behaviors and HIV/AIDS prevention education among IDUs in drug treatment in Shanghai. *J Urban Health* **82**(3 Suppl 4):iv84–91.

52. Schooley RT. (2005). HIV and hepatitis C virus coinfection: bad bedfellows. *Top HIV Med* **13**:112–6.

53. Levy V, Grant RM. (2006). Antiretroviral therapy for hepatitis B virus-HIV-coinfected patients: promises and pitfalls. *Clin Infect Dis* **43**:904–10.

54. Lieber E, Li L, Wu Z, Rotheram-Borus MJ, Guan J. (2006). HIV/STD stigmatization fears as health-seeking barriers in China. *AIDS Behav* **10**:463–71.

55. Anderson AF, Zheng Q, Wu G, Li Z, Liu W. (2003). Human immunodeficiency virus knowledge and attitudes among hospital-based healthcare professionals in Guangxi Zhuang Autonomous Region, People's Republic of China. *Infect Control Hosp Epidemiol* **24**:128–31.

56. Zhang FJ, Pan J, Yu L, Wen Y, Zhao Y. (2005). Current progress of China's free ART program. *Cell Res* **15**:877–82.

57. Zhang F, Hsu M, Yu L, Wen Y, Pan J. (2006). Initiation of the National Free Antiretroviral Therapy Program in Rural China. In: Kaufman J, Kleinman A, Saich T, eds. *AIDS and Social Policy in China.* Cambridge, MA: Harvard University Asia Center. p96–124.

58. Wu Z, Sullivan SG, Wang Y, Rotheram-Borus MJ, Detels R. (2007). Evolution of China's response to HIV/AIDS. *Lancet* **369**:679–90.

59. Ministry of Health, National Planning Committee, Ministry of Education, Ministry of Science and Technology, Ministry of Public Security, Ministry of Justice, Ministry of Finance, and State Administration of Broadcast, Film and Television of P.R. China. (2001). *Implementation Guideline for China's Medium and Long Term Plan for HIV/AIDS Prevention and Control (1998–2010).* Beijing: Government of P. R. China.

60. Shen J, Yu DB. (2005). Governmental policies on HIV infection in China. *Cell Res* **15**:903–7.

61. Médecins Sans Frontières. (2006). *The Cost of AIDS Care in China: Are Free Antiretroviral Drugs Enough?* Beijing: Médecins Sans Frontières.

62. Liu ZM, Yang YS, Wang XL, Wen RX. (2006). Recent progress on anti-HIV research of traditional Chinese medicine and components. *Zhongguo Zhong Yao Za Zhi* **31**:1753–8.

63. Liu JP, Manheimer E, Yang M. (2005). Herbal medicines for treating HIV infection and AIDS. *Cochrane Database Syst Rev* 2005(3):CD003937.

64. United Nations Health Partners Group in China. (2005). *A Health Situation Assessment of the People's Republic of China.* Beijing: United Nations Health Partners Group in China. p 6–7.

65. World Bank. (2005). *Health Service Delivery in China: A Review. World Bank Rural Health in China Briefing Notes.* Available at http://web.worldbank.org/WBSITE/EXTERNAL/COUNTRIES/ EASTASIAPACIFICEXT/EXTEAPREGTOPHEANUT/0,contentMDK:20717431~pagePK:34004173~piPK: 34003707~theSitePK:503048,00.html (accessed 23 March 2007).

66. World Bank. (2005). *Rural Health Insurance – Rising to the Challenge. World Bank Rural Health in China Briefing Notes.* Available at http://web.worldbank.org/WBSITE/EXTERNAL/COUNTRIES/ EASTASIAPACIFICEXT/EXTEAPREGTOPHEANUT/0,contentMDK:20717431~pagePK:34004173~piPK: 34003707~theSitePK:503048,00.html (accessed 23 March 2007).

67. Grace C. (2005). *A Briefing Paper for DFID: Update on China and India and Access to Medicines.* Available at http://www.dfidhealthrc.org/publications/access_medicines.html (accessed 23 March, 2005).

68. Cai T. (2006). Perspectives on Stigma and the Needs of People Living with AIDS in China. In: Kaufman J, Kleinman A, Saich T, eds. *AIDS and Social Policy in China.* Cambridge, MA: Harvard University Asia Center. p170–174.

Chapter 18

Country review: South Africa

Robin Wood* and Des Martin

Epidemiology

South Africa is a middle-income country with a population of 47 million and a gross domestic product (GDP) of US$160 billion. Although the GDP per capita (PPP) is US$10,346, there is an unequal distribution of wealth, with 34% of the population living on less than US$2 per day [1]. About 57% of South Africa's population lives in urban areas.

Prior to 1990, the HIV epidemic was largely limited to men who had sex with men (MSM), with the predominant HIV-1 subtypes being B and D [2]. Following the new political dispensation in South Africa, regional transport routes between South Africa and its neighbouring countries were reopened. The initial epidemic has subsequently been overshadowed by a predominantly heterosexually transmitted epidemic with a central African subtype C HIV-1 [3]. The heterosexually transmitted epidemic has been monitored since 1990 by annual antenatal seroprevalence surveys, which have shown a steady increase of HIV-1 prevalence from 0.8% in 1990 to 15% in 1996, and with a further increase to 30% in 2005 (all data from the antenatal clinic surveys) [4].

Demographic modelling, together with the results of antenatal surveys, estimated there were 5.5 million HIV-infected individuals in South Africa in 2005, of whom 3.1 million (56%) were adult women over the age of 15 years [4]. There are now an estimated 240,000 children under the age of 14 years living with AIDS [5]. To date, intravenous drug use (IVDU) has not been reported as a significant mode of HIV transmission within South Africa.

There are more than 600,000 individuals in immediate need of antiretroviral therapy (ART), and there have been an estimated accumulated total of 2 million deaths related to AIDS up to 2006. Life expectancy in 2004 was estimated to be 48.5 years for males and 52.7 years for females, with an infant mortality rate of 56 per 1000 live births. In 2010 there will be an estimated 2 million maternal orphans under the age of 18 years, 1.5 million of whom will be AIDS orphans. Without ART, the estimated annual number of AIDS-related deaths in South Africa will increase to 495,000 by 2010 [6].

Government policy on universal access to ART

In South Africa, political agendas have obscured scientific facts. Prior to 2002, the national government vacillated by questioning the link between HIV and AIDS [7] and exaggerating the toxicities of antiretroviral (ARV) drugs [8,9]. Meanwhile, it briefly encouraged the use of local products such as virodene, a topically applied formulation of dimethylformamide, a known hepatotoxic carcinogen [10] and, more generally, a wide variety of herbal extracts and other natural products, including African potato, candelabra tree, glory bower, polyanthus, peach, grapefruit, olive, senna,

* Corresponding author.

sunflower seed and honey [11]. The government's HIV/AIDS/STD Strategic Plan for South Africa 2000–2005 [12], however, did envisage limited use of antiretroviral drugs for occupational post-exposure prophylaxis (PEP) and undertook to review data on the utility of ART for post-sexual assault and the prevention of mother-to-child transmission (PMTCT) of HIV. In 2002, following a petition from civil society groups, including the Treatment Action Campaign (TAC), a constitutional court ruling instructed the Department of Health to make single-dose nevirapine (NVP) universally accessible to pregnant women for PMTCT within the public health system. By 2004–5, the PMTCT programme had extended to a total of 3064 facilities offering services to 55% of South African HIV-infected mothers [4].

In 2002, the Department of Health acknowledged that ART could improve the quality of life of people living with HIV/AIDS (PLWHA) [13] but still considered universal access to ARV drugs too costly [14]. The government policy on the non-affordability of universal access to ARV drugs was based on a costing study financed by the World Bank and performed by Abt Associates in 2000 [15]. This model produced very high estimates for both non-ARV and ARV treatments, but by 2003 the original modelled calculations of ARV drug costs were no longer considered to be suitable for policy making [11]. An alternative costing analysis based on the ASSA2000 demographic model and lowered ARV drug costs became available in 2002, which again explored the feasibility of a national ART programme [16].

The South African Cabinet asked the Department of Health to develop an ART programme as a matter of urgency, and the Minister of Health established a task team to develop an operational plan for implementation of an ART programme [17]. The task team produced a full report on 8 August 2003 [11]. An operational plan was published on 19 November 2003 and included an estimate of the number of new cases projected to start ART over the following six years. An estimated 1,470,510 patients were expected to be on ART by 2008–9 [18].

National treatment guidelines were published in early 2004. These recommended using two scheduled ARV regimens together with laboratory monitoring including safety, CD4 counts and viral load measurement every six months [19]. By September 2005, an estimated 85,000 patients had been enrolled for ART at 199 facilities within the public sector [20].

Treatment access in South Africa

Treatment access has evolved in three phases (Figure 18.1). Between 1996 and 2000, access to ART was limited to those who could afford the out-of-pocket expense of commercially available

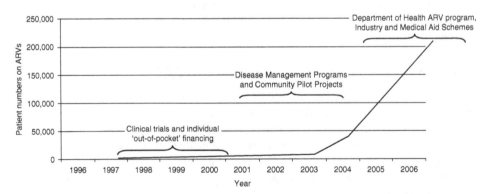

Fig. 18.1 Estimated number of individuals receiving antiretroviral therapy in South Africa between 1996 and 2006.

drugs or to those who could enter ART trials, which largely took place in academic centres located in the major metropolitan areas [21–24]. The period between 2001 and 2003 saw the development of the first community-based ART programmes in the Western Cape Province [25,26] and the development of HIV disease management programmes by a few private medical aid schemes [27].

In 2002, the largest of these schemes reimbursed treatment costs for approximately 10,500 clients [31]. Initially, reimbursements were for dual nucleoside reverse transcriptase inhibitor (NRTI) therapy only, but with the decline in antiretroviral drug costs in South Africa, triple-drug therapy became the standard of care (Figure 18.2).

The latest period, from 2003 to 2006, saw a major expansion in treatment access from 12,000 to 210,000 individuals. This was due to a combination of increased antiretroviral drug availability in the public sector and ART being included in the minimum package of benefits that medical aid schemes are required by legislation to provide. These schemes, however, frequently have caps on the maximum reimbursement for HIV care, which may result in out-of-pocket expenses for those who have exhausted their medical benefits. Those who have exhausted their private medical aid benefits and are unable to afford extra out-of-pocket expenses frequently transfer their HIV care responsibility to the state sector [32].

The Department of Health treatment guidelines developed in 2004 [19] largely parallel the World Health Organization's 2002 treatment guidelines as outlined in *Scaling Up Antiretroviral Therapy in Resource-Limited Settings: Guidelines for a Public Health Approach* [33].

The scale of need for HIV/AIDS treatment in South Africa is such that demand is likely to continue to far exceed the supply of ART. In order to address the possible inequalities in access to care, the Department of Health plan envisaged public sector access to HIV services including ART in at least one site within each of the 162 health districts of the country. By early 2006, the number of nationally accredited service points delivering ART had increased to 210 [28].

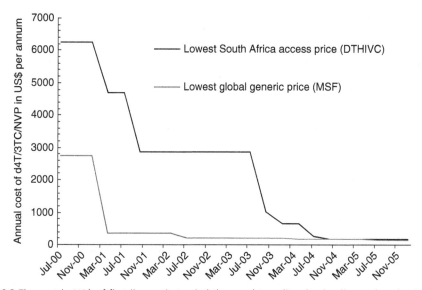

Fig. 18.2 The cost in US$ of first-line antiretroviral therapy (stavudine, lamivudine and nevirapine), as registered with the South African Medicines Council, and the lowest world price of generic formulations.

A few large South African companies have led the corporate response to HIV infection in their workforce. In 2001, DaimlerChrysler, in partnership with the German Technical Cooperation Agency (GTZ) and Medscheme, a South African medical insurer, offered a package of comprehensive HIV medical care, including ART, to 23,000 workers and their families [29]. Other corporations joined the Medscheme 'AID for AIDS' programme, and by early 2003, approximately 8000 patients had accessed ART via this programme [29]. In 2002, two large South African mining corporations, Anglo American and Goldfields of South Africa [29, 30], extended their existing wellness clinic services to include ART for their workforce. However, by 2006 only 38% of South African companies surveyed had implemented an HIV/AIDS workplace policy [4].

With substantial additional financial support from the US President's Emergency Plan for AIDS Relief (PEPFAR), the Anglo American programme was extended in 2006 to 5500 employees and individuals in those communities from which workers were recruited [30]. Similar funding from PEPFAR has allowed the Catholic Relief Services, a faith-based organization, to rapidly extend ART services in their mission hospitals to more than 15,000 individuals in poorly served rural areas.

By May 2006, a total of 200,000 individuals were estimated to be receiving ART in South Africa, of whom 110,000 were in the public sector and 90,000 were in the non-governmental and private sectors [28].

Southern African HIV Clinicians Society

With the growing number of HIV-infected patients in the country, the need arose for educational initiatives and networking within the medical profession. In 1998, the Southern African HIV Clinicians Society (SAHIVS) was founded. This is an organization that falls within the South African Medical Association's (SAMA) Special Interest Groups (SIG). It has now become the largest SIG within South Africa, with approximately 12,000 members, the majority of whom are general practitioners. The SAHIVS's main objective is to support the provision of quality clinical care for PLWHA.

Since its inception in 1998, the SAHIVS has witnessed a sustained growth in its membership. While the majority of its members are still within South Africa, there is an ever increasing membership throughout neighbouring African countries. It has fostered and supported the growth of branches in Namibia, Botswana, Zimbabwe, Zambia, Swaziland and Lesotho. Branches carry out a number of functions, including monthly educational meetings, dissemination of information, organization of continuing medical education courses and provision of teaching faculty for education initiatives in both the public and private sectors. Almost 10,000 healthcare professionals, mostly doctors and nurses, have been trained and have participated in the entry-level course. A number of alumni of the entry courses have returned for further updates and refresher courses. Donor funding has enabled the courses to be offered at affordable prices, thus promoting wider access.

The role of activism

Activism has played a major role in promoting access to ART to those who require treatment. Sadly, South Africa has lacked leadership from prominent political leaders, and this has contributed greatly to the delay in ART roll-out. President Thabo Mbeki is a denialist, and his Minister of Health, Manto Tshabala-Msimang, has been influenced by his views. The persistence of the Treatment Action Campaign (TAC), the AIDS Law Project, the SAHIVS and various overseas organizations, as well as disclosure by some very high profile South Africans—Justice Edwin Cameron and activist Zackie Achmat—ultimately influenced the government to commence a public sector roll-out of ART in 2004. The AIDS Law Project and TAC have used direct negotiations with pharmaceutical companies and the South African competition legislation to effect significant reductions in antiretroviral drug costs, which in turn has had a major influence in promoting access to treatment (Figure 18.2). In late 2006, while the incumbent Minister of Health was on sick leave, the Deputy Minister of Health, Nozizwe Madlala-Routledge, moved away from the existing confrontational relationship with civil society and began a constructive engagement with TAC and other civil society groups. She is largely credited with the launch of the National Strategic Plan for HIV/AIDS and Sexually Transmitted Infections for 2007–2011, as well as the relaunch of the South African National AIDS Council. However, Mbeki unceremoniously sacked her in August 2007 for making an allegedly unauthorized trip to an AIDS conference held in Madrid, which many activists view as a pretence to mask his discontent with the combination of her more active engagement with civil society, as well as her expressions of regret over the government's failure to do more to combat HIV/AIDS in South Africa.

Treatment strategies

National public sector guidelines recommend initiation of ART in adults at a CD4 cell count of less than 200 cells/mm^3 or at the occurrence of an AIDS diagnosis. Paediatric ART initiation is based on either a WHO clinical stage 3 diagnosis or a CD4 cell count percentage of less than 15% of the total lymphocyte count. Two scheduled regimens are made available. The initial adult regimen consists of a non-nucleoside reverse transcriptase inhibitor (NNRTI) together with the NRTIs stavudine (d4T) and lamivudine (3TC). NVP is the preferred NNRTI in women of child-bearing age, with efavirenz (EFV) as the preferred NNRTI when ART is combined with rifampicin-containing tuberculosis (TB) therapy. The second protease inhibitor (PI)-based regimen consists of zidovudine (ZDV), didanosine (ddI) and ritonavir (RTV)-boosted lopinavir (LPV). A limited number of antiretroviral drug switches are allowed within each regimen for toxicity, intolerance, pregnancy and TB. Monitoring for safety and efficacy is performed every six months, and a confirmed viral load of greater than 5000 copies/mL after adherence intensification is a justification for change to the second regimen. No viral load monitoring is performed on second-line therapy because at present there is no salvage option available in the public sector programme [19].

Laboratory monitoring

Laboratory support for patients on ART has varied according to the setting in which antiretroviral drugs have been used. In the first instance, for patients funding their own therapy or those who belong to health insurance schemes, a full range of laboratory tests is available. These include viral load tests, CD4 counts and monitoring for drug toxicities. Genotypic resistance testing is available in the instance of treatment failure. Therapeutic drug monitoring (TDM) is not widely available.

Frequency of virologic and immunologic monitoring in the private setting occurs at intervals of three to four months and more frequently if indicated. For paediatric HIV treatment, specialized testing for polymerase chain reaction (PCR) diagnosis and virologic and immunological monitoring are readily available.

In South Africa's National ART roll-out programme, the frequency of viral load monitoring is reduced to six-monthly intervals with no allowances made for specialized testing such as genotypic resistance testing. Viral load monitoring is limited to the first treatment regimen and is not performed routinely during the second-line regimen. The laboratory support for the national programme resides in the National Health Laboratory Services, which requires specimens for viral load and PCR-based technologies to be transported to the larger centres. There is an increasing use of portable, hand-held lactate meters in primary care clinics as a result of increasing awareness of lactic acidaemia and acidosis as complications of prolonged d4T use.

A locally developed flow cytometry-based assay for CD4 cell counting has markedly increased the affordability of CD4 count monitoring within South Africa [34]. The panleucogated assay (PLG) uses a generic CD45 monoclonal antibody for flow cytometry gating rather than total lymphocyte population gating. The use of the PLG assay in combination with improved blood sample transport media has allowed accurate CD4 cell measurement to be performed on samples from remote rural clinics that cannot reach a central laboratory within 24 hours. The central laboratories servicing the public sector ART programme have adopted the PLG assay as their standard assay in centralized laboratories.

Centralized laboratories rely on well-developed pathology sample transport infrastructures, which may be lacking in rural areas. The use of newer transport media and modalities such as dried blood spots for PCR assays increases the peripheral reach of central laboratories. An alternative strategy that has been explored is to develop peripheral laboratory capacity; alternative initiatives that are currently being evaluated include peripheral monitoring laboratories situated in primary healthcare clinics or HIV treatment centres. A self-contained laboratory housed in a modified shipping container utilized best-of-breed, US Food and Drug Administration (FDA)-approved technologies to provide viral load testing, CD4 counts and toxicity monitoring to the Gugulethu programme in Cape Town over a three-year period of rapid expansion in numbers of patients on ART [35]. These types of laboratories can provide significant capacity development and overcome some of the logistical problems of specimen transport, turnaround times and delayed result reporting associated with centralization of laboratory services.

Therapeutic drug monitoring capacity is restricted to a very few centres in the public or private sectors and is neither widely used nor a part of routine patient management.

In 2002, a study of the molecular characteristics of the prevalent South African HIV-1 established that, while there was considerable genetic diversity and polymorphism within HIV-1 subtype C, there was little evidence of drug resistant mutations prior to the availability of widespread ART [36]. There is, as yet, no national registry to monitor the frequency and patterns of resistance to antiretroviral drugs. The scheduled regimen approach as outlined in the national treatment guidelines has been taken up by the managed care segment of the private health sector, and non-governmental organizations (NGOs) such as Médecins Sans Frontières (MSF) have modified treatment regimens to harmonize with the guidelines.

Importance of HAART on control of viraemia, opportunistic infections, and survival

Results from early pilot projects show remarkably low levels of loss to follow-up and high levels of adherence to therapy, with a reported 88% of patients in the Khayelitsha pilot ART programme and more than 90% of patients in the Gugulethu programme maintaining viral suppression below 400 copies/mL after one year of ART [25, 26]. In the early phases, when ART availability was very limited, some programmes had strict entry criteria, including proven regular clinic attendance, disclosure of HIV diagnosis to friends or family, and demonstrated adherence to prophylactic medication [26]. The early reported successes of these programmes may have been partly influenced by entry criteria, which introduced a selection bias for populations with better adherence. As ART availability has improved, the numbers accessing treatment have increased and these strict rationing strategies have fallen away.

In contrast to hospital-based services, the early pilot programmes in the Western Cape were community-based and located in primary care facilities, thereby reducing the need for patient transport and the resultant losses to follow-up of patients with insufficient funds. Differing strategies to maintain adherence to therapy were explored, including a designated 'treatment buddy' system [26] and the use of HIV-infected 'therapeutic counsellors' from the same locality [25]. Although it is difficult to attribute which specific components of any programme are responsible for success, the combination of locally based services and targeted adherence strategies has been associated with high rates of viral suppression (<400 copies/mL) in 90% of patients maintained over three years [37].

Following on from the experience of the early pilot projects, the national treatment guidelines have also stressed the importance of structured adherence counselling and support within the ART roll-out programme [19]. In contrast, a large work-based ART programme operating across 70 different healthcare sites was able to identify health system factors associated with worse virologic outcomes, which included: long waiting times for clients; use of staff without specialized HIV care training; lack of active follow-up of defaulting clients; and poor communication between medical and pharmacy staff [38].

Antiretroviral therapy is associated with considerable improvement in survival probability, and early pilot projects have reported 80–85% cohort survival after one to three years of therapy in those programmes with active follow-up [26,34]. Early mortality is high but declines rapidly [39]. Risk of death in ART programmes has three distinct phases, namely, the combination of mortality that precedes the commencement of ART, that which occurs soon after starting ART, and that occurring in patients late in ART [40]. Extremely high pre-treatment (33 per 100 patient-years (PY)) and early mortality (19 per 100 PY) reflect the advanced stage of HIV disease in those accessing therapy. Risk factors for early death include male gender, an AIDS diagnosis and a low baseline CD4 count. Late mortality is much lower (2.9/100 PY) and is related to virologic and immunologic response to treatment rather than baseline characteristics [40].

Of particular concern is the early mortality rate, which reflects the very high pre-treatment mortality of patients qualifying for ART in South Africa. The causes of pre- and early-ART mortality are similar. Major causes of death include wasting syndrome, acute infections, TB, Kaposi's sarcoma, cryptococcal meningitis, chronic pulmonary disease, and drug toxicity [39]. The median CD4 count of patients accessing ART in South Africa is less than 100 cells/mm^3 (25, 34), and unless patients can be encouraged to access therapy earlier, the majority of deaths will continue to occur before individuals can start ART [40].

Tuberculosis is the most common opportunistic infection (OI) in South Africa [41–43], and the World Health Organization (WHO) has identified HIV/TB co-infection as a regional emergency in sub-Saharan Africa [4]. In newly urbanized populations in Cape Town, TB disease notification rates are over 1000 per 100,000 and are increasing [44, 45]. Tuberculosis notification rates among HIV-infected individuals living in a Cape Town township have been reported to be as high as 5000 per 100,000 [46]. Notification data are based on passive case finding that may significantly underestimate the true community burden of TB disease, which can more accurately be identified by active case finding [46]. In South Africa, patients with advanced HIV infection accessing ART programmes have exceptionally high burdens of TB disease, with more than 50% having been treated for TB in the preceding three years, and 25% having a new diagnosis of TB requiring treatment either immediately prior to or during the ART screening process [42].

Primary multi-drug resistance to isoniazid and rifampicin among new cases of TB in South Africa has been low in the past, ranging from 0.8% to 2.6% [47]. Re-treatment of TB, however, has been associated with increased rates of multi-drug resistance. The national TB control programme has not routinely tested for resistance to second-line TB drugs. Recently, an outbreak of extensively drug resistant (XDR) TB was reported from a rural area of Kwa-Zulu Natal [48]. In this outbreak over a 15-month period, the prevalence of multi-drug resistant (MDR)-TB among culture-confirmed TB cases was 39%, and XDR-TB was confirmed in 6%. Only 55% of patients with XDR-TB had been previously treated for TB. There was a strong association between

XDR-TB and HIV infection, as all individuals tested for HIV were confirmed to be co-infected. Mortality was 98% among XDR-TB cases, with a median survival of only 16 days [48]. Since publication of the details of this outbreak, there has been increased testing for resistance to second-line agents, with subsequent recognition of XDR-TB cases throughout the country.

Antiretroviral therapy has been shown to decrease the incidence of TB in HIV infection significantly in a South African hospital-based cohort study [49]. Tuberculosis incidence has been also shown in the Gugulethu ART programme to decrease from 22 per 100 patient-years during the first three months of ART to approximately 4.5 per 100 patient-years after three years [42]. While ART has a positive impact on TB risk at an individual level, its future impact on TB control is less clear [50]. The observed rate of TB in patients receiving ART for three years is still four to seven times higher than in HIV-negative individuals living in the same communities. With increased survival as a result of effective ART programmes, the numbers of individuals at increased susceptibility for TB in South African communities will continue to increase and will pose a future challenge to the TB control programme.

Side effects

The South African ART roll-out plan utilizes a public health approach using an initial scheduled regimen of d4T, 3TC and an a NNRTI, followed by a second regimen of ZDV, ddI and LPV/r (LPV/RTV). There has been an increased awareness of serious metabolic complications associated with the first-line regimen, and calls have been made to substitute the nucleotide reverse transcriptase inhibitor (NtRTI) tenofovir (TDF) with d4T.

Two ART pilot programmes [25,26] were launched in the Western Cape in 2002 and represent the longest experience of public health system use of ART. Virologic suppression rates were high, and analysis of regimen switches in this cohort (n=2679) shows that 70% of patients remained on their first-line therapy at three years (Figure 18.3). Time-dependent analyses of switches from

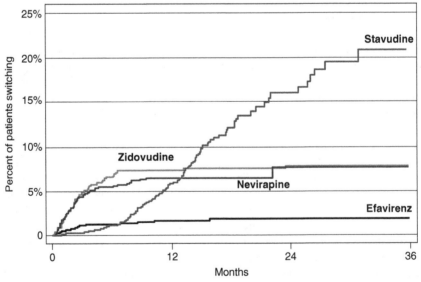

Fig. 18.3 A Kaplan-Meier estimate of time to first switch, from stavudine, zidovudine, nevirapine or efavirenz, within first-line antiretroviral therapy. Data combined from two public sector antiretroviral treatment programmes in Cape Town, South Africa.

initial NRTIs demonstrate an approximate 7% switching from ZDV in the first six months, which was CD4+ cell count-dependent. Although initially well tolerated, there was an increasing switching rate from d4T due to toxicity and intolerance after the first six months of therapy, predominantly due to lipodystrophy, peripheral neuropathy and symptomatic hyperlactataemia, with peripheral neuropathy presenting earlier in treatment than lipodystrophy. Symptomatic hyperlactataemia occurred most frequently in African females with high body mass indices, at a rate of 175 per 1000 patient-years. Early switching was greater from NVP than EFV, but there were few toxicity switches of these drugs after six months. At present, there are a limited number of NRTI options for the public sector, as TDF is not registered for use in South Africa, and abacavir (ABC) use has been restricted due to its high cost relative to other NRTI options. These toxicity profiles, therefore, have major implications for both the initial choice of regimens and costing for both antiretroviral drugs and programme safety monitoring.

HIV and hepatitis B and C co-infections

Chronic hepatitis B virus (HBV) infection predisposes to hepatoma, hepatic cirrhosis and increased drug toxicities. It is estimated that there are approximately 50 million HBV carriers in sub-Saharan Africa, and that 2.5 million of these reside in South Africa. Seroprevalence studies have demonstrated that the overall HBsAg carrier rate is 9%; however, there is a marked difference in prevalence between urban and rural settings [51]. The carrier rate can be as high as 15% in rural areas and 1% or less in urban areas. [52].

The transmission of HBV in Africa is predominantly horizontal, by pathways that are not clearly understood, and occurs during the first few years of life. It is clear, therefore, that HBV infection and its sequelae may be present for some time prior to the acquisition of the HIV infection. This is in contrast to the developed world, where the majority of HBV transmission occurs in adulthood by sexual intercourse and IVDU.

Of particular concern is that occult HBV infection can be present in HIV-infected patients. A recent study [53] showed that an increased proportion of hepatitis B surface antigen antibody positives (20.5%) in the HIV-infected compared to the HIV-uninfected (8.2%) had evidence of HBV as measured by hepatitis B DNA levels. Of added concern is that evidence of hepatitis B replication was found in hepatitis B surface antigen-negative patients. Once again this occurred with increased frequency among HIV-positive subjects (22.1% versus 2.4%). Additionally, 33.3% of sera with isolated hepatitis B core antibody positivity were viraemic in the HIV-positive group compared to 0% in the HIV-negative group.

The interaction between these viral pathogens has a number of far-reaching implications, including: alteration of the natural history of both viral diseases; potential for increasing the risk of hepatotoxicity of antiretroviral and other drugs; possible influence on the choice of drug regimens, which has cost implications (e.g. TDF); potential for immune reconstitution disease on commencing ART; and screening of patients for chronic HBV infection at baseline before commencing ART.

Hepatitis C virus (HCV) infection is less prevalent in South Africa than in many industrialized settings, and IVDU is not currently a common HIV acquisition risk behaviour. In a retrospective analysis of samples from a large multinational ART study performed in 1996, HIV/HCV co-infection was highest (48.6%) in Italy and lowest (1.9%) in South Africa [54]. HCV genotype 5 is the prevalent genotype in South Africa [55]. This genotype has been reported to be an 'easy to treat' virus with response rates similar to those of genotypes 2 and 3. However, availability of HBV- and HCV-specific therapies is limited to only a few research centres located in tertiary institutions within the country's larger metropolitan areas.

The presence of significant numbers of patients with chronic viral hepatitis adds a further complexity to the public health approach to HIV management, particularly in a population using d4T, 3TC and an NNRTI as first-line treatment, together with high rates of TB necessitating frequent use of potentially hepatotoxic antituberculous therapy.

Economics

The cost of antiretroviral drugs in South Africa has decreased markedly over the last 10 years, and these price reductions have been fundamental to the increased access to ART in both the public and private health sectors (see Figures 18.1 and 18.2). Private sector medical aid schemes conducted cost-per-patient/by-disease analyses, which showed as early as 2001 that the use of ART could avoid the high costs of hospitalization associated with OI treatment. Since 2001, HIV disease management organizations have subsequently become responsible for an increasing proportion of private sector HIV care [4].

Macroeconomic studies have projected highly variable impacts of AIDS on South African per capita income, but they have uniformly predicted a negative impact on GDP growth, due to decreased productivity resulting from employee illness and death [56–58]. Unemployment in South Africa is high, and the initiation of ART programmes in the larger South African corporations, many of which are dependent on relatively low-skilled labour, was due to social, trade union and shareholder pressures rather than economic cost-effectiveness studies. Significant improvements in absenteeism and productivity have, however, been reported in the mining industry following ART programme initiation [30].

Prior to 2003, there were few published cost-benefit analyses of ART from resource-poor settings on which to base public sector policy [59], and government policy was strongly influenced by a modelled economic evaluation conducted in 2000 [11] that concluded ART was unaffordable [15]. By 2002, the cost of first-line therapy registered in South Africa had declined by 50% (Figure 18.2), and generic formulations were available in other countries at less than 10% of South African costs in 2000 [16]. The feasibility of a national ART programme using different coverage scenarios was therefore explored again [11]. Modelled estimates for 2010 expenditure were US$1 billion for HIV care without ART and US$2 billion for a programme scenario with 50% ART coverage. The national ART programme has been linked to considerable increases in central government budget allocation; the HIV and AIDS budget allocation in 2005/6 had increased to US$0.5 billion from US$5 million in 1994 [12].

Subsequent South African cost-effectiveness studies have shown that even in the public sector, ART is a cost-effective intervention, although the incremental cost-effectiveness ratios are very sensitive to drug costs and to the clinical stage or CD4 count at which therapy is initiated [60,61].

Healthcare delivery

South Africa's health system consists of a large, underfunded public sector and a smaller, well-funded private sector. The state provides approximately 40% of healthcare expenditure in order to deliver services to 80% of the population in the public sector. The private sector meets the needs of the remaining 20% of the population. Private sector medical scheme membership has remained stable at 7 million beneficiaries since 1996, despite population growth of 4 million over the period to a present population of 45 million, thus increasing the proportion of the population dependent on the state sector. The Medical Schemes Act (1998) came into effect on 1 January 2000 with the express aim of reversing this increasing inequality. It promoted more equitable access to healthcare resources and legislated against discrimination against the aged and chronically ill by either 'risk rating' or denial of membership. The Act has also expanded the prescribed minimum scheme benefits to include treatment of chronic medical conditions including HIV infection [2,31]. Membership in medical aid schemes can no longer be denied to individuals on the basis of an HIV-positive diagnosis.

The majority of doctors and pharmacists in South Africa are employed in the private sector. In the public sector, community care nurses deliver most of the primary care medical services, especially in rural areas, using a limited range of medication that is included in a national essential drug list. In contrast, the model of HIV care in the private sector has been based on the individual practitioner, usually a doctor, selecting a patient's treatment and medication. However, ART is expensive and individual difficulties in making payment for ART have led to suboptimal treatment of many patients. Medical insurance schemes have therefore increasingly contracted HIV care to specialized disease management programmes, which have developed limited treatment algorithms and give telephone support to individual doctors. The SAHIVS has developed guidelines for initiation and monitoring of ART for independent private practitioners. Drug procurement and distribution in the private sector is via a sophisticated network of community pharmacies, each with online ordering and stock control facilities.

The operational difficulty of delivering ART rapidly to large numbers of individuals in a variety of geographical settings within an underfunded and understaffed public health sector has resulted in a failure to reach the treatment targets outlined in the national treatment plan [12]. Each of the stages of the patient management cycle — drug selection, procurement, delivery, and use — has been confronted with a variety of different challenges. The WHO's 2002 guidelines for ART delivery in resource-limited settings were used for the initial selection of recommended regimens [33]. However, drug selection has been made in the absence of data on: efficacy in similar settings; effect of regimen choice on emergence of resistant viruses; and the intensity of laboratory monitoring necessary to avoid treatment complications. Antiretroviral drug procurement has been made in the absence of any historical record of drug consumption, and needs estimates have been based on a combination of modelled population HIV prevalence and an estimate of the proportion qualifying for therapy. Although centralized procurement was entertained in the first year in order to monitor uptake of ART [11], a decentralized procurement policy at provincial level has been used to date, resulting in a lack of accurate national reporting of numbers on treatment. Drug distribution in the public sector utilizes provincial depots, which are subject to thefts and stock-outs, and most of which are equipped with only basic inventory systems. Finally, appropriate use of ART requires standardized protocols, training and retention of medical staff. A national standardized protocol was developed in 2003 [19]; however, there has been no national training programme in the use and implementation of the protocol.

Staff retention has been a major constraint to ART programmes, which have required an expansion of service delivery due to pre-existing national shortages of physicians, nurses and pharmacists [25, 35]. These shortages of medical personnel have been exacerbated by competition from both the private sector and the 'brain drain' of medical professionals to Europe and other developed countries. The magnitude of the challenge to provide ART to over a million South Africans within the present human resource constraints will require an innovative harnessing of both public and private sector resources.

Summary

The HIV pandemic reached South Africa later than its neighbouring countries in Central and Southern Africa. The South African epidemic developed rapidly in a country undergoing political upheaval and unprepared for the HIV onslaught. Over the last decade, treatment efforts have consistently lagged far behind the needs of the HIV-infected population. In the early era of

HAART, from 1996–2000, access to therapy was limited to the wealthy and those who could access a few research studies. From 2000 to 2003, community pilot projects in the public sector and managed care programmes in the private sector extended access somewhat and did serve to show that ART was a feasible, effective and affordable healthcare intervention. The period since 2004 has seen the development of ambitious plans to develop the world's largest ART programme, but both logistical constraints and poor political leadership have hampered those plans. The medical system has failed those 2 million South Africans who have already succumbed to their illness, but the challenge remains to address the treatment needs of the 5 million HIV-infected in South Africa today.

References

1. United Nations Development Programme (UNDP). (2006). *UNDP Human Development Reports, South Africa. UNDP.* Available at http://hdr.undp.org/hdr2006/statistics/countries/default.cfm (accessed 12/03/2007).

2. van Harmelen J, Wood R, Lambrick M, Rybicki EP, Williamson A-L, Williamson C. (1997). An association between HIV-1 subtype and mode of transmission in Cape Town, South Africa. *AIDS* **11**:81–88.

3. van Harmelen J, van der Ryst E, Loubser AS, *et al.* (1999). A predominantly HIV Type 1 Subtype C-Restricted Epidemic in South African Urban Population. *AIDS Research and Human Retroviruses* **15**:395–8.

4. Republic of South Africa. (2006). *Progress-report on declaration of commitment on HIV and AIDS, March 2006 United Nations General Assembly Special Session on HIV and AIDS.* Available at http://www.doh.gov.za/docs/reports/2006/ungass/index.html (accessed August 2006).

5. The Joint United Nations Programme on HIV/AIDS (UNAIDS). (2006). *Report on the Global AIDS epidemic. A UNAIDS 10th anniversary special edition.* Geneva: UNAIDS. Available at http://www.unaids.org/en/hiv_data/2006GlobalReport/default.asp (accessed 28 August 2006).

6. Dorrington RE, Bradshaw D, Johnson L, Budlender D. (2004). *The demographic impact of HIV/AIDS in South Africa. National indicators for 2004.* Cape Town: Centre for Actuarial Research Unit, South African Medical Research Council and Actuarial Society of South Africa.

7. Government of South Africa. (2001). *National press club luncheon with South African President Thabo Mbeki, 27 June 2001.* Pretoria: Government of South Africa. Available at http://www.info.gov.za/speeches/2001/010716245p1002.htm (accessed 28 August 2006).

8. Government of South Africa. (2000). *Press briefing by Minister of Health, 10 July 2000.* Pretoria: Government of South Africa. Available at http://www.info.gov.za/speaches/2000/000720110p1002.htm (accessed 28 August 2006).

9. Government of South Africa. (1999). *Address to the National Council of Provinces, Cape Town 28 October 1999.* Pretoria: Government of South Africa. Available at http://www.dfa.gov.za/docs/speeches/1999/mbek1028.htm (accessed 28 August 2006).

10. Sidley P. (1997). Miracle AIDS cure hits the South African press. *BMJ* **314**:450.

11. Government of South Africa, Ministry of Health. (2003). *Full report of the joint health and treasury task team charged with examining treatment options to supplement comprehensive care for HIV/AIDS in the public sector. 8 August 2003.* Pretoria: Government of South Africa. Available at http://www.info.gov.za (accessed 28 August 2006).

12. Government of South Africa. (2000). *HIV/AIDS/STD strategic plan for South Africa 2000–2005.* Pretoria: Government of South Africa. Available at http://www.info.gov.za/otherdocs/2000/aidsplan2000.pdf (accessed 28 August 2006).

13. Government of South Africa. (2002). *Summary of Government's position on HIV/AIDS. 17 April 2002.* Pretoria: Government of South Africa. Available at http://www.info.gov.za/issues/hiv/govposition02.htm (accessed 28 August 2006).

14. Government of South Africa. (2002). *Update on Cabinet's statement of 17th April 2002 on fighting HIV/AIDS*. Available at http://www.info.gov.za/issues/hiv/updateoct02.htm (accessed 28 August 2006).

15. Abt Associates. (2000). *HIV facts, figures and the future: South African Health Review 2000*. Cambridge, Massachussetts: Abt Associates Inc. Available at http://www.hst.org.za/sahr/2000/chapter15.htm.

16. Boule A, Kenyon C, J Skordis, Wood R. (2002). Exploring of the costs of a limited public sector antiretroviral treatment program in South Africa. *S Afr Med J* **92**:811–817.

17. Government of South Africa. (2003). *Statement by the Minister of Health, Dr ME Tshabalala-Msimang, on the establishment of a national task team to develop a detailed operational plan for an antiretroviral treatment programme for South Africa, 20th August 2003*. Pretoria: Government of South Africa. Available at http://www.info.gov.za/speaches/2003/03082209331015.htm (accessed 28August 2006).

18. Government of South Africa. (2003). *Operational plan for comprehensive HIV and AIDS care, management and treatment for South Africa*. Pretoria: Government of South Africa. Available at http://www.info.gov.za/issues/hiv/careplan.htm (accessed 28August 2006).

19. Government of South Africa, National Department of Health. (2004). *National antiretroviral treatment guidelines*. Pretoria: Government of South Africa. Available at http://www.doh.gov.za (accessed 28 August 2006).

20. Government of South Africa. (2005). *Implementation of the comprehensive plan on prevention, treatment and care of HIV and AIDS: Fact sheet*. Pretoria: Government of South Africa. Available at http://www.info.gov.za/issues/hiv/implementation2006.htm (accessed 28 August 2006).

21. CAESAR coordinating committee. (1997). Randomised trial of addition of lamivudine or lamivudine plus loviride to zidovudine-containing regimens for patients with HIV-1 infection: the CAESAR trial. *Lancet* **349**:1413–21.

22. Wood R. (2000). Sustained efficacy of Nevirapine (NVP) in combination with two nucleosides in advanced, treatment-naïve HIV infected patients with high viral load. A BI 1090 sub-study. XIII International Conference on AIDS, July 2000, Durban, South Africa. [Abstr WeOrB607]

23. Blanckenberg DH, Wood R, Horban A, *et al*. (2004). Compact Highly Active Antiretroviral Medication Study. Evaluation of nevirapine and/or hydroxyurea with nucleoside reverse transcriptase inhibitors in treatment-naïve HIV-1 infected subjects. *AIDS* **18**:631–640.

24. van Leth F, Phanuphak P, Ruxrungtham K, Baraldi E, *et al*. (2004). The 2NN Study: Comparison of first-line antiretroviral therapy with regimens including nevirapine, efavirenz or both drugs combined, together with stavudine and lamivudine: A randomised open-label trial, the 2NN Study. *Lancet* **363**:1248–50.

25. Bekker L-G, Orrell C, Reader L, *et al*. (2003). Antiretroviral Therapy in A Community Clinic: Early Lessons from a Pilot Project. *S Afr Med J* **93**:458–462.

26. Coetzee D, Hildebrand K, Boulle A, *et al*. (2004). Outcomes after two years of providing antiretroviral treatment in Khayelitsha, South Africa. *AIDS* **18**:887–95.

27. McCleod HD, Achmat Z, Stein AM. (2003). Minimum benefits for HIV/AIDS in South African Medical Schemes. *South African Actuarial Journal* **3**:77–112.

28. AIDS Law Project. (2006). *Resolutions of the 7th meeting of the Joint Civil Society Monitoring Forum*. Braamfontein, South Africa: AIDS Law Project. Available at http://www.alp.org (accessed 28 August 2006).

29. d'Adesky A-C. (2003). *Global AIDS – The private sector starts to take notice*. Available at http://www.healthgap.org/press_releases/a03/013003_AmfAR_MNC_HGAP.html (accessed 12 March 2007).

30. Charalambous S, Grant AD, Day JH, *et al*. (2007). Establishing a workplace antiretroviral therapy programme in South Africa. *AIDS Care* **19(1)**:34–41.

31. Health Systems Trust. (2002). *South African Health Review 2002*. Durban: Health Systems Trust. Available at http://www.hst.org.za (accessed 28August 2006).

32. Health Systems Trust. (2004). *South African Health Review 2003/4*. Durban: Health Systems Trust. Available at http://www.hst.org.za (accessed 28 August 2006).

33. World Health Organization (WHO). (2002). *Scaling up antiretroviral therapy in resource-limited settings. Treatment guidelines for a public health approach.* Geneva: WHO.

34. Janossy G, Jani IV, Bradley NJ, *et al.* (2002). Affordable CD4(+)-T-cell counting by flow cytometry: CD45 gating for volumetric analysis. *Clin Diagn Lab Immunol* **9**:1085–94.

35. Bekker L-G, Myer L, Orrell C, Wood R. (2006). A South African Community-based Antiretroviral program: Outcomes during 3 years of Scale-up. *S Afr Med J* **96**:315–320.

36. Gordon M, De Oliveira T, Bishop K, *et al.* (2003). Molecular characteristics of human immunodeficiency virus type-1 subtype C virus from KwaZulu-Natal, South Africa: Implications for vaccine and antiretroviral control strategies. *J Virol* **77**:2587–2599.

37. Orrell C, Harling G, Lawn SD, *et al.* (2007). Conservation of first line antiretroviral treatment regimen where therapeutic options are limited. *Antiviral Therapy* **12**:83–88.

38. Fielding KL, Charalambous S, Pemba L, *et al.* 12-month outcomes in a work-based antiretroviral therapy programme in South Africa. (Manuscript in preparation).

39. Lawn SD, Myer L, Orrel C, Bekker L-G, Wood R. (2005). Early mortality among patients accessing a community-based antiretroviral service in South Africa: Implications for program design. *AIDS* **19**:2141–2148.

40. Lawn SD, Myer L, Harling G, Orrell C, Bekker L-G, Wood R. (2006). Determinants of mortality and non-death losses from an antiretroviral treatment service in South Africa: implications for program evaluation. *Clin Inf Dis* **43**:770–776.

41. Holmes CB, Wood R, Badri M, *et al.* (2006). CD4 decline and incidence of opportunistic infections in Cape Town, South Africa. Implications for prophylaxis and treatment. *JAIDS* **42**:464–469.

42. Lawn SD, Badri M, Wood R. (2005). Tuberculosis among HIV-infected patients receiving HAART: long term incidence and risk factors in a South African cohort. *AIDS* **19**:2109–2116.

43. Lawn SD, Bekker L-G, Middelcoup K, Myer L, Wood R. (2006). Impact of HIV on age-specific tuberculosis notification rates in a peri-urban community in South Africa. *Clin Inf Dis* **42**:1040–1047.

44. World Health Organization. (2005). *WHO declares TB an emergency in Africa. Call for "urgent and extraordinary actions" to halt a worsening epidemic.* Geneva: WHO. Available at http://www.who.int/mediacentre/news/2005/africa_emergency/en/ (accessed 06/09/2005).

45. Health Systems Trust. (2005). *Cape Town TB Control: Progress report 1997–2003.* Cape Town: Health Systems Trust. Available at www.hst.org.za

46. Wood R, Middelkoop K, Myer L, *et al.* (2006). The burden of undiagnosed tuberculosis in an African community with high HIV-prevalence: implications for TB control. *Am J Resp Crit Care Med* (Epub, 14 September 2006).

47. World Health Organization, IUATB Global Project on Anti-Tuberculosis Drug Resistance Surveillance. (2004). *Anti-tuberculosis drug resistance in the world: third global report.* Geneva: World Health Organization.

48. Gandhi NR, Moll A, Sturm AW, *et al.* (2006). Extensively drug-resistant tuberculosis as a cause of death in patients co-infected with tuberculosis and HIV in a rural area of South Africa. *Lancet* **368**:1575–1580.

49. Badri M, Wilson D, Wood R. (2002). Effect of highly active antiretroviral therapy on incidence of tuberculosis in South Africa: a cohort study. *Lancet* **15**:2059–2064.

50. Williams B, Dye C. (2003). Antiretroviral drugs for tuberculosis control in the era of HIV/AIDS. *Science* **301**:1535–1537.

51. Kiire CF. (1996). The epidemiology and prophylaxis of hepatitis B in sub-Saharan Africa: a view from tropical and subtropical Africa. *Gut* **38**(Suppl 2):S5–12.

52. Kew MC. (1996). Progress towards the comprehensive control of hepatitis B in Africa: a view from South Africa. *Gut* **38**(Suppl 2):S31–36.

53. Mphahlele MJ, Lukhwareni A, Burnett RJ, *et al.* (2006). High risk of occult hepatitis B infection in HIV-positive patients from South Africa. *J Clin Virol* **35**:14–20.

54. Amin J, Kaye M, Skidmore S, Pillay D Cooper DA, Dore GJ. (2004). HIV and hepatitis C co-infection within the CAESAR study. *HIV Med* **5**:174–9.

55. Nguyen MH, Keefe EB. (2005). Prevalence and treatment of hepatitis C virus genotypes 4, 5 and 6. *Clin Gastroenterol Hepatol* **3**(10 Supp12):S97-S101.

56. Quattek K. (2000). *The economic impact of AIDS in South Africa: A dark cloud on the horizon.* Johannesburg, South Africa: Konrad Adenaur Stiftung (KAS). Available at http://www.kas.org.za/Publications/ (accessed 29August 2006).

57. Arndt C, Lewis J. (2001). The HIV/AIDS pandemic in South Africa. Sectoral impacts and unemployment. *Journal of International Development* **13**:427–449.

58. Bell C, Devarajan S, Gersbach H. (2003) *The long run economic costs of AIDS: Theory and an application to South Africa.* Available at http://www1.worldbank.org/hiv_aids/docs/BeDeGe_BP_total2.pdf (accessed 29 August 2006).

59. Harling G, Wood R, Beck EJ. (2005). Review of the efficiency of interventions in HIV infection: 1994–2004. *Disease Management & Health Outcomes* **13**:71–94.

60. Badri M, Mandalia S, Maartens G, *et al.* (2006). Cost-effectiveness of highly active antiretroviral therapy in South Africa. *PLoS Med* **3**(1):e4.

61. Badri M, Cleary S, Maartens G, *et al.* (2006). When to initiate HAART in sub-Saharan Africa: a cost-effectiveness study. *Antiviral Therapy* **11**:63–72.

Chapter 19

Country review: Thailand

Praphan Phanuphak*, Sanchai Chasombat and
Jintanat Ananworanich

Thailand and the HIV Epidemic

Thailand is the size of France in geographical and population terms. In 2006, its population was
estimated to be approximately 64 million, and its gross national income (GNI) was US$8,020 per
capita [1]. Thailand is considered a medium-income or medium human development country.

The first cases of AIDS in Thailand were documented in 1984–5 [2,3]. The epidemic initially
appeared in men who have sex with men (MSM), then spread to injection drug users (IDUs),
female sex workers, clients of female sex workers and, finally, into the heterosexual population
and newborns [4]. There were an estimated 580,000 people living with HIV/AIDS (PLWHA)
in Thailand in 2006, with a similar number having already died since the beginning of the
epidemic [1]. Up to 90% of infected individuals acquired HIV through heterosexual transmission.
HIV prevalence among pregnant women at present is between 1.3% and 1.4%. The current rate
of new infection is 16,000–18,000 per year, with about 21,000 HIV-related deaths per year [1].

In terms of paediatric HIV infection, a total of 50,620 Thai children were diagnosed with HIV
infection between 1988 and 2005, only 20,000 of whom are still living [5]. The HIV epidemic in
Thai children has changed drastically in recent years, primarily for two reasons. First, in 1998 the
Ministry of Public Health (MOPH) initiated a nationwide programme for the prevention of
mother-to-child transmission (PMTCT) of HIV using voluntary counselling and testing (VCT),
antiretroviral therapy (ART) and the provision of infant formula. The transmission risk
to infants decreased from 18% without any intervention, to 8% with zidovudine (ZDV) (or azidothymidine (AZT)) monotherapy, and to 5% with AZT monotherapy and single-dose nevirapine (NVP) [6,7]. The number of newly infected babies declined from over 1000 in 1997 to fewer
than 300 in 2005. Second, the production of a generic triple-drug formulation by Thailand's
Government Pharmaceutical Organization (GPO), which began in 2002 and enabled the government to offer highly active antiretroviral therapy (HAART) to all children, resulted in a significant decrease in child mortality and morbidity. As of June 2006, there were over 6000 children
receiving ART within the government programme, and it is estimated that another 1500 children
are receiving care in the private sector. There is, however, a worrying increase in new cases being
reported among 15–19 year-olds; these new infections are more common in teenage girls than
boys. Thai teenagers commonly begin having sexual intercourse at age 14, and less than 20%
report using condoms [8].

The MOPH responded to the HIV epidemic relatively early, starting with serosurveillance of
high-risk groups, followed by targeted as well as broad educational campaigns. The well known,
nationwide campaign on condom use among sex workers was launched in 1991–2, resulting in

* Corresponding author.

an impressive decrease in sexually transmitted diseases (STDs) and HIV prevalence in all risk groups except IDUs since 1996 [9,10]. HIV prevalence among IDUs has not decreased over time, remaining at around 35–40% [11]. However, it is alarming to note that HIV prevalence among MSM in Thailand has increased rapidly in recent years. The 2003 survey of MSM in Bangkok who were not sex workers showed an HIV prevalence of 18% [12], which then increased to 28% in 2005 [13]. In addition, it has been observed that STDs have been steadily rising recently. This may signal an impending second wave of the HIV epidemic in Thailand.

Thailand has relatively good healthcare infrastructure. Healthcare workers are well trained, and district hospitals are well equipped, although the overall health expenditure, only US$80 per capita (about 4% of gross domestic product (GDP)) in 2004, is not very high [1]. HIV counselling and testing, as well as treatment and prevention of opportunistic infections (OIs), can be done at district hospital level. All of the early antiretroviral drugs were registered in Thailand within 12 months of their registration in the United States. All patients are required to be tested for CD4 count before ART is started. Initially, CD4 counts were done manually using fluorescent microscopes, but this was later replaced by flow cytometry. Facilities for CD4 determination were gradually expanded, partly through support from the Global Fund to Fight AIDS, Malaria and Tuberculosis (Global Fund). At present, almost all of the 75 provincial hospitals in Thailand have a flow cytometer, and district hospitals are well connected with the provincial hospital for CD4 testing services.

Early use of antiretrovirals in Thailand

Although the first antiretroviral drug, AZT, was registered in Thailand in 1988, its initial use was limited mainly to university hospitals and to private hospitals where patients could pay for the drugs. The MOPH began providing free AZT to Thai patients in 1992 (Table 19.1). The programme started with 150 patients, increasing to 4200 patients by 1995. However, the AZT monotherapy programme was later judged ineffective by an evaluation team from the World Health Organization (WHO) due to the lack of long-term benefit and a high rate of loss to

Table 19.1 Antiretroviral therapy provided by the Thai Government treatment programmes

Year	Regimens	Data
1992	AZT monotherapy	4200 Thais received this regimen by year 1995 when the programme was stopped due to lack of long-term benefit and a high rate of loss to follow-up and death [14]
1995	AZT/ddI or AZT/ddC	1500 Thais received these regimens as part of a comparative network trial of 58 hospitals up to year 2000 [15]
2000	Triple-drug combinations with 2 NRTIs and one NNRTI or one PI	The triple-ART was used in selected centres as a way for clinicians to gain experience [48]
2003	Generic d4T/3TC/NVP fixed-dose combination (GPO-virS)	Provided free of charge nationwide. As of August 2006, a total of 103,861 patients had entered the programme, 6118 of whom were children [52]
2007	Both GPO-virS and GPO-virZ (AZT/3TC/NVP)	It is expected that first-line HAART in Thailand will soon be changed to GPO-VirZ in accordance with the 2006 WHO Guidelines [25]

Sources: [14,15,25,48,52].

follow-up and death [14]. As a result, in 1995, the government's budget allocation for antiretroviral drugs was shifted to a 1500-patient comparative trial of AZT/ddI (didanosine) and AZT/ddC (zalcitabine) among several government hospitals. Such a research-based programme was intended to strengthen the infrastructure of government and university hospitals for AIDS care through the HIV/AIDS Clinical Research Network (CRN) [15]. Participation in the CRN increased from 45 hospitals in 1996 to 58 hospitals in 1999. In 2000, this government funding was reallocated to buy triple-drug combinations as a way for Thai doctors to gain some experience with HAART. The widespread use of HAART in Thailand began in 2002, when triple-drug therapy became available at a low price due to the local production of generic drug formulations.

Early use of HAART in Thailand

HAART was first used in Thailand around 1997–8, when protease inhibitors (PIs) were registered in the country. These new and potent antiretroviral drugs were primarily used as rescue or second-line therapy for those whose pre-existing antiretroviral regimens had failed. By that time, many high- and middle-income Thai patients had already been treated for several years with AZT or ddI monotherapy, or with AZT/ddI and AZT/ddC, and many of these regimens had already failed. Lamivudine (3TC) and stavudine (d4T) became available later on, but were mainly used as substitutes for failing AZT/ddI or AZT/ddC regimens. As a consequence, when a PI was added to construct a three-drug combination, the regimen was more or less PI monotherapy. Thanks to the high potency of the early PIs, most patients showed dramatic clinical and immunologic improvement when PIs were added to the double nucleoside combination. The choice of which dual NRTIs to add to the PI was usually made by an experienced physician based on a patient's history with NRTIs.

The early PIs (saquinavir (SQV), indinavir (IDV) and ritonavir (RTV)) were registered in Thailand in 1997–8, while the non-nucleoside reverse transcriptase inhibitors (NNRTIs) (NVP and efavirenz (EFV)) were not registered until 1999. Largely because of the more aggressive marketing strategy of the PI-manufacturing companies (Roche Laboratories, Merck & Co. and Abbott Laboratories) in Thailand, PIs were preferred over NNRTIs as the third component of the triple-drug regimen in the early years of HAART in the country. A compassionate access programme was established by certain PI manufacturers, and some PI drugs were offered to physicians as 'professional samples' with which to treat HIV patients. As a result, many unskilled practitioners prescribed the free PI samples to their patients as 'PI monotherapy'. In addition, when the supply of these free PIs ran out, many patients went back to their original, failing double NRTI regimen since they could not afford the price of the PIs. Eventually, some pharmaceutical companies offered their PIs at half price so that patients could continue to use them. However, such offers were for a limited time only.

Viral load assays became available in Thailand in 1996, but the initial price was very high. The test was used as a marketing strategy by many PI manufacturers, who offered a free viral load test for every three or four bottles of PIs that patients bought, i.e. one every three to four months. Again, this was a limited-time offer. Nevertheless, it familiarized treating physicians in Thailand with the use of viral load technology to monitor patients' response to HAART.

All the scenarios described above demonstrate how patients, physicians and pharmaceutical companies struggled during the early years of HAART in Thailand. But while each party might have had its own agenda, the common goal was for patients to gain access to HAART.

Thai patients were extremely adherent and tolerant to early PI dosing regimens that were very difficult to take—for example, 600 mg of RTV twice daily, or 800 mg of IDV thrice daily before meals, with abundant water intake during the day—because it was the only way they could obtain the free drugs that could make them better after experiencing failure with dual NRTIs for an extended period of time.

Driving forces in the scale-up of HAART in Thailand

HAART has been provided free of charge by the MOPH nationwide since 2003 (Table 19.1). It was evident that the single most important factor driving this national policy was the availability of the generic fixed-dose combination of d4T/3TC/NVP (GPO-Vir S) at an affordable price of US$1 a day. The drug is produced by the GPO, which is a government enterprise. GPO-Vir S30 (30 mg d4T) and GPO-Vir S40 (40 mg d4T) were made available in Thailand in 2002. Prior to that, the GPO had also produced generic AZT, d4T, 3TC, AZT/3TC, NVP and ddI powder to treat patients at prices much lower than their brand name counterparts. The indirect benefit of having cheap, generic antiretroviral drugs in Thailand was to drive the price of some of their branded counterparts down even if their generic versions were not available, for example with EFV and IDV.

The next important driving force was demand and pressure from networks of PLWHA and various non-governmental organizations (NGOs) in Thailand. They began a dialogue with government officials as early as 2001, with rounds of face-to-face meetings and large-scale demonstrations that finally caught the serious attention of the government. It was fortunate that the Thai government at that time was undertaking the 'pro-people policy' as their political strategy to get support from the poor, who make up the majority of voters in Thailand. One initiative launched under this policy was the '30 Baht Scheme' for medical care, whereby patients would have to pay only 30 Baht, or about US$0.75, for each medical visit to their assigned hospitals. Therefore, it was not too surprising when the MOPH announced its intention to treat 10,000 patients with HAART in 2003. Coverage was increased to 50,000 patients in 2004 in order to boost the status of Thailand in the eyes of the international community on the occasion of Thailand's hosting the XV International AIDS Conference in Bangkok that year. Finally, HAART was included in the '30 Baht Scheme' in 2006, which theoretically meant universal coverage for HAART throughout Thailand. In practice, however, this reality will take some years to reach. Nevertheless, such a national policy serves to reflect the Thai government's strong commitment to HIV care.

There have been many other driving forces behind the scale-up of HAART in Thailand. Experiences gained by the developed world, as reported in the literature and at various international conferences, aroused the interest of Thai physicians in the use of HAART to treat their patients. The most convincing reports concerned the dramatic reduction of HIV-related morbidity and mortality following the initiation of HAART [16,17], as well as its cost-effectiveness [18]. Increasing numbers of Thai physicians have learned how to use HAART appropriately and efficiently, particularly from internationally prominent clinicians/researchers who have come to Thailand to give lectures on HAART.

Besides lectures, round-table discussions with Thai experts have been most useful, permitting practical questions to be put directly to those with the most expertise. One such educational opportunity is the Bangkok Symposium on HIV Medicine, which has been held annually since 1997 by the HIV Netherlands-Australia-Thailand Research Collaboration (HIV-NAT), an international unit of the Thai Red Cross AIDS Research Centre. Local clinical trials such as those carried out by HIV-NAT have helped convince Thai physicians of the efficacy of HAART for their patients [19–21]. Such trials also put indirect pressure on the MOPH and the Department of Disease Control, which is responsible for HIV/AIDS, to provide ART to patients outside the trials. Financial support from international donors like the Global Fund [22], and ART advocacy support from the WHO—for example, the WHO/UNAIDS '3 by 5' initiative—have also contributed to the ART scale-up in Thailand [23].

Current use of HAART in Thailand

HAART is now the standard of care in Thailand for patients put on ART. Criteria for ART initiation follow the 2003 WHO guidelines for ART delivery in resource-limited settings [24]. CD4 counts are used to guide ART initiation in Thailand, as they are widely available and not too expensive. According to the recent 2006 WHO guidelines, HAART should be started in asymptomatic patients before CD4 counts drop below 200 cells/mm^3 [25]. Whether the threshold should be below 350 cells/mm^3 or between 200–250 cells/mm^3 is a question that has not yet been settled for the country's treatment guidelines.

As mentioned above, the first-line antiretroviral regimen in the Thai treatment guidelines has been GPO-Vir S. Although 40 mg of d4T is recommended for patients weighing over 60 kg, most experts recommend a 30 mg dose in order to avoid or delay d4T-related side effects, since a lower dose of d4T has been found effective in Thai studies [26]. However, with the availability of a fixed-dose combination of AZT/3TC/NVP (GPO-Vir Z250, as it contains only 250 mg of AZT) in 2005, it is expected that first-line HAART in Thailand will soon be changed to GPO-Vir Z250 in accordance with the 2006 WHO guidelines. Nevertheless, many physicians still prefer to start with GPO-Vir S for three to six months before switching to GPO-Vir Z250 in order to avoid the early side effects of AZT in immunocompromised patients who may also need other concurrent medications.

There is no doubt that 250 mg AZT twice a day is appropriate and safe for Thai patients, as has been previously reported [27]. In fact, during the era of monotherapy and dual NRTI therapy, 200 mg twice-daily AZT was used in Thailand because the 250 mg preparation was not available. The result was satisfactory, but was not well documented until a recently published pharmacokinetic study of 200 mg twice daily AZT as part of HAART in Thai patients weighing under 60 kg, which showed plasma exposure similar to 300 mg twice a day in heavier patients [28]. This finding is important, since it supports the use of lower-dose AZT (200 mg twice a day) in patients who develop anaemia from the high-dose AZT (300 mg BID), although anaemia may still recur in a minority of those using lower-dose AZT.

Patients taking HAART through the government access programme are allowed a free CD4 count every six months to monitor treatment outcomes. Free semi-annual viral load testing is to be included in Thailand's ART package as of 2007, as well as genotypic resistance testing if indicated.

It is estimated that some 20,000 of the 100,000 patients taking HAART in Thailand in 2006 were buying the drugs using their own financial resources. These would be the more well-to-do patients, or those who had been on ART for several years and whose regimens had been modified to the point where the current government first-line regimen is unlikely to be effective. Treatment for experienced patients is not a priority for the government ART roll-out programme, as these patients are viewed by the MOPH as wealthier and more fortunate, whereas, in fact, many are strangled by debts incurred due to treatment costs. There are also patients who find it difficult to get to the health posts to which they are assigned for free medical care, including ART; the assigned hospital may be far away from where they live or work, or ART services may not be readily available there. Many patients opt to pay for their own first-line regimen, since it is relatively inexpensive, in order to avoid risks, including disclosure of their condition; this is particularly true for government or private company employees for whom reimbursement of medical costs is contingent on a physician's certificate and requires many approval steps. When second-line treatment is needed, however, it will be more difficult for these patients to continue paying for their medications out of pocket.

There are more choices of first-line regimens for those who can afford it, depending on how much the patient is prepared to pay and on the physician's preference. The regimen most preferred is AZT/3TC/EFV, since it is still relatively inexpensive and is easy to administer. Some physicians choose a ddI/3TC/EFV regimen to avoid thymidine analogue-related mitochondrial toxicity and because it only needs to be taken once a day, but this regimen is more expensive. Alternatively, some physicians may choose a PI, particularly RTV-boosted lopinavir (LPV) or atazanavir (ATV), instead of an NNRTI for their wealthier patients, in order to obtain more prolonged viral suppression. Tenofovir (TDF), which became available in 2007, is expected to have an increasing role as a component in first-line regimens, since Gilead Sciences has offered this drug to Thailand for only US$1 a day.

The response to GPO-Vir S in Thai patients has been found to be as good as the response to other regimens using brand-name drugs in developed countries [29]. These findings support the 2006 WHO recommendations to use NVP-containing ART as a first-line regimen in resource-limited settings [25], since NNRTIs are generally cheaper than PIs. For cost reasons, NVP is preferred over EFV, but EFV is made available for those who cannot tolerate NVP.

The question of when to switch regimens, as well as what to switch to, based on viral load criteria, is still controversial in Thailand. Many experts feel that the viral load cut-off level to allow for free genotypic resistance testing should be around 5,000–10,000 copies/mL instead of 1000 copies/mL, since genotypic resistance could not be identified in a significant proportion of patients with a viral load of 1000–5000 copies/mL, thus wasting resources. This recommendation is consistent with recent findings that patients with sustained low-level viraemia will not experience disease progression [30]. The only value for resistance testing in GPO-Vir S or GPO-Vir Z failure is to determine the number of nucleoside analogue mutations (NAMs) the patient's virus has developed. With early resistance testing and early switching, the NRTI class may still be recycled [31,32]. On the other hand, once AZT/d4T/3TC/NVP fails, there is almost certain to be 3TC and NNRTI resistance. Therefore, if the second-line regimen is to be TDF/abacavir(ABC)/ritonavir-boosted lopinavirLPV/r, as currently recommended in the WHO guidelines, the need for resistance testing or an early switch may not be so critical. This latter argument favours no resistance testing and late switching when immunologic failure becomes evident.

The question of which is the most cost-effective second-line regimen after failure of AZT (or d4T/3TC/NVP) is a common one among countries with limited resources, and one that cannot be answered until an exhaustive comparison of various regimens has been done. Durability, cost, long-term side effects, and future options for third-line (salvage) regimens all have to be taken into consideration. Controversy will remain until proof is evident. Some conservative experts in Thailand recommend the use of ddI/3TC/IDV/r as a second-line regimen, since it is the least expensive, while keeping the door open for future salvage regimens. Other experts recommend the use of sole double-boosted PIs, namely SQV plus LPV/r. Now that TDF has become available in Thailand at an affordable price, it remains to be seen what to combine it with in a second-line regimen. ABC and LPV/r are still very expensive, even though TDF is not.

Antiretroviral regimens for PMTCT are still controversial in Thailand. The MOPH recommends the use of 12-week AZT plus single-dose NVP by all pregnant women, followed by one-week AZT and single-dose NVP for newborns, whereas many experts are pushing for HAART for all PMTCT regimens since the country has the resources and healthcare infrastructure to support its implementation. Which regimen is most cost-effective—i.e. AZT/3TC/NVP or AZT/3TC/nelfinavir (NFV)—is still to be determined. The experience of the Thai Red Cross AIDS Research Centre revealed that, although AZT/3TC/NVP may cause higher incidence of hepatotoxicity in pregnant women with a high CD4 count, the side effects can be managed with close liver function test monitoring [33]; this view is echoed in a safety report from an African cohort study [34]. Adherence and tolerance to thrice-daily NFV may be a problem, as is its variable pharmacokinetics in pregnant women [35]. The WHO recommendation to administer one week of AZT to the newborn if the mother has received a 12-week AZT plus single-dose NVP [36] also needs to be re-examined, since many of the women receiving 12-week AZT will still have detectable viral load at delivery, and the effectiveness of one-week, post-exposure AZT prophylaxis has never been documented in either humans or animals [37,38]. One can argue that single-dose NVP added to one-week AZT may work, but proof is needed before it can be recommended in international guidelines.

ART in Thai children

Early studies suggested that Thai children not treated with ART, or treated only with AZT monotherapy, suffered a more rapid HIV disease progression than Caucasian children similarly treated. Almost half the Thai children in these studies died by age three [39–41]. Fortunately, with more experience, subsequent studies using more potent regimens in Thai children have shown good prognoses and outcomes similar to those in Western cohorts [42–44].

The Thai government's Access to Care (ATC) programme began providing free ART to a small number of children in 2000. Initially, the children were treated with dual NRTIs, mostly AZT/ddI. Dual therapy was lifesaving, and was especially effective clinically and immunologically for children who did not have AIDS and had a baseline CD4 percentage above 15% [42]. Unfortunately, this dual NRTI regimen did a poor job in maintaining HIV RNA suppression. In a cross-sectional study of 95 dual NRTI-treated Thai children with a median baseline CD4 percentage of 16% and a mean duration on dual NRTI of 3.8 years, 96.8% had resistance to at least one NRTI, and 40% had multi-NRTI resistance [45].

In 2002, the ATC programme began providing HAART with two NRTIs and one NNRTI as the first-line regimen of choice. The most commonly used regimen is GPO-vir S, which has been shown to have acceptable pharmacokinetic parameters and excellent treatment outcomes [43,46].

The Thai government's policy on HAART

Although ART has been provided free of charge by the government of Thailand since 1992, its provision actually began in the year 2000 through the ATC programme, which uses a multi-sectoral approach involving PLWHA and members of the community on the care teams [47]. The target of the ATC was set at 3000 patients, with at least the same budget allocation earmarked for the programme every year. Guidelines for the treatment and care of HIV/AIDS-infected adults and children in Thailand were developed even before the era of HAART and have been updated almost every year. These guidelines were used as a guiding principle for the ART scale-up in Thailand.

During the early phase of the ATC, when demand far exceeded supply, criteria for selecting patients who would be given priority access to HAART were developed by joint hospital-community committees established in each hospital. In general, medical criteria came first, i.e., patients with CD4 counts less than 200 cells/mm^3, or with CD4 counts less than 250 cells/mm^3 in symptomatic patients. In addition, patients had to be ART-naïve. The non-medical selection criteria included giving priority to heads of families, community leaders and non-drug users, as well as patients exhibiting a cooperative attitude. Good adherence was another important aim. Non-adherent patients without satisfactory explanations faced the threat of losing their treatment opportunity. In addition, in order to maximize the number of patients who could be treated within the fixed budget available, co-payments were introduced in parallel with the ATC for those who could afford certain drugs or diagnostic tests. The co-payment scheme was later discontinued however, since no clear benefit to patients was demonstrated; nevertheless, there was a trend toward better adherence under the co-payment scheme.

The availability of fixed-dose combination GPO-Vir S in 2002 was a great turning point for HAART scale-up in Thailand. The number of patients receiving HAART through the ATC programme increased from 1710 in 2001 to 19,551 in 2003, well above the target of 13,000 set for that year [48]. Many training sessions were given to all levels of healthcare providers, including NGOs and PLWHA, and a positive change in attitude on their part towards providing HAART could be observed during this period. Relevant policy makers were well aware of the ATC programme, which led to greater financial and political support. Key ART programme managers and NGOs were involved in several rounds of discussions that led to the policy of access for all starting in October 2003. Financial resources were secured in 2004 and have been increasing every year. However, the major portion of the budget has been spent on treatment and care, while the prevention budget has not increased.

MOPH policies on quality and comprehensive ART services

The Thai government's ART programme is called The National Access to Antiretroviral Programme for People Living With HIV/AIDS (NAPHA). The following MOPH policies regarding ART have been widely disseminated to all government health facilities:

- HAART is the standard treatment for all HIV-positive individuals with clinical indications.
- Every government hospital should be able to provide ART service packages according to MOPH guidelines.
- The healthcare facility must prepare and update core components of ART services on a regular basis.
- All patients enrolled in the programme shall receive services free of charge.
- All hospitals are required to submit relevant treatment data periodically.
- Technical support, financial support and supervision mechanisms will be made available to all healthcare facilities.

In addition to NAPHA, the Social Security Office (SSO) provides ART to all employees who are registered in the Social Security Health Care Scheme. Viral load and genotypic testing are available if indicated and are approved through a peer consultation system. Patients who fail the first-line regimen will receive second-line regimens based on a co-payment principle in which the SSO will cover up to 5,000 Baht (US$152) per month for second-line drugs [49]. In addition, the MOPH's Department of Health provides ART for PMTCT and to mothers after delivery, if needed, as well as to their husbands; this is called the CARE programme.

By the end of 2004, 58,133 patients were being treated through these three ART programmes (NAPHA, SSO and CARE). In 2005, this increased to 88,261 patients. NAPHA data from January 2000 to March 2005 revealed that 47.8% of the patients were female and the median age was 34.1 years. At baseline, 49.3% had clinical AIDS and the median CD4 count was 46 cells/mm^3. Nevirapine-based regimens constituted 90.2% of all initial regimens, whereas EFV-based regimens accounted for only 8.1%. During this follow-up period, 85.1% of patients remained on treatment, while 2.6% stopped ART, 5.4% were lost to follow-up, 6.2% died of AIDS-related complications and 0.7% died of other causes. The risk of AIDS-related death was significantly increased with lower baseline CD4 counts. Among 13,192 patients with 12 months of follow-up, 89.9% remained on the baseline regimen [50].

From NAPHA to Universal Health Care Coverage

The provision of HAART has now become the MOPH's flagship programme. The real challenge remains how to manage the programme to meet increasing need and maintain its quality. In view of demands from various sources, the MOPH finally integrated NAPHA into its popular Universal Health Care Coverage programme ('30 Baht scheme') in 2006, although there remains some concern as to how to manage NAPHA under this programme [51]. The Department of Disease Control and the National Health Security Office have jointly taken active roles in managing NAPHA under the Universal Health Care Coverage programme. Key service components of the ART package have expanded beyond just treatment, and now include:

♦ *HIV counselling and testing*: HIV testing is provided free of charge to both walk-in patients or inpatients who meet one of the following criteria: medically indicated; high-risk behaviour as evaluated by a trained counsellor; spouse of an HIV-positive individual; couple engaged to be married; individual who has been raped; post-exposure to HIV. Frequency of testing depends on the risks evaluated by healthcare providers. In addition, all children born to HIV-positive mothers are to receive DNA-polymerase chain reaction (PCR) testing through a network of PCR services run by the Department of Medical Science. It is estimated that over 8000 children a year will benefit from the test.

♦ *Provision of asymptomatic care*: Every asymptomatic HIV-positive individual benefits from a physical examination, health education and regular follow-up visits, which include biannual CD4 testing. Every province has already put a CD4 testing facility in place.

♦ *Provision of flexible first-line ART regimens*: More alternative regimens for first-line ART, such as a fixed-dose combination of AZT/3TC/NVP and TDF, are being made available to treating physicians. Antiretroviral drugs available in the hospital pharmacy may be used interchangeably among patients. Patients are allowed to have viral load testing at six and 12 months after initiation of HAART, and annually thereafter. Patients can also have genotypic resistance testing if the first-line regimen fails.

♦ *Provision of flexible second-line regimens*: A regional ART expert committee will review patients' data and make recommendations to the treating physicians in the region about the proper second-line ARV regimens; LPV/r, ATV, and TDF are included in the list of drugs for second-line regimens. Physicians may choose between NRTIs and NNRTIs available in the programme as backbone drugs, while IDV, SQV, RTV, LPV and ATV are the available choices for PIs.

♦ *Raising awareness of secondary prevention in HIV-positive individuals*: An HIV-positive individual can receive, on a voluntary basis, condoms and health education on how to live his or her life normally without spreading HIV to others.

♦ *Enhancing collaboration between healthcare providers and PLWHA*: Selected groups of PLWHA will receive financial support from the government to synergize the work of healthcare providers both inside and outside hospital.

♦ *Strengthening patients' adherence to medication and clinic visits*: Adherence strategies such as medication logbooks, visual analogue scale and pill boxes are being put in place in every hospital under the Universal Health Care Coverage programme. In addition, measures to enhance patient follow-up will also be implemented.

Other ART programmes also have to be modified to comply with the Universal Health Care Coverage programme. For example, the SSO ART programme will join NAPHA in providing coverage under the '30 Baht Scheme'. There will be no co-payment, even with costly regimens.

As of September 2006, a total of 23,373 employees had registered and received ART in 269 contracted hospitals, of which 119 were private and 150 were public facilities. The CARE programme will also be integrated into NAPHA under the '30 Baht Scheme' eventually.

The latest reported figures on NAPHA enrolment showed that, as of August 2006, a cumulative total of 103,861 patients had entered the programme, 6118 of whom were children. The monthly enrolment rate was approximately 100–200 cases. Only 82,340 patients (79.3%) remained on the treatment at that date [52].

The impact of HAART on the control of viraemia and survival

The efficacy of GPO-vir S in Thais with advanced HIV disease has been confirmed by several studies. In a cohort of 90 adults, two-thirds of whom had had previous OIs, the median baseline CD4 count and viral load were 52 cells/mm³ and 280,000 (5.4 log$_{10}$) copies/mL, respectively. At one year, over 90% had achieved either viral load <50 copies/mL or a 50% increase in their CD4 count [53]. Another study of 101 advanced HIV-positive patients indicated an 80% viral load undetectability rate below 400 copies/mL by intention-to-treat analysis and 97.6% by on-treatment analysis after six months of GPO-vir S. There was also a remarkable 100 CD4 cells/mm³ rise at six months [29]. A third study further confirmed these results when, after one year of GPO-vir S, patients with a median CD4 count of only 13 cells/mm³ and a high viral load of 363,500 copies/mL had a median CD4 count increase to 191 cells/mm³, and 64% and 82% had viral loads below 50 copies/mL by intention-to-treat and on-treatment analyses, respectively. All three studies showed similar virological suppression rates in patients with baseline viral loads below and above 100,000 copies/mL [54]. A recent study showed that the efficacy and safety of GPO-vir S did not differ in patients with baseline CD4 counts below or above 50 cells/mm³ [55].

A study of 107 children on NNRTI-based treatment, including half with GPO-vir S, showed that despite their low baseline CD4 percentage of 3% and high viral load of 5.4 log, the children had a good virologic response, with 76% having a viral load below 50 copies/mL at week 72. Similarly, the CD4 percentage rose to 21% during the same period of time [43].

With these immunologic and virologic outcomes following HAART, it is not surprising that the survival rates in Thais have improved significantly. In a large cohort of 1003 adults with HIV/tuberculosis (TB) co-infection, half of whom were treated with HAART and half not, the survival rates were significantly higher in the HAART-treated group. At one, two, and three years after TB diagnosis, the survival rates were 96%, 94%, and 88%, respectively, for the HAART group, and 44%, 19%, and 9% for the non-HAART group (p<0.001). Within the HAART-treated group, patients who delayed treatment for six months or more after TB diagnosis also had a higher mortality rate than those who were initiated on earlier treatment (p=0.018) [56]. A retrospective cohort study evaluated the survival in adults with baseline CD4 counts of less than 200 cells/mm3 and found that survival rates did not differ between those treated with Thai-produced generic versus branded NNRTI-based regimens [57]. In a cohort of 417 patients enrolled in a series of randomized trials, it was found that the HAART-treated Thai patients had a low HIV disease progression rate comparable to that of patients in developed countries [58].

In a study of 192 children with advanced HIV disease, the hospitalization rate decreased from 31% during the first six months to 2% three years after HAART. The mortality rate decreased from 6% during the first six months of HAART to less than 1% afterwards [59]. The country census showed that there are now fewer reported AIDS cases in children below 15 years of age: 74 cases in 2006 compared with 937 in 2003 and 11,161 during the early years of the epidemic.

The average age of children living with HIV has increased; almost half are now 10 years of age or older.

Challenges for large-scale ART coverage in Thailand

Many challenges lie ahead for universal access to HAART in Thailand. Continued political commitment is essential, particularly as an increasing number of treated patients require second-line therapy, which is far more expensive. The budget for HIV care will certainly continue to increase. How this will affect the HIV prevention budget remains to be seen. The level of commitment of the next Thai government is also an unknown. Treatment advocacy groups need to remain strong, and evidence must be gathered to convince policy makers that treatment and care are cost-effective, and that care and prevention are inextricably linked and of equal importance. Since such evidence will only be available if Thailand's national programme is well monitored, there is an urgent need for a substantial portion of the country's ART budget to be allocated to stringent monitoring and evaluation, preferably by one or more independent organizations.

Adherence to treatment is essential, particularly for regimens containing 3TC and NNRTIs, where a single mutation can cause a high level of drug resistance [60,61]. Several global studies have shown that adherence to ART in patients from developing countries is as good as, or better than, that in developed countries [62]. One reason for this could be that patients from developing countries have greater respect and trust in their healthcare providers. Another possible reason is that they know the value of ART because of the huge effort it requires to obtain it. Notwithstanding evidence of dropout rates as high as 50% in populations that pay for their ART services out of pocket [63], there is some concern in Thailand that free access for all, as opposed to a co-payment scheme, may actually jeopardize the level of adherence.

Good adherence to lifelong treatment of diseases such as HIV/AIDS requires close and serious attention from all members of the healthcare team. Doctors, nurses, counsellors, pharmacists, social workers and others need to emphasize the importance of adherence to their patients as often as possible. This approach has been found to be especially critical during the first two months of ART. Patients may have to come back to the clinic every week or two, and adherence is stressed at each visit by every healthcare provider they encounter. Our experience from the MTCT-Plus clinic indicates that having PLWHA working as volunteers in the clinic, as well as being accessible by telephone 24 hours a day, is of great help in enhancing adherence. Such an approach is costly and time-consuming, but it will pay off by reducing the likelihood of treatment failure.

The need for cheaper monitoring tools for ART (viral load, resistance assay) is another challenge in Thailand, as is the need for affordable second-line regimens and for human resources for scaling up ART. Doctors are limited in number and in their attitudes towards HIV/AIDS care; they are generally busy with many other patients and have rapid turnover. On the other hand, nurses have a better attitude, since they have more experience in caring for HIV-positive patients. There is therefore an urgent need in developing countries to train nurses to assist or replace doctors in busy HIV clinics. They need training that is practical and applicable to their work [64]. In addition, their legal and social status needs to be improved, since in many countries, including Thailand, nurses are not allowed to write prescriptions, when that is in fact what clinics need.

Like patients from the developed world, Thai patients, after becoming healthier with ART, may resume their original lifestyle, potentially including unprotected sex and drug use. This can result in the further spread of HIV and STDs as well as unplanned pregnancy. Continuous counselling on secondary HIV prevention, STDs and family planning is thus needed along the care continuum.

In addition, some HIV-infected couples may decide to have children, calling for appropriate counselling on child bearing and approaches for PMTCT. Intrauterine insemination for discordant couples who decide to have children is also needed in order to avoid the risk of infecting the seronegative partner.

Metabolic complications are well-known, long-term clinical challenges associated with ART [65,66]. As well as switching antiretroviral regimens, lifestyle modifications, including dietary changes and exercise, can be needed. Additionally, facilities for annual check-ups, annual cervical smears for infected women and annual rectal PAP smears for MSM need to be established with easy accessibility.

Challenges in ART treatment of Thai children

Thailand is facing many challenging issues in treating children with HIV infection. Thai researchers have responded by generating locally relevant scientific data to guide practices. These challenges, and the relevant data, are described below.

When to start ART

The appropriate time to start ART in children is unknown. Traditionally, because of limited resources and a scarcity of second-line regimens, ART has been initiated later in developing countries than in developed countries. With no cure in sight, many current guidelines from both resource-rich and resource-limited settings suggest waiting until there is evidence of advanced or severe immune suppression before initiating ART [67,68]. The 2007 Thai Ministry of Public Health Guidelines recommendations are similar to those of the WHO [68]: children with severe or advanced HIV symptoms, or with CD4 counts in the severe immunosuppression range, should start ART (CD4 percentage <25% for age <1 year, CD4 percentage <20% for ages 1–3 years, and CD4 percentage <15% for ≥3 years) [69].

An attempt has been made in Thailand to answer the question of when to start ART. HIV-NAT carried out a randomized study, HIV-NAT 010, of 43 children with mild or moderate HIV symptoms and CD4 counts in the moderate immune suppression (15–24%) range, using either immediate (CD4 percentage 15–24%) or deferred (CD4 percentage <15%) treatment with AZT/3TC/NVP. At almost three years, it was found that none of the children had disease progression or had died. Half of the deferred arm had to start ART because their CD4 percentage had dropped below 15%. The CD4 percentage was significantly lower and the HIV RNA was significantly higher in the deferred arm, but both were in the acceptable ranges (median CD4 percentage 24% and median viral load 3.2 log). Moreover, when comparing only the children on ART, the HIV RNA suppression responses and CD4 percentages were the same in both arms [70].

The PREDICT study, a follow-up study funded by the US National Institutes of Health (NIH), has the same study design as HIV-NAT 010 and will enrol 300 children in Thailand and Cambodia [71]. An important issue that will be addressed in the PREDICT study is the effect of the time of ART initiation on neurodevelopment impairment, as there is growing evidence that neurocognitive impairment may not be reversed by ART and is associated with high baseline HIV RNA and low baseline CD4 percentage [72].

Formulations

There are limited formulations of generic, liquid antiretroviral drugs, and most pills are too large for children to take. The most common regimen for children, GPO-Vir S, may deliver too little NVP in some weight bands and consequently promote the development of resistance [46,73].

The current practice of using adult antiretroviral drugs for Thai children by opening capsules or crushing pills is widely employed with good tolerability and outcome, but there are no data to support the pharmacokinetics of this practice.

Resistance and second-line treatment

Because the country is faced with growing numbers of children experiencing failure on NNRTI-based regimens, there is a need to find appropriate second-line treatments. The HIV-NAT 017 study enrolled 50 children with NRTI/NNRTI failure and treated them with double-boosted PIs—LPV/r and SQV hard gel capsules—at regular dosing. This regimen was effective in suppressing HIV RNA and increasing CD4 counts; however, the regimen was burdensome because of the large pill sizes. Furthermore, the occurrence of hyperlipidaemia in 44% of children at week 48 caused concern [74,75]. The virologic failures experienced by eight of the 50 children were mostly due to poor adherence. Fortunately, no failing children were found to have PI mutations [76].

There are few choices for second-line therapy available. Aside from LPV/r, no other RTV-boosted PI dosing is known. LPV is the drug of choice for second-line therapy because of its efficacy [77,78], but the cost is approximately US$200 per child per month and is not widely affordable. While IDV is the least expensive and most commonly used PI in Thailand, the dosing of IDV boosted with RTV in children is not known. Thai experts found that the dosing proposed in a Dutch study of IDV 400 mg/m^2 with RTV 125 mg/m^2 twice daily [79] resulted in high rates of nephrotoxicity and intolerability. A more recent study in Thai children supported the efficacy, safety and pharmacokinetics of a lower dose of 230–300 mg/m^2 IDV with RTV 100 mg twice daily [80].

Complications after ART

With the increasing use of d4T as first-line therapy and PIs as second-line therapy, the occurrence of hyperlipidaemia and lipodystrophy is becoming more common [65,66,81]. There is no treatment for these conditions in children, as no lipid-lowering agents are licensed for use in children under 12 years of age. Consequently, there is a push toward the use of AZT in first-line regimens instead of d4T; for second-line therapy, there is unfortunately no easy solution. Because the majority of children accessing ART through the ATC programme have advanced HIV disease, immune reconstitution syndrome is seen in about 20% of cases, mostly from *Mycobacterium spp.* and occurring within the first four weeks of therapy [82]. There is an effort by government as well as NGOs to encourage caregivers to seek care for children earlier and to educate caregivers and healthcare workers on this condition.

Psychosocial impacts

A large proportion of children with HIV in Thailand are reaching their teenage years and entering adulthood. As a result, issues of coping and living with HIV, which can affect children's treatment compliance, have become increasingly important. The disclosure of an HIV diagnosis to a child is an issue of particular concern. It has been found that the majority of children, even those over 10 years of age, have not been informed of their diagnosis. The most common reason for non-disclosure is the fear that the knowledge of his or her HIV-positive status might have negative psychological consequences for the child [83,84]. The caregivers are unprepared, have limited understanding about disclosure, and are willing to deceive the child [84]. There are now attempts to develop guidelines to help healthcare personnel provide support to Thai children and caregivers in disclosing an HIV diagnosis.

Many children and teenagers in Thailand lack the necessary life skills to make informed and rational choices. This might be due to the expectations of Thai society, and of their families. Thai children generally have difficulties expressing themselves, as they are taught from an early age not to disagree with or question adults, particularly their parents. Thai society values the ability to hide disagreeable feelings, and Thai teenagers may therefore have many unresolved issues that they are unable to express and deal with, which can potentially result in harmful behaviours towards themselves and others.

Conclusion

Antiretroviral therapy in any country has its own story. Knowing the background or reasoning behind the initiation of ART, how it has been scaled up, and the successes or failures faced in each country is important not only to historians, but to the policy makers of national programmes or international agencies planning large-scale ART programmes in developing countries. Lessons learned will minimize failures and enhance successes.

The story from Thailand shows that implementing a large-scale ART programme is not easy and requires many steps to achieve success. There are many stakeholders behind a successful roll-out effort, and each party performs its role on a voluntary basis rather than as a duty. Nevertheless, there are many challenges still to face in making such a programme sustainable and of enduring benefit to HIV-infected and HIV-affected individuals, and to the country as a whole.

References

1. Joint United Nations Programme on HIV/AIDS (UNAIDS). (2006). *2006 report on the global AIDS epidemic*. Geneva, Switzerland: UNAIDS. Available at http://www.unaids.org/en/hiv_data/2006global-report/default.asp

2. Phanuphak P, Locharoenkul C, Panmuang W, Wilde H. (1985). A report of three cases of AIDS in Thailand. *Asian Pacific J Allerg Immunol* **3**:195–199.

3. Limsuwan A, Kanapa S, Siristonapun Y. (1986). Acquired immune deficiency syndrome in Thailand. A report of two cases. *J Med Ass Thai* **60**:164–169.

4. Brown T, Sittitrai W, Vanichseni S, Thisyakorn U. (1994). The recent epidemiology of HIV and AIDS in Thailand. *AIDS* **8**(Suppl 2):S131–S141.

5. AIDS Cluster. Bureau of AIDS, TB and STIs Department of Diseases Control Ministry of Public Health, Thailand. Available at http://www.aidsthai.org/aidsenglish (accessed 3 October 2006).

6. Kanshana S, Simonds RJ. (2002). National programme for preventing mother-to-child HIV transmission in Thailand: successful implementation and lessons learned. *AIDS* **16**:953–959.

7. Lallemant M, Jourdain G, Le Coeur S, *et al.* (2004). Perinatal HIV Prevention Trial (Thailand). Single-dose perinatal nevirapine plus standard zidovudine to prevent mother-to-child transmission of HIV-1 in Thailand. *N Engl J Med* **351**:217–228.

8. Thato S, Charron-Prochownik D, Dorn LD, Albrecht SA, Stone CA. (2003). Predictors of Condom Use Among Adolescent Thai Vocational Students. *Journal of Nursing Scholarship* **35** (2): 157–163.

9. Hanenberg RS, Rojanapithayakorn W, Kunasol P, Sokal DC. (1994). Impact of Thailand's HIV-control programme as indicated by the decline of sexually transmitted diseases. *Lancet* **344**:243–245.

10. Punpanich W, Ungchusak K, Detels R. (2004). Thailand's response to the HIV epidemic: yesterday, today, and tomorrow. *AIDS Educ Prev* **16**:119–136.

11. Vanichseni S, Kitayaporn D, Mastro TD, *et al.* (2001).Continued high HIV-1 incidence in a vaccine trial preparatory cohort of injection drug users in Bangkok, Thailand. *AIDS* **15**:397–405.

12. Van Griensven F, Thanprasertsuk S, Jommaroeng R, *et al.* (2005). Bangkok MSM Study Group. Evidence of a previously undocumented epidemic of HIV infection among men who have sex with men in Bangkok, Thailand. *AIDS* **19**:521–526.

13. Van Griensven F, Varangrat A, Wimonsate W, *et al.* (2006). HIV prevalence among populations of men who have sex with men – Thailand, 2003 and 2005. *MMWR* **55**:844–848.

14. Kunanusont C, Phoolcharoen W, Rojanapitayakorn W. (1996). The preliminary report on formulating rational use of antiretrovirals in Thailand. In: Boonmee Sathapatayavongs, ed. *HIV/AIDS in Thailand 1996: Adults & Pediatrics.* Bangkok: Infectious Disease Association of Thailand. p82–99.

15. Kunanusont C, Phoolcharoen W, Bodaramik Y. (1999). Evolution of medical services for HIV/AIDS in Thailand. *J Med Assoc Thai* **82**:425–433.

16. Murphy EL, Collier AC, Kalish LA, *et al.* (2001). Viral Activation Transfusion Study. Highly active antiretroviral therapy decreases mortality and morbidity in patients with advanced HIV disease. *Ann Intern Med* **135**:17–26.

17. Bonnet F, Morlat P, Chene G, *et al.*, Groupe d' Epidemiologie Clinique du SIDA en Aquitaine (GECSA). (2002). Causes of death among HIV-infected patients in the era of highly active antiretroviral therapy, Bordeaux, France, 1998–1999. *HIV Med* **3**:195–199.

18. Freedberg KA, Losina E, Weinstein MC, *et al.* (2001). The cost effectiveness of combination antiretroviral therapy for HIV disease. *N Engl J Med* **344**:824–831.

19. Cardiello PG, van Heeswijk RP, Hassink EA, *et al.* (2002). Simplifying protease inhibitor therapy with once-daily dosing of saquinavir soft-gelatin capsules/ritonavir (1600/100 mg): HIV-NAT 001.3 study. *J Acquir Immune Defic Syndr* **29**:464–470.

20. Burger D, Boyd M, Duncombe C, *et al.* (2003). Pharmacokinetics and pharmacodynamics of indinavir with or without low-dose ritonavir in HIV-infected Thai patients. *J Antimicrob Chemotherapy* **51**:1231–1238.

21. Safreed-Harmon K, Cooper DA, Lange JM, Duncombe C, Phanuphak P. (2004). The HIV Netherlands Australia Thailand research collaboration: lessons from 7 years of clinical research. *AIDS* **18**:1971–1978.

22. The Global Fund to Fight AIDS, Tuberculosis and Malaria. (2005). *The Global Fund Annual Report 2005.* Geneva, Switzerland: The Global Fund. Available at http://www.theglobalfund.org/en/about/publications/annualreport2005

23. World Health Organization. (2006). *Working with countries to achieve the 3 by 5 target.* Geneva, Switzerland: WHO. Available at http://www.who.int/3by5/publications/briefs/countries/en/print.html

24. World Health Organization. (2004). *Scaling up antiretroviral therapy in resource-limited settings: Treatment guidelines for a public health approach, 2003 edition.* Geneva, Switzerland: WHO.

25. World Health Organization. (2006). *Antiretroviral therapy for HIV infection in adults and adolescents in resource-limited settings: Towards universal access, recommendations for a public health approach (2006 revision).* Geneva, Switzerland: WHO.

26. Ruxrungtham K, Kroon ED, Teeratakulpisarn S, *et al.* (2000). A randomized, dose-finding study with didanosine plus stavudine versus didanosine alone in antiviral-naïve, HIV-infected Thai patients. *AIDS* **14**:1375–1382.

27. Phanuphak P, Grayson ML, Sirivichayakul S, *et al.* (2000). A comparison of two dosing regimens of zidovudine in Thai adults with early symptomatic HIV infection. Conducting clinical HIV trials in South-East Asia. *Aust NZ J Med* **30**:11–20.

28. Cressey TR, Leenarsirimakul P, Jourdain G, Tawon Y, Sukrakanchana P, Lallemant M. (2006). Intensive pharmacokinetics of zidovudine 200 mg twice daily in HIV-1-infected patients less than 60 kg on highly active antiretroviral therapy. *J Acquir Immune Defic Syndr* **42**:386–388.

29. Anekthananon T, Ratanasuwan W, Techasathit W, Sonjai A, Suwanagool S. (2004). Safety and efficacy of a simplified fixed-dose combination of stavudine, lamivudine and nevirapine (GPO-Vir) for the treatment of advanced HIV-infected patients: a 24-week study. *J Med Assoc Thai* **87**:760–767.

30. Alatrakchi N, Duvivier C, Costagliola D, *et al.* (2005). Persistent low viral load on antiretroviral therapy is associated with T cell-mediated control of HIV replication. *AIDS* **19**:25–33.

31. Miller V, Larder BA. (2001). Mutational patterns in the HIV genome and cross-resistance following nucleoside and nucleotide analogue drug exposure. *Antivir Ther* **6**(Suppl 3):25–44.

32. Hirsch MS, Brun-Vezinet F, D'Aquila RT, *et al.* (2000). Antiretroviral drug resistance testing in adult HIV-1 infection: recommendations of an international AIDS Society-USA Panel. *JAMA* **283**:2417–2426.

33. Phanuphak N, Apornpong T, Intarasuk S, Teeratakulpisarn S, Phanuphak P. (2005). Toxicities from nevirapine in HIV-infected males and females, including pregnant females with various CD4 cell counts. 12th Conference on Retroviruses and Opportunistic Infections, 2005, Boston,USA. [Abstract 21]

34. Marazzi MC, Germano P, Liotta G, *et al.* (2006). Safety of nevirapine-containing antiretroviral triple therapy regimens to prevent vertical transmission in an African cohort of HIV-infected pregnant women. *HIV Medicine* **7**:338–344.

35. US Public Health Service. (2006). *Public Health Service Task Force recommendation for use of antiretroviral drugs in pregnant HIV-1-infected women for maternal health and interventions to reduce perinatal HIV-1 transmission in the United States*, July 6 2006 Washington DC: US Public Health Service.. Available at http://AIDSinfo,nih.gov

36. World Health Organization. (2005). *Antiretroviral drugs and the prevention of mother-to-child transmission of HIV infection in resource-limited settings. Recommendations for a public health approach (2005 revision)*. Geneva, Switzerland: WHO.

37. Jackson JB, Musoke P, Fleming T, *et al.* (2003). Intrapartum and neonatal single-dose nevirapine compared with zidovudine for prevention of mother-to-child transmission of HIV-1 in Kampala, Uganda: 18-month follow-up of the HIVNET 012 randomized trial. *Lancet* **362**:859–868.

38. Shih C-C, Kaneshima H, Rabin L, *et al.* (1991). Postexposure prophylaxis with zidovudine suppresses human immunodeficiency virus type 1 infection in SCID-hu mice in a time-dependent manner. *J Infect Dis* **163**:625–627.

39. Galli L, de Martino M, Tovo PA, Gabiano C, Zappa M. (2000). Predictive value of the HIV paediatric classification system for the long-term course of perinatally infected children. *Int J Epidemiol* **29**:573–578.

40. Chearskul S, Chotpitayasunondh T, Simonds RJ, *et al.*, The Bangkok Collaborative Perinatal HIV Transmission Study Group. (2002). Survival, disease manifestations, and early predictors of disease progression among children with perinatal human immunodeficiency virus infection in Thailand. *Pediatrics* **110**:e25.

41. Vanprapar N, Chearsakul S, Chokephaibulkit K, Phongsamart W, Lolekha R. (2002). High CD4+ T-cells percentage and/or low viral load are predictors of 1–5 years survival in HIV-1 vertically infected Thai children. *J Med Assoc Thai* **85**(Suppl 2):S690–693.

42. Chokephaibulkit K, Chearskul S, Vanprapar N, *et al.* (2002). Early initiation of antiretroviral therapy with dual nucleoside reverse transcriptase inhibitors in HIV-infected infants: A multicenter study in Bangkok. First Asian Congress of Paediatric Infectious Diseases, 10–13 November 2002, Pattaya, Thailand. [Abstract TU-FP11-B3]

43. Puthanakit T, Oberdorfer A, Akarathum N, *et al.* (2005). Efficacy of highly active antiretroviral therapy in HIV-infected children participating in Thailand's National Access to Antiretroviral Program. *Clin Infect Dis* **41**:100–107.

44. Resino S, Resino R, Bellon JM, *et al.*, Spanish Group of Pediatric Infection. (2006). Clinical Outcomes Improve with Highly Active Antiretroviral Therapy in Vertically HIV Type-1-Infected Children. *Clin Infect Dis* **43**:243–252.

45. Lolekha R, Sirivichayakul S, Siangphoe U, *et al.* (2005). Resistance to dual nucleoside reverse-transcriptase inhibitors in children infected with HIV clade A/E. *Clin Infect Dis* **40**:309–312.

46. Chokephaibulkit K, Plipat N, Cressey TR, *et al.* (2005). Pharmacokinetics of nevirapine in HIV-infected children receiving an adult fixed-dose combination of stavudine, lamivudine and nevirapine. *AIDS* **19**:1495–1499.

47. Thailand Ministry of Public Health, AIDS Division, Department of Communicable Disease Control. (2001). *Operational Guideline of Access to Care Programme in Thailand*. Bangkok, Thailand: Ministry of Public Health.

48. Chasombat S, Lertpiriyasuwat C, Thanprasertsuk S, Saubsaeng L, Lo RY. (2006). The National Access to Antiretroviral Program for PHA (NAPHA) in Thailand. *Southeast Asian J Trop Med Public Health* **37**:704–715.

49. Thai Ministry of Labour, Medical Coordination and Rehabilitation Division, Social Security Office. (2004). *Announcement of Rules and Regulations for HIV Benefits*. Nonthaburi, Thailand: Ministry of Labour.

50. Ningsanond P, Lertpiriyasuwat C, McConnell M, *et al.* (2006). Rapid expansion of the national antiretroviral treatment program in Thailand: program outcomes and patient survival, 2000–2005. XVI International AIDS Conference, August 13–18, 2006, Toronto, Canada. [Abstract THLB 0209]

51. Thailand Ministry of Public Health, Bureau of AIDS, TB and STIs, Department of Disease Control. (2005). *Study and analysis of policy and administration of integrating ART into the universal health care coverage*. Bangkok, Thailand: Thailand Ministry of Public Health.

52. Thailand Ministry of Public Health, Department of Disease Control. (2006). *Departmental Monthly Report*. Bangkok, Thailand: Thailand Ministry of Public Health.

53. Kiertiburanakul S, Khongnorasat S, Rattanasiri S, Sungkanuparph S. (2007). Efficacy of a generic fixed-dose combination of stavudine, lamivudine and nevirapine (GPO-VIR) in Thai HIV-infected patients. *J Med Assoc Thai* **90**:237–243.

54. Getahun A, Tansuphasawadikul S, Desakorn V, Dhitavat J, Pitisuttithum P. (2006). Efficacy and safety of generic fixed-dose combination of stavudine, lamivudine and nevirapine (GPO-vir) in advanced HIV infection. *J Med Assoc Thai* **89**:1472–1478.

55. Manosuthi W, Chimsuntorn S, Likanonsakul S, Sungkanuparph S. (2007). Safety and efficacy of a generic fixed-dose combination of stavudine, lamivudine and nevirapine antiretroviral therapy between HIV-infected patients with baseline CD4 <50 versus CD4 >/= 50 cells/mm³. *AIDS Res Ther* **4**:6.

56. Manosuthi W, Chottanapand S, Thongyen S, Chaovavanich A, Sungkanuparph S. (2006). Survival rate and risk factors of mortality among HIV/tuberculosis-coinfected patients with and without antiretroviral therapy. *J Acquir Immune Defic Syndr* **43**:42–46.

57. Chaovavanich A, Chottanapund S, Ausavapipit J, Adulyawat N, Ubonsai W. (2006). Survival time of AIDS patients in Bamrasnaradura Institute. *J Med Assoc Thai* **89**:1859–1863.

58. Duncombe C, Kerr SJ, Ruxrungtham K, *et al.* (2005). HIV disease progression in a patient cohort treated via a clinical research network in a resource limited setting. *AIDS* **19**:169–178.

59. Puthanakit T, Aurpibul L, Oberdorfer P, *et al.* (2007). Hospitalization and mortality among HIV-infected children after receiving highly active antiretroviral therapy. *Clin Infect Dis* **44**:599–604.

60. Schuurman R, Nijhuis M, van Leeuwen R, *et al.* (1995). Rapid changes in human immunodeficiency virus type 1 RNA load and appearance of drug-resistant virus populations in persons treated with lamivudine (3TC). *J Infect Dis* **171**:1411–1419.

61. Quiros-Roldan E, Airoldi M, Moretti F, *et al.* (2002). Genotype resistance profiles in patients failing an NNRTI-containing regimen, and modifications after stopping NNRTI therapy. *J Clin Lab Anal* **16**:76–78.

62. Ivers LC, Kendrick D, Doucette K. (2005). Efficacy of antiretroviral therapy programs in resource-poor settings: A meta-analysis of the published literature. *Clin Infect Dis* **41**:217–224.

63. Hosseinipour MC, Neuhann FH, Kanyama CC, *et al.* (2006). Lessons learned from a paying antiretroviral therapy service in the public health sector at Kamuzu Central Hospital. *Journal of the International Association of Physicians AIDS Care* **5**:103–108.

64. Teeratakulpisarn S, Phanuphak N, Phanuphak P. (2006). A training initiative to empower nurses to assist doctors in managing HIV patients in Thailand. XVI International AIDS Conference, August 13–18, 2006, Toronto, Canada. [Abstract THPE 0946]

65. Carr A. (2003). HIV lipodystrophy: risk factors, pathogenesis, diagnosis and management. *AIDS* **17**(Suppl 1):S141–S148.

66. Cherry CL, Lal L, Wesselingh SL. (2005). Mitochondrial toxicity of nucleoside analogues: mechanism, monitoring and management. *Sexual Health* **2**:1–11.

67. World Health Organization. (2006). *Antiretroviral therapy of HIV infection in infants and children in resource-limited settings, towards universal access: Recommendations for a public health approach.* Geneva: WHO. Available at http://www.who.int/hiv/mediacentre/fs_2006guidelines_paediatric/en/index.html

68. Sharland M, Blanche S, Castelli G, Ramos J, Gibb DM. (2004). PENTA guidelines for the use of anti-retroviral therapy, 2004. *HIV Med* **5**(Suppl 2):61–86.

69. Thailand Ministry of Public Health. (2007). *National guidelines for the clinical management of HIV infection in children and adult.* Bangkok: Ministry of Public Health. English version, *In press.*

70. Ananworanich J, Kosalaraksa P, Pancharoen C, *et al.* (2006). Randomized Study of Immediate versus Deferred Highly Active Antiretroviral Therapy (HAART) in children. 13th Conference on Retroviruses and Opportunistic Infections, February 5–9, 2006, Denver, USA. [Abstract 701]

71. PREDICT Study. Available at http://www.clinicaltrials.gov/ct/show/NCT00234091 (accessed November 2007).

72. Jeremy RJ, Kim S, Nozyce M, *et al.*, the Pediatric AIDS Clinical Trials Group (PACTG) 388 & 377 Study Teams. (2006). Neuropsychological functioning and viral load in stable antiretroviral therapy-experienced HIV-infected children. *Pediatrics* **115**:380–387.

73. Verweel G, Sharland M, Lyall H, *et al.* (2003). Nevirapine use in HIV-1-infected children. *AIDS* **17**:1639–1647.

74. Kosalaraksa P, Bunupuradah T, Engchanil C, *et al.*, the HIV-NAT 017 Study Team. (2006). Efficacy and Safety of Double boosted saquinavir (SQV)/lopinavir/ritonavir (LPV/r) in nucleoside pre-treated children at 48 weeks. XVI International AIDS Conference, August 13–18, 2006, Toronto, Canada. [Abstract MOPE 0201]

75. Ananworanich J, Kosalaraksa P, Hill A, *et al.*, the HIV-NAT 017 Study Team. (2005). Pharmacokinetics and 24-week efficacy/safety of dual boosted saquinavir/lopinavir/ritonavir in nucleoside-pretreated children. *Pediatr Infect Dis J* **24**:874–879.

76. Bunupuradah T, Kosalaraksa P, Engchanil C, *et al.*, The HIV-NAT 017 Study Team. (2006). Lack of PI resistance in children failing double boosted saquinavir (SQV)/ lopinavir/ ritonavir (LPV/r) combination, XVI International AIDS Conference, August 13–18, 2006, Toronto, Canada. [Abstract MOPE 0202]

77. Ramos JT, De Jose MI, Duenas J, *et al.*, The Spanish Collaborative Group on HIV Infection in Children. (2005). Safety and antiviral response at 12 months of lopinavir/ritonavir therapy in human immunodeficiency virus-1-infected children experienced with three classes of antiretrovirals. *Pediatr Infect Dis J* **24**:867–873.

78. Resino S, Bellon JM, Munoz-Fernandez MA. (2006). Antiretroviral activity and safety of lopinavir/ritonavir in protease inhibitor-experienced HIV-infected children with severe-moderate immunodeficiency. *J Antimicrob Chemother* **57**:579–582.

79. Bergshoeff AS, Fraaij PL, van Rossum AM, *et al.* (2004). Pharmacokinetics of indinavir combined with low-dose ritonavir in human immunodeficiency virus type 1-infected children. *Antimicrob Agents Chemother* **48**:1904–1907.

80. Plipat N, Cressey TR, Vanprapar N, Chokephaibulkit K. (2007). Efficacy and plasma concentrations of indinavir when boosted with ritonavir in human immunodeficiency virus-infected Thai children. *Pediatr Infect Dis J* **26**:86–88.

81. Lapphra K, Vanprapar N, Phongsamart W, Chearskul P, Chokephaibulkit K. (2005). Dyslipidemia and lipodystrophy in HIV-infected Thai children on highly active antiretroviral therapy (HAART). *J Med Assoc Thai* **88**:956–966.

82. Puthanakit T, Oberdorfer P, Akarathum N, Wannarit P, Sirisanthana T, Sirisanthana V. (2006). Immune reconstitution syndrome after highly active antiretroviral therapy in human immunodeficiency virus-infected Thai children. *Pediatr Infect Dis J* **25**:53–58.

83. Oberdorfer P, Puthanakit T, Louthrenoo O, Charnsil C, Sirisanthana V, Sirisanthana T. (2006). Disclosure of HIV/AIDS diagnosis to HIV-infected children in Thailand. *J Paediatr Child Health* **42**:283–288.

84. Apateerapong W, Pancharoen C, Eggermont L, *et al.* (2004). HIV Disclosure in children. XV International AIDS Conference, July 11–16, 2004, Bangkok, Thailand. [Abstract TuPeB 4408]

Chapter 20

Cohort studies in Brazil: Projeto Praça Onze

Mauro Schechter* and Suely Hiromi Tuboi

Introduction

The first AIDS case in Brazil was diagnosed in 1982. By 1990, the number of cases had risen to 10,000, leading the World Bank to predict that Brazil would face an estimated 1.2 million cases of HIV/AIDS within a decade. However, by the year 2000, the estimated number of HIV-infected individuals was half what had been predicted, leading the Brazilian response to its HIV epidemic to be seen as an example to other developing countries.

With a population of approximately 185 million, Brazil is the fifth most populous country in the world. Based on the estimated gross national income (GNI) per capita in 2005 of US$3,460, Brazil is at the bottom of the list of upper middle-income countries according to the World Bank classification. In 2004, based on the Human Development Index (HDI), Brazil was ranked 69th in the world, a measure of the large inequalities that exist within the country [1].

Brazil was the first developing country to provide free and universal access to antiretroviral therapy (ART) to all who need it. The Brazilian response to HIV/AIDS was based on a multi-sectoral strategy involving national and provincial governments, civil society, comprehensive prevention measures and health system enhancement. In 1991, zidovudine (ZDV) was made available on a very limited scale. In 1996, a bill was passed guaranteeing free and universal access to treatment through the public healthcare system to all HIV-infected individuals who qualify for treatment according to locally developed guidelines. In order to provide this unprecedented access to treatment, the healthcare system needed to be scaled up, and treatment guidelines needed to be developed and periodically updated. Thus, an external and independent expert advisory committee was created and given the responsibility of establishing treatment criteria. This committee was (and still is) composed of local experts who meet periodically to review the latest scientific developments in order to develop and adjust treatment guidelines accordingly. At present, approximately 180,000 patients are receiving free antiretroviral drugs from the National AIDS Program (NAP). In addition to a countrywide network of drug dispensaries based in primary care facilities, outpatient clinics and hospitals, the NAP has established networks of laboratories for viral load measuring, CD4 lymphocyte counting and genotyping, all of which are also available to all patients at no cost.

In the early 1980s, the vast majority of HIV-infected individuals were well-educated men aged 20–44, with the main transmission routes being male homosexual sex and the use of contaminated needles by injection drug users (IDUs). Over time, however, the epidemic has shifted into the general population. In 1981–6, for example, the incidence rate of AIDS was

* Corresponding author.

1.4 per 100,000 inhabitants, but for the period 1995–6, the mean annual incidence had reached 29.2 per 100,000 in men and 11.3 per 100,000 in women. At present, new HIV infections and AIDS cases are increasingly frequent in women and in individuals with fewer years of formal education, a marker for lower socio-economic status.

The HIV/AIDS mortality rate peaked in 1995, when it reached 9.7 per100,000 inhabitants. As was the case in the developed world, there was an initial precipitous drop in mortality rates immediately after the implementation of universal access to treatment, followed by a relative stability in these rates, which have remained at around 6.4 per 100,000 since 1999. The median survival time after the diagnosis of AIDS increased from five months in 1989 to nearly five years in 2002, and the occurrence of common HIV-related opportunistic infections (OIs) declined by 60–80% in the same period. According to official government estimates, from 1996 to 2004 the policy of universal access to treatment prevented 90,000 deaths, and over 600,000 AIDS-related hospital admissions were averted, resulting in savings of more than US$1.8 billion in that period.

According to official government reports, the estimated national prevalence of HIV infection among adults in 2005 was 0.6%, a rate that is similar to that in the United States and which is fairly modest when compared with other developing countries. From the beginning of the epidemic, Brazil implemented a comprehensive prevention strategy, including promotion of condom use and behavioural changes, encouraging voluntary counselling and testing, providing harm reduction programmes for IDUs, preventing mother-to-child transmission of HIV, and providing support and education programmes for people living with HIV/AIDS (PLWHA). Paramount to the success of Brazil's AIDS programme was the active involvement of civil society, balanced prevention and treatment efforts, direct and consistent messages and a practical, locally developed public health approach.

In short, Brazil has been widely praised for being the first developing country to provide free and universal access to ART, as well as for realizing from the start that prevention and treatment are inextricably intertwined. Unfortunately, Brazilian scientific output is not commensurate with its successes in treatment and prevention. In this chapter we review published data on the contribution of cohort studies to documenting the epidemiology of HIV infection in Brazil, the natural history of the disease, the role of co-infections and the effectiveness of highly active antiretroviral therapy (HAART), as well as its effect on mortality patterns.

Epidemiology and prevention studies

Men who have sex with men

The *Projeto Praça Onze* was a prospective cohort study conducted in Rio de Janeiro between 1995 and 1998 to estimate the incidence of HIV infection in high-risk seronegative men who have sex with men (MSM), and to determine whether this population would be suitable for vaccine and non-vaccine intervention studies. Inclusion criteria for the study were male gender, reported homosexual or bisexual behaviour, age 18–50 years, and either documented HIV seronegativity or a lack of previous testing for HIV infection. Subjects were excluded if they reported injection drug use, but not illicit drugs taken by other methods of administration. Subjects who were confirmed to be HIV-seronegative and met the other eligibility requirements were enrolled and asked to return every six months for repeat evaluation.

Among the 700 eligible individuals who were followed for a mean of 1.5 years, the seroincidence was 3.1 per 100 person-years of follow-up. The incidence was quite high (8.0%) among subjects under 20 years of age at enrolment, while no seroconversions were observed among participants aged 40 and above at enrolment [2]. A large proportion of members of this high-risk cohort declared a willingness to participate in an HIV vaccine trial, even one with a placebo arm. Factors independently associated with willingness to participate in HIV vaccine trials included seroconversion during follow-up, a low education level, and exchanging sex for room, board or clothing [3].

Heterosexual populations

In the early stages of the epidemic, the vast majority of AIDS cases in Brazil occurred in MSM and in IDUs. From the mid- to late 1980s onwards, the proportion of cases in women and heterosexual men started to steadily increase. Following the advance of the epidemic into the heterosexual population, the *Projeto Praça Onze* group conducted a study to assess the suitability of an HIV testing site in Rio de Janeiro for recruitment of high-risk heterosexual males and females into intervention trials. The study was conducted at one of the largest testing sites in Rio de Janeiro, with more than 700 patient visits per month and an overall HIV seroprevalence of approximately 10%. Sera from heterosexual men and women attending the HIV testing site between March and December 1998 were analyzed using the sensitive/less sensitive (S/LS) assay. The estimated HIV seroincidence was 1.9 per 100 person-years and 2.8 per 100 person-years for heterosexual women and men, respectively. This was similar to reports from other heterosexual cohorts in developing countries in the western hemisphere and was sufficiently high for HIV vaccine trials. In a survey on willingness to participate in future placebo-controlled HIV vaccine trials, approximately 55% of heterosexual men and women indicated that they would definitely be willing to participate [4].

A similar study was conducted at the same HIV testing site, investigating men and non-pregnant women aged 18 years or older who were first-time visitors to the site from February to July 2002. The overall estimated HIV seroincidence was 2.46 per 100 person-years, or approximately 1.5%, in both heterosexual men and women, suggesting the incidence in these populations had remained relatively stable [5].

Post-exposure prophylaxis

Between December 1998 and May 2001, another study was conducted by *Projeto Praça Onze* involving former participants of the cohort study to estimate the incidence of HIV infection in high-risk seronegative MSM. At the time, there were virtually no data on the acceptability, tolerability, safety, impact on sexual behaviour and HIV seroincidence among people taking post-sexual exposure chemoprophylaxis or post-exposure prophylaxis (PEP). Hence, the purpose of the study was to examine these issues in a cohort of homosexual men who were provided with ready access to PEP.

Participants were given a four-day supply of ZDV and lamivudine (3TC) at enrolment and instructed to begin PEP immediately after sexual exposure of a mucous membrane to blood or semen, and to report for evaluation within 96 hours. If the exposure was deemed to fulfill study criteria, a further 24-day supply was given. All participants were interviewed semi-annually concerning sexual exposures in the preceding six months.

Two hundred subjects were enrolled and followed for a median of 24.2 months. Post-exposure prophylaxis was initiated 109 times by 68 (34.0%) participants. In comparison with reported behaviour at baseline, reported high-risk sexual activities, on average, declined over time for both PEP and non-PEP users. There were no serious drug-related adverse events. There were 11 HIV seroconversions, 10 among non-PEP users and one that was a PEP failure. The overall seroincidence was 2.9 per 100 person-years. The expected number of new HIV infections and the corresponding expected seroincidence based on the risk profile were 11.8 and 3.1, respectively (p>0.97). The most commonly reported reasons for not initiating PEP among seroconverters were sex with a steady partner and not considering the exposure to be of sufficiently high risk to warrant PEP.

Despite the ease of access, use of PEP was uncommon and was not associated with an increase in reported high-risk behaviour. On the other hand, ready access to PEP did not appear to have substantially affected HIV transmission, suggesting a limited public health impact of this intervention [6].

Mother-to-child transmission

In São Paolo, a retrospective cohort study involving 485 HIV-positive women who delivered in seven different hospitals between 1993 and 1995 found an overall risk of mother-to-child transmission (MTCT) of 16% (95% confidence interval (CI):13–20) [7]. These results are in marked contrast with subsequent studies performed after ZDV was made available for prevention of mother-to-child transmission (PMTCT) of HIV. For example, in a prospective study conducted in Rio de Janeiro between 1996 and 2000, the transmission rate in consecutive children born to HIV-infected mothers was 4 out of 145 (2.75%) (95% CI:0.1–5.4), an almost sixfold reduction in the rate of transmission. In this study, HIV-infected women were offered ZDV as early as the fourteenth week of pregnancy. Mother-to-infant transmission was more frequent in women whose duration of membrane rupture was greater than four hours, but no association was found with mode of delivery, birth weight or prematurity [8].

Another study conducted in Rio de Janeiro between 1996 and 2001 reported a similar MTCT rate (3.1%; 95% CI:1.6–5.5) in a cohort of 297 women. A significant association was found between low birth weight and HIV status of the infant (OR (odds ratio)=27.4; 95% CI:2.7–272.7), and treatment during pregnancy was associated with reduced risk of transmission (OR=0.75; 95% CI:0.61–0.93) [9].

In summary, available data indicate that mother-to-child transmission in Brazil declined by approximately 75% after antiretroviral drugs became available in the public health sector for PMTCT.

Prevention studies in other populations

One study assessed the efficacy of an intervention on behavioural changes in night school students. Of 394 young adults who took part in the baseline survey, 304 (77%) completed a post-intervention questionnaire. At baseline, 87% had been sexually active at some time, and 76% had had sex in the previous six months. Among those who reported vaginal and/or anal intercourse, condom use was low. After the intervention, statistically significant behavioural changes were demonstrated only for women, who reported improved communication with partners about sex and AIDS and fewer instances of unprotected sex with non-monogamous partners [10].

Another study assessed changes in risk behaviours among workers at the port of Santos, the largest port in Latin America. A random sample of 395 male employees at Santos Port Authority were enrolled in a three-wave cohort. An intervention was directed toward the community of 20,000 port workers immediately after wave 2, and consisted of face-to-face contact between peer educators and port workers, and free provision of condoms. AIDS-related knowledge, attitudes and practices were measured before and after the intervention, and participants were tested for HIV and syphilis. No evidence of decreasing heterosexual risk behaviour prior to the intervention (between waves 1 and 2) was found. In contrast, a substantial and significant drop in risk behaviour after the intervention (between waves 2 and 3) was observed. Men who had negative attitudes about condoms and/or a history of drug use were most likely to engage in risky behaviours after the intervention (OR=1.9; 95% CI:1.1–3.5 and OR=2.9; 95% CI:1.2–7.2, respectively) [11].

Natural history of HIV infection

Viral subtypes and the natural history of HIV infection

HIV-1 is characterized by marked genetic variability, which is largely dependent on its high replication and mutation rates. Phylogenetic analyses have shown that HIV-1 can be divided into several subtypes and that geographical variations exist in the distribution of these subtypes [12]. There are also data to indicate that genetic variability may be associated with different transmission rates and rates of disease progression, which, in turn, can affect the dynamics of the epidemic. Additionally, it is possible that protection afforded by vaccines may be subtype-specific.

Early studies using molecular techniques identified the presence of subtypes B, F, and C in Brazil [13–15]. Subsequent studies described the dynamics and the distribution of these subtypes and of recombinant forms in different regions of the country. Although subtype B remains the most common in Brazil, other subtypes such as F, C, D, A and B/F have also been shown to circulate in various parts of the country [16–20]. Recombinant forms of subtypes B and C have also been increasingly reported, particularly in southern Brazil [21].

Few studies have looked at the epidemiological and clinical implications of this diversity. For example, Pinto et al., using restriction-fragment length polymorphism, investigated genetic variability in a convenience sample of participants in the HIV cohort of the Federal University of Rio de Janeiro [21]. Of 95 individuals investigated, 69 (72.6%) were subtype B, 10 (10.5%) were subtype F, 8 (8.4%) were subtype D, and 8 (8.4%) had patterns of mixed homotypic infections. According to the authors, clinical and epidemiological data suggested the intermittent introduction of these subtypes into Brazil, with subtype F probably being introduced more recently than subtype B [22].

In Brazil, subtype B comprises two variants. The first one corresponds to the B subtype variant that predominates in the United States and Europe. The second variant (B-Br) bears a characteristic motif at the tip of the V3 loop (GWGR) that substitutes for the GPGR usually present in the first variant. In addition, serotype B-Br differs from serotype B in the amino acid composition of the V1 and V2 regions of the viral envelope. In a prospective study, the rate of disease progression between patients infected with the HIV-1 V3 serotypes B and B-Br was determined in the cohort of patients followed at the Federal University of Rio de Janeiro. Among 445 HIV-infected patients who were tested with a specific enzyme immune assay, 204 (46%) had serotype B-Br and 127 (28%) serotype B infection. Both groups were similar with regard to baseline CD4 count, serum HIV RNA viral load, initial clinical stage and the proportions that were treated with antiretroviral drugs. Patients with serotype B infection were significantly younger and tended to report homosexual behaviour more frequently. Mean follow-up was 30±13.5 months. During the study period, 41 (32%) patients infected with serotype B and 44 (22%) infected with serotype B-Br developed AIDS (p=0.03). In a regression model adjusted for age and risk factor for HIV infection, progression to AIDS was faster in patients infected with serotype B (hazard ratio (HR)=1.59; 95% CI:1.03–2.43; p=0.03). A similar trend was observed in a model that considered AIDS or death as the outcome (HR=1.43; 95% CI:0.95–2.0; p=0.09). These results suggested that infections with closely related HIV-1 serotypes may differ in the rate of progression to AIDS [23].

Acute infection

Two studies conducted in Rio de Janeiro have reported on early events associated with HIV seroconversion.

A nested case-control study involving participants in the previously mentioned *Projeto Praça Onze* seroincidence study was conducted by Hofer et al. [24]. In the seroincidence study, at each return visit participants were submitted to an extensive interview on risk behaviour, signs and symptoms generally associated with HIV seroconversion, and sexually transmitted diseases, focusing on the preceding six-month period. For the purpose of the case-control study, cases were defined as participants with confirmed HIV seroconversion during the study period; controls were all individuals who remained HIV-seronegative throughout the follow-up period. Data for these analyses referred to the visit in which seroconversion was documented for cases, or to the second study visit for controls. There were 34 HIV seroconversions during the follow-up period. Among the seroconverters, 11 (34%) denied any symptoms attributable to HIV seroconversion, and 22 (66%) described one or more symptoms. Sexually transmitted diseases (STDs) in the preceding six months were more common among seroconverters then among controls. Although among HIV seroconverters, symptoms consistent with the HIV seroconversion syndrome were relatively common, the authors were unable to identify a sensitive case definition that could be used as a screening tool [24].

The same group described virologic and immunologic events among seroconverters from the *Projeto Praça Onze* seroincidence study and from the PEP study previously cited. Thirty-nine individuals with a median of 4.0 (1–16) laboratory measurements and a median follow-up time of 301 (99–1098) days after seroconversion were analyzed. An unusual finding was the relatively low HIV RNA viral load shortly after seroconversion, as compared with similar patients in developed countries. Median viral load increased substantially at around 600 days after the estimated date of seroconversion. As for CD4 count, the initial period of HIV infection was characterized by an increase, followed by a steep decline at approximately 200 days, after which a gradual decrease was observed in the median CD4 count, reaching 281 cells/mm^3 (95% CI:100–466) at 1000 days after the estimated date of seroconversion. Although viral load dynamics resembled those observed in developed countries, CD4 counts appeared to decline at a faster rate than in similar cohorts previously reported from developed countries at comparable points in time [25].

Prognostic models

In 1990, the World Health Organization (WHO) proposed a staging system for HIV infection in adults and adolescents to help design and evaluate drug and vaccine trials [26]. Staging systems are important because they 'facilitate communication between practitioners and researchers, assist clinicians in selecting appropriate therapeutic interventions and allow appropriate prognostic stratification for clinical studies' [27]. Nonetheless, the usefulness of any staging system will depend on its applicability in various settings, as well as its ability to provide clinically relevant prognostic information.

Using retrospective data from the cohort of patients followed at the Federal University of Rio de Janeiro between 1988 and 1992, Lima *et al.* [28] assessed the capacity of the WHO staging system and of a modified version, which included lymphocyte count, to predict survival of HIV-infected patients. Although both systems could efficiently differentiate between early and late disease, the modified system was more capable than the original system of predicting survival among patients at more advance stages [28].

The WHO staging system and the modified version were then assessed as predictors of CD4 count in a prospective study involving 106 patients, using data from the first visit of the patients to the outpatient clinic. The two models differed only in that the original WHO system treated clinical staging and total lymphocytes independently, whereas the second model, using the modified staging system, integrated both variables. The sensitivity of the first model was 95.7%, and its specificity was 83.3%. The second model had a sensitivity of 91.3% and a specificity of 86.1%. This study, which was conducted in the early 1990s, was the first to show that, although clinical and laboratory parameters individually are relatively poor predictors of absolute CD4 counts, the use of the WHO staging system together with simple and widely available laboratory tests could predict CD4 counts of <200 cells/mm^3 with high sensitivity and specificity [29]. These findings formed the basis for the WHO treatment recommendations for resource-constrained settings where CD4 counts are not available [30].

HIV and STDs in women

The prevalence of HIV infection among women of reproductive age is increasing worldwide, particularly among adolescent girls. According to the Brazilian Ministry of Health, in 2004, for every HIV-infected boy aged 13–19 there were six infected girls of the same age group.

To determine the prevalence of HIV infection and other STDs in Brazilian women who seek HIV testing, a cross-sectional study was conducted in 2002 of 200 consecutive women aged 14 to 29 years who attended the HIV testing site previously mentioned. Participants completed a questionnaire and received testing for HIV, syphilis, chlamydia and gonorrhoea. HIV and other STDs were common (HIV 8%, syphilis 6.5%, chlamydial infection 8% and gonorrhoea 9.5%). HIV was significantly associated with lower education and with having an HIV-infected partner. Other STDs were significantly associated with young age at first intercourse, heavy alcohol consumption, and marijuana use [31].

As suggested by the study of Cook *et al.* [31], factors other than sexual behaviour may be associated with female vulnerability to HIV and other STDs. A prospective study conducted in Rio de Janeiro between 1996 and 2004, involving 458 HIV-infected women, found a history of STDs in 220 women (48.0%), with 128 patients (27.9%) reporting a history of herpes, 86 (18.8%) a history of human papilloma virus (HPV) lesions, 58 (12.7%) a history of syphilis, and 19 (4.1%) a history of gonorrhoea. Moreover, 28.4% reported a history of domestic violence, nearly half reported having lost a partner with HIV/AIDS, and 62 reported having a child with HIV/AIDS [32].

Gender, disease progression and survival

A study was conducted to assess the association of gender and survival among incident AIDS cases in the cohort of patients followed at the Federal University of Rio de Janeiro. Among 617 patients (425 men and 192 women) who attended the outpatient clinic during the study period (January 1991–July 1995) and who had not had a prior diagnosis of AIDS, 124 incident cases of AIDS (20%) were diagnosed. There was no significant difference between the proportion of men and women who developed AIDS. The median time elapsed between the first medical visit and the diagnosis of AIDS, the median CD4 count at the first clinic visit, and the interval between the date of AIDS diagnosis and the previous outpatient visit were also similar for men and women. However, women tended to be less symptomatic at their first visit to the outpatient clinic. There were no significant differences by gender in the proportion of patients who eventually developed AIDS who had used primary prophylaxis for *Pneumocystis carinii* pneumonia (PCP) or ART. In addition, the proportion of patients who began treatment only after the diagnosis of AIDS was similar for men and women. After adjustment for age and AIDS-defining condition, survival after a diagnosis of AIDS was shorter among women (HR=4.43; p<0.001). Adjusting for CD4+ and CD8+ counts reduced the difference between genders (HR=3.33; p=0.017). These results suggested that survival after an AIDS diagnosis may be shorter among women then men in Brazil [33].

Co-infections

Human T-cell lymphotropic virus type I

Human T-cell lymphotropic virus type I (HTLV-I) is associated with adult T-cell leukaemia and the neurological disorder tropical spastic paraparesis, also referred to as HTLV-I-associated myelopathy.

Studies in the United States and Europe, as well as in other developing countries, have shown a high prevalence of HTLV-I/II co-infection among HIV-infected individuals [34,35]. Data about long-term outcomes of co-infected patients are conflicting and suggest variable outcomes, including delayed progression to AIDS in some reports and accelerated disease progression in others [36–38].

In Brazil, a high prevalence of HTLV-I/II has been reported among HIV-infected patients, particularly in the north-eastern part of the country [39,40]. However, few studies have assessed the impact of the co-infection on HTLV or HIV disease progression. A case-control study conducted in the north-eastern city of Salvador, comparing 63 HTLV-I/HIV co-infected patients with 135 HIV-monoinfected controls followed between 1989 and 1999, found a shorter survival time among co-infected individuals. Co-infection with HTLV-1 was strongly associated with parenteral exposure (OR=4.77; 95% CI:2.3–9.0) [38].

In patients enrolled in the HIV cohort at the Federal University of Rio de Janeiro in the early 1990s, the prevalence of HIV and HTLV-I/II co-infection was found to be 6.3%. In a nested case-control study, 27 patients seropositive for HIV and HTLV-I were compared to 99 age-matched HIV-monoinfected controls. Co-infected individuals had higher CD4 counts, more advanced clinical disease and higher β_2 microglobulin levels than those with HIV infection only. Co-infection was associated with both a higher CD4 count and more advanced HIV disease, suggesting that a higher CD4 count did not offer immunologic benefit [41]. A subsequent analysis of these patients using HIV RNA plasma viral load showed that this marker did not differ between cases and controls [42]. Co-infected individuals had an estimated 78% higher CD4 count than those with single infection after adjustment for serum HIV RNA plasma viral load, supporting the argument that CD4 count cut-offs used in making clinical decisions in HIV infection might not be appropriate in co-infection [43].

In the same cohort, it was also determined that a high proportion of co-infected patients (73%) had some evidence of myelopathy, and 60% had relatively severe myelopathy. Peripheral neuropathy was also more common among co-infected individuals compared with subjects infected solely with HIV. These findings raised the hypothesis that HIV enhances HTLV-1-associated disease, and, conversely, that HTLV-1 increases the risk of HIV-associated vacuolar myelopathy [44].

Tuberculosis

Tuberculosis (TB) and HIV/AIDS are inextricably linked. HIV infection has been shown to be the single most important risk factor for the development of active TB among individuals infected with *M. tuberculosis*. Tuberculosis, in turn, is the leading cause of death amongst people with HIV infection in most parts of the world. Studies conducted in Brazil have assessed the usefulness of purified protein derivative (PPD) skin test reactivity as a predictor for the development of active TB in HIV-infected individuals, the impact of chemoprophylaxis for TB on the survival of HIV-infected patients, and the impact of ART on the risk of developing active TB.

Chemoprophylaxis can effectively prevent the development of active TB in patients latently infected with *M. tuberculosis* [45, 46]. In general, recommendations for TB prophylaxis are based on PPD skin test reactivity, which, in turn, depends on previous exposure to *M. tuberculosis* and on the integrity of the cellular immune response. Since the latter is compromised in HIV-infected patients, skin reactivity might not be the best marker for the institution of prophylaxis, especially in populations with high rates of *M. tuberculosis* infection.

The relationship between reactivity to PPD and risk of developing TB in the pre-ART era was assessed in the HIV cohort at the Federal University of Rio de Janeiro. Although the overall incidence of TB was statistically similar in reactors and non-reactors, the association only became apparent after three years of follow-up, indicating the need for a relatively preserved immune system for PPD reactivity to occur. The discriminatory power of PPD was poor for patients with asymptomatic HIV infection, suggesting the limited predictive ability of PPD for screening patients to receive chemoprophylaxis [47].

A subsequent study assessed the impact of chemoprophylaxis on survival of PPD-positive patients. Patients potentially eligible for the study were those admitted to the HIV cohort of the Federal University of Rio de Janeiro between January 1991 and December 1994 and followed until 30 September 1998. Patients were included in the study if they had a positive tuberculin skin test, defined as cutaneous induration of >5 mm. Patients were excluded if they had a previous diagnosis of TB or if they developed tuberculosis in the first 30 days of follow-up. For this study, the start of the follow-up period was defined as the date of the first positive tuberculin skin test. Patients were considered to be lost to follow-up if their last visit took place less than six months before the end of the follow-up period. During the study period, 617 patients were admitted to the cohort. Of these, 72 (12%) were excluded from further analyses. Reasons for exclusion were a diagnosis of TB before admission (eight patients) or during the first 30 days of follow-up (14 patients), or not having a PPD test performed (50 patients). Among the 545 patients potentially eligible, 306 (56%) who had a PPD reaction >5 mm were included in this study. Of these, 131 (43%) were prescribed anti-tuberculous chemoprophylaxis. The median follow-up time was 49.1 months. The annual incidence of TB among patients who did not use prophylaxis was 4.8%, whereas the annual rate after the prescription of chemoprophylaxis was 2.0%. Chemoprophylaxis was associated with a reduction in risk for tuberculosis (hazard ratio (HR)=0.34; 95% CI:0.14–0.85, p=0.01). In a regression model adjusted for differences in ART, chemoprophylaxis was associated with longer survival (HR=0.50; 95% CI:0.27–0.93, p=0.023) [48].

The impact of ART on the risk of developing active TB was also investigated in an observational study that involved participants in the HIV cohort of the Federal University of Rio de Janeiro. At the time the study was conducted, ART in Brazil was generally reserved for patients with advanced HIV infection, according to contemporary recommendations of the Brazilian Ministry of Health. Thus, only patients with advanced immunodeficiency, defined as at least one CD4+ lymphocyte percent measurement of <15%, were included in the study. After a median follow-up of 22 months, there were 48 cases of TB among the 255 patients included in the study, corresponding to an incidence rate of 8.4 cases per 100 person-years. In crude regression analyses, the use of ART was associated with a reduction in the risk of TB after adjustment for PPD status (HR=0.2; 95% CI:0.04–1.13; p=0.06). Although limited power and follow-up time precluded definitive conclusions, this was the first study to suggest that ART could reduce the risk of developing active TB in patients with more severe immunodeficiency in a setting with a high incidence of TB [49].

Antiretroviral therapy

Effectiveness of ART

Despite being the first developing country to provide free and universal access to ART, there are scarce data on its effectiveness in Brazil. Studies conducted in developed countries have indicated that, in therapy-naïve patients, virologic response at six months of ART is an important independent predictor of progression to AIDS or death, irrespective of pre-treatment clinical or laboratory parameters. Predictors of virologic response six months after initiation of ART were investigated in a retrospective cohort study that included treatment-naïve patients attending an HIV clinic in southern Brazil for whom ART was prescribed between January 1996 and January 2004, and for whom there was information on plasma viral load three to nine months after treatment was initiated. Among 454 patients who met the inclusion criteria, 72% had an undetectable viral load three to nine months after starting therapy. When analyses were restricted to those who started treatment in 1999 or later, the overall success rate was close to 90%, and even higher for patients in the higher CD4 strata. In univariate analysis, virologic failure was associated with younger age, prior diagnosis of AIDS, higher baseline viral load, lower baseline CD4 count, non-adherence, regimen containing a single protease inhibitor (PI) as compared with ritonavir (RTV)-boosted PIs, and year that therapy was initiated (if before 1999). To minimize the systematic effect of therapy indication, a subset of 158 patients with a CD4 count <200 cells/mm^3, who started therapy after 1999, was analyzed separately. After adjusting for age, education, adherence, regimen, and baseline viral load, non-adherence and fewer years of education remained associated with virologic failure. The authors concluded that a significant improvement was found in virologic suppression over time, consistent with the introduction of non-nucleoside reverse transcriptase inhibitors (NNRTIs) and RTV-boosted PIs into clinical practice [50].

Time to diagnosis and survival time of paediatric AIDS cases were analyzed in a retrospective cohort study that was conducted in 10 cities. The study included all patients younger than 13 years of age at the time of diagnosis who were registered in the Brazil National AIDS registry, whose diagnosis occurred between 1983 and 1998, and who had been followed until 2002 (N=1154). Data were censored on the date of last clinical contact for children not known to have died. Among children infected through MTCT, the median time from birth to diagnosis was 12.2 months. Survival time increased steadily and substantially. Prior to 1988, the probability of surviving for five years for children infected through mother-to-child transmission was 0.246, but by 1998 it had risen to 0.605. Similarly, the median survival increased from 20 months in 1988–92 to more than four years by 1998, with the probability of subjects surviving for five years after diagnosis increasing every year from 1992 onward [51].

Adherence to treatment

Adherence to therapy is widely considered the most important predictor of response to ART. Since 1998, Brazil's NAP has conducted periodic evaluations on the quality of care provided in public clinics. Based on several indicators, clinics were classified into four levels based on the quality of care provided. An initial survey assessed 322 public clinics located in 10 states, which provided care to 87,000 patients (corresponding to 72% of all patients on treatment through the public health system in Brazil at the time). A nationally representative sample of 60 clinics was then randomly selected based on these levels. Subsequently, 1972 patients on ART receiving these services were interviewed using a structured questionnaire. Patients who reported taking more than 95% of the prescribed pills in the preceding three days were considered to be adherent. Using this criterion, approximately 75% of the patients were considered to be adherent to treatment. The level of quality of care was not associated with non-adherence. Predictors of non-adherence included services that cared for fewer than 100 patients, missed appointments, the complexity of the prescribed regimen, the number of pills in the regimen, and fewer than two years of formal education [52].

Factors associated with undetectable viral load were investigated in a cross-sectional study that involved 244 non-pregnant adults who were receiving ART in a clinic in southern Brazil, 48% of whom had an undetectable viral load. In multivariate analyses, sex, clinical status, current immune status, and treatment regimen were not associated with an undetectable viral load. Nonetheless, adherence to treatment was strongly associated with having an undetectable viral load [53].

Patient-related factors associated with ART failure were investigated in a cross-sectional study of adults who had been on antiretroviral therapy for six to 24 months in five public clinics in Rio de Janeiro. Patients were interviewed and their charts reviewed. Patients who did not experience at least one log decline in viral load and did not have a CD4 increase of ≥50 cells/mm³ in comparison to pre-treatment levels were considered to be non-responders. Of 211 patients enrolled, 38 (18%) were non-responders. In multivariate analysis, less than 80% adherence, lack of trust in the healthcare provider, not having a friend with HIV, and perceptions about ART were independently associated with lack of response to therapy, as well as baseline CD4 count, interval between starting ART and first viral load/CD4 testing, and having opportunistic disease after starting ART [54].

In Minas Gerais, a prospective study involving 306 patients found a 36.9% cumulative incidence of non-adherence during the first year of therapy (incidence rate=0.21 per 100 person-days). Independent risk factors for non-adherence were unemployment, alcohol use in the month prior to the baseline interview, use of more than one health service, high pill count, reporting of three or more adverse reactions, switching regimens, and longer time between HIV test results and first ART prescription [55].

Sexual transmission of HIV has been shown to correlate with blood plasma HIV viral load and is likely to be mediated through shedding of HIV in genital secretions. Nonetheless, relatively little is known about factors responsible for persistent shedding of HIV in semen among people on treatment. To determine predictors of seminal HIV RNA suppression after six months of therapy, 93 treatment-naïve participants of the Federal University of Rio de Janeiro's HIV cohort whose primary physician had prescribed antiretroviral therapy had their seminal HIV RNA measured at baseline and at one, two, three and six months after the introduction of therapy. Adherence to therapy was self-reported. Inability to adhere to therapy was found to be strongly and independently associated with persistent shedding of HIV RNA in semen. The association was strengthened by the demonstration of a dose-response effect between adherence and shedding of HIV in semen [56].

Adverse effects associated with ART

Despite the unquestionable efficacy of ART, several limitations have become increasingly evident, including concerns about the long-term safety of antiretroviral drugs and their impact on quality of life. At licensing, relatively little is known about the safety profile of each drug since, in general, only about 1000 patients will have been exposed to the drug, most of them for a period of less than 96 weeks. Thus, adverse events that occur in a low percentage of patients and/or are associated with long-term use of the drug will only become apparent after licensing.

Additionally, there are data to suggest a considerable influence of host genetics on pharmacokinetics of various drugs, which in turn can lead to geographical variations in the frequency of adverse events. For example, plasma levels of efavirenz (EFV) are higher in non-Caucasian patients, who appear to be at higher risk for drug-induced toxicity [57]. Susceptibility to a potentially life-threatening hypersensitivity syndrome associated with abacavir (ABC) use also has a strong genetic component. Since the presence of a particular haplotype (HLA-B*5701) strongly predicts hypersensitivity to ABC, it is not surprising that marked geographical variations in the frequency of this side effect have been reported. There are also marked geographical variations in the frequency of lactic acidosis, another potentially life-threatening adverse event associated with some nucleoside reverse transcriptase inhibitors (NRTIs) [58]. Like most developing countries, Brazil lacks effective pharmacovigilance mechanisms. Thus, despite the fact that over 200,000 Brazilians have received antiretroviral drugs that were provided by the government, there are extremely few data on adverse events associated with their use. Furthermore, there are no published reports of prospective studies investigating incident adverse events on Brazilian patients receiving ART.

One retrospective study reported on adverse events associated with antiretroviral drugs during the first 12 months following initiation of ART in approximately 400 patients treated between 2001 and 2003. The cumulative incidence of adverse events attributed to antiretroviral drugs was 33.7%. Most adverse events occurred before the fourth month of treatment and were common in women and in patients using indinavir (IDV)-containing regimens [59].

HIV shedding in genital secretions

The effectiveness of ART on HIV shedding in semen was evaluated in a study conducted from November 1996 to May 1998 that included patients being followed in the HIV cohort of the Federal University of Rio de Janeiro. At the time it was conducted, it was the largest prospective study examining the impact of therapy on genital shedding of HIV. Ninety-three HIV-infected men were recruited when they decided to start ART. The decision to start, change or stop therapy was made by study patients and their physicians according to contemporary guidelines of Brazil's Ministry of Health, without input from the study investigators. The baseline visit occurred before the introduction of ART. Follow-up visits were scheduled for one, two, three and six months after initiation of therapy. Patients with genital ulcerations or urethral discharge were excluded from the analysis. At baseline, HIV RNA was detected in 69 semen samples (74%) and 89 blood samples (96%). Six months after introduction of therapy, HIV RNA was detected in 29 semen samples (33%) and 33 blood samples (38%). The mean reduction in levels of HIV RNA in semen at six months was 1.65 $\log_{10}$ units. Thus, after six months on therapy, a substantial proportion of patients may still be infectious and may be shedding drug resistant strains [60]. As discussed earlier in the chapter, lack of adherence to the prescribed regimen was found to be the most important factor contributing to persistent shedding of HIV in semen at six months [56].

The same group conducted a study to evaluate the correlation of HIV-1 blood plasma viral load and cervicovaginal HIV-1 viral load, as well as the effect of ART on cervicovaginal HIV-1 viral load. Twenty-seven women were recruited for the study. Viral load was undetectable in three (11%) blood plasma samples and seven (26%) cervicovaginal lavage samples. Four women (15%) had detectable HIV-1 in blood plasma but not in cervicovaginal lavage. A significant correlation was found between HIV-1 viral load in cervicovaginal lavage fluid and blood plasma levels. A longitudinal study that included 11 women who initiated antiretroviral therapy was also performed. In these 11 women, HIV-1 viral load was detected at baseline in 10 (91%) blood and cervicovaginal samples. After one month on therapy, most of the women had a significant reduction in viral load in both blood and cervicovaginal samples. Nevertheless, HIV-1 was still detected in seven (64%) blood samples and three (27%) cervicovaginal samples [61].

Survival before and after ART

In the developed world, the rapid introduction and widespread use of ART led to dramatic changes in morbidity and mortality associated with HIV infection [62,63]. In Brazil, one study documented the decline in mortality trends before ART became widely available. In São Paolo, a cohort of 145 asymptomatic patients followed between 1985 and 1997 was investigated to determine the probability of remaining AIDS-free at two and four years of follow-up, as well as the one-year estimated cumulative probability of survival for the AIDS incident cases. The cumulative probability of remaining AIDS-free was 79% at two years and 64.4% at four years after first known positive anti-HIV serology. Women had a marginally higher probability of remaining AIDS-free after both two and four years of known seropositivity, compared with men. The only single parameter associated with better prognosis was an initial CD4 count >350 cells/mm³. The probability of survival one year after the diagnosis of AIDS was 78%, and the 50% estimated probability of survival was 19 months. The probability of survival with AIDS observed in this study was higher than in previously published estimates for Brazil. However, since the time frame was so long, these results may not be entirely comparable with earlier studies. Possible explanations for this potentially better prognosis could include more efficient prophylaxis for opportunistic diseases, as well as an increase in the availability of antiretroviral drugs [64].

A retrospective cohort study examined survival among patients diagnosed with AIDS in 1995 and 1996, the latter being the year that Brazil began providing free and universal access to ART. Thus, these two years were chosen as the earliest in which a substantial proportion of patients would have received ART and the latest for which follow-up time would be sufficient to determine median survival. The sample was drawn from 40,587 adult AIDS cases that had been reported to the country's NAP as having been diagnosed in 1995 and 1996. A nationally representative sample of 18 cities was selected, and adult cases in these 18 cities were randomly selected for inclusion in the final sample. Sampling fractions in the selected cities were weighted to provide a demographically representative sample of all reported cases in Brazil and 3930 cases were selected for medical record review. AIDS cases diagnosed in 1995 had a median survival of 18 months, while survival at one and two years was 60% and 45%, respectively. Cases diagnosed in 1996 showed much increased survival; median survival was 58 months, with one-year survival of 72% and two-year survival of 63%. For cases diagnosed in 1995 and 1996 combined, the median survival was 36 months. The study of cases diagnosed in 1982–9 found a median survival of 5.1 months and survival at one and two years of 32% and 21%, respectively. When patients who had not survived at least seven days after diagnosis were excluded from the analysis (for better comparability with the 1995–6 data), median survival increased to 6.8 months. These results compared favourably to contemporary data from industrialized countries [65].

Using data from the same cohort, Marins et al. investigated mortality rates of patients co-infected with the hepatitis C virus (HCV). Of 2821 cases studied, only 29.5% had been tested for HCV infection. Although co-infected individuals had a 26% higher crude mortality rate, the difference disappeared after adjusting for ART and the severity of illness at the time of AIDS diagnosis [66].

Another retrospective cohort study compared survival rates using the Brazilian Ministry of Health's 2004 and the US Centers for Disease Control and Prevention (CDC) 1993 case definitions in a cohort of patients being followed at a referral center in Rio de Janeiro. The study included 1415 cases diagnosed up to 31 December 2003. Of these, 445 patients (31%) had died, 205 (14%) were lost to follow-up, and 765 (55%) were alive as of the end of the study. Of the cases that progressed to death, 393 (88%) were AIDS-related and 52 (12%) were from unrelated or unknown causes. The Ministry of Health case definition identified 289 cases that did not meet the CDC criteria, with the opposite occurring in only 16 cases. Three-quarters of patients were still alive 22 months after AIDS diagnosis according to the CDC case definition, and 31 months after diagnosis according to the Ministry of Health case definition. Because the vast majority of AIDS patients were still alive at the end of the study, it was not possible to estimate the median length of survival using either case definition. A temporal increase in survival over time was observed in bivariate analysis. Compared with the period after 1996, the risk of death was more than nine times higher for cases diagnosed up to 1990, and four times higher for the period 1991–9, for both case definitions. In multivariate analysis, the absence of a baseline clinical syndrome and any use of ART were predictors of longer survival for both case definitions. The authors concluded that, although the choice of criteria for case definition can influence findings, prognosis in this cohort was also comparable to reported results from developed countries [67].

Although a decrease in overall mortality has been documented, as of early 2007 there were no published data on the impact of ART on causes of death among Brazilian HIV/AIDS patients. Therefore, Pacheco et al. assessed temporal trends of overall mortality and of cardiovascular diseases

(CVD), diabetes mellitus (DM) and non HIV-related conditions in Brazil between 1999 and 2004 utilizing data from the Brazilian Mortality System. The authors compared causes of death in individuals for whom HIV/AIDS was mentioned on the death certificate (the exposed group) with those for whom HIV/AIDS was not mentioned (the non-exposed group) using a mortality odds ratio analysis approach. Separate analyses were done for three distinct outcomes: DM, CVD and non HIV-related causes. A total of 5,856,056 deaths were reported in Brazil between 1999 and 2004. Of these, 67,249 (1.15%) had HIV/AIDS mentioned on the death certificate, corresponding to a stable rate of about 6.4 cases per 100,000 inhabitants per year (p=0.67). The adjusted yearly increases for the exposed and non-exposed groups were 8% and 3% (p<0.001) for non HIV-related causes of death, 8% and 0.8% for CVD (p<0.001), and 12% and 2.8% for DM (p<0.001), respectively. This study was thus the first to document changes in causes of death in HIV-infected individuals at a population level in a developing country after the introduction of ART. Since the introduction of ART in Brazil, the frequency of CVD, DM, and other conditions generally not associated with HIV/AIDS, when assessed as contributory causes of death, has increased significantly among HIV-infected individuals compareds to the general population [68] (Figure 20.1).

Drug resistance in antiretroviral-naïve patients

In 2001, the NAP established a national network to monitor transmission of drug resistant strains in Brazil. A survey involving 535 samples collected in 2001 from eight states found a relatively low prevalence of primary drug resistant mutations: 4.42% for NRTIs and NNRTIs, and 2.24% for PIs [69].

In another study, trends in prevalence of drug resistance were assessed in newly infected patients identified by a standardized algorithm for recent HIV seroconversion (STARHS) in a sample of blood donors in São Paolo. After adjustment for year of collection and infection subtype,

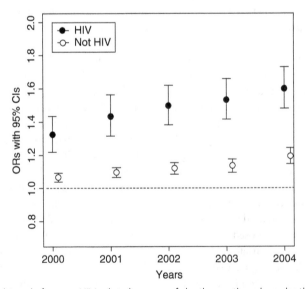

Fig. 20.1 Temporal trends for non-HIV-related causes of death mentioned on death certificates of patients who had or did not have HIV mentioned on the death certificate. OR and 95% CI in comparison to 1999.

Notes: Slopes of trends are significantly different between the two groups (p<0.001)
Source: [68]

the proportion of strains with evidence of resistance was significantly higher among newly infected donors (12.7%; 95% CI:5.2–24.5%) than in those with long-standing infections (5.0%; 95% CI:2.8–8.2%; p=0.02), suggesting that transmission of drug resistant viruses may be increasing [70].

Conclusion

It is widely recognized that the Brazilian response to the HIV epidemic set an example to be followed by other developing countries. Particularly important was the decision made in 1996 to provide free and universal access to ART, as well as the realization from the very beginning that prevention and treatment were inextricably intertwined. Although the success of the Brazilian response to HIV/AIDS is evident, its impact remains largely undocumented due to a scientific output that is not commensurate with its achievements. In this chapter, data from cohort studies conducted in Brazil were reviewed, some of which have made considerable contributions to our present knowledge of HIV infection, treatment and prevention.

References

1. UNDP. (2006). *Human Development Report 2006*. Available at http://hdr.undp.org/hdr2006/statistics/countries/data_sheets/cty_ds_BRA.html (accessed 11 May 2007).

2. Harrison LH, do Lago RF, Friedman RK, *et al.* (1999). Incident HIV infection in a high-risk, homosexual, male cohort in Rio de Janeiro, Brazil. *J Acquir Immune Defic Syndr* **21**:408–12.

3. Perisse AR, Schechter M, Moreira RI, *et al.* (2000). Willingness to participate in HIV vaccine trials among men who have sex with men in Rio de Janeiro, Brazil. Projeto Praca Onze Study Group. *J Acquir Immune Defic Syndr* **25**:459–63.

4. Schechter M., do Lago RF, de Melo MF, *et al.* (2000). Identification of a high-risk heterosexual population for HIV prevention trials in Rio de Janeiro, Brazil. Projeto Praco Onze Study Group. *J Acquir Immune Defic Syndr* **24**:175–7.

5. Barroso PF, Harrison LH, de Fatima Melo M, *et al.* (2004). Identification of a high-risk heterosexual cohort for HIV vaccine efficacy trials in Rio de Janeiro, Brazil, using a sensitive/less-sensitive assay: an update. *J Acquir Immune Defic Syndr* **36**:880–1.

6. Schechter M, do Lago RF, Mendelsohn AB, *et al.* (2004). Behavioral impact, acceptability, and HIV incidence among homosexual men with access to postexposure chemoprophylaxis for HIV. *J Acquir Immune Defic Syndr* **35**:519–25.

7. Tess BH, Rodrigues LC, Newell M-L, *et al.* (1998). Breastfeeding, genetic, obstetric and other risk factors associated with mother-to-child transmission of HIV-1 in Sao Paulo State, Brazil. Sao Paulo Collaborative Study for Vertical Transmission of HIV-1. *AIDS* **12**:513–20.

8. Nogueira SA, Abreu T, Oliveira R, *et al.* (2001). Successful prevention of HIV transmission from mother to infant in Brazil using a multidisciplinary team approach. *Braz J Infect Dis* **5**:78–86.

9. Joao EC, Cruz ML, Menezes JA, *et al.* (2003). Vertical transmission of HIV in Rio de Janeiro, Brazil. *AIDS* **17**:1853–5.

10. Antunes MC, Stall RD, Paiva V, *et al.* (1997). Evaluating an AIDS sexual risk reduction program for young adults in public night schools in Sao Paulo, Brazil. *AIDS* **11**(Suppl 1):S121–7.

11. Hearst N, Lacerda R, Gravato N, *et al.* (1999). Reducing AIDS risk among port workers in Santos, Brazil. *Am J Public Health* **89**:76–8.

12. Robertson DL, Anderson JP, Bradac JA, *et al.* (2000). HIV-1 nomenclature proposal. *Science* **288**:55–6.

13. Potts KE, Kalish ML, Lott T, *et al.* (1993). Genetic heterogeneity of the V3 region of the HIV-1 envelope glycoprotein in Brazil. Brazilian Collaborative AIDS Research Group. *AIDS* **7**:1191–7.

14. Louwagie J, Delwart EL, Mullins JI, et al. (1994). Genetic analysis of HIV-1 isolates from Brazil reveals presence of two distinct genetic subtypes. AIDS Res Hum Retroviruses 10:561–7.

15. Morgado MG, Sabino EC, Shpaer EG, et al. (1994). V3 region polymorphisms in HIV-1 from Brazil: prevalence of subtype B strains divergent from North American/European prototype and detection of subtype F. AIDS Res Hum Retroviruses 10:569–76.

16. Bongertz V, Bou-Habib DC, Brigido LF, et al. (2000). HIV-1 diversity in Brazil: genetic, biologic, and immunologic characterization of HIV-1 strains in three potential HIV vaccine evaluation sites. Brazilian Network for HIV Isolation and Characterization. J Acquir Immune Defic Syndr 23:184–93.

17. Caride E, Brindeiro R, Hertogs K, et al. (2000). Drug-resistant reverse transcriptase genotyping and phenotyping of B and non-B subtypes (F and A) of human immunodeficiency virus type I found in Brazilian patients failing HAART. Virology 275:107–15.

18. Couto-Fernandez JC, Silva-de-Jesus C, Veloso VG, et al. (2005). Human immunodeficiency virus type 1 (HIV-1) genotyping in Rio de Janeiro, Brazil: assessing subtype and drug-resistance associated mutations in HIV-1 infected individuals failing highly active antiretroviral therapy. Mem Inst Oswaldo Cruz 100:73–8.

19. Soares EA, Santos RP, Pellegrini JA, et al. (2003). Epidemiologic and molecular characterization of human immunodeficiency virus type 1 in southern Brazil. J Acquir Immune Defic Syndr 34:520–6.

20. Vicente AC, Otsuki K, Silva NB, et al. (2000). The HIV epidemic in the Amazon Basin is driven by prototypic and recombinant HIV-1 subtypes B and F. J Acquir Immune Defic Syndr 23:327–31.

21. Santos AF, Sousa TM, Soares EA, et al. (2006). Characterization of a new circulating recombinant form comprising HIV-1 subtypes C and B in southern Brazil. AIDS 20:2011–2019.

22. Pinto ME, Tanuri A, Schechter M. (1998). Molecular and epidemiologic evidence for the discontinuous introduction of subtypes B and F into Rio de Janeiro, Brazil. J Acquir Immune Defic Syndr Hum Retrovirol 19:310–2.

23. Santoro-Lopes G, Harrison LH, Tavares MD, et al. (2000). HIV disease progression and V3 serotypes in Brazil: is B different from B-Br? AIDS Res Hum Retroviruses 16:953–8.

24. Hofer CB, Harrison LH, Struchiner CJ, et al. (2000). Acute retrovirus syndrome among prospectively identified homosexual men with incident HIV infection in Brazil. Projecto Praca Onze Study Group. J Acquir Immune Defic Syndr 25:188–91.

25. Djomand G, Duerr A, Faulhaber JC, et al. (2006). Viral Load and CD4 Count Dynamics After HIV-1 Seroconversion in Homosexual and Bisexual Men in Rio de Janeiro, Brazil. J Acquir Immune Defic Syndr 43:401–404.

26. World Health Organization. (1990). Acquired immunodeficiency syndrome (AIDS): interim proposal for a WHO staging system for HIV infection and disease. Wkly Epidemiol Rec 65:221–8.

27. Montaner JS, Le TN, Le N, et al. (1992). Application of the World Health Organization system for HIV infection in a cohort of homosexual men in developing a prognostically meaningful staging system. AIDS 6:719–24.

28. Lima LA, May SB, Perez MA, et al. (1993). Survival of HIV-infected Brazilians: a model based on the World Health Organization staging system. AIDS 7:295–6.

29. Schechter M., Zajdenverg R, Machado LL, et al. (1994). Predicting CD4 counts in HIV-infected Brazilian individuals: a model based on the World Health Organization staging system. J Acquir Immune Defic Syndr 7:163–8.

30. World Health Organization. (2006). WHO case definitions of HIV for surveillance and revised clinical staging and immunological classification of HIV-related disease in adults and children 2006. Geneva: WHO.

31. Cook RL, May S, Harrison LH, et al. (2004). High prevalence of sexually transmitted diseases in young women seeking HIV testing in Rio de Janeiro, Brazil. Sex Transm Dis 31:67–72.

32. Grinsztejn B, Bastos FI, Veloso VG, et al. (2006). Assessing sexually transmitted infections in a cohort of women living with HIV/AIDS, in Rio de Janeiro, Brazil. Int J STD AIDS 17:473–8.

33. Santoro-Lopes G, Harrison LH, Moulton LH, *et al.* (1998). Gender and survival after AIDS in Rio de Janeiro, Brazil. *J Acquir Immune Defic Syndr Hum Retrovirol* **19**:403–7.

34. Khabbaz RF, Onorato IM, Cannon RO, *et al.* (1992). Seroprevalence of HTLV-1 and HTLV-2 among intravenous drug users and persons in clinics for sexually transmitted diseases. *N Engl J Med* **326**:375–80.

35. Quinn TC, Zacarias FR, St John RK. (1989). HIV and HTLV-I infections in the Americas: a regional perspective. *Medicine (Baltimore)* **68**:189–209.

36. Chavance M, Neisson-Vernant C, Quist D, *et al.* (1995). HIV/HTLV-I coinfection and clinical grade at diagnosis. *J Acquir Immune Defic Syndr Hum Retrovirol* **8**:91–5.

37. Gotuzzo E, Escamilla J, Phillips IA, *et al.* (1992). The impact of human T-lymphotrophic virus type I/II infection on the prognosis of sexually acquired cases of acquired immunodeficiency syndrome. *Arch Intern Med* **152**:1429–32.

38. Brites C, Alencar R, GusmaoR, *et al.* (2001). Co-infection with HTLV-1 is associated with a shorter survival time for HIV-1-infected patients in Bahia, Brazil. *AIDS* **15**:2053–5.

39. Moreira ED Jr, Ribeiro TT, Swanson P, *et al.* (1993). Seroepidemiology of human T-cell lymphotropic virus type I/II in northeastern Brazil. *J Acquir Immune Defic Syndr* **6**:959–63.

40. Guimaraes ML, Bastos FI, Telles PR, *et al.* (2001). Retrovirus infections in a sample of injecting drug users in Rio de Janeiro City, Brazil: prevalence of HIV-1 subtypes, and co-infection with HTLV-I/II. *J Clin Virol* **21**:143–51.

41. Schechter M, Harrison LH, Halsey NA, *et al.* (1994). Coinfection with human T-cell lymphotropic virus type I and HIV in Brazil. Impact on markers of HIV disease progression. *JAMA* **271**:353–7.

42. Harrison LH, Schechter M. (1997). Human T cell lymphotropic virus type II and human immunodeficiency virus type 1 disease progression. *J Infect Dis* **176**:308–9.

43. Schechter M, Moulton LH, Harrison LH. (1997). HIV viral load and CD4+ lymphocyte counts in subjects coinfected with HTLV-I and HIV-1. *J Acquir Immune Defic Syndr Hum Retrovirol* **15**:308–11.

44. Harrison LH, Vaz B, Taveira DM, *et al.* (1997). Myelopathy among Brazilians coinfected with human T-cell lymphotropic virus type I and HIV. *Neurology* **48**:13–8.

45. Woldehanna S, Volmink J. (2004). Treatment of latent tuberculosis infection in HIV infected persons. *Cochrane Database Syst Rev* **1**:CD000171.

46. Bucher HC, Griffith LE, Guyatt GH, *et al.* (1999). Isoniazid prophylaxis for tuberculosis in HIV infection: a meta-analysis of randomized controlled trials. *AIDS* **13**:501–7.

47. Zajdenverg R., Valle SO, Silva DR, *et al.* (1993). Reactivity to purified protein derivative and the risk of tuberculosis in HIV-infected Brazilian patients. *Chest* **104**:646.

48. de Pinho AM, Santoro-Lopes G, Harrison LH, *et al.* (2001). Chemoprophylaxis for tuberculosis and survival of HIV-infected patients in Brazil. *AIDS* **15**:2129–35.

49. Santoro-Lopes G, de Pinho AM, Harrison LH, *et al.* (2002). Reduced risk of tuberculosis among Brazilian patients with advanced human immunodeficiency virus infection treated with highly active antiretroviral therapy. *Clin Infect Dis* **34**:543–6.

50. Tuboi SH, Harrison LH, Sprinz E, *et al.* (2005). Predictors of virologic failure in HIV-1-infected patients starting highly active antiretroviral therapy in Porto Alegre, Brazil. *J Acquir Immune Defic Syndr* **40**:324–8.

51. Matida LH, Novaes A, Moncau JEC, *et al.* (2006). Impact of free and universal access to antiretroviral treatment on the survival among Brazilian children with AIDS. XVI International AIDS Conference,13–18 August 2006, Toronto, Canada. [Abstract MOAB0202]

52. Nemes MI, Carvalho HB, Souza MF. (2004). Antiretroviral therapy adherence in Brazil. *AIDS* **18** (Suppl 3):S15–20.

53. Silveira MP, Draschler Mde L, Leite JC, *et al.* (2002). Predictors of undetectable plasma viral load in HIV-positive adults receiving antiretroviral therapy in Southern Brazil. *Braz J Infect Dis* **6**:164–71.

54. Hofer CB, Schechter M, Harrison LH. (2004). Effectiveness of antiretroviral therapy among patients who attend public HIV clinics in Rio de Janeiro, Brazil. *J Acquir Immune Defic Syndr* **36**:967–71.

55. Bonolo Pde F., Cesar CC, Acurcio FA, *et al.* (2005). Non-adherence among patients initiating antiretroviral therapy: a challenge for health professionals in Brazil. *AIDS* **19** (Suppl 4):S5–13.

56. Barroso PF, Schechter M, Guptav P, *et al.* (2003). Adherence to antiretroviral therapy and persistence of HIV RNA in semen. *J Acquir Immune Defic Syndr* **32**:435–40.

57. Burger D, van der Heiden I, la Porte C, *et al.* (2006). Interpatient variability in the pharmacokinetics of the HIV non-nucleoside reverse transcriptase inhibitor efavirenz: the effect of gender, race, and CYP2B6 polymorphism. *Br J Clin Pharmacol* **61**:148–54.

58. Boulle A. (2006). Regimen Durability and Tolerability to 36-month Duration on ART in Khayelitsha, South Africa. 13th Conference on Retroviruses and Opportunistic Infections, 5–8 February 2006, Denver, CO, USA. [Abstract 66]

59. Padua CA, Cesar CC, Bonolo PF, *et al.* (2006). High incidence of adverse reactions to initial antiretroviral therapy in Brazil. *Braz J Med Biol Res* **39**:495–505.

60. Barroso PF, Schechter M, Gupta P, *et al.* (2000). Effect of antiretroviral therapy on HIV shedding in semen. *Ann Intern Med* **133**:280–4.

61. Vettore MV, Schechter M, Melo MF, *et al.* (2006). Genital HIV-1 viral load is correlated with blood plasma HIV-1 viral load in Brazilian women and is reduced by antiretroviral therapy. *J Infect* **52**:290–3.

62. Hogg RS, Heath KV, Yip B, *et al.* (1998). Improved survival among HIV-infected individuals following initiation of antiretroviral therapy. *JAMA* **279**:450–4.

63. Palella FJ Jr, Delaney KM, Moorman AC, *et al.* (1998). Declining morbidity and mortality among patients with advanced human immunodeficiency virus infection. HIV Outpatient Study Investigators. *N Engl J Med* **338**:853–60.

64. Fonseca LA, Reingold AL, Casseb JR, *et al.* (1999). AIDS incidence and survival in a hospital-based cohort of asymptomatic HIV seropositive patients in Sao Paulo, Brazil. *Int J Epidemiol* **28**:1156–60.

65. Marins JR, Jamal LF, Chen SY, *et al.* (2003). Dramatic improvement in survival among adult Brazilian AIDS patients. *AIDS* **17**:1675–82.

66. Marins JR, Barros MB, Machado H, *et al.* (2005). Characteristics and survival of AIDS patients with hepatitis C: the Brazilian National Cohort of 1995–1996. *Aids* **19** (Suppl 4):S27–30.

67. Campos DP, Ribeiro SR, Grinsztejn B, *et al.* (2005). Survival of AIDS patients using two case definitions, Rio de Janeiro, Brazil, 1986–2003. *AIDS* **19** (Suppl 4):S22–6.

68. Pacheco AGF, Tuboi SH, Faulhaber JC, Harrison LH, Schechter M. (2008). Significant increases in cardiovascular diseases and diabetes as causes of death in HIV-infected individuals in the HAART era in Brazil: a population based analysis. *PLoS one* **3**(1): e1531.

69. Brindeiro RM, Diaz RS, Sabino EC, *et al.* (2003). Brazilian Network for HIV Drug Resistance Surveillance (HIV-BResNet): a survey of chronically infected individuals. *AIDS* **17**:1063–9.

70. Barreto CC, Nishyia A, Araujo LV, *et al.* (2006). Trends in antiretroviral drug resistance and clade distributions among HIV-1–infected blood donors in Sao Paulo, Brazil. *J Acquir Immune Defic Syndr* **41**:338–41.

Chapter 21

The HIV Netherlands-Australia-Thailand research collaboration (HIV-NAT)

Kiat Ruxrungtham

Introduction

The HIV-1 epidemics in Asia have shown great diversity, both in severity and in timing. While significant progress has been made in stemming new HIV infections, especially in the so-called 'prevention successful' countries of Thailand and Cambodia, several countries, including China, Indonesia and Vietnam, have growing epidemics.

Three major HIV-1 subtypes are dominant in Asia: C, CRF_01AE, and B. In Southeast Asian countries such as Thailand, Cambodia, Myanmar (Burma) and Vietnam, the circulating recombinant form CRF_01AE predominates [1]. Thus, clinical trials of antiretroviral drugs relevant to the Asian population and to the development of appropriate highly active antiretroviral therapy (HAART) guidelines and HIV care programmes in the region are needed [1].

The HIV Netherlands-Australia-Thailand Research Collaboration (HIV-NAT) is an HIV-related clinical trials research centre under the aegis of the Thai Red Cross AIDS Research Centre (TRC-ARC). It was established in 1996 by collaboration between three organizations: the Thai Red Cross AIDS Research Centre in Bangkok; the National Centre in HIV Epidemiology and Clinical Research (NCHECR) in Sydney; and the International Antiviral Therapy Evaluation Centre (IATEC) in Amsterdam. HIV-NAT is located in Bangkok. Its main missions are to conduct clinical trials of antiretroviral drugs according to the International Conference on Harmonisation/WHO Good Clinical Practice (ICH GCP) standards and to address research questions that are relevant and have a high impact on developing countries. Over the past decade, HIV-NAT has conducted at least 50 clinical trials and is still conducting several other studies; it is also following up cohorts of adults and paediatric patients on HAART. In this chapter, some findings from the relevant studies for Asia and developing countries are highlighted.

Lower-dose optimization of antiretroviral drugs for Asian and resource-limited settings

Low-dose nucleoside reverse transcriptase inhibitors (NRTIs)

Dual NRTIs had been widely used in Thailand prior to 2003. HIV-NAT 001 and 002 were conducted to see if NRTIs could be halved for Asian patients. HIV-NAT 001 explored whether the dosage of azidothymidine (AZT)/zalcitabine (ddC) could be reduced (see Table 21.1). One hundred and eleven patients (n=111) with mean body weight of 56.4 kg, mean CD4 count of 324 cells/mm^3, and mean HIV RNA of 4.7 $\log_{10}$ copies/mL were randomized to AZT 200 mg thrice daily/ ddC 0.75 mg thrice daily versus AZT 100 mg thrice daily/ ddC 0.375 mg thrice daily. They were followed up for 48 weeks and no significant differences in adverse events were seen.

Table 21.1 Summary of major HIV-NAT and other collaborative study results

Study	Regimen	Sample size	Trial design	Baseline CD4, VL	% undetectable pVL	CD4 increased from baseline	Remarks
Nucleoside RT inhibitor studies							
HIV-NAT 001	AZT/ddC standard doses versus AZT/ddC half dose[2]	116 (45% female)	Randomized, open-label	Mean BW 56 kg CD4 =324 cells/mm³ VL = 4.7 log10c/mL	**Week 48** % pVL <400: the standard dose AZT/ddC =52% Half-dose arm = 20%	**Week 48** 52 and 78 cells/mm³, respectively	Half dose AZT/ddC is not recommended[2]
HIV-NAT 002	ddl alone d4T/ddl: standard (H/H) d4T/ddl H/L d4T/ddl L/H d4T/ddl L/L (H=standard dose, L=half-a-dose)[3]	78	Randomized, open-label	Mean CD4 =255 cells/mm³ VL= 4.3 log10 c/mL	**Week 24** % pVL <500 ddl alone =78% Combined d4T/ddl = 20%[3]	**Week 24** 101 and 76 cells/mm³ for ddl alone and combined d4T/ddl, respectively	Receiving high dose ddl but not d4T may correlate with a better viral suppression.[3]
HIV-NAT 003	AZT/3TC AZT/3TC/ddl[14]	106	Randomized, open-label		**Week 48** % pVL <50 55% vs 11%, found in triple vs dual NRTIs, respectively (ITT).[14]	Maximal mean change of CD4 from baseline found at **Week 24:** +125 vs +81 cells/mm³ (p =ns)	The majority (80%) of patients who failed either dual or triple NRTIs showed NAMs[57] (see **Fig. 21.5a**)
Protease inhibitor studies							
HIV-NAT 005	AZT/3TC plus IDV 800 mg tid versus IDV/r 800/100 mg bid[17]	103	Randomized, open-label in NRTI-experienced patients (median 29 months)	Median pVL = 4.0 log10 Median CD4=166 cells/mm³	**Week 112** the mean ± SD change in timeweighted average HIV RNA from baseline: −1.6 ± 1.1 in three times daily arm versus −1.4 ±1.1 HIV RNA copies/week/mL in the twice daily arm (p =ns)[17]	Mean ± SD changes in time-weighted CD4+ T-cell count from baseline were 88 ± 84 cells/week /mm³ in the IDV three times daily arm; and 70 ±109 cells/week/mm³ in the IDV/rtv twice daily arm (p =ns)	Both arms were associated with substantial toxicity expressed as serious adverse events and study drug interruptions. The twice daily arm experienced greater dyslipidaemia.[17]

Study	Regimen	N	Design	Baseline	Efficacy	CD4 change	Comments
HIV-NAT 009	EFV/IDV/r EFV 600 mg qd IDV 800 mg bid RTV 100 mg bid[19]	61 (38% female)	Single arm prospective study in NRTI-experienced patients	Median CD4 = 169 cells/mm^3 pVL = 4.1 log10	Week 48 and 96 % pVL<50 =87 and 69%, respectively[19]	Week 48 and 96 74 and 103 cells/mm^3, respectively[19]	RTV boosted IDV and EFV provides a robust and durable efficacy in extensive NRTIs-experienced patients. 20% experienced nephrotoxicity required IDV dose reduction.
SQV/r qd study in naïve patients	2NRTIs/SQV/r[12]	200 treatment naïve	Single arm prospective study	Median CD4= 267 cells/mm^3 pVL = 4.7 log10	Week 24 96% pVL,400 89% pVL<50[12]	Week 24 Median rise = 122 cells/mm^3	Only 3.3% with virologic failure found and without resistance mutants detected[12]
HIV-NAT 001.3	Switching from well viral suppression of 2NRTIs+ SQV-SQC 1400 mg bid regimen to 2NRTIs+ SQV/r 1600/100 qd[10]	69	Open-label single arm		Week 24 93% maintained pVL<50 Week 48 91% sustained pVL<50[10]	Median increased CD4+ cell= 134 cells/mm^3,	2NRTIs+ SQV/r 1600/100 qd may be used as a maintenance regimen in well-virologically suppressed patients even though had been experienced 2 NRTIs therapy
IDV/r low dose	IDV/r 400/100 mg bid Plus d4T/3TC[8]	19 (50% female) median BW 51 kg	PK and short-term efficacy trial	Median CD4=13 cells/mm^3, pVL=5.22 log10	Week 24 % pVL<400 was 89%[8]	NA	Our observation has been confirmed by the other study with a total of 80 patients of which 69% (ITT), and 89% (OT) of patients had pVL<50 at 96 weeks.[9]

Sources: as indicated in superscript within the Table.

Week 48 data showed the proportion with HIV RNA <400 copies/mL was significantly higher in the standard-dose arm, at 52%, than in the half-dose arm, at 20%, (intent-to-treat (ITT) analysis, p=0.001). The results indicate that AZT/ddC should not be reduced to half-dose [2].

Stavudine (d4T), although associated with a risk of mitochondrial toxicity, remains a key NRTI being used in Asia and other developing countries. The HIV-NAT-002 study investigated whether half-dose d4T and didanosine (ddI) are efficacious. Seventy-eight patients were randomized to four regimens of high (standard dose) and low (half of the recommended dose) doses of ddI and d4T combinations, or to ddI alone (see Table 21.1). The mean baseline CD4 count was 255 cells/mm^3 and mean plasma HIV-1 RNA was 4.3 log$_{10}$ copies/mL. In the ITT analysis, 78% of patients in the pooled combination d4T/ddI arms, and 20% of patients in the ddI alone arm, showed plasma HIV-1 RNA <500 copies/mL at week 24 (p<0.001), and 59% (d4T/ddI arm) versus 53% (ddI alone arm), at week 48 (d4T was added to the ddI alone arm after 24 weeks). There was no significant difference in median CD4 count increases from baseline at week 24 (101 cells/mm^3 versus 76 cells/mm^3, respectively) between the groups. Logistic regression modelling suggested that receiving high-dose (standard recommended doses) ddI, but not d4T, may correlate with better viral suppression [3].

Another, larger-scale study of 327 patients (the ARV065 study) was coordinated by HIV-NAT with the support of the Thailand's Center for Diseases Control. This multi-centre, randomized open-label study evaluated the efficacy and safety of half-dose d4T. Patients were randomly assigned to either:

- low-dose d4T 30 or 40 mg/day (weight adjusted) plus ddI 250 or 400 mg/day (n=109) (group A);
- standard dose d4T 60 or 80 mg/day plus ddI (n=110) (group B); or
- AZT 300 or 400 mg/day plus ddI (n=108) (group C).

Of 327 patients, the mean body weight was 54.4 kg, and baseline characteristics were comparable. The ITT analysis at 96 weeks showed 33%, 47.3%, and 9.3% of patients had a viral load <500 copies/mL, respectively. Multivariate logistical regression showed the likelihood of a viral load <500 copies/mL was significantly greatest in group A. Both d4T groups compared to the AZT group (p<0.01, odds ratio (OR)=5 (2.3–11.2)). In group B, the baseline viral load was <10,000 copies/mL (OR=4; p<0.01); in group C, the baseline CD4 count was between 200–350 versus <200 cells/mm^3 (OR=2.3; p=0.03). There was no significant difference between groups A and B, though serious lactic acidosis was found in three patients in group B. This study confirmed that half-dose d4T is comparable in efficacy to full-dose d4T, and that it is superior to AZT when combined with ddI [4].

A meta-analysis based on four randomized trials (n=377) and three cohort studies (n=631) was performed [5]. Of those 1008 patients, 56% were on standard d4T dose, 32% on a low dose, and 12% switched from standard to low-dose d4T. In the largest comparative cohort study (n=508), the proportion with peripheral neuropathy was 26% for d4T 40 mg versus 13% for d4T 30 mg (p=0.001). Lipoatrophy, measured in one randomized trial and two cohorts, was more pronounced for d4T 40 mg versus 30 mg. It was concluded that d4T 40 mg and 30 mg twice daily show equivalent antiviral efficacy, but with higher adverse event rates for d4T 40 mg twice daily (see Figure 21.1) [5].

Thus, although all developed countries have stopped recommending d4T for first-line regimens, d4T remains widely used in most Asian countries due to its low cost. Until tenofovir (TDF) becomes available and affordable, the recommended first-line antiretroviral regimen in Thailand begins with d4T at a low dose—i.e. 30 mg—for the first three to six months, followed by a switch to AZT. This is to avoid severe AZT-induced anaemia, which can be seen in 10–20% of advanced HIV-infected patients treated with AZT as their first-line regimen.

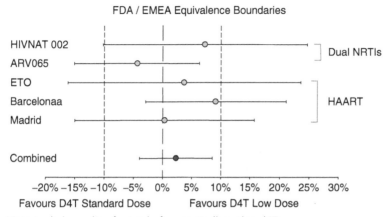

Fig. 21.1 Meta-analysis results of a total of seven studies using d4T.

Low-dose ritonavir (RTV)-boosted indinavir (IDV): pharmacokinetics and efficacy

Current treatment guidelines for adult patients in the United States and Europe recommend four boosted protease inhibitors (PIs) as preferred PI-based regimens, including lopinavir (LPV), RTV-boosted fosamprenavir (fAPV), atazanavir (ATV) and saquinavir (SQV) [6]. For resource-limited settings, however, the most affordable PI is RTV-boosted IDV, which unfortunately carries a unique risk of nephrotoxicity. The risk has been shown to be associated with plasma IDV level; patients with an indinavir area under the curve (AUC) greater than 30 (eight-hour regimen) or 60 (12-hour regimen) mg/L/h were at increased risk of developing nephrotoxicity [7]. Moreover, there is some anecdotal evidence of lower-dose boosted IDV 400 mg/ RTV 100 mg every 12 hours showing promising results in terms of pharmokinetic profiles and efficacy.

In light of the above, a study was conducted to examine the pharmacokinetics of IDV 400 mg boosted with RTV 100 mg twice daily in treatment-naïve patients. This study was carried out in collaboration with the Srinagarind Hospital in Khon Kaen, Thailand, and was a steady-state, open-label pharmacokinetic study of 19 patients. A pharmacokinetic curve of 12 was recorded after an overnight fast. Median baseline values for CD4 count and plasma viral load were 13 cells/mm^3 and 167,000 copies/mL, respectively. The results indicated that IDV exposure in this reduced-dose regimen of 400 mg with 100 mg RTV twice daily was dose-proportionally lower than that previously observed with the IDV/RTV regimen dosed at 800/100 mg twice daily. Therapeutic minimum concentration (C_{min}) levels of IDV were achieved in 84% of the subjects, and short-term virologic response was satisfactory; 89% had a viral load <400 copies/mL at 12 weeks. It is worth noting that these patients started this two-NRTIs plus a low-dose RTV-boosted IDV regimen at an advanced disease stage with high baseline viral loads [8] (Table 21.1).

The efficacy of this low-dose RTV-boosted IDV has been further confirmed with an open-label, non-randomized single-arm study of 80 patients with median CD4 count of 19 cells/mm^3 (range 2–197) and median baseline plasma HIV RNA of 174,000 copies/mL (range 16,800–750,000). The efficacy results of d4T/lamivudine (3TC) plus RTV-boosted IDV (IDV 400 mg/RTV 100 mg twice daily) were 84% and 69% (ITT) at 48 and 96 weeks, respectively. Ninety-eight percent and 88.7% (on-treatment) of patients had plasma HIV RNA <50 copies/mL at 48 and 96 weeks, respectively [9]. Nevertheless, hyperglycaemia, hypercholesterolaemia and hypertriglyceridaemia were found in 8.3%, 33.3%, and 37.0% of the patients, respectively.

Thus, IDV/RTV 400/100 mg plus d4T/3TC twice daily—the least expensive RTV-boosted PI—appears to be effective and safe up to 96 weeks despite high baseline viraemia and low CD4 count in treatment-naive patients.

Low-dose, once-daily RTV-boosted SQV

The efficacy and safety of once-daily SQV soft gel capsules (SGCs) (1600 mg) boosted with a 100 mg dose of RTV plus dual NRTIs, was first investigated in HIV-infected patients with plasma viral load (pVL) <50 HIV-1 RNA copies/mL following three years of antiretroviral therapy (ART) [10]. A total of 69 patients with pVL <50 copies/mL after 162 weeks of ART started this SQV-based regimen once daily while continuing dual NRTIs. After 48 weeks, 63 of 69 patients (91%) had pVL <50 copies/mL; five of the six remaining patients had pVL <400 copies/mL, and one patient had an unexplained rise to 39,500 copies/mL, which decreased to <50 copies/mL 12 weeks later. These data support the use of this regimen as a maintenance regimen in patients who have been virologically well controlled (Table 21.1).

To further investigate whether such a regimen can be also used among treatment-naïve patients, another, larger prospective study was carried out. This study was preparatory to the Staccato study, a structured treatment interruption trial [11,12] with an enrolment of 200 patients (n=200) [12]. At 24 weeks, 89% of patients had plasma HIV RNA <50 copies/mL (ITT analysis), with a median rise in CD4 count of 122 cells/mm^3. Only 3.3% had viral rebound. However, no major protease mutations were detected following virologic failure [13] (Table 21.1).

HAART trials in treatment-naïve patients

Triple NRTI-based regimen

The results of HIV-NAT 003 (n=106) had shown that triple NRTI therapy with AZT, 3TC and ddI was more effective in inducing sustained virologic responses than the double combination of AZT and 3TC, as evidenced by the fact that 54.7% and 11.3% of patients, respectively, had HIV RNA <50 copies/mL in an ITT analysis at 48 weeks (p=0.001) [14]. There was, however, no significant difference in increase of CD4 count.

Based on a long-term retrospective analysis, when compared with to the dual NRTI group, the triple NRTI group had a higher proportion of patients with pVL<50 copies/mL at 144 weeks (60% versus 18%; p<0.001), higher median CD4 count (388 cells/mm^3 versus 346 cells/mm^3; p<0.05), and longer duration of response, defined as the time from onset of viral suppression (<500 copies/mL) to the time of treatment failure or withdrawal from the study (144 weeks versus 104 weeks; p=0.002).

Multivariate regression analyses showed that significant predictors for treatment success, defined as a pVL <50 copies/mL at week 144, were: asymptomatic clinical status at enrolment; baseline plasma viral load <30,000 copies/mL; treatment with triple nucleosides; and a viral load response of <500 copies/mL by week 12 [15] (Table 21.1). Nevertheless, although triple NRTIs were significantly superior to dual NRTI regimens, it is clear that they resulted in a significantly lower proportion of patients with pVL and durable viral suppression than other currently recommended triple combination therapies, such as two NRTIs plus a non-nucleoside reverse transcriptase inhibitor (NNRTI) or two NRTIs plus an RTV-boosted PI [16]. It is therefore not recommended as one of the preferred first-line regimens [16].

RTV-boosted PI-based regimen

In the studies mentioned above, once-daily RTV-boosted SQV-based therapy and low-dose RTV-boosted IDV both showed high rates of undetectable viral load (see Table 21.1).

ART in NRTI-experienced patients

IDV and RTV-boosted IDV

As IDV is the most affordable PI and is therefore widely used in resource-limited Asian countries, three IDV-related studies were carried out:

- HIV-NAT 005: boosted IDV 800 mg /RTV 100 mg twice daily versus IDV 800 mg thrice daily (see next paragraph);
- HIV-NAT-009: IDV/RTV 800/100 mg twice daily plus efavirenz (EFV) (see next section); and
- low-dose RTV-boosted IDV (see earlier section).

HIV-NAT 005 (n=103) was a randomized, open-label trial of RTV-boosted IDV (as described in the list above), with AZT and 3TC, in patients who had been previously treated with dual NRTIs for at least three months (median of 29 months) [17]. The baseline median (interquartile range) $\log_{10}$ HIV RNA was 4.0 (3.3–4.5) and baseline CD4 count was 166 (40–323) cells/mm^3. An ITT analysis at week 112 showed 64% and 59% of patients had plasma viral load <50 copies/mL, respectively. However, both arms were associated with substantial toxicity. The twice-daily RTV-boosted arm experienced greater dyslipidaemia [17] (see Table 21.1). This study led to a further investigation of the use of lower doses of RTV-boosted IDV to improve better tolerability without loss of efficacy. Our recent reports indicate that IDV down-dosing in patients taking RTV-boosted IDV (800 mg IDV plus 100 mg RTV) twice daily has been shown to be effective in minimizing kidney toxicity while maintaining viral suppression [18].

RTV-boosted SQV-based regimen

As mentioned above, based on 69 patients who were NRTI-experienced and had pVL <50 copies/mL for 162 weeks of ART (two NRTIs plus SQV- soft gel capsules twice daily), it was found that switching to a lower-dose once-daily SQV-SGC boosted with RTV 1600/100 mg plus two NRTIs produced a high virologic suppression rate; after 48 weeks, 91% had pVL <50 copies/mL) [10].

RTV-boosted IDV plus EFV in patients who have failed dual-NRTI therapy

HIV-NAT 009 (n=61), a open-label, single-arm prospective study, has shown that IDV boosted with RTV (800/100 mg twice daily) plus EFV 600 mg once daily gave a potent, durable response in patients whose NRTI therapy had failed [19]. In this study, the baseline median interquartile range NRTI exposure was 4.4 years, baseline median viral load was 4.09 $\log_{10}$ HIV-1 RNA copies/mL, and baseline median CD4 count was 169 cells/mm^3. ITT analyses at 48 and 96 weeks showed 87% and 69% of patients with HIV RNA <50 copies/mL, respectively. However, adverse effects on renal, metabolic and blood pressure parameters were observed. Sixteen per cent of patients permanently ceased therapy, and 26% underwent temporary drug interruptions because of drug-related adverse events in the study. Fasted-lipid values rose significantly over the 96 weeks of the study, as did median blood glucose and median serum creatinine levels. Twelve patients (20%) underwent IDV dose reduction, mainly because of nephrotoxicity [19] (see Table 21.1).

In this cohort, the changes in mitochondrial DNA and lipodystrophy after the switch from NRTI-based therapy to an RTV-boosted PI plus EFV were also investigated. A predominantly adverse metabolic profile developed, in terms of triglyceride, total cholesterol, estimated low-density lipoprotein (LDL) cholesterol, ratio of total cholesterol to high-density lipoprotein (HDL) cholesterol, and blood glucose levels. These had increased by 206%, 67%, 58%, 19% and 6%, respectively, at week 96 [20].

Antiretroviral drug-related adverse events

Overall adverse effects among patients on ART

Of 417 patients with a median 3.7 years of observation, 24% had grade III/IV toxicities, which included 8% with hepatic toxicity, 14% with hypercholesterolaemia, 6% with hypertriglyceridaemia and 4% with anaemia [21]. Antiretrovirals used were AZT, d4T, 3TC, ddC, ddI, EFV, SQV, RTV and IDV. These results suggest that for a resource-limited setting, simple and inexpensive monitoring of alanine aminotransferase (ALT) and haemoglobin could prevent serious short-term toxicity. Long-term toxicity can be addressed with a yearly monitoring of triglycerides, cholesterol, glucose and creatinine if nephrotoxic drugs such as IDV are used [21].

NNRTI-related rash

An analysis was made of 202 HIV-positive, treatment-naïve patients who had enrolled in the 2NN study in Thailand and been followed for at least one week [22]. Patients were randomized to:

♦ once-daily EFV 600 mg versus
♦ twice-daily nevirapine (NVP) 200 mg versus
♦ once-daily NVP 400 mg versus
♦ once-daily NVP 400 mg plus EFV 800 mg, all four groups with d4T/ 3TC.

It was found that 34.2% developed a rash from NNRTI, with 20% of rashes related to EFV, 21% to twice-daily NVP, and 38% to once-daily NVP. The proportions of grade III rash were: EFV 2.9%; twice-daily NVP 2.3%; and once-daily NVP 6.4%. Multivariate analyses showed the risk factors for developing the rash were being female with a CD4 count $\geq$250 cells/mm^3, a high body mass index of >21.3 kg/m, and a rise in CD4 count of $\geq$53 cells/mm^3 and ALT of $\geq$34 U/l at week 4 [22]. Thai patients treated with NVP twice daily had the same rash incidence as those treated with EFV for rash of all grades. Females and individuals with earlier HIV disease or with a large rise in CD4 count after starting therapy were found to be at greater risk for NNRTI-related rash.

ART-related hepatotoxicity

The incidence of severe hepatotoxicity observed was 6.1 per 100 person-years (95% confidence interval (CI):4.3–8.3/100) among 692 patients on ART in the HIV-NAT cohort. In a multivariate analysis, predictors of severe hepatotoxicity were hepatitis B virus (HBV) or hepatitis C virus (HCV) co-infection and NNRTI-containing therapy. Incidence of severe hepatotoxicity was particularly high among patients receiving NVP (18.5 per 100 person-years; 95% CI:11.6–27.8) [23]. These findings indicate that incidence and risk factors for severe hepatotoxicity appear similar among Thai patients when compared with those in other racial groups.

Indinavir-related hyperbilirubinaemia and UDP-glucuronosyltransferase 1A1 (UGT1A1) polymorphism among Thai patients were investigated, and it was found that, in contrast to Caucasian HIV-infected patients treated with IDV, the promoter polymorphism (UGT1A1*28) is of less significance than the coding region (UGT1A1*6) mutation as a risk factor for hyperbilirubinaemia [24].

Nephrotoxicity associated to IDV

Although IDV is the least expensive PI and is still being widely used in Asia and other settings where resources are constrained, a major disadvantage of treating with IDV is nephrotoxicity. From the analysis of 204 IDV-treated patients (88% on RTV-boosted IDV) and with a median follow-up of 216 weeks, 52% had leukocyturia, and 35% had symptoms such as flank pain or dysuria. Almost half of the patients had significant loss of renal function. However, patients experiencing nephrotoxicity were safely maintained on IDV by means of therapeutic drug monitoring. Parameters of renal function improved but did not return to baseline values, at least in the short term [25]. In settings where other, less toxic PIs are available and more affordable, IDV should no longer be included in a PI regimen, and these less toxic PIs need to be made available in resource-limited countries.

HIV co-infection

HIV and viral hepatitis

The prevalence of HBV, HCV and HBV/HCV co-infection was found to be 8.7%, 7.2% and 0.4%, respectively, among 692 patients (48% of whom were female) in the HIV-NAT cohort. HIV and viral hepatitis co-infection was not associated with increased HIV disease progression. Delayed CD4 count recovery among HIV patients co-infected with viral hepatitis was observed in the early stages of the study; however, it was not sustained. By week 48, CD4 cell increases were similar to those found in patients without co-infection [26].

HIV and active tuberculosis (TB)

EFV and rifampicin co-administration

While rifabutin is not available in Thailand and other resource-limited settings, rifampicin is the key anti-TB medication in the treatment regimen. Rifampicin, however, is a strong cytochrome p450 inducer and has been shown to reduce plasma levels of EFV and NVP to approximately 25% and 40%, respectively [27,28]. There have been small studies suggesting that an increase in dosage of EFV to 800 mg once daily and of NVP to 300 mg twice daily [28,29] might be advisable. However, the results of studies conducted by Manosuthi *et al.* in collaboration with HIV-NAT did not support such dosage adjustments, especially for Asian patients with low average body weight [30–33].

To address the question of whether EFV dosage should be adjusted in Asian patients from 600 mg to 800 mg when taken with rifampicin, 84 active TB/HIV co-infected patients were randomized to receive EFV 600 or 800 mg once daily plus d4T/3TC twice daily [30–33]. Both study groups had advanced HIV disease with very low median CD4 counts of 32 cells/mm^3 and 37.5 cells/mm^3. Mean body weight was 51 kg and median plasma HIV-1 RNA was 5.5 log$_{10}$ copies/mL. The results showed median plasma EFV levels were 3.02 mg/L and 3.39 mg/L, respectively (p=0.6). Plasma EFV levels were <1 mg/L in 8% of patients (3 of 42) and in 0% of patients, respectively (p=0.3) (see Figure 21.2) [30].

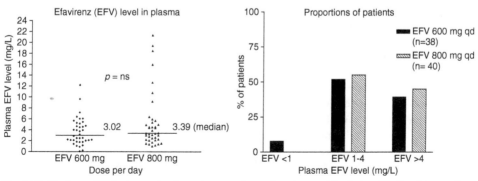

Fig. 21.2 Efavirenz (EFV) plasma levels and proportions of patients with plasma EFV level <1 mg/L, 1–4 mg/L and >4 mg/L, at two EFV doses.

Interestingly, after 24 weeks of ART, all three patients who showed a suboptimal EFV level had plasma HIV RNA levels <50 copies/mL. Plasma EFV levels >4 mg/L occurred in 15 of the patients in the group receiving 600 mg EFV, and in 18 patients in the 800 mg group; one patient receiving 600 mg had to discontinue ART owing to severe headache. At 48 weeks, 34 patients (81.0%) in the 600 mg group and 31 patients (73.8%) in the 800 mg group had continued EFV-based ART up to 48 weeks [34]. Thirty-one out of 34 patients (91.2%) in the 600 mg group and 27 out of 31 patients (87%) in the 800 mg group had viral loads <50 copies/mL [31]. Overall, similar virologic and immunologic outcomes at both 24 and 48 weeks were observed. Thus, 600 mg/day EFV should be sufficient when taken with rifampicin among patients with a body weight of approximately 50 kg [31,32] (see Table 21.2).

NVP and rifampicin co-administration

A recent cross-sectional study demonstrated that NVP plasma concentrations were 3.3 mg/L lower when co-administered with rifampicin (mean NVP concentration 5.47 ± 2.66 mg/L versus 8.72 ± 3.98 mg/L in the control group). Nevertheless, more than 86% of these patients had optimal plasma NVP concentrations >3.1 mg/L [32]. Manosuthi *et al.*, in collaboration with HIV-NAT, have further shown the efficacy of standard-dose NVP administered concomitantly with rifampicin, based on a study comparing 70 HIV-infected patients receiving rifampicin to 70 HIV-infected patients not receiving rifampicin. Mean plasma NVP levels at 8 and 12 weeks were significantly lower in patients receiving rifampicin (p<0.05). However, virologic and immuno-logic outcomes at 24 weeks were no different between the two groups [33]. After discontinuation of rifampicin therapy, mean NVP levels (± standard deviation) increased from 5.4 ± 3.5 mg/L to 6.4 ± 3.4 mg/L (p<0.05), but no NVP-related adverse events occurred. There was no statistically significant difference in 60-week antiviral efficacy between these patients and those receiving NVP-based ART alone [34] (see Table 21.2).

To address whether NVP dosage needs to be increased from 400 mg to 600 mg per day when administered with rifampicin, and whether a lead-in of 200 mg of NVP in the first two weeks is advantageous, another randomized study of NVP 400 mg versus NVP 600 mg in patients treated concomitantly with rifampicin was recently conducted. A total of 30 HIV-infected patients (15 per arm) with CD4 counts of <200 cells/mm^3 and active TB, and who had been receiving rifampicin for two to six weeks, were randomized to receive 400 mg or 600 mg of NVP per day, plus AZT and 3TC. An NVP lead-in was given to both groups at 200 mg and 400 mg/day, respectively. Plasma NVP level was obtained at weeks two, four, and 12. Twelve-hour pharmacoki-netic profiles for NVP were obtained for 19 patients (10 in the 400 mg arm and 9 in the 600 mg arm) at week four using high-performance liquid chromatography (HPLC). The results demon-strated that up to 80% of patients in the 400 mg arm had suboptimal levels of plasma NVP two weeks after the lead-in period (77% versus 13% of patients with NVP C_{min} <3.1 mg/L in the 400 mg and 600 mg arms, respectively; p=0.01). In contrast, 600 mg/day NVP was associated with a high rate of NVP hypersensitivity (four of 15 patients, or 27%, versus none in the 400 mg group). A full pharmacokinetic review at week four showed that the median (interquartile range) NVP AUC 0–12 hour was comparable between groups (64.8 (54–78.3) mg/L versus 85.2 (72.6–107.2) mg/L; p=0.05). Immune reconstitution inflammatory syndrome (IRIS) occurred in 33% (5:5) of patients, and 30% had severe AZT-induced anaemia. The 12-week efficacy showed no differences in proportion of HIV RNA (ITT) <50 copies/mL (53% versus 50%) or the median CD4 cell rise (76 cells/mm^3 versus 88 cells/mm^3) [35].

Therefore, in settings where EFV and rifabutin are not affordable or accessible, or where patients cannot tolerate EFV, NVP can be recommended as an alternative NNRTI to co-administer with rifampicin. In fact, NVP has been widely used in developing countries, co-administered with rifampicin. Based on the HIV-NAT studies, NVP at a standard dose of 200 mg administered

Table 21.2 Rifampicin and NNRTI drug interaction studies

Study	NNRTI	Sample size	Study design	Drug levels	Virologic suppression	Summary
Efavirenz (EFV)-rifampicin (RIF) interaction study[30, 31]	EFV 600 vs 800 mg in RIF treating patients	84	Randomized open-label	Median plasma EFV levels were 3.02 mg/L in the 600 mg group and 3.39 mg/L in the 800 mg group ($p = 0.6$). 10% vs 0% had EFV level <1 mg/L, respectively	There was no significant difference in time to HIV RNA <50 copies/mL at 24 weeks. The efficacy was comparable up to 48 weeks	EFV 600 mg/day should be sufficient for concurrent use with RIF, especially in patients with mean BW <60 kg[30, 31]
Cross-sectional nevirapine (NVP)-RIF study[34]	NVP 200 mg bid in patients taking or not taking RIF	148	Cross-sectional case-control	Mean NVP concentration was 5.47 ± 2.66 mg/L, and 8.72 3.98 mg/L, respectively 7 vs 0 cases had NVP level <3.1 mg/L, respectively ($p = 0.2$).	NA	Although NVP plasma level were 3.3 mg/L lower when taking with RIF, still more than 86% patients had NVP level > 3.1 mg/L.[34]
Prospective NIF-RIF study[32, 33]	NVP	140	Prospective case-control	Mean plasma NVP levels at 8 and 12 weeks were lower in patients receiving RIF ($p=.048$).	Virological and immunological outcomes at 24 weeks were not different between the 2 groups ($P>.05$).	NVP can be an alternative NRTI in patients taking RIF

Sources: as indicated in superscript within the Table.

twice daily, concomitantly with rifampicin is efficacious. However, the lead-in strategy of 200 mg NVP once daily for the first two weeks should be avoided as it was associated with suboptimal NVP level among most of the patients. In addition, an increase in NVP dosage to 600 mg per day was shown to be associated with a high risk of NVP-related hypersensitivity syndrome and is therefore not recommended.

Pharmacokinetics and drug-drug interaction studies in adults

Pharmacokinetics of IDV

HIV-NAT has carried out pharmacokinetic studies on IDV 800 mg, IDV/RTV 800/100 mg, and IDV/RTV 400/100 mg. In a study of 36 patients (18 in each group; 11 females and 25 males), receiving IDV 800 mg every eight hours and IDV 800 mg plus a boosting dose of RTV (100 mg) twice daily, the median (interquartile range) body weight was 60 (54–72) kg. The median and interquartile range values for IDV AUC, maximum plasma concentration (C_{max}) and C_{min} were not largely different from values found in Caucasian patients, with the exception of relatively high peak levels of IDV in Thai subjects. Cut-off values for optimal virologic efficacy were an IDV C_{min} of 0.10 and 0.25 mg/L for the thrice-daily (every eight hours) and the twice-daily (every 12 hours) regimens, respectively. Patients with an IDV AUC greater than 30 (every eight hours) or 60 (every 12 hours) mg/L/h were at increased risk of developing nephrotoxicity [7].

The study of low-dose RTV-boosted IDV twice daily was a steady-state, open-label pharmacokinetic study of 19 patients. A 12-hour pharmacokinetic curve was recorded after an overnight fast. Median baseline values for CD4 count and viral load were 13 cells/mm^3 and 167,000 copies/mL, respectively. The median (interquartile ranges) for IDV AUC, C_{max}, and C_{min} were 18.1 (15.3–23.8) mg/L/h 4.1 (3.6–4.8) mg/L, and 0.17 (0.12–0.30) mg/L, respectively. Short-term virologic response was satisfactory. We found that therapeutic C_{min} levels of IDV were achieved in 84% of the subjects and that short-term virologic response was satisfactory, as indicated by 89% having a viral load <400 copies/mL, even in a cohort of patients starting HAART at an advanced disease stage with high baseline viral loads [8].

The other study investigating the phamacokinetics of RTV-boosted IDV in combination with EFV was conducted in a total of 20 patients (10 males and 10 females) [19]. The geometric mean AUC versus time curve, C_{min}, and maximum plasma concentration of IDV were 45.7 mg/L/h (95% CI:39.8–52.5), 0.32 mg/L (95% CI:0.24–0.44), and 11.1 mg/L (95% CI:9.4–13.0), respectively. A >10-fold variation in IDV C_{min} was observed. The geometric mean concentration at 12 hours and C_{min} of EFV were 3.1 mg/L (95% CI:2.5–3.7) and 2.1 mg/L (95% CI:1.6–2.6), respectively. The findings indicate that despite the known pharmacokinetic interaction between EFV and RTV-boosted IDV, the combination of IDV/RTV at 800/100 mg twice daily and EFV at 600 mg once daily results in adequate minimum concentrations of both IDV and EFV for treatment-naïve patients [19]. The results are summarized in Table 21.3.

Pharmacokinetics of SQV

HIV-NAT has studied the pharmacokinetics of SQV 2000 mg boosted with RTV 100 mg once daily, SQV 1000/ RTV 100 mg twice daily, and SQV 1600/ RTV 100 mg once daily (see Table 21.3). One pharmacokinetic substudy evaluated 13 randomly selected HIV-1-infected subjects taking once-daily SQV-SGC/RTV (1600/100 mg), plus dual NRTIs. Subjects took one week of RTV-boosted SQV in hard-gel capsule (HGC) format plus NRTIs, followed by steady-state SQV pharmacokinetic determinations. Subjects then changed to SQV-SGC/RTV plus NRTIs for one week, followed again by steady-state SQV pharmacokinetic determinations. The results showed no significant difference in AUC values between HGCs and SGCs, with a median (interquartile range) of

50.0 (42.6–71.5) versus 35.5 (28.0–50.2) mg/L/h, respectively. Inter-subject variability resulted in four of 13 subjects on the SQV-SGCs, and two of 13 subjects on the SQV-HGCs having a C_{min} below the minimum effective concentration of 0.05 mg/L. The results indicate that once-daily 1600 mg SQV-HGCs boosted with once-daily 100 mg RTV resulted in pharmacokinetic parameters that were similar to those observed with 1600 mg of SQV-SGC/100 mg RTV once daily. The HGC regimen is easier to use in developing countries and may increase access because the drug cost is reduced, the capsule size is smaller, and there is less need for refrigeration [36].

It is worth noting that the pharmacokinetic profiles of RTV-boosted SQV in Thailand (HIV-NAT studies) and in the United Kingdom showed that RTV AUC and study site (Thailand versus United Kingdom) were significantly related to SQV AUC (p<0.01) [27]. Higher SQV AUCs, C_{max} and C_{min} were seen in Thai patients than in UK patients. In the multivariate analysis, the RTV AUC and study site appeared to be related to exposure to SQV [37].

Can ketoconazole or itraconazole be used to boost SQV?

There is evidently a need to find an alternative pharmacokinetic booster for PIs besides RTV to minimize RTV-associated metabolic adverse effects and, if possible, to minimize cost for resource-limited settings. Ketoconazole and itraconazole have theoretically been considered potential candidates. A study of SQV-SGC 800 mg or 1200 mg twice daily boosted with 100 mg of itraconazole once daily resulted in adequate SQV pharmacokinetics not significantly different from SQV-SGC 1400 mg twice daily. However, the pharmacokinetic enhancement was significantly lower than that of RTV [38]. Whether itraconazole is efficacious as a PI booster and whether it is cost-effective needs further investigation (see Table 21.3).

Previous studies have suggested that ketoconazole inhibits CYP3A and transport systems such as P-glycoprotein or MRP-1 [39]. When ketoconazole was co-administered with SQV, it enhanced the AUC of SQV by 37–69% in HIV-infected subjects [39]. We have therefore investigated whether SQV-HGC could be boosted with ketoconazole instead of RTV in a once-daily regimen [40]. Sixteen adults infected with HIV-1 were switched from a regimen of 2000/100 mg SQV/RTV taken once daily to a 2000/400 mg SQV/ketoconazole regimen. A full pharmacokinetic steady-state analysis was conducted for both regimens. Using RTV as the pharmacoenhancer resulted in median SQV AUC, C_{max} and C_{min} values of 56.21 mg/L/h, 8.4 mg/L and 0.31 mg/L, respectively. When given with ketoconazole, median SQV AUC, C_{max}, and C_{min} values were 12.6 mg/L/h, 2.01 mg/L, and 0.04 mg/L, respectively. The AUC, C_{max}, and C_{min} were all four to six times lower in the ketoconazole phase. Although SQV AUCs were potentially adequate for treatment when administered with ketoconazole, trough concentrations were below target (0.1 mg/L), which may cause therapy failure. Thus, SQV should not be boosted with ketoconazole in a once-daily regimen unless future efficacy data suggest otherwise [41].

Other antiretroviral drug-drug interaction studies

A study was conducted to investigate whether dosages of LPV and SQV-HGC can be reduced in Thai patients when administered in a double-boosted PI regimen [42] (see Table 21.3 and Figure 21.3). Forty-eight treatment-naïve patients were randomized in a 24-week prospective study to either:

- LPV 400/100 mg plus SQV 1000 mg twice daily (arm A);
- LPV 400/100 mg plus SQV 600 mg twice daily (arm B);
- LPV 266/66 mg plus SQV 1000 mg twice daily (arm C); or
- LPV 266/66 mg plus SQV 600 mg twice daily (arm D).

Table 21.3 Pharmacokinetics of protease inhibitors (PIs) and boosted PI studies in adults

Study	Population	Sample size	Body weight Median (IQR), Kg	Cmin Median (IQR), mg/L	Cmax Median (IQR), mg/L	AUC Median (IQR), mg.h/L	Comments
IDV 800 mg q 8 hr[7] versus	HIV-infected individuals with NRTI experienced[7]	36 (11 female)	60 (54–72)	0.13 (0.09–0.27)	8.1 (6.6–9.4)	20.9 (13.1–27.0)	IDV cut-off values for optimal virological efficacy C_{min} of 0.10 and 0.25 mg/L for the every 8 h and the every 12 h regimen, respectively.
IDV/r 800/100 q 12 hr[7]				0.68 (0.43–0.77)	10.6 (8.5–13.2)	49.2 (42.5–60.4)	IDV AUC >30 (q 8 h regimen) or 60 (q 12 h regimen) mg/L/h were at increased risk of developing nephrotoxicity.
IDV/r 400/100 BID[8]	Treatment naïve	19 (8 female)	51 (50–53)	0.17 (0.12–0.30)	4.1 (3.6–4.8)	18.1 (15.3–23.8)	Therapeutic C_{min} levels of indinavir were achieved in >80% of the subjects and short-term virological response was satisfactory.
IDV/r 800/100 mg BID plus EFV 600 mg qd[19]	HIV-infected individuals with NRTI experienced	20 (10 female)	54.5 kg (49–62)	Mean 0.32 (95% CI, 0.24–0.44)	Mean11.1 (95% CI, 9.4–13.0)	Mean: 47.5 (95% CI, 39.8–52.5)	Indinavir/ritonavir at 800/100 mg BID plus efavirenz at 600 mg qd results in adequate minimum concentrations of both indinavir and efavirenz for treatment-naïve patients.
SQV/r 1600/100 mg oral qd[36]	HIV-infected patients were taking 2NRTIs BID + SVQ/rtv 1600/100 mg QD with stable CD4+T cell counts and viral load	20 (16 female)	Approximately 50 kg	0.32 ± 0.28	6.5 ± 3.59	53.95 ± 29.92	Our short-term efficacy results of 200 treatment-naïve patients at week 24 showed that SQV/rtv 1600/100 mg qd plus 2 NRTIs had 96% of patients with pVL<400 and 89% pVL<50.

Regimen	Patients	n	Weight				Comments
SQV/r 1000/100 mg oral BID[36]	HIV-infected patients were taking 2NRTIs BID + SVQ/rtv 1600/100 mg QD with stable CD4+ T cell counts and viral load	10 (9 female)	54.5 kg	1.02 ± 0.74	3.89 ± 2.30	55.33 ± 35.08	
SQV/r 2000/100 mg oral qd[36]	HIV-infected patients were taking 2NRTIs BID + SVQ/rtv 1600/100 mg QDwith stable CD4+ T cell counts and viral load	10 (7 female)	44.3 kg	0.46 ± 0.23	8.85 ± 3.40	82.00 ± 30.01	
SQV 800 and 1200 mg + itraconazole 100 mg oral BID versus SQV 1400 mg BID[38]	HIV-infected Patients	SQV 800/itraconazole 100 BID: n=9;	51 Kg (47-58)	0.08 (0.06-0.08)	0.98 (0.84-1.21)	4.07 (2.76-4.49)	A controlled trial to compare to SQV 1600/rtv 100 mg qd plus 2 NRTIs in term of efficacy and tolerability is warranted.
		SQV 1200/itracon azole 100 mg BID: n=8; SQV 1400 mg BID, n=17		0.11 (0.06-0.14) 0.09 (0.04-0.13)	1.42 (0.6-2.19) 1.05 (0.69-2.48)	4.29 (3.14-7.67) 3.33 (1.96-7.34)	
SQV 2000 mg + ketoconazole 400 mg qd versus SQV 2000/100 mg+ RTV 100 mg qd[41]	HIV-infected patients on stable SQV/rtv 2000/100 mg qd plus 2 NRTIs	16	NA	0.04	2.01	12.6	saquinavir should not be boosted with ketoconazole in a once-daily regimen unless future efficacy data suggest otherwise.

Table 21.3 (continued) Pharmacokinetics of protease inhibitors (PIs) and boosted PI studies in adults

Study	Population	Sample size	Body weight Median (IQR), Kg	C_{min} Median (IQR), mg/L	C_{max} Median (IQR), mg/L	AUC Median (IQR), mg/L/h	Comments
HIV-NAT 019: Various dosing of double boosted PI: Kaletra/ritonavir/saquinavir in adults[42] **Arm A:** LPV/RTV 400/100 mg BID + SQV 1000 mg BID **(n=13)** **Arm B:** LPV/RTV 400/100 mg BID + SQV 600 mg BID **(n=11)** **Arm C:** LPV/RTV 266/66 mg BID + SQV 1000 mg BID **(n=11)** **Arm D:** LPV/RTV 266/66 mg BID +SQV 600 mg BID **(n=13)**	Treatment-naïve Patients	48 (28 female)	BW Mean 53-59 kg	**Arm A** Mean ± SD **LPV C_{min}** 6.5 ± 1.11 **SQV C_{min}** 1.2 ± 0.3 **Arm B** **LPV C_{min}** 6.4 ± 1.2 **SQV C_{min}** 0.9 ± 0.3 **Arm C** **LPV C_{min}** 2.9 ± 0.6 **SQV C_{min}** 0.9 ± 0.2 **Arm D** **LPV C_{min}** 3.1 ± 0.6 **SQV C_{min}** 0.5 ± 0.1	Mean ± SD **LPV C_{max}** 14.9 ± 1.30 **SQV C_{max}** 5.3 ± 0.8 **LPV C_{max}** 13.3 ± 1.9 **SQV C_{max}** 3.4 ± 0.7 **LPV C_{max}** ± 1.1 **SQV C_{max}** 4.0 ± 0.8 **LPV C_{max}** 9.1 ± 0.7 **SQV C_{max}** 2.3 ± 0.4	Mean ± SD **LPV AUC_{0-12h}** 129.0 ± 14.9 **SQV AUC** 35.3 ± 6.3 **LPV AUC_{0-12h}** 121 ± 18.2 **LPV AUC_{0-12h}** 26.2 ± 6.2 **LPV AUC_{0-12h}** 63 ± 10 **SQV AUC_{0-12h}** 26.0 ± 6.1 **LPV AUC_{0-12h}** 73.3 ± 6.6 **SQV AUC_{0-12h}** 15.5 ± 3	There was no significant difference of mean C_{min} and AUC_{0-12h} of SQV among the arms, whereas the PK profiles of LPV were significantly lower at LPV/r 266/66 mg BID as compared to the standard doses. Nevertheless, our results suggested that when LPV/r and SQV-HGC are combined, the LPV/r at 266/66mg BID PK profile should confer more than adequate coverage in PI-naïves. It is therefore warranted to further investigate whether the new formulation LPV/r 'Maltrex tablet' can be dosed at 200/50 mg BID for Thai or Asian patients.

Sources: as indicated in superscript within the Table.

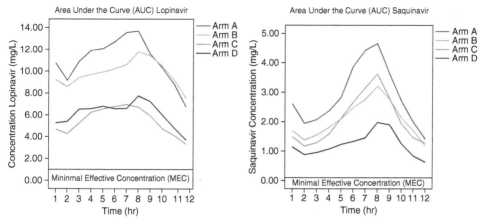

Fig. 21.3 Area under the curves (AUC$_{0-12h}$) of LPV and SQV, results from the HIV-NAT 019 study to address proper doses of LPV/RTV (Kaletra®) and SQV-HGC as a double-boosted PI regimen in Thai patients.

A 12-hour pharmacokinetic analysis was carried out at week two of treatment. Mean (standard deviation (SD)) values for LPV and SQV AUC, C$_{max}$, and C$_{min}$ of each arm are summarized in Table 21.3, and the AUC curves are shown in Figure 21.3 [42].

The results showed that the mean C$_{min}$ of both LPV and SQV in the low-dose arms were greater than the optimal level for PI-naïve patients. Sub-therapeutic C$_{min}$ values were observed in four patients (one in each group, all for LPV). There were no significant differences in the first and second phases of viral decline between arms. In phase I, the overall mean half-life (SD) was 5.67 (0.05) days. The proportion of patients with a viral load <50 copies/mL at week 24 was 38.5% for arm A, 77.7% for arm B, 60.0% for arm C, and 61.5 % for arm D (by ITT) [42]. These observations have led to a plan to conduct further low-dose pharmacokinetic studies at HIV-NAT to explore a cost-effective dose for RTV-boosted PIs in Thai and Asian patients.

Antiretroviral drug-drug interaction studies

Our studies showed no relevant drug-drug interaction between enfuvirtide (ENF) and RTV, RTV-boosted SQV, or rifampicin [43,44]. Tenofovir did not alter SQV trough levels [45].

Disease progression and death in HIV-NAT cohorts

Based on an HIV-NAT treated cohort of 1677 person-years of follow-up in a total of 417 patients, the rate of progression to combined endpoint was 1.7 per 10 person-years, and to death alone was 0.7 per 10 person-years. Compared to patients with baseline CD4 cell counts ≥350 cells/mm^3, the adjusted hazard ratio (HR) for progression was 3.67 (95% CI:1.31–10.27) for patients with <200 cells/mm^3. Responses to six months of therapy were the strongest predictors of disease progression; the HR for progression was 4.95 (pVL>4 log$_{10}$ versus undetectable viral load; 95% CI:2.14–11.46) (Figure 21.4) [46]. Observations indicate that in settings like Thailand or other Asian countries, ART initiation could generally be delayed until the CD4 count approaches 200 cells/mm^3. Based on a larger sample size and much longer-term following-up cohort, further study is under way to investigate a more narrow stratum of CD4 counts ranging from 201–250 cells/mm^3 to 250–350 cells/mm^3 to see whether early initiation of HAART (at a CD4 count of 200 cells/mm^3) is relevant and cost-effective for the Thai population.

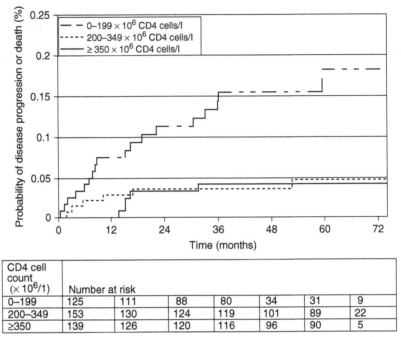

CD4 cell count ($\times 10^6$/1)	Number at risk						
0–199	125	111	88	80	34	31	9
200–349	153	130	124	119	101	89	22
≥350	139	126	120	116	96	90	5

Fig. 21.4 Kaplan-Meier curves of probability for disease progression according CD4 cell count, based on HIV-NAT cohort of 417 patients with 1677 person-years of follow-up.

Immune-based therapeutic study

To investigate safety and tolerability as well as identify optimal dose of subcutaneous inter-leukin 2 (scIL-2) in Thai patients, a randomized, controlled 24-week scIL-2 study was carried out [47]. This study provides the most extensive experience of subcutaneous IL-2 (scIL-2) therapy in HIV-1-infected women and Asians, and demonstrates the immunologic efficacy, tolerability and feasibility of scIL-2 therapy in this population. In this study, a total of 72 patients with a CD4 count ≥350 cells/mm³ and without history of opportunistic infections (OIs) were randomized into four arms:

♦ 1.5 million International Units (MIU) of scIL-2 twice daily for five days every eight weeks (one cycle) for three cycles over a 24-week study period (12 patients);

♦ 4.5 MIU of scIL-2 twice daily for five days every eight weeks (one cycle) for three cycles over a 24-week study period (12 patients);

♦ 7.5 MIU of scIL-2 twice daily for five days every eight weeks (one cycle) for three cycles over a 24-week study period (12 patients); and

♦ control arm (36 patients).

The time-weighted mean change in CD4 count from baseline was 252 cells/mm³ over 24 weeks for the combined scIL-2 groups compared with 42 cells/mm³ over 24 weeks for the control group (p=0.0001). The highest doses at 7.5 MIU BID showed a significant increase in CD4 count compared to the control group (p<0.0001). Furthermore, 75% of patients who were treated at 7.5 MIU attained CD4 count increases up to >1000 cells/mm³ compared to 0% in the control arm. The frequency and severity of toxicities was dose-dependent; patients who received 7.5 MIU experienced more severe fatigue, fever, myalgias and arthralgias compared with the other dosing groups. There were no grade IV toxicities, and no clinical or laboratory toxicities were dose-limiting. There was no significant difference in time-weighted mean change in viral load between the overall scIL-2 and control groups over 24 weeks. The dose at 7.5 MIU BID of scIL-2 has therefore been chosen for Thai patients enrolling in the ongoing clinical endpoint phase III trial, ESPRIT.

Structured treatment interruptions

To explore the safety of CD4 count-guided structured treatment interruptions and week-on/week-off therapy, a pilot randomized prospective study, HIV-NAT 001.4, was carried out. The study enrolled a total of 74 individuals who had been pre-treated with ART, consisting of two NRTIs for one year followed by three years of HAART containing a PI. All patients had CD4 counts $\geq$350 cells/mm^3 and a plasma viral load of <50 copies/mL and were randomized to three therapy arms:

+ continuous therapy (arm A);
+ CD4 count-guided theory (arm B); and
+ week-on/week-off (WOWO) therapy. The study endpoints were percentage of patients who developed an AIDS-defining condition or who died, and a CD4 count of $\geq$350 cells/mm^3 (arm C).

At week 48, one patient in arm C had an AIDS-defining condition. The proportion of patients with a CD4 count $\geq$350 cells/mm^3 was 100%, 87%, and 96% in treatment arms A, B, and C, respectively. Notably, 30% of patients in the WOWO group (arm C) experienced virologic failure. Weeks of antiretroviral drug use were 100%, 41.1% and 69.8% in arms A, B and C, respectively, and adverse events were not significantly different among the three arms. The HIV RNA suppression rate was similar in patients treated with continuous HAART and in those re-treated with 12 to 24 weeks of HAART after CD4 count-guided therapy [48,49].

A larger-scale multinational scheduled treatment interruption (STI) study called 'Staccato' was conducted with a similar study design [50]. A total of 430 HIV-infected patients with CD4 counts greater than 350 cells/mm^3 and viral load less than 50 copies/mL were randomized to continued therapy (n=146) or scheduled treatment interruptions (n=284). The results showed that drug savings with scheduled treatment interruption were substantial, and no evidence of increased treatment resistance emerged. Treatment-related adverse events were more frequent with continuous treatment, but low CD4 counts and minor manifestations of HIV infection were more frequent among patients on CD4 count-guided interruptions [50].

Although the Staccato study has shown a positive result favouring the CD4 count-guided strategy, the Strategies for Management of Antiretroviral Therapy (SMART) study, a much larger randomized, clinical endpoint, CD4 count-guided trial (including 2720 patients across several countries) has recently reported problems associated with the structured treatment interruption approach [51]. Thus, such an approach is not currently recommended in clinical practice pending further trials [52].

Two (PI plus NRTI) versus three (PI, NRTI, plus viral entry inhibitor) HIV targets

In a 12-week study of 22 patients randomized to receive either: RTV-boosted SQV and EFV with the fusion inhibitor ENF (the three-target arm); or the same without ENF (the two-target arm), there were no differences observed in the mean ±SD elimination rate constant for overall HIV viral decay. Therefore, ART that inhibits HIV reverse transcriptase and protease exerts potent antiviral effects that might not be increased by the addition of an HIV fusion inhibitor. The limitation of this study is, however, its small sample size [53].

Paediatric studies

Neonatal pharmacokinetics

Nelfinavir (NFV)

The pharmacokinetics of NFV in neonates younger than four weeks old was assessed [54]. Three cohorts of HIV-exposed neonates were enrolled to receive 15, 30, or 45 mg of NFV/kg twice daily in combination with d4T and ddI for four weeks after birth. Trough NFV concentrations or C_{min} were measured at one and seven days of age. Intensive pharmacokinetic evaluations were performed at 14 and 28 days of age. The systemic exposure of NFV decreased after seven days of age, possibly because of hepatic enzyme maturation, autoinduction of NFV metabolism, and/or changes in NFV absorption. The highly variable systemic exposure observed in the study indicates that therapeutic drug monitoring seems warranted to ensure adequate NFV dosing in this population [54].

d4T and ddI

The pharmacokinetics of d4T and ddI in neonates were evaluated [55]. Eight neonates born to HIV-infected mothers were enrolled to receive 1 mg of d4T per kg of body weight twice daily and 100 mg of ddI per $m^{(2)}$ once daily in combination with NFV for four weeks after birth. Pharmacokinetic evaluations were performed at 14 and 28 days of age and demonstrated that systemic levels of exposure to d4T were comparable to those seen in older children, suggesting that the paediatric dose of 1 mg per kg twice daily is appropriate for neonates at 2–4 weeks of age. Levels of exposure to ddI were modestly higher than those seen in older children. Whether this observation warrants a reduction of the ddI dose in neonates remains unclear [55].

Dual boosted PIs pharmacokinetics and efficacy in children

Currently, the best second-line antiretroviral regimen for HIV-infected children who have failed NNRTI-based therapy is unknown. Dual boosted PIs may be an option, but optimal doses are also unknown. We therefore conducted a pilot pharmacokinetics and efficacy study on double-boosted PIs. A total of 12 NRTI-pre-treated children (median age 8.5 years) received 50 mg per kg twice-daily SQV (230 mg/m) and LPV (57.5 mg/m) twice daily. Plasma drug concentrations of SQV, LPV and RTV were at the higher limits of expected ranges for adult treatment at approved dosages [56]. After 24 weeks of treatment, HIV RNA was suppressed below 400 copies/mL for 16 of 20 (80%) children (ITT analysis) and below 50 copies/mL for 12 of 20 children (60%), and CD4 counts rose by a median of 6% (216 cells/mm³) (see Table 21.4). However, there are no evidence-based data to support whether double-boosted PIs versus recycling two NRTIs plus an RTV-boosted PI or versus mono-boosted PIs are suitable options in this population. Therefore, larger controlled trials to find a suitable second-line regimen for NRTI-experienced children are warranted.

HIV-1 drug resistance in Thailand, where subtype CRF_01 AE is predominant

Adult studies

Dual and triple NRTI treatment failure

Multi-NRTI resistance (thymidine analogue-associated mutations (TAMs) and Q151M complexes) and M184V (only in 3TC treatment failure) were commonly found in HIV-1 subtype A/E infections associated with NRTI failure in adults [57]. As shown in Figure 21.5a [57], TAMs

Table 21.4 Pharmacokinetics of protease inhibitors (PI) and boosted PI studies in children

Study	Population	Sample size	Body weight Kg	C_{min} Median , mg/L	C_{max} Median , mg/L	AUC Median , mg.h/L	Comments
nefinavir (NFV) 15, 30, and 45 mg/kg twice daily in neonates[54]	HIV-exposed infant	26 (age <4 weeks, 17 female)	Mean 3.3-3.5 ± 3 kg	**NFV 15 mg/kg** (n=6) C_{min} = 0.19, 1.21, 0.51, and 0.33 at 1, 7, 14, and 28 days of age	C_{max} =1.82 and 1.13 at 14 and 28 days of age	AUC_{0-12h}= 14.4 and 8.7 at 14 and 28 days of age	The systemic exposure of NFV decreased after 7 days of age, possibly because of hepatic enzyme maturation, autoinduction of NFV metabolism, and/or changes in NFV absorption.
				NFV 30 mg/kg (n=5) C_{min} =1.02, 3.18, 0.73, and 0.55 at 1, 7, 14, and 28 days of age	C_{max} = 2.64 and 1.73 at 14, and 28 days of age	AUC_{0-12h}= 19.4 and 15.8 at 14 and 28 days of age	
				NFV 45 mg/kg (n=11) C_{min} =0.67, 3.21, 0.70, and 0.73 at 1, 7, 14, and 28 days of age	C_{max} = 2.81 and 2.09 at 14, and 28 days of age	AUC_{0-12h}= 23.4 and 18.5 at 14 and 28 days of age	
stavudine (d4T) 1 mg/kg bid[55]	HIV-exposed infant	8	3.3 (mean)	NA	0.46 (day 14 PK)	1.87 (day 14 PK)	The results suggesting that the paediatric dose of 1 mg/kg twice daily is appropriate for neonates at 2-4 weeks of age.
didanosine (ddl) 100 mg of ddl per m2 once daily[55]				NA	1.57 (day 14 PK)		Levels of exposure to ddl were modestly higher than those seen in children. Whether requiring for ddl dose reduction in neonates is unclear.
double boosted PI: Kaletra/ ritonavir/saquinavir in children[56]	NNRTI-failure	20 (female 14, median age 8.5 years old)	Median (IQR) 19.5 (17.3–24.5)	SQV 1.4 LPV 5.9	SQV 1.4	SQV 39.4 LPV 118	At week 24, 16 of 20 (80%) children had HIV RNA <400 copies/mL and 12 of 20 (60%) <50 copies/mL

Sources: as indicated in superscript within the Table.

were detected in 80% of patients (or more) who failed any dual or even triple NRTI treatment. In our studies, 20% of patients who failed d4T/ddI treatment had Q151M complexes. Thus, suboptimal and dual NRTI therapy is not recommended for global application [56,57].

NNRTI treatment failure

The resistance profiles of NNRTI-based first-line treatment failure among Thai patients, who are predominantly infected with recombinant subtype CRF_01 AE infection, were investigated [59] (Figure 21.6a and 21.6b) [59]. The prevalence of drug resistance was found to be high among the 64 HIV-infected Thai patients who failed NNRTI-based regimens. Eighty-nine per cent of patients had one or more NNRTI mutation resistances, almost all patients had resistance to at least one NRTI, and 42% had multiple-NRTI resistance (with >3 TAMs and/or Q151M complexes) [57]. Patients who had a longer treatment exposure, i.e., more than 48 weeks, had a higher risk of multi-drug resistant (MDR) mutation (relative risk 5.12; 95% CI:1.035–25.316, p=0.045). This observation suggests that in patients with longer-term NNRTI-based treatment failure, it will not be feasible to have an active NRTI backbone available for approximately 40% of patients. The optimal second-line regimen for these patients remains unknown. Determining whether recycled 3TC with or without AZT in combination with an RTV-boosted PI, or whether a mono-boosted PI is efficacious in such circumstances, requires a controlled study.

There are few data on the selection of resistance by RTV-boosted SQV, particularly in treatment-naïve patients. A study to assess the incidence of virologic failure and the evolution of resistance in treatment-naïve individuals receiving RTV-boosted SQV was conducted in the induction phase of the Staccato trial. Treatment-naïve subjects (n=272) received SQV (1600 mg) boosted with RTV (100 mg) once daily with two NRTIs for at least 24 weeks. Patients were defined as having virologic failure when there were two consecutive HIV-1 RNA measurements >500 copies/mL after week 12. Viral genotypes (reverse transcriptase (RT) and protease (PRO)) were determined at baseline in all patients and as close as possible to the time of initial failure in patients experiencing virologic failure. It was found that RTV-boosted SQV plus two NRTIs (1600/100 mg once daily) resulted in a low rate of viral rebound (3.3%). Among patients with virologic failure, no major HIV protease mutations were detected, but two out of eight patients (25%) displayed single new minor PRO substitutions (M36I, L10I) at the time of virologic failure that were known or suspected not to have been present at baseline; both these substitutions exist as natural polymorphisms. A third patient displayed a single new RT mutation (M184I). Our observations were similar to other reports suggesting that early virologic failure in RTV-boosted PIs is unlikely to be associated with major PI-associated mutations and may preserve future treatment options [13].

Paediatric study: dual NRTI failure

A very high prevalence of NRTI mutations among 95 HIV-infected Thai children who were treated with dual NRTIs was observed, i.e. almost all children had resistance to at least one NRTI, and approximately half of the children had resistance to multiple NRTIs [58] (see Figure 21.5b).

Conclusions

Thailand is a country in which the prevalence of HIV infection is high, the common circulating HIV-1 infection is subtype CRF_01AE, and patients are non-Caucasian and have low body weight on average. In Asian countries with high rates of HIV infection, where the common HIV-1 subtype is non-B and the ethnic population differs from those studied in most of the pharmacokinetics and clinical trials conducted in the West, it is essential to generate population-specific, evidence-based clinical and therapeutic information to guide national practice guidelines, and,

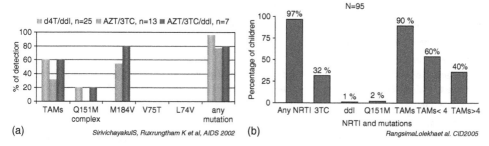

(a)

SirivichayakulS, Ruxrungtham K et al, AIDS 2002

(b)

RangsimaLolekhaet al. CID2005

Fig. 21.5 (a) Thymidine analogue-associated mutations (TAMs) were commonly detected among HIV-1-infected adults who had failed dual NRTI regimens·
(b) Thymidine analogue-associated mutations (TAMs) were commonly detected among HIV-1-infected children who had failed dual NRTI regimens.

therefore, committed research organizations need to play a significant role in collecting such data. HIV-NAT, under the Thai Red Cross AIDS Research Centre, one of the collaborating international research organizations in Thailand, has generated a number of HIV-related clinical research studies relevant to Thai, Asian and global applications (see Table 21.5).

Based on results from several HIV-NAT studies and collaborating cohorts, key observations include:

- HIV-1 CRF01_AE subtype has a similar virologic response rate and genotypic resistance profile to subtype B;

- due to generally low average body weights of Thai patients, some antiretroviral drugs, such as d4T, RTV-boosted IDV, and possibly other boosted PIs such as SQV and LPV, can be administered at a lower dose than those recommended in other settings;

- in TB/HIV co-infection where patients are treated with rifampicin, there is no need to increase EFV from 600 to 800 mg per day; and

- NVP can also be used effectively as an alternative if EFV cannot be prescribed.

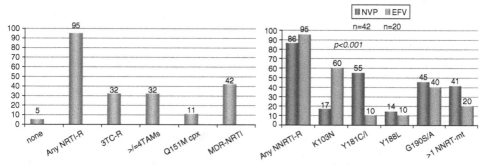

Fig. 21.6 NNRTI-based treatment failure and resistance profiles. High rates of multiple NRTI drug resistances were observed in adult patients who failed NNRTI regimens·

Table 21.5 Highlights of HIV-NAT trials and cohort studies

1. HIV-1 CRF01AE, the most common subtype prevalence in Thailand, showed a similar response and drug resistance mutations profile to subtype B.

2. In resource-limited settings, dose d4T and low-dose IDV/r (400/100 mg bid) have been shown to be efficacious and more tolerable, and may be a suitable alternative treatment options while waiting for more tolerable ARVs such as TDF and other bPI to be accessible. However, the major trade-off is adverse events i.e., d4T-related lipodystrophy and IDV-related nephrotoxicity.

3. Antiretroviral-related adverse effects:

   a. The incidence of NNRTI-related rash were high, i.e., 20% EFV-related, 21% NVP twice daily-related, and 38% NVP once daily-related. The proportions of grade III rash were EFV 2.9%; NVP BID 2.3%; and NVP QD 6.4%. Females, and persons with earlier HIV disease or with a large rise in CD4+ cell count after starting therapy are at greater risk for NNRTI-related rash.

   b. Approximately one-fifth of patients had grade III/IV toxicities. Thus, in a resource-limited setting, the simple and inexpensive monitoring of ALT and haemoglobin could prevent the most serious short-term toxicity. Long-term toxicity can be addressed with a yearly monitoring of triglycerides, cholesterol, glucose and creatinine if nephrotoxic drugs such as indinavir are used.

   c. The predictors of ARV-related severe hepatotoxicity were HBV or HCV co-infection, and NNRTI-containing therapy.

4. Tuberculosis and HIV co-infection:

   a. In advanced HIV patients with tuberculosis, immune recovery syndrome (IRIS) occurred in 33%, and 30 % had severe AZT induced anaemia.

   b. For patients with tuberculosis and HIV co-infection and taking rifampicin, our studies did not support dose increase of either EFV or NVP. EFV 600 mg/day should be sufficient when taken with RIF by patients with body weight of approximately 50 kg.

   c. In settings where EFV and rifabutin are not affordable or accessible, or when patients can not tolerate EFV, NVP can be recommended as an alternative NNRTI to co-administer with RIF. However, the lead-in strategy at 200 mg once daily for the first two weeks should be avoided because it was associated with suboptimal NVP level among most of the patients. An increase in NVP dose to 300 mg twice daily was shown to be associated with a high risk of NVP-related hypersensitivity syndrome and hence should not be recommended.

5. There is clearly a need to find an alternative booster for PIs beside ritonavir to minimize ritonavir-associated metabolic adverse effects and, if possible, to minimize cost for resource-limited settings. However, our PK studies conclude that ketoconazole showed no significant boosting effect, whereas itraconazole showed a significant boosting effect to SQV; however, the PK enhancement was significantly lower than that of ritonavir.

6. HIV-1 drug resistance in high-prevalence CRF_01 AE infection:

   a. Almost all patients who failed dual NRTIs or first-line 2NRTIs+NNRTI carried at least one thymidine-analogue-associated mutation (TAM). Almost a half of patients carried multi-drug resistance (MDR) against NRTIs.

   b. And almost all patients who failed a first-line NNRTI-based regimen developed at least one NNRTI-associated resistant mutation, and one-third showed more than one NNRTI mutation. These observations lead to the challenges of choosing a second-line in majority of first line NNRTI-based antiretroviral treatment failure.

   c. Similar to other observations, patients treated with boosted protease inhibitors (in our case saquinavir boosted with ritonavir) who had an early virologic failure showed no findings of new major PI-associated resistant mutations.

Table 21.5 (continued) Highlights of HIV-NAT trials and cohort studies

7. Low-dose boosted PIs such as SQV/r 1600/100mg once daily and IDV/r 400/100 mg twice daily have been shown efficacious in treatment-naïve patients. Further studies to investigate other low-dose bPIs appropriate for Asian population i.e., LPV/r 200/100 mg BID and ATV/r 200/100 mg BID in adults, are under way.
8. Boosted PI pharmacokinetics study in children has shown that currently recommended doses were associated with a high-level exposure, particularly for LPV/r. Thus, studies on lower-dose boosted PIs are being carried out.

In addition, NNRTI-associated sensitivity—skin reaction, in particular—is much more common among Thai patients when compared against Western reports (see Table 21.5).

Finally, a most significant development in Thailand has been the establishment of the Universal Coverage (UC) Programme for HIV Prevention and Care implemented in mid-2007 through the National Health Security Office. Conducting more relevant operational research as well as high-quality clinical research will further strengthen and provide policy and clinical management guidance to this important national HIV/AIDS programme.

Acknowledgements

The author wishes to thank Professors Praphan Phanuphak, David A Cooper and Joep MA Lange for their guidance and support. Thanks, too, to our key collaborators: David Burger, Bernard Hirschel, Reto Nuesch, Andrew Hills, Sean Emery, Ploenchan Chetchotisakd, Weerawat Manosuthi, Surapol Suwanagool, Sunee Sirivichayakul and Supranee Burnaprditkul. And finally, thanks to all HIV-NAT trial coordinating physicians: Drs Jintanat Ananworanich, Chris Duncombe, Mark Boyd, Anchalee Avihingsanon, Eugene Kroon, Chaiwat Ungsedhapand, Saskia Autar, Peter Cardiello, Chokechai Rongkavilit and Jasper Van der Lugt, and to all the HIV-NAT teams.

References

1. Ruxrungtham K, Brown T, Phanuphak P. (2004). HIV/AIDS in Asia. *Lancet* **364**:69–82.

2. Kroon ED, Ungsedhapand C, Ruxrungtham K, Chuenyam M, *et al.* (2000). A randomized, double-blind trial of half versus standard dose of zidovudine plus zalcitabine in Thai HIV-1-infected patients (study HIV-NAT 001). HIV Netherlands Australia Thailand Research Collaboration. *AIDS* **14**:1349–56.

3. Ruxrungtham K, Kroon ED, Ungsedhapand C, Teeratakulpisarn S, *et al.* (2000). A randomized, dose-finding study with didanosine plus stavudine versus didanosine alone in antiviral-naive, HIV-infected Thai patients. *AIDS* **14**:1375–82.

4. Siangphoe U, Srikaew S, Waiwaravuth C, *et al.* (2004). Efficacy and safety of half dose compared to full dose stavudine (d4T) and zidovudine (AZT) in combination with didanosine (ddI) in Thai HIV-infected patients: 96 week results of ACTT002/ARV065 study. The XV International AIDS Conference, 11–16 July 2004, Bangkok, Thailand. [Abstract WePeB5952]

5. Hill A, Ruxrungtham K, Havanich M, *et al.* (2006). Meta-analysis of efficacy and safety for clinical studies of d4T 40 mg versus 30 mg BID in 1008 patients. The XVI International AIDS Conference, 13–18 August 2006, Toronto, Canada. [Abstract THPE0120]

6. Hammers SM, Saag MS, Schechter M, *et al.* (2006). Treatment for Adult HIV Infection 2006 Recommendations of the International AIDS Society–USA Panel. *JAMA* **296**:827–843.

7. Burger D, Boyd M, Duncombe C, *et al.* (2003). Pharmacokinetics and pharmacodynamics of indinavir with or without low-dose ritonavir in HIV-infected Thai patients. *J Antimicrob Chemother* **51**:1231–8.

8. Boyd M, Mootsikapun P, Burger D, *et al.* (2005). Pharmacokinetics of reduced-dose indinavir/ritonavir 400/100 mg twice daily in HIV-1-infected Thai patients. *Antivir Ther* **10**:301–7.

9. Mootsikapun P, Chetchotisakd P, Anunnatsiri S, Boonyaprawit P. (2005). Efficacy and safety of indinavir/ritonavir 400/100 mg twice daily plus two nucleoside analogues in treatment-naive HIV-1-infected patients with CD4+ T-cell counts <200 cells/mm3: 96-week outcomes. *Antivir* Ther **1**:911–6.

10. Cardiello P, Srasuebkul P, Hassink E, *et al.* (2005). The 48-week efficacy of once-daily saquinavir/ritonavir in patients with undetectable viral load after 3 years of antiretroviral therapy. *HIV Med* **6**:122–8.

11. Ananworanich J, Gayet-Ageron A, Le Braz M, *et al.* (2006). Staccato Study Group. CD4-guided scheduled treatment interruptions compared with continuous therapy for patients infected with HIV-1: results of the Staccato randomised trial. *Lancet* **368**:459–65.

12. Ananworanich J, Hill A, Siangphoe U, *et al.* (2005). Staccato Study Group. A prospective study of efficacy and safety of once-daily saquinavir/ritonavir plus two nucleoside reverse transcriptase inhibitors in treatment-naive Thai patients. *Antivir Ther* **10**:761–7.

13. Ananworanich J, Hirschel B, Sirivichayakul S, *et al.* (2006). Staccato Study Team. Absence of resistance mutations in antiretroviral-naïve patients treated with ritonavir-boosted saquinavir. *Antivir Ther* **11**:631–5.

14. Ungsedhapand C, Kroon ED, Suwanagool S, *et al.* (2001). A randomized, open-label, comparative trial of zidovudine plus lamivudine versus zidovudine plus lamivudine plus didanosine in antiretroviral-naïve HIV-1-infected Thai patients. *J Acquir Immune Defic Syndr* **27**:116–23.

15. Ungsedhapand C, Srasuebkul P, Cardiello P, *et al.*, on behalf of the HIV-NAT 002 and HIV-NAT 003 Study Team. (2004). Three-year durability of dual-nucleoside versus triple-nucleoside therapy in a Thai population with HIV infection. *J Acquir Immune Defic Syndr* **36**:693–701.

16. Gulick RM, Ribaudo HJ, Shikuma CM, *et al.* (2004). Triple-nucleoside regimens versus efavirenz-containing regimens for the initial treatment of HIV-1 infection. *N Engl J Med* **350**:1850–61.

17. Boyd MA, Srasuebkul P, Khongphattanayothin M, *et al.* (2006). Boosted versus unboosted indinavir with zidovudine and lamivudine in nucleoside pre-treated patients: a randomized, open-label trial with 112 weeks of follow-up (HIV-NAT 005). *Antivir Ther* **11**:223–32.

18. Boyd MA, Siangphoe U, Ruxrungtham K, *et al.* (2006). The use of pharmacokinetically guided indinavir dose reductions in the management of indinavir-associated renal toxicity. *J Antimicrob Chemother* **57**:1161–7.

19. Boyd MA, Siangphoe U, Ruxrungtham K, *et al.* (2005). Indinavir/ritonavir 800/100 mg bid and efavirenz 600 mg qd in patients failing treatment with combination nucleoside reverse transcriptase inhibitors: 96-week outcomes of HIV-NAT 009. *HIV Med* **6**:410–20.

20. Boyd MA, Carr A, Ruxrungtham K, *et al.* (2006). Changes in body composition and mitochondrial nucleic acid content in patients switched from failed nucleoside analogue therapy to ritonavir-boosted indinavir and efavirenz. *J Infect Dis* **194**:642–50.

21. Nuesch R, Srasuebkul P, Ananworanich J, Ruxrungtham K, Phanuphak P, Duncombe C, HIV-NAT Study Team. (2006). Monitoring the toxicity of antiretroviral therapy in resource limited settings: a prospective clinical trial cohort in Thailand. *J Antimicrob Chemother* **58**:637–44.

22. Ananworanich J, Moor Z, Siangphoe U, *et al.* (2005). Incidence and risk factors for rash in Thai patients randomized to regimens with nevirapine, efavirenz or both drugs. *AIDS* **19**:185–92.

23. Law WP, Dore GJ, Duncombe CJ, *et al.* (2003). Risk of severe hepatotoxicity associated with antiretroviral therapy in the HIV-NAT Cohort, Thailand, 1996–2001. *AIDS* **17**:2191–9.

24. Boyd MA, Srasuebkul P, Ruxrungtham K, *et al.* (2006). Relationship between hyperbilirubinaemia and UDP-glucuronosyltransferase 1A1 (UGT1A1) polymorphism in adult HIV-infected Thai patients treated with indinavir. *Pharmacogenet Genomics* **16**:321–9.

25. Avihingsanon A, Avihingsanon Y, Darnpornprasert P, *et al.* (2006). High prevalence of indinavir-associated renal complications in Thai HIV-infected patients. *J Med Assoc Thai* **89**:S21–7.

26. Law WP, Duncombe CJ, Mahanontharit A, *et al.* (2004). Impact of viral hepatitis co-infection on response to antiretroviral therapy and HIV disease progression in the HIV-NAT cohort. *AIDS* **18**:1169–77.

27. Ribera E, Pou L, Lopez RM, *et al.* (2001). Pharmacokinetic interaction between nevirapine and rifampicin in HIV-infected patients with tuberculosis. *J Acquir Immune Defic Syndr* **28**:450–3.

28. Lopez-Cortes LF, Ruiz-Valderas R, Viciana P, *et al.* (2002). Pharmacokinetic interactions between efavirenz and rifampicin in HIV-infected patients with tuberculosis. *Clin Pharmacokinet* **41**:681–90.

29. Ramachandran G, Hemanthkumar AK, Rajasekaran S, *et al.* (2006). Increasing nevirapine dose can overcome reduced bioavailability due to rifampicin coadministration. *J Acquir Immune Defic Syndr* **42**:36–41.

30. Manosuthi W, Sungkanuparph S, Thakkinstian A, *et al.* (2005). Efavirenz levels and 24-week efficacy in HIV-infected patients with tuberculosis receiving highly active antiretroviral therapy and rifampicin. *AIDS* **19**:1481–6.

31. Manosuthi W, Kiertiburanakul S, Sungkanuparph S, *et al.* (2006). Efavirenz 600 mg/day versus efavirenz 800 mg/day in HIV-infected patients with tuberculosis receiving rifampicin: 48 weeks results. *AIDS* **20**:131–132.

32. Autar RS, Wit FW, Sankote J, *et al.* (2005). Nevirapine plasma concentrations and concomitant use of rifampin in patients coinfected with HIV-1 and tuberculosis. *Antivir Ther* **10**:937–43.

33. Manosuthi W, Sungkanuparph S, Thakkinstian A, *et al.* (2006). Plasma nevirapine levels and 24-week efficacy in HIV-infected patients receiving nevirapine-based highly active antiretroviral therapy with or without rifampicin. *Clin Infect Dis* **43**:253–5.

34. Manosuthi W, Ruxrungtham K, Likanonsakul S, *et al.* (2007). Nevirapine levels after discontinuation of rifampicin therapy and 60-week efficacy of nevirapine-based antiretroviral therapy in HIV-infected patients with tuberculosis. *Clin Infect Dis* **44**:141–4.

35. Avihingsanon A, Manosuthi W, Kantipong P, *et al.* (2007). Pharmacokinetics and 12 Weeks Efficacy of Nevirapine, 400 mg vs 600 mg per day in HIV-infected Patients with Active TB Receiving Rifampicin: A Multicenter Study. The 14th Conference on Retroviruses and Opportunistic Infections (CROI), 25–28 February 2007, Los Angeles, CA, USA. [Abstract 576]

36. Autar RS, Ananworanich J, Apateerapong W, *et al.* (2004). Pharmacokinetic study of saquinavir hard gel caps/ritonavir in HIV-1-infected patients: 1600/100 mg once-daily compared with 2000/100 mg once-daily and 1000/100 mg twice-daily. *J Antimicrob Chemother* **54**:785–90.

37. Autar RS, Boffito M, Hassink E, *et al.* (2005). Interindividual variability of once-daily ritonavir boosted saquinavir pharmacokinetics in Thai and UK patients. *J Antimicrob Chemother* **56**:908–13.

38. Cardiello PG, Samor T, Burger D, *et al.* (2003). Pharmacokinetics of lower doses of saquinavir soft-gel caps (800 and 1200 mg twice daily) boosted with itraconazole in HIV-1-positive patients. *Antivir Ther* **8**:245–9.

39. Khaliq Y, Gallicano K, Venance S, *et al.* (2000). Effect of ketoconazole on ritonavir and saquinavir concentrations in plasma and cerebrospinal fluid from patients infected with human immunodeficiency virus. *Clin Pharmacol Ther* **68**:637–46.

40. Grub S, Bryson H, Goggin T, *et al.* (2001). The interaction of saquinavir (soft gelatin capsule) with ketoconazole, erythromycin and rifampicin: comparison of the effect in healthy volunteers and in HIV-infected patients. *Eur J Clin Pharmacol* **57**:115–21.

41. Autar RS, Sankote J, Wit F, *et al.* (2005). Boosting of saquinavir with ritonavir or ketoconazole. The 6th International Workshop on Clinical Pharmacology of HIV Therapy, 28–30 April 2005, Québec, Canada. [Abstract 8.1]

42. Van der Lugt J, Autar S, Ubolyam S, *et al.* (2007). Pharmacokinetics and Pharmacodynamics of a Double-boosted PI Regimen of Saquinavir and Lopinavir/Ritonavir in Treatment-naive HIV-1-infected Adults. The 14th Conference on Retroviruses and Opportunistic Infections (CROI), February 25–28 2007, Los Angeles, CA, USA. [Abstract 578]

43. Ruxrungtham K, Boyd M, Bellibas SE, *et al.* (2004). Lack of interaction between enfuvirtide and ritonavir or ritonavir-boosted saquinavir in HIV-1-infected patients. *J Clin Pharmacol* **44**:793–803.

44. Boyd MA, Zhang X, Dorr A, *et al.* (2003). Lack of enzyme-inducing effect of rifampicin on the pharmacokinetics of enfuvirtide. *J Clin Pharmacol* **43**:1382–91.

45. Ananworanich J, Siangphoe U, Mahanontharit A, *et al.* (2004). Saquinavir trough concentration before and after switching NRTI to tenofovir in patients treated with once-daily saquinavir hard gel capsule/ritonavir 1600 mg/100 mg. *Antivir Ther* **9**:1035–6.

46. Duncombe C, Kerr SJ, Ruxrungtham K, *et al.* (2005). HIV disease progression in a patient cohort treated via a clinical research network in a resource limited setting. *AIDS* **19**:169–78.

47. Ruxrungtham K, Suwanagool S, Tavel JA, *et al.* (2000). A randomized, controlled 24-week study of intermittent subcutaneous interleukin-2 in HIV-1 infected patients in Thailand. *AIDS* **14**:2509–13.

48. Cardiello PG, Hassink E, Ananworanich J, *et al.* (2005). A prospective, randomized trial of structured treatment interruption for patients with chronic HIV type 1 infection. *Clin Infect Dis* **40**:594–600.

49. Ananworanich J, Siangphoe U, Hill A, *et al.* (2005). Highly active antiretroviral therapy (HAART) retreatment in patients on CD4-guided therapy achieved similar virologic suppression compared with patients on continuous HAART: the HIV Netherlands Australia Thailand Research Collaboration 001.4 study. *J Acquir Immune Defic Syndr* **39**:523–9.

50. Ananworanich J, Gayet-Ageron A, Le Braz M, *et al.* Staccato Study Group; Swiss HIV Cohort Study. (2006). CD4-guided scheduled treatment interruptions compared with continuous therapy for patients infected with HIV-1: results of the Staccato randomised trial. *Lancet* **368**:459–65.

51. The Strategies for Management of Antiretroviral Therapy (SMART) Study Group. (2006). CD4+ Count–Guided Interruption of Antiretroviral Treatment. *N Engl J Med* **355**:2283–96.

52. Sledge M. (2006). Structured treatment interruptions: after SMART. *BETA* **18**:30–6.

53. Boyd MA, Dixit NM, Siangphoe U, *et al.* (2006). Viral decay dynamics in HIV-infected patients receiving ritonavir-boosted saquinavir and efavirenz with or without enfuvirtide: a randomized, controlled trial (HIV-NAT 012). *J Infect Dis* **194**:1319–22.

54. Rongkavilit C, van Heeswijk RP, Limpongsanurak S, *et al.* (2002). Dose-escalating study of the safety and pharmacokinetics of nelfinavir in HIV-exposed neonates. *J Acquir Immune Defic Syndr* **29**:455–63.

55. Rongkavilit C, Thaithumyanon P, Chuenyam T, *et al.* (2001). Pharmacokinetics of stavudine and didanosine coadministered with nelfinavir in human immunodeficiency virus-exposed neonates. *Antimicrob Agents Chemother* **45**:3585–90.

56. Ananworanich J, Kosalaraksa P, Hill A, *et al*, the HIV-NAT 017 Study Team. (2005). Pharmacokinetics and 24-Week Efficacy/Safety of Dual Boosted Saquinavir/Lopinavir/Ritonavir in Nucleoside-Pretreated Children. *Pediatr Infect Dis J* **24**:874–879.

57. Sirivichayakul S, Ruxrungtham K, Ungsedhapand C, *et al.* (2003). Nucleoside analogue mutations and Q151M in HIV-1 subtype A/E infection treated with nucleoside reverse transcriptase inhibitors. *AIDS* **17**:1889–96.

58. Lolekha R, Sirivichayakul S, Siangphoe U, *et al.* (2005). Resistance to dual nucleoside reverse-transcriptase inhibitors in children infected with HIV clade A/E. *Clin Infect Dis* **40**:309–12.

59. Chetchotisakd P, Anunnatsiri S, Kiertiburanakul S, *et al.*, HIV-NAT Study Team. (2006). High rate multiple drug resistances in HIV-infected patients failing non-nucleoside reverse transcriptase inhibitor regimens in Thailand, where subtype A/E is predominant. *J Int Assoc Physicians AIDS Care* **5**:152–6.

Part 4

HAART in low human development countries

Chapter 22

Country review: Haiti

Serena Koenig*, Julia Carney, Peter Bendix and Jean William Pape

Introduction

Haiti is the poorest country in the western hemisphere and one of the poorest in the world. It ranks 154th of 177 countries on the human development index [1] and has the worst health statistics in the Caribbean. Life expectancy is less than 52 years, the per capita income is under US$1 per day, and more than 60% of the population is unemployed [2]. Poverty and illiteracy are rampant, and there are only 25 physicians for every 100,000 people [1]. These statistics make Haiti more closely identified with African nations than aligned with countries in its region.

The history of HIV/AIDS and Haiti is complicated; it is largely the story of stigma, discrimination, poverty and racism. Early in the epidemic, the US Centers for Disease Control and Prevention (CDC) classified Haitians as a risk group. While studies later showed that Haitians share the same risks as others, the damage was done; HIV/AIDS and Haiti were married in the minds of the public. Such national stigmatization had immediate social and psychological consequences and agitated an already precarious economic state.

After two decades of a generalized epidemic, Haiti has the highest prevalence of HIV outside of sub-Saharan Africa. The outbreak has been fuelled by poor socio-economic status and inadequate health and social services, areas that are difficult to improve given the country's chronic political instability and high internal migration rates. Nevertheless, Haiti has waged one of the world's most successful campaigns against the disease. It is one of the few countries with a declining disease prevalence; the percentage of Haitian adults living with HIV decreased from 6.2% to 3.1% between 1993 and 2003 [3], and the most recent survey of adults in 2006 (10,757 women and 4958 men), found it to be 2.2% [unpublished data, 2006 from *l'Institut Haitien de l'Enfance* (IHE)/ *Groupe Haitien d'Étude du Sarcome de Kaposi et des Infections Opportunistes* (GHESKIO)].

Haiti was one of the first countries in the developing world to offer widespread access to highly active antiretroviral therapy (HAART). By the end of 2006, almost 9500 people had received HAART and experienced outcomes rivalling those of the United States [4]. Haiti's innovative strategies have served as a model for other nations, as they provide social support, women's health services, and treatment for tuberculosis (TB) and other co-morbid conditions [5]. Many of these successes can be attributed to strong non-governmental organizations (NGOs), nationwide prevention efforts and high-level government commitment early in the country's HIV epidemic.

---

* Corresponding author

Epidemiology

The early years of the epidemic

The CDC created a national surveillance task force for Kaposi's sarcoma (KS) and *Pneumocystis carinii* pneumoniae (PCP) in 1981, as these diseases were reported in a very unusual pattern among otherwise healthy, young homosexual men [6]. Subsequent cases were described in haemophiliacs, heterosexual partners of people with AIDS, injection drug users (IDUs), and recipients of blood transfusions. Thirty-four cases were also noted in Haitians who lived in Florida and New York [7].

Physicians could not categorize the Haitian patients by the classic HIV risk factors. The patients denied any history of homosexual sex, and none said they had used drugs, shared needles, or received a blood transfusion [8–10]. The CDC thus inferred that Haitians, as a group, had unique risk factors for the syndrome. The CDC Task Force on AIDS argued that certain factors—such as being Haitian—could help organize future cases: 'AIDS cases may be separated into groups based on these risk factors: homosexual or bisexual males—75 percent, intravenous drug abusers with no history of male homosexual activity—13 percent, Haitians with neither a history of homosexuality nor a history of intravenous drug abuse—6 percent, persons with haemophilia A who were not Haitians, homosexuals or intravenous drug abusers— 0.3 percent, and persons in none of these groups—5 percent' [11]. Haitians were labelled a risk group, while the racial identities of other patients were never revealed.

The association between Haitians and HIV/AIDS spread rapidly through the American public, and Haiti and AIDS became inextricably linked in people's minds. The US news at the time was already rife with articles about the thousands of Haitians who had fled to Miami to escape extreme poverty and the regime of deposed President Jean-Claude Duvalier. The media was not sympathetic; Haitians were blamed for causing the epidemic and for bringing it to the United States. They were depicted as impoverished 'boat people' and as exotic worshipers of sorcery and voodoo. Some suggested that Haitians had become infected by 'monkeys as part of bizarre sexual practices in Haitian brothels,' even though the country had no such animal in the wild or in captivity [12]. Reputable medical journals published theories that buttressed these claims. A letter to the editor of the *Journal of the American Medical Association* (*JAMA*) in 1986, for example, described the correlation between Haiti and HIV/AIDS: 'Even now, many Haitians are voodoo serviteurs and partake in its rituals (*New York Times*, May 15, 1985, pp1,6). (Some also are members of secret societies such as Bizango or "impure" sects, called "cabrit thomazo", which are suspected to use human blood itself in sacrificial worship)' [13].

The stigmatization of Haitians and Haiti wrought devastating consequences. The tourism industry was severely crippled. The number of visitors to the country dropped dramatically. During the winter of 1981–2, the Bureau of Tourism estimated that there were 75,000 foreign travellers. By the following year, the figure was fewer than 10,000 [14]. The tourist industry had been a major employer of Haitians and a generator of foreign currency. Its abrupt collapse aggravated a fragile situation: 'Already suffering from an image problem, Haiti has been made an international pariah by AIDS. Boycotted by tourists and investors, it has lost millions of dollars and hundreds of jobs at a time when half the work force is jobless. Even exports are being shunned by some' [15]. The economy never recovered.

Shortly after being reported in the United States, KS was diagnosed in Haiti among 11 previously healthy young people [16]. The emergence of HIV/AIDS in Haiti caused great consternation among native medical professionals, who were already concerned about the country's declining image, depleting resources and worsening political situation. The presence of the disease created fears that a new and worrying epidemic had developed, and prompted 13 physicians and scientists to form the Haitian Study Group on Kaposi's Sarcoma and Opportunistic Infections (GHESKIO) in 1982—an organization they immediately affiliated with the Weill Medical College of Cornell University. GHESKIO sought to study the syndrome in its own country and focused its efforts towards operational research, patient care and the training of community leaders and medical personnel for the treatment of HIV/AIDS, TB and other communicable illnesses.

GHESKIO published the first series of case studies on HIV/AIDS in a developing nation in 1983. In their report, they retrospectively diagnosed 61 instances of AIDS from June 1979 to October 1982 using CDC criteria [17]. The cases mirrored those detailed in the United States. They occurred during the same time periods, and it was clear that the patients in both countries were from the same populations. In the Haitian cohort, 85% were men, and 80% lived in Port-au-Prince—largely in the suburb of Carrefour, the hub for male and female sex workers. GHESKIO, however, observed fewer cases of PCP and atypical mycobacteria, more TB, and lower rates of mean survival after diagnosis than the cases in the United States (less than six months mean survival in Haiti compared with more than one year in the United States).

GHESKIO researchers wanted to determine and better understand the risk factors for HIV/AIDS among Haitians. To achieve this, they conducted a variety of studies that elicited specific information about their patients. The results were arresting. In one cohort, GHESKIO found that 22 of the 34 patients (65%) could be classified by HIV/AIDS indicators identified by US physicians: 13 (39%) were bisexual, seven (21%) had received a blood transfusion, and two (6%) had either a history of injection drug use or a spouse with AIDS. The others (35%) probably acquired the disease through heterosexual transmission [18]. By 1988, GHESKIO researchers observed these characteristics among 72% of their HIV-infected patients.

This research indicated that Haitians shared the same HIV/AIDS risk factors as other groups [17–19]. GHESKIO inferred that the studies of HIV/AIDS-infected Haitians in the United States did not account for important cultural considerations. They underscored that Haitians in a foreign place were probably uncomfortable disclosing information regarding sexual orientation, as homosexuality was widely stigmatized in Haiti. The patients, they argued, gave more reliable responses in their own country and language [20].

Other research early in the epidemic also refuted the widespread notion that HIV/AIDS developed in Haiti. Epidemiology studies suggested that the virus travelled first to the United States and then to Haiti via US tourists or natives returning home. Moreover, there was no evidence that HIV was present in Haiti before being reported in the United States. Blood samples from Haitian adults during a 1977–9 outbreak of dengue fever were tested for HIV and found to be negative [21]. No cases were ever documented in Americans who used a blood banking company that purchased Haitian blood in the 1970s. Haitian pathologists also completed thousands of post-mortem studies of people who had died during the 1970s at the Albert Schweitzer Hospital and the General Hospital (*l'Hôpital de l'Université d'Etat d'Haiti*), and found not a single AIDS-defining illness before 1978.

The CDC finally removed Haitians from the risk group category for HIV/AIDS in 1985 [22]. This action, however, was never publicized. The stigma still exists, and many people continue to associate AIDS and its origins with Haiti.

Risk factors

The risks identified for HIV in Haiti quickly changed after the first three years of the epidemic. The proportion of cases attributed to homosexuality/bisexuality plummeted from 50% in 1983 to 1% in 1987 [21]. Since 1985, heterosexual contact has been the predominant route of transmission, and each year more women are infected. In 1983, HIV was five times more common among males than females, but by 1985, the ratio had dropped to 3:1, and then to 2.3:1 in 1987, and to 1.6:1 in 1990. An equal number of men and women were infected in 2000, but by 2006, the prevalence in adults was higher among women [3].

Poverty and gender inequality have made Haitian women particularly vulnerable to HIV/AIDS exposure; multiple studies have shown that these conditions enhance susceptibility to this disease and to other sexually transmitted diseases (STDs) [14,23,24]. In Haiti, researchers at the Albert Schweitzer Hospital have found that economically unstable patients have an increased risk of infection [25]; nearly 30% of women who attended the hospital's antenatal clinics in late 1996 said they had entered a sexual relationship out of economic necessity. These women had more than six times the risk of contracting HIV (odds ratio (OR)=6.3; confidence interval (CI): 2.0–19.7) and more than twice the risk of developing syphilis seropositivity (OR=2.3; CI:1.0–5.2) compared to others. Women observed in antenatal clinics in a Haitian slum were also studied for risk factors of HIV and other STDs [26]. The researchers concluded that illiteracy and low socio-economic status were strongly correlated with a positive syphilis test, and that HIV seropositivity was associated with an unemployed partner.

Females in rural areas are also at risk. Researchers at the *Clinique Bon Sauveur*, the Partners in Health (PIH) medical complex in the village of Cange, for example, conducted a case-control study of HIV/AIDS in rural Haitian women in the mid-1980s [24]. They found that HIV-positive women were more likely to have worked as servants than HIV-negative women (72% versus 4%). They also found that HIV-positive women had a similar number of partners to HIV-negative women (2.7 versus 2.4), but that their partner was far more likely to be a truck driver (48% versus 8%) or a soldier (36% versus 0%) than that of an HIV-negative woman. These studies indicated that men with relative economic security tended to engage in high-risk sexual behaviours and that females in rural areas, who lacked employment opportunities, were forced into sexual relationships because of their financial disadvantages. These women did not have the power to demand that their partners remain monogamous or use a condom.

Another PIH study of women in Cange between 1999 and 2001 had equally grim results. Researchers found that only 51% of the females who presented to the women's health clinic had attended school; 16% had completed the sixth grade. Twenty-three per cent reported that their partners were involved at the time with other women, and 57% said that they had been forced or pressured to have sex. Only 11% had ever used a condom. Two-thirds said that it was not difficult to procure a condom, but a quarter said they had trouble convincing their partners to use one [27]. PIH also found that women who lacked employment opportunities were more susceptible to STDs. Those who worked as domestic servants quadrupled their likelihood of contracting an STD, while those who worked as market vendors and had personal incomes reduced their risk by half.

HIV prevalence in Haiti

The Caribbean has the second highest HIV prevalence in the world, and 65% of cases are located in Haiti, which thus bears the overwhelming burden in the region. Disease prevalence has been carefully monitored with studies conducted at regular intervals. The best methods of surveillance have been observations of the general population, in particular of pregnant women who present for antenatal visits.

Once introduced into Haiti, the virus quickly spread throughout the country. As noted earlier, blood samples from a dengue fever outbreak showed no instances of HIV before 1978 [21]. Within a decade, however, the rate of prevalence had soared. It was 8.4 % in 1990 among women who sought antenatal care in Cité Soleil, a slum in the outskirts of Port-au-Prince [28]. This figure rose to 9.9% in 1987 and to 10.5% by 1989. Women appeared to acquire the infection shortly after becoming sexually active, with pregnant women from ages 14 to 19 having a prevalence of 8%. These patients had only had one sexual partner in the prior year, but had a slightly higher occurrence when compared with other groups. This suggests that they were infected by their first and only partner [28].

GHESKIO researchers described similar rates in the population they examined in Port-au-Prince. In 1986 and 1987, they surveyed sera from 801 healthy adults and reported that the overall prevalence was 8% [29], and in 1988, they observed that 7% of women who sought antenatal care at the General Hospital were infected with HIV [30]. These findings catalyzed a series of cohort and case-control studies that yielded important information about subgroups of patients. In these groups, high prevalence was found among people with low socio-economic status (13%), those who worked in hotels that catered to tourists (12%), and mothers of sick infants (12%). Male and female spouses of HIV-positive patients (55%), and female sex workers (53%) had the highest prevalence in the capital [29].

Rates were somewhat lower in the rural areas. In 1998, 4% of unscreened blood donors from rural Haiti were HIV-positive, as well as 3% of mothers of infants admitted for diarrhoea [20]. Another study conducted in rural Haiti concluded that 6.1% of patients who presented for surgery and 4% of pregnant women were HIV-positive [31].

HIV infection remained widespread through the 1980s and 1990s. Two GHESKIO studies showed that between 1986 and 1992, prevalence in Port-au-Prince increased from 6% to 8%, and from 2% to 4% in the rural areas (Deschapelles and Leogane) [30]. Sentinel surveillance surveys in 1993 and 1996 by the IHE and GHESKIO showed similar statistics. They detected the prevalence of HIV, syphilis and hepatitis B among pregnant women who sought antenatal care in each of Haiti's medical departments. In 1993, HIV/AIDS prevalence was 6.2% among pregnant women, and in 1996, it remained elevated at 5.9 % [32,33]. AIDS had become the leading cause of death among adults in Haiti by 1993.

Shortly thereafter, the prevalence rate dropped (see Figure 22.1). In the sentinel surveillance survey conducted in 2000, HIV/AIDS prevalence was 4.5%, but by 2004, it had decreased to 3.1%. This figure was 50% lower than at the peak of the disease 10 years earlier [3]. The most recent assessment conducted in 2006 illustrates further progress, showing that HIV prevalence among Haitian adults was down to 2.2% [Enquête Mortalité, Morbidité et Utilisation des Services (EMMUS–IV), 2005–2006. Unpublished data].

The reduction of HIV prevalence in Haiti can be explained by a combination of factors. One reason is the Haitian government's commitment to the fight against HIV/AIDS. The government developed a nationwide prevention and treatment plan, supported countrywide efforts to fight

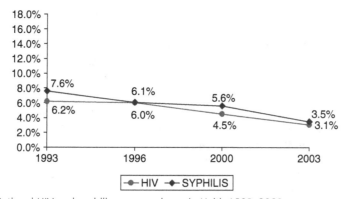

Figure 22.1 National HIV and syphilis seroprevalence in Haiti, 1993–2003
Source: MOH, IHE, GHESKIO

the disease, and secured the blood bank early in the epidemic—a move that prevented countless infections. Strong NGOs have also played a major role. They bolstered a Ministry of Health (MOH) campaign to increase condom use and encourage other safe sex practices, provided countrywide HIV testing and treatment, and expanded access to reproductive health services. Their success is reflected in the concurrent decline in syphilis [34].

Mathematical models have been developed as another way to explain Haiti's decline in prevalence. Hallet et al. found that the decrease in prevalence could only be replicated through decreases in HIV risk associated with safer sexual behaviours [35]. Gaillard et al. attributed the major reasons for the decline in HIV prevalence in Haiti to the more rapid progression from the acquisition of HIV infection to death, as well as the government's early interventions to secure the blood supply. They also found an increase in abstinence, fidelity and condom use [34].

Presenting illnesses among HIV-1 patients

Of the first 61 cases of HIV/AIDS described in Haiti in 1983, 16 had KS and 31 had confirmed diagnoses of opportunistic infections (OIs) as follows: 26 had candida esophogitis, one had aspergillosis, two had disseminated cryptococcosis, six had PCP pneumonia, two had central nervous system toxoplasmosis, three had cryptosporidiosis, 11 had TB, five had anogenital herpes infection, and six had disseminated cytomegalovirus. The 15 people with probable HIV/AIDS had candida esophogitis. All presented with weight loss. Ninety-one per cent had diarrhoea at the time of diagnosis, while all patients experienced it during the course of the illness [17].

Additional studies confirmed these findings. A review of 42 patients showed that 39 (95%) had chronic diarrhoea for up to 33 months. Among those diagnosed with OIs, 88% had oesophogeal candidiasis, 31% had intestinal cryptosporidiosis, and 22% had TB. Significant weight loss (in 95%), fatigue (in 95%), chronic fever (in 90%), and skin lesions (in 54%) were also common [36]. In a later case study, GHESKIO documented 144 more patients with HIV/AIDS; 13 had KS and 131 had OIs. Of patients with such infections, 68% had candidiasis, 48% had cryptosporidiosis, 31% had mycobacterium, 16% had genital herpes, 16% had isospora, 8% had cytomegalovirus, 7% had toxoplasmosis, 7% had PCP pneumonia, 5% had salmonella, 5% had Cryptococcus, and 2% had aspergillus. Among the same group, 84% had chronic or recurrent watery diarrhoea, 71% had intermittent or continuous fever, and 70% had progressive weight loss. An AIDS diagnosis was established within two months of presentation in 89% of patients, and 50% died within four months of their initial visit, with 90% dying within a year [37].

Skin rashes were also common. Liautaud et al. [38] observed that nearly 50% of people with HIV/AIDS had pruritic skin lesions without a clearly defined etiology. The lesions were erythematous, round macules, papules, and nodules affecting the arms, legs, trunk and face. In 80% of the patients, these lesions were the presenting manifestation of HIV/AIDS, and they appeared within a mean of eight months before signs of more advanced immunosuppression (KS or an OI). Such lesions did not improve with treatment at the time—the pre-HAART era—and usually persisted throughout the illness.

PIH conducted a study of 200 patients consecutively diagnosed with HIV from 1993 to 1995. More than half the patients presented with TB (46% with pulmonary TB and 8% with extrapulmonary TB). Ten per cent of patients were diagnosed during antenatal screening, and 5% were tested because they had another STD or because their partner had HIV. Eight per cent of patients presented with chronic enteropathies, 6% had weight loss without localizing symptoms, 5% had bacterial pneumonia, 5% had herpes zoster, 4% had strongyloidiasis or Loeffler's syndrome, 2% had enteric fever, and 1% had PCP [39].

In Haiti, progression to AIDS and death occurs more rapidly than in developed country settings. Studies from industrialized nations suggest that the average time from acquisition of

HIV infection to AIDS is 10 years, and from infection to death is 12 years. From 1985 to 1997, GHESKIO conducted a longitudinal study of 42 patients with documented dates of HIV sero-conversion and found that the median time from seroconversion to first HIV symptoms was three years, to AIDS diagnosis was 5.2 years, and to death was 7.4 years [40].

HIV and TB

The TB burden in Haiti is one of the highest in the western hemisphere. The World Health Organization (WHO) estimated the figure at 306 individuals per 100,000 in 2004. Eighty per cent of the adult population is latently infected with *Mycobacteria tuberculosis* and thus tests positive on the purified protein derivative (PPD) skin test. HIV/AIDS has exacerbated the TB epidemic in Haiti. More than 10% of patients co-infected with HIV and latent TB develop active TB each year. GHESKIO conducted a randomized trial that demonstrated that isoniazid prophylaxis could prevent the development of active TB in the majority of these patients [41,42]. They also showed that isoniazid prophylaxis delayed the onset of HIV-associated signs and symptoms, AIDS, and death.

Until recently, multi-drug resistant (MDR)-TB rates were believed to be low in Haiti. A cross-sectional survey of MDR-TB prevalence at GHESKIO's HIV testing centre between January 2000 and December 2002, however, showed a higher than anticipated figure [43]. Every patient in the study with TB symptoms was screened for TB with a sputum culture, and all *Mycobacteria tuber-culosis* isolates (n=330 patients) underwent drug susceptibility testing. MDR-TB was documented in 16 (6%) of 281 patients with primary TB. Of the 115 patients who were HIV-positive with primary TB, 11 (10%) had MDR, and of the 49 with recurrent TB, 10 (20%) had MDR.

For the past decade, PIH has been the only organization treating MDR-TB in Haiti. They serve as the national referral centre for all cases and have had impressive results. Treatment outcomes have been outstanding, equal or superior to those in industrialized nations. GHESKIO is now initiating an MDR-TB treatment programme based on the PIH model in collaboration with PIH, the MOH and the National Tuberculosis Programme.

HIV/AIDS prevention

Efforts to secure the blood supply in Haiti early in the epidemic have prevented significant disease transmission. GHESKIO researchers found, in 1985, that blood transfusions were an important mode of HIV transmission; nearly 4% of all blood donors were HIV-infected, and 40% of HIV-positive Haitian women had a history of blood transfusion [19]. These findings prompted the MOH to establish safer blood-banking procedures. In 1986, it closed the Public Blood Bank, which bought and sold blood, and established the Red Cross as the only authorized organization to give transfusions. It also instituted mandatory behavioural and laboratory screening of all blood products for HIV and other transmissible infections. Blood transfusion, as a result, has not been an important mode of HIV transmission in Haiti.

Nationwide prevention strategies were otherwise limited until 1986, when the Duvalier regime collapsed. In 1987, the first National AIDS Commission was formed, and AIDS was declared to be a priority disease. A year later, the commission expanded to include representatives of the press, the clergy, and the country's ministries of health, education, information, social affairs and transportation. The AIDS Coordination Bureau was created within the MOH to coordinate the actions of NGOs and direct the implementation of national HIV prevention strategies. Many of these state endeavours were unfortunately short-lived, hindered by political strife and frequent changes in administration. The AIDS Coordination Bureau operated the longest—until 1991, when Haiti's president, Jean-Bertrand Aristide, was forced from power and all foreign aid was stopped.

The nationwide prevention campaign continued despite being burdened by the country's internal conflicts. More than 30 NGOs worked to augment the weak governmental response to the disease in the 1990s. They broadcast their messages via radio, television advertisements and billboards, and created counselling services for high-risk individuals. They supplied nutritional resources and micronutrients to HIV-infected patients and their families, and established extensive health and reproductive services. They launched initiatives for safe sex practices and enlisted sex workers and brothel owners in Haitian cities to encourage their clients to use condoms. They also educated school children about equality, sexual violence, STD and HIV prevention, and contraception, and opened centres for hundreds of thousands of youths.

One of the most important of these NGOs was PIH, a group affiliated with Harvard Medical School and Brigham and Women's Hospital in Boston, Massachusetts. As described later in this chapter, PIH sought to provide interventions in Haiti as soon as they became available in the United States. They developed models for TB and HIV care that have been replicated around the world, effectively linked the patient with the clinic, and showed that high adherence rates in resource-poor settings were attainable with the right programme structure [44]. PIH first opened a small community clinic and hospital complex in the rural village of Cange in 1985 with its sister Haitian organization, Zanmi Lasante. There, they provided comprehensive medical care and worked with local community leaders to develop and disseminate HIV prevention messages that reflected HIV risks in the rural areas. One video, created by community members and activists, was particularly successful. It was called *Chache Lavi, Detwi Lavi* (Looking for Life, Destroying Life), and it was the first film that candidly portrayed HIV in Haiti.

While the Haitian government has been committed to the HIV/AIDS fight, political and economic instability in recent years has paralyzed its efforts to adequately address the epidemic. However, they have had some significant successes despite difficult conditions. The sale of male condoms, for instance, increased from 2 million in 1990 to almost 12 million in 2000. Moreover, in 2000, an interim HIV/AIDS strategic plan for 2001–2 was developed, and in 2001, the Aristide government launched a five-year strategic plan for a government-led national response to HIV/AIDS. Mildred Aristide, the First Lady of Haiti, outlined the mission of the plan that year in her presentation to the United Nations General Assembly Special Session on HIV/AIDS (UNGASS):

> Despite limited resources, Haiti has been able to mount a defense against AIDS. They include an aggressive prevention campaign, a programme to prevent mother-to-child transmission, the launching of a trial vaccination programme, and a limited anti-retroviral drug treatment for people with HIV .... The goals of the 5-year strategic plan that Haiti will begin to prepare has been set: reduce the HIV/AIDS infection rate by 33 percent, reduce the level of sexually transmitted disease by 50 percent, and reduce mother-to-child transmission by 50 percent. The approach is multi-sectoral, under the leadership of our Ministry of Health with the close collaboration of NGOs active in the treatment and prevention of HIV/AIDS and activist Haitians living with HIV/AIDS. [45]

In 2002, the HIV/AIDS National Strategic Plan for 2002–6 was created to strengthen the national response to the epidemic. It focused on the prevention of HIV/AIDS, STDs and mother-to-child transmission (MTCT) of HIV, and aimed to ensure blood safety and give care and support to people with HIV/AIDS. This initiative provided the foundation for the successful grant application to the Global Fund to Fight AIDS, Tuberculosis and Malaria (Global Fund) in 2002.

The HIV/AIDS prevention campaign in Haiti has had remarkable success, given the country's political upheavals. The sale of condoms has dramatically increased, the prevalence of syphilis has declined, and, most importantly, the prevalence of HIV among adults has been reduced by more than 50% in the last 10 years. Although it is theoretically simple for behavioural changes to occur with improved education and availability of condoms, it is difficult to change behaviours in the midst of desperate poverty, political instability and gender inequality.

Co-infection

It has been well documented that transmission of HIV is enhanced by concurrent infection with other STDs [46–49]. In Haiti, GHESKIO showed in one study, for instance, that a genital ulcer in the HIV-negative partner increased the likelihood of acquiring HIV sevenfold. A positive syphilis test in either the HIV-negative or the HIV-infected partner was proven to be associated with relative risks of 2.9% and 2.25%, respectively, and a positive syphilis test in both partners increased the risk to 4.47%. GHESKIO also found that seronegative women with abnormal vaginal discharge were three times more likely to seroconvert [50].

To address this situation, the MOH and a network of NGOs and donor organizations worked to develop a national plan in the 1990s for the management of STDs. As part of that effort, GHESKIO organized studies in 1992 to determine the type of infection responsible for a presenting genital symptom. They found that in men, 45% had urethral discharge, 34% had genital ulcers, and 18% reported swollen or inflamed inguinal lymph nodes. The majority of females had vaginal discharge (85%). The likely cause for urethral discharge in men was gonorrhoea, which was identified in 48% of the patients. Among women with vaginal discharge, an STD was recognized in only 36% of cases (gonorrhoea, trichomoniasis or chlamydia), while 64% of cases were presumed to result from non-infectious sources. Of all the cases with symptomatic STDs, HIV was the disease most commonly diagnosed in patients who sought medical consultation for an STD (26%), followed by syphilis (18%) [51].

These data were used to develop a strategy hoped to prevent STD-related complications and to stop further transmission. Diagnoses were based on presenting symptoms, due the limited laboratory infrastructure in the county. Using this syndromic approach, healthcare providers treated patients for the STD most likely to be causing their symptoms. Each patient was also given detailed education about prevention and treatment of the infection [52], and patients' partners were notified and offered care.

Infant mortality and prevention of MTCT

As more women became infected with HIV, the number of children with the disease increased. Before antiretroviral therapy (ART) became available, about 25% of infants contracted HIV through vertical transmission. In 1987, children accounted for 3.6% of AIDS cases in Haiti. This figure rose to 6.6% in 1990. These statistics probably underestimated the actual rate of paediatric infection, as the surveillance system was weak, HIV-infected infants had a high rate of early death, and it was difficult to establish an HIV diagnosis within the first 15 months of life [53].

Mortality in HIV-infected children was high in the pre-HAART era. Halsey et al. [54] found that among 4588 pregnant women who lived in an urban slum, 443 (9.7%) were HIV-positive. Infants born to HIV-positive mothers in Haiti were more likely to be premature, of low birth weight and malnourished. By one year of age, 23.4 % of infants born to HIV-positive mothers had died, compared with 10.8% of those born to HIV-negative women. At 24 months, these rates were 31.3% and 14.2 %, respectively.

GHESKIO researchers surveyed a variety of paediatric groups during 1987 and 1988 and found that HIV prevalence was significantly higher in subgroups of children at risk for infection. For example, the prevalence of HIV among 558 infants in the dehydration unit of the General Hospital was 8%. It was 16% among 75 children in the paediatric TB hospital and 33 % among 135 children in an urban orphanage [21]. The prevalence in the orphanage increased to 55% within two years.

Medications for MTCT were made available through PIH and GHESKIO shortly after they were shown to be effective in other settings. Progressive MTCT programmes were implemented starting in 1996, in collaboration with the MOH. They provided antenatal, perinatal and postnatal care for mothers and infants, 'short course' zidovudine (ZDV) monotherapy, infant formula, cotrimoxa-zole prophylaxis, early paediatric diagnosis of HIV, and HAART for mothers and infants who met clinical or laboratory indications for therapy. HIV-positive pregnant women initially received ZDV in the third trimester of pregnancy, but since 2003, with the broader introduction of three-drug ART in Haiti and evidence that HAART is more effective than ZDV monotherapy, HAART has been used for MTCT whenever feasible. Family planning services are also offered. Condoms and/or hormonal contraception are available after delivery, and women are given ferrous sulfate, folic acid and tetanus toxoid vaccination in accordance with MOH guidelines.

Screening to determine HIV status in infants is initiated at two months of age. Since 2004, infants diagnosed with HIV infection have started HAART when clinically indicated. Mothers are also given formula. Immunizations recommended by the Ministry of Health, as well as *Pneumococcus* and *Haemophilus influenzae* vaccines, are supplied, and the infant's weight is obtained at each visit. Cotrimoxazole treatment is initiated at six weeks and continued until the infant's HIV status is resolved.

Treatment

History of HIV treatment in Haiti

HIV/AIDS mortality in the industrialized world plummeted in 1996 with the provision of HAART. The medications were nevertheless deemed too expensive and complicated for use in resource-poor settings, so most efforts in these countries were focused on prevention. PIH vehemently disagreed with this line of thought. They argued that everyone was entitled to treatment, regardless of ability to pay or country of residence. They launched the 'HIV Equity Initiative' in 1998 to treat the sickest patients with HAART. People were selected exclusively according to their clinical status, and a clinical algorithm was used to identify those in the greatest need. Patients subsequently received an uninterrupted supply of HAART. Patients were monitored clinically, as laboratory services were limited; CD4 counts were not available for the first five years of the programme.

Community health workers, called *accompagnateurs*, were the backbone of this initiative. They linked the clinic with the villages scattered throughout the region and visited patients once or twice per day to provide directly observed treatment (DOT) with HAART. This successful model was developed 10 years earlier for the provision of DOT for TB. The *accompagnateurs* were well respected in their communities. They were trained monthly about clinical management and treatment of HIV infection, as well as being educated about the importance of confidentiality, and were advised about the most effective ways to provide emotional support: 'During the program review, we learned that *accompagnateurs* were sharing food with their patient-neighbors, babysitting, and running errands. Some of the *accompagnateurs* were themselves receiving anti-retrovirals from their own *accompagnateurs*. Something far more complex and beneficial than DOT—a "virtuous social cycle"—occurs when neighbors are enlisted in the struggle against tuberculosis and HIV infection' [55].

The clinic staff also provided other important services. Before HAART was initiated, a social worker conducted a detailed assessment of a patient's household financial situation, evaluated the patient's support network and identified potential barriers to adherence or to treatment response. Monthly meetings were conducted to exchange information and strengthen pro-gramme reception.

Outcomes were excellent, with the clinical response to therapy favourable in 59 of the first 60 patients. In a subset of 21 patients whose viral loads were monitored, 18 (86%) had no detectable virus in their blood [39]. The scope of the project was limited solely by the inability to find significant funding. It was very hard to garner support for the treatment of HIV in rural Haiti.

Potential donors often said that HAART was too complicated and expensive for such an under-developed country. They said the medications would not be used properly and were better suited for more highly developed nations.

The services offered by GHESKIO were also constrained by a lack of financial resources, mean-ing physicians had to prioritize. They had to somehow cope with the high cost of HAART and the large number of patients—between 5000 and 8000—who sought care. Physicians believed that the most cost-effective strategy was to focus on the treatment and prevention of OIs, such as TB, because the medications for such illnesses prolonged and improved the quality of life of HIV-infected patients. They also treated STDs, which were the major co-factors for HIV transmission, as well as providing intense counselling, distributing free condoms and creating a family plan-ning unit. HAART came into use after 1998 for rape victims, mothers at risk for MTCT and people with occupational exposure; HAART for chronic care was given only to patients with enough money to pay for the drugs, or to patients who could obtain the medicine privately or from family members abroad.

Antiretroviral therapy

Impact of the Global Fund to Fight AIDS, Tuberculosis and Malaria (Global Fund)

Nationwide access to HIV/AIDS prevention and treatment services was widely expanded after the establishment of the Global Fund. Haiti submitted an application in 2002 to the newly formed organization for a nationwide HIV prevention and treatment programme and was awarded funding for a nationwide HIV/AIDS programme in 2003. Consequently, the widespread use of HAART in Haiti finally became feasible. A meeting was held in early April 2003 to discuss how to scale up treatment in the country. 'From Models to Implementation' was organized by PIH, Brigham and Women's Hospital, GHESKIO, Cornell University and Harvard Medical School's Division of AIDS. More than 100 HIV experts from Haiti, the United States and other nations attended. There were also members of the US President's Emergency Plan for AIDS Relief (PEPFAR), the Global Fund, the US National Institutes of Health (NIH), the International AIDS Society (IAS), the Joint United Nations Programme on HIV/AIDS (UNAIDS), the WHO and the Haitian MOH. Physicians at GHESKIO and PIH presented posters and delivered lectures about the clinical management of HIV in Haiti. After discussing diagnosis and treatment outcomes, the group then devised important plans and outlined strategies to improve HIV care.

In March 2003, Haiti received the first installment of the US$67 million grant to be distributed over a five-year period. HIV and HIV-related services were widely implemented, and the country's First Lady was appointed head of Haiti's Country Coordinating Mechanism. Access to HAART was widely expanded [5] under the guidance of PIH, GHESKIO and the Ministry of Health.

PIH and the MOH revitalized eight clinic-hospital complexes in the rural Central Plateau. These clinics offered DOT-HAART, delivered through community health workers—the system developed in Cange. Extensive renovations were made at each location, with every site receiving a functioning pharmacy and laboratory, a space for clinical examinations, and a generator-pow-ered electricity supply. The administrators secured teams to provide comprehensive medical, paediatric and obstetric care. They also hired additional staff: physicians, nurses, pharmacists and support personnel. Within three months of completion, each site experienced an approximate 10-fold increase in ambulatory visits [44].

The results from one clinic illustrate the health improvements that immediately followed the scale-up [56]. In Lascahobas, general medical visits went from fewer than 20 to more than 200 per day within the first 14 months of the site's expansion. The number of patients diagnosed and treated for TB also increased from nine to more than 200 by the next year. HIV tests were widely conducted, and anyone diagnosed positive received care. In the first year, HAART was initiated in 120 patients in Lascahobas. Antenatal services were added, vaccination access was improved, a small inpatient unit was built, and staff morale and community participation was high. These changes occurred at every PIH facility. Overall, PIH provided 885,853 patient encounters (clinic visits or hospital admissions) and coordinated community health workers and other medical staff to visit 895,766 patients at home in the year 2006 alone.

GHESKIO and the MOH created a network of public and private hospitals in 25 locations around the country with the Global Fund monies. They sought to implement an integrated healthcare programme to prevent and treat HIV, and to manage STDs and TB. Their strategy was based on evidence that an individual at risk for HIV, or who was already infected, could be identified by any of a number of factors. When patients presented to local health centres, the teams could quickly recognize conditions and subsequently provide appropriate care [57]. Voluntary counselling and testing (VCT) centres, screening for syphilis and other STDs, screening and treatment for TB, counselling and family planning services, nutritional support and comprehensive HIV treatment were all provided. Access to HAART also continues to expand rapidly (see Figure 22.2).

In addition to clinical services, GHESKIO facilitates ongoing education for healthcare workers in Haiti. In 2006, for instance, they trained 630 laboratory technicians, 258 social workers, 2186 nurses, 785 physicians, 39 pharmacists and 6478 community leaders. GHESKIO also provides information about HIV testing and other prevention services, and about the management of TB, the treatment of OIs, MTCT and the use of HAART.

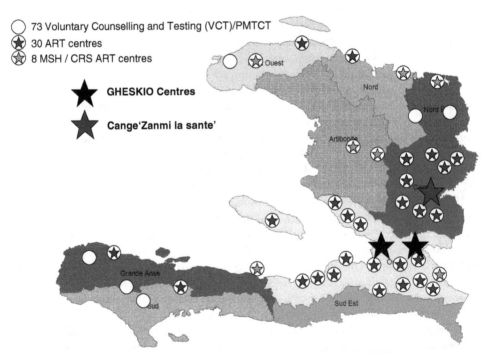

Fig. 22.2 National plan for expansion of care and prevention in Haiti, 2005–2006
Source: GHESKIO, 2006

Guidelines for ART delivery in Haiti

HAART is currently provided in Haiti as recommended by both the MOH and WHO guidelines. Treatment is based on the clinical stage of the patient's disease and the CD4 count [58]. Patients with CD4 counts below 200 cells/mm^3 and those with WHO Stage 4 (advanced) disease are given HAART as soon as possible. HAART is also considered in patients with Stage 3 disease and in those with CD4 counts ranging from 200 to 350 cells/mm^3. The preferred first-line ART regimen for adults and adolescents is ZDV, lamivudine (3TC) and efavirenz (EFV). Stavudine (d4T) is substituted for ZDV in patients with severe anaemia, and nevirapine (NVP) is substituted for EFV in women who could become pregnant, while EFV is used for patients with TB and HIV co-infection [4]. For patients who fail first-line treatment, tenofovir (TDF), abacavir (ABC) and lopinavir (LPV) are available. This is, however, not common, and most patients (>97%) remain on first-line therapy [4,5,44].

Clinical outcomes with ART

Treatment results in Haiti have been outstanding. The first 1004 patients to receive HAART at GHESKIO experienced outcomes that rivalled those in the United States. Eighty-seven per cent of the 910 adults and adolescents, and 98% of 94 children, were alive after one year. In adults and adolescents, the median increase in the CD4 count at six months was 128 cells/mm^3 (interquartile range (IQR):62–197 cells/mm^3), and was greater than the baseline value in 459 of 504 patients (91%). The median increase in the CD4 count at 12 months was 163 cells/mm^3 (IQR:77–251 cells/mm^3), and was greater than the baseline value in 360 of 397 patients (91%). In children, the median CD4 cell percentage rose from a baseline value of 13% (IQR:8–20%) to 21% (IQR:16–29%) at six months, and to 26 % (IQR:22–36 %) at 12 months [4].

Most of the first GHESKIO patients on HAART gained weight. At six months, adult and adolescent patients had gained a median of 4.0 kg (IQR:0.9–7.7), and 639 of 759 patients (84%) had increased their weight overall. At 12 months, they had gained a median of 5.5 kg (IQR:1.4–10.5), and 396 of 466 patients (85%) had gained overall.

Of the 910 adult and adolescent patients, 113 (12%) received concurrent treatment for TB while on HAART. Of the 113 patients, 89 (79%) were cured, 20 (18%) died, one (1%) did not respond to TB therapy, and three (3%) were lost to follow-up. Two patients with CD4 counts of 50–200 cells/mm^3 started TB treatment but died before HAART was initiated. Among the 94 children, 13 (14%) received HAART with concurrent treatment for TB. Eleven of these patients appeared clinically cured, while two (15%) were lost to follow-up. None of the children died.

Of the 113 adults and adolescents treated for TB and HIV/AIDS, 72 received TB medication before HAART, while 41 began TB treatment after HAART. Of the 72 patients who started TB treatment before HAART, 11 (15%) had a suspected immune reconstitution syndrome, which caused a temporary worsening of TB symptoms after HAART was initiated. These patients experienced a recurrent fever, an increased cough and a drained lymph-node fistula. Four were treated with corticosteroids, but none of the 11 stopped HAART. Of the 41 patients (63%) diagnosed with TB after HAART was initiated, 26 developed TB symptoms within three months of ART. Patients who lost more than 5% of their body weight by the third month of HAART were significantly more likely to be diagnosed with TB (OR=2.62; 95% CI:1.17–5.86; p=0.04) [4]. There was no significant difference in survival between patients with TB and those without TB in either the adult or paediatric populations.

The one-year survival rate after HAART was initiated was 87% for adults and adolescents, and 98% for children (see Figure 22.3). In contrast, the one-year survival rate for adults with AIDS in the pre-HAART era in Haiti had been just 30% [40]. Of the 910 adult and adolescent patients in the first GHESKIO cohort, 127 (14%) died. Of these, 55 deaths (43%) were due to persistent

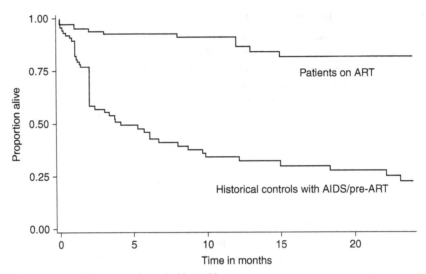

Fig. 22.3 Antiretroviral therapy and survival in Haiti

Notes: Kaplan-Meier Estimate of survival in 1996 HIV-infected adults treated with antiretrovival therapy (ART) by GHESKIO, compared to survival of 99 historical controls diagnosed with AIDS before ART was available.

Source: Unpublished presentation by D. Fitzerald, 'Lessons Learned from the use of ARVs in Haiti. Workshop on Antiretrovival Therapy Use in Resource-constrained Settings. Institute of Medicine of the National Academies Washington, DC, 27 January 2004.

wasting syndrome, 20 (16%) to TB, six (5%) to bacterial pneumonia, five (4%) to toxoplasmosis, four (3%) to cancer, four (3%) to cryptosporidiosis, four (3%) to sepsis syndrome, three (2%) to congestive heart failure, three (2%) to trauma and 23 (18%) to an unknown cause. One hundred of the deaths (79%) occurred within six months of initial ART. In the overall group of 1004 patients, 90% were alive at six months and 87% were alive at 12 months. Predictors of death included the presence of an AIDS-defining illness, a CD4 count <50 cells/mm^3 and a body weight before HAART was initiated in the lowest quartile for sex. Two of the 94 children died within one month of enrolment. One child died from a sepsis-like syndrome and the other from a respiratory tract infection of unknown origin.

GHESKIO researchers evaluated the outcomes of 236 children treated with HAART in another study. The patients were followed for a median of 20 months (range 0–36 months). At the time of study publication, 191 (81%) were still monitored, 21 (9%) had died, and 24 (10%) were lost in follow-up. Kaplan-Meier survival analysis demonstrated that 80% of the children were alive and under care after 24 months of follow-up. Of the 21 children who died, 15 (71%) died within six months of HAART initiation. The median time to death was 48 days. Nine children (45%) died of respiratory failure, four (20%) of gastroenteritis and hypovolemic shock, three (15%) of severe anaemia, and five (24%) of unknown etiology. Baseline predictors were age <18 months, a CD4 cell percentage of ≤5% and a weight-for-age Z-score of ≤3.

Side effects of HAART

HAART is tolerated well among Haitians. In the GHESKIO outcomes study described in the previous section, 229 (25%) of the 910 adult and adolescent patients required changes to their first-line regimen. One hundred and two (11%) switched because of toxic effects, 29 (3%) because they were sexually active women of reproductive age, 11 (1%) due to suspected treatment failure and 21 (2%) due to TB. Sixty-six (7%) altered their regimen because of medication stock-outs, which occurred when international suppliers delivered drugs months after the scheduled delivery. Thus, while all patients received an uninterrupted supply of HAART, some underwent temporary substitutions for drugs of equal efficacy.

Anaemia and central nervous system (CNS) symptoms were the most common side effects of HAART. Among the 910 adults and adolescents in the GHESKIO cohort, ZDV caused anaemia in 5% of patients. EFV caused CNS symptoms in 6%, gynaecomastia in 3%, and rash and nausea in less than 1% of patients. NVP caused rash in 3%, and nausea and hepatitis in less than 1% of patients. NVP was also suspected to cause the two cases of Stevens–Johnson syndrome that developed in the cohort (one of which was fatal). ABC caused rash in about 2% of patients. Of the 94 children, nine (10%) required a medication change. Five of these required ART modification because of side effects, one because of a drug stock-out and three because of concurrent TB treatment. Of the children who switched drugs due to side effects, two developed anaemia on ZDV, one developed a rash on NVP, one developed hepatitis on EFV, and one developed gynecomastia on EFV [4]. At PIH, HAART was also well tolerated; less than 5% of patients required medication changes [39,44].

Monitoring patients on ART

At GHESKIO and PIH, patients are clinically monitored every month for signs or symptoms of medication toxicity. Patients with side effects or with evidence of an OI undergo a targeted diagnostic work-up and are given appropriate treatment. Weight is scrutinized at each visit, as it can be a predictor of improved outcomes for those who gain. Patients who lose weight, however, receive a further work-up, such as a CD4 count and evaluation for other infections.

Laboratory capacity is unfortunately very limited in Haiti. This makes it extremely difficult to determine if patients are failing treatment. Viral load and resistance testing is not available; only a few sites, such as the GHESKIO clinic in Port-au-Prince and the PIH centres in the Central Plateau, follow a patient's CD4 count every six months, although the CDC is working to scale up countrywide access to CD4 count technology. Without sophisticated laboratory tests, early signs of treatment failure, such as a bump in viral load, cannot be recognized. For this reason, it is critical that patients receive support to maintain a high level of treatment adherence.

It is expected that in Haiti, as in other developing countries, patients who fail HAART may have extensive resistance mutations. It is also anticipated that patients with viraemia will develop the M184V mutation, which confers resistance to 3TC, and the K103N mutation, which causes resistance to EFV and NVP. As these patients remain on failing regimens, they are also likely to develop thymidine analogue-associated mutations (TAMs) and the K65R mutation, which can cause resistance to drugs they have not yet been exposed to (ABC, didanosine (ddI), TDF). It is critical to delay the development of drug resistance by ensuring an uninterrupted supply of medication and providing social and adherence support to all patients.

PEPFAR in Haiti

US President George W Bush unveiled PEPFAR in 2003, which is the largest financial commitment ever made by a nation to a single disease or international health initiative. Haiti is one of the programme's recipient countries, receiving more than US$40 million per year to bolster the ongoing expansion of HIV-related prevention and treatment services. Many of the organizations who are part of the Global Fund grant are given PEPFAR money as well. Among other things, PEPFAR helps them develop laboratory infrastructure, improve counselling and testing services, and expand access to treatment. It assists NGOs to care for orphans and vulnerable children, and to develop important data-collection tools, such as medical record systems, and gives technical assistance. PEPFAR also supports efforts to prevent MTCT, encourage safe sex, secure condoms and expand access to HAART. It has financed mobile HIV counselling and testing clinics and provider training programmes, and has helped refurbish hospitals.

GHESKIO, PIH and the MOH provide the majority of HIV-related services in Haiti, but access to treatment is increasing at other sites as well (see Figure 22.3). In 2006, 166,000 (86%) of the 193,000 Haitians tested for HIV were in the PIH-GHESKIO-MOH network. Twenty-seven per cent of these patients were pregnant women. All women who tested positive were given comprehensive services to prevent MTCT. In 2006, 8955 patients (8.9%) tested positive for HIV in the GHESKIO network, and 2987 (4.6%) tested positive in the PIH network. HAART was initiated for all patients who met WHO clinical eligibility criteria. At the end of 2006, more than 9400 people were being treated with HAART in Haiti. Of this group, 7240 (77%) received treatment in the PIH-GHESKIO-MOH network. By April 2007, the cumulative number of patients who had been treated with HAART in Haiti had increased to 12,316 [PEPFAR, unpublished data, 2007].

Conclusion

Despite ongoing political difficulties and limited resources, Haiti has launched one of the world's most effective responses to the HIV epidemic. The decline in prevalence and the countrywide scale-up of services are laudable achievements. International funding has played a contributing role in these programmatic successes, but more recent advances would not have been possible without the strong network of institutions that were firmly established and already providing prevention and treatment services for HIV/AIDS at the time that funding became available. These organizations have proven that treatment outcomes rivalling those of developed countries can be attained, even in the midst of adverse conditions or in deeply impoverished settings. Now that funding has become more widely available with support from the Global Fund and PEPFAR, the number of institutions involved in the prevention and care of HIV has increased exponentially, and we expect that this will be reflected in further declines in prevalence and ongoing expansion of access to HAART in Haiti.

In order to continue lowering HIV prevalence in Haiti, the public health and medical infrastructure must be strengthened under MOH guidance. HIV services must be further expanded with the goal of providing HAART to 20,000 people by the end of 2008. As HAART is scaled up, adherence must be monitored to delay the development of drug resistance, and the TB programme must be strengthened. Human resources must be augmented with innovative delivery models, such as the training of nurses to work as physicians' assistants, and the network of community health workers must be expanded. Social services such as nutritional supplementation and transportation subsidies must be included in order for HIV/AIDS treatment programmes to reach the most vulnerable patients, and it will be critical to improve women's economic and educational opportunities. Though there are challenges ahead, Haiti is well on the way to providing universal treatment for all who are afflicted with HIV.

References

1. United Nations Development Programme. (2006). *United Nations Development Index, 2006.* Geneva: United Nations.
2. World Bank. (2004). *Haiti at a Glance.* Washington DC: World Bank.
3. UNAIDS. (2006). *UNAIDS Epidemic Update.* Geneva: UNAIDS.
4. Severe P, Leger P, Charles M, *et al.* (2005). Antiretroviral therapy in a thousand patients with AIDS in Haiti. *N Engl J Med* **353**:2325–34.

5. Mukherjee JS, Ivers L, Leandre F, Farmer P, Behforouz H. (2006). Antiretroviral therapy in resource-poor settings. Decreasing barriers to access and promoting adherence. *J Acquir Immune Defic Syndr* **43**(Suppl 1):S123–6.

6. US Centers for Disease Control. (1981). Kaposi's sarcoma and *Pneumonocystis* pneumonia. *MMWR* **30**:409–410.

7. US Centers for Disease Control (1982). Opportunistic Infections and Kaposi's Sarcoma among Haitians in the United States. *MMWR* **31**:353–354, 360–361.

8. Moskowitz LB, Kory P, Chan JC, Haverkos HW, Conley FK, Hensley GT. (1983). Unusual causes of death in Haitians residing in Miami. High prevalence of opportunistic infections. *JAMA* **250**:1187–91.

9. Jaffe HW, Bregman DJ, Selik RM. (1983). Acquired immune deficiency syndrome in the United States: the first 1,000 cases. *J Infect Dis* **148**:339–45.

10. Pitchenik AE, Fischl MA, Dickinson GM, *et al.* (1983). Opportunistic infections and Kaposi's sarcoma among Haitians: evidence of a new acquired immunodeficiency state. *Ann Intern Med* **98**:277–84.

11. Centers for Disease Control Task Force on Kaposi's Sarcoma and Opportunistic Infections. (1982). Epidemiologic aspects of the current outbreak of Kaposi's sarcoma and opportunistic infections. *N Engl J Med* **306**:248–252.

12. Sabatier R. (1988). *Blaming Others: Prejudice, Race, and Worldwide AIDS*. London: Pamos Publications.

13. Greenfield WR. (1986). Night of the living dead II: slow virus encephalopathies and AIDS: do necromantic zombiists transmit HTLV-III/LAV during voodooistic rituals? *JAMA* **256**:2199–200.

14. Farmer PE. (1992). *AIDS and Accusations*. Berkeley: University of California Press.

15. Chaze W. (1983). In Haiti, a view of life at the bottom. *US News and World Report*. **95**:41–42.

16. Liautaud B, Laroche C, Duvivier J, Pean-Guichard C. (1983). Kaposi's sarcoma in Haiti: unknown reservoir or a recent appearance?. *Ann Dermatol Venereol* **110**:213–9.

17. Pape JW, Liautaud B, Thomas F, *et al.* (1983). Characteristics of the acquired immunodeficiency syndrome (AIDS) in Haiti. *N Engl J Med* **309**:945–50.

18. Pape JW, Liautaud B, Thomas F, *et al.* (1986). Risk factors associated with AIDS in Haiti. *Am J Med Sci* **291**:4–7.

19. Pape JW, Liautaud B, Thomas F, *et al.* (1985). The acquired immunodeficiency syndrome in Haiti. *Ann Intern Med* **103**:674–8.

20. Pape JW, Stanback ME, Pamphile M, *et al.* (1990). Prevalence of HIV infection and high-risk activities in Haiti. *J Acquir Immune Defic Syndr* **3**:995–1001.

21. Pape JW, Johnson WD Jr. (1988). Epidemiology of AIDS in the Caribbean. In: Piot P and Mann J, eds. *Clinical Tropical Medicine and Communicable Diseases, AIDS and HIV Infection in the Tropics*, Vol. 3, Na 1. London: Ballière Tindall Limited, Harcourt Brace Jovanovic, p.31–42.

22. US Centers for Disease Control and Prevention. (1985). Update: acquired immunodeficiency syndrome—United States. *MMWR Morb Mortal Wkly Rep* **34**:245–8.

23. Farmer PE, Connor M and Simmons J. (1996). *Women, Poverty, and AIDS*. Monroe, ME: Common Courage Press.

24. Farmer PE. (1999). *Infections and Inequalities. The Modern Plagues*. Berkeley: University of California Press.

25. Fitzgerald DW, Behets F, Caliendo A, *et al.* (2000). Economic hardship and sexually transmitted diseases in Haiti's rural Artibonite Valley. *Am J Trop Med Hyg* **62**:496–501.

26. Behets FM, Desormeaux J, Joseph D, *et al.* (1995). Control of sexually transmitted diseases in Haiti: results and implications of a baseline study among pregnant women living in Cite Soleil Shantytowns. *J Infect Dis* **172**:764–71.

27. Smith Fawzi MC, Lambert W, Singler JM, *et al.* (2003). Prevalence and risk factors of STDs in rural Haiti: implications for policy and programming in resource-poor settings. *Int J STD AIDS* **14**:848–53.

28. Boulos R, Halsey NA, Holt E, *et al.* (1990). HIV-1 in Haitian women 1982–1988. The Cite Soleil/JHU AIDS Project Team. *J Acquir Immune Defic Syndr* **3**:721–8.

29. Johnson WD Jr, Pape J. (1989). AIDS in Haiti. In: Levy J, ed. *AIDS: Pathogenesis and Treatment.* New York: Marcel Dekker.

30. Pape JW, Deschamps MM, Verdier RI, *et al.* (1992). The urge for an AIDS vaccine: perspectives from a developing country. *AIDS Res Hum Retroviruses* **8**:1535–7.

31. Allain JP, Hodges W, Einstein MH, *et al.* (1992). Antibody to HIV-1, HTLV-I, and HCV in three populations of rural Haitians. *J Acquir Immune Defic Syndr* **5**:1230–6.

32. Institut Haitien de l'Enfance, Centres GHESKIO. (1994). *Resultat d'une étude de surveillance serosentinelle: Prévalence du VIH, du VHB et de la Syphilis chez les femmes enceintes dans cinq (5) sites de surveillance serosentinelle en Haiti.* Haiti: Pan American Health Organization, World Health Organization.

33. Institut Haitien de l'Enfance, Centres GHESKIO. (1996). *Evolution Globale des prévalences de l'infection au VIH, de la syphilis et de l'hépatite B chez les femmes Haitiennes enceintes.* Haiti: Pan American Health Organization, World Health Organization.

34. Gaillard EM, Boulos LM, Cayemittes MP, **et al.** (2006). Understanding the reasons for decline of HIV prevalence in Haiti. *Sex Transm Infect* **82**(Suppl 1):i14–20.

35. Hallett TB, Aberle-Grasse J, Bello G, *et al.* (2006). Declines in HIV prevalence can be associated with changing sexual behaviour in Uganda, urban Kenya, Zimbabwe, and urban Haiti. *Sex Transm Infect* **82**(Suppl 1):i1–8.

36. Guerin JM, Malebranche R, Elie R, *et al.* (1984). Acquired immune deficiency syndrome: specific aspects of the disease in Haiti. *Ann N Y Acad Sci* **437**:254–63.

37. Desvarieux M, Pape JW. (1991). HIV and AIDS in Haiti: recent developments. *AIDS Care* **3**:271–9.

38. Liautaud B, Pape JW, DeHovitz JA, *et al.* (1989). Pruritic skin lesions. A common initial presentation of acquired immunodeficiency syndrome. *Arch Dermatol* **125**:629–32.

39. Farmer P, Leandre F, Mukherjee J, *et al.* (2001). Community-based approaches to HIV treatment in resource-poor settings. *Lancet* **358**:404–9.

40. Deschamps MM, Fitzgerald DW, Pape JW, Johnson WD Jr, *et al.* (2000). HIV infection in Haiti: natural history and disease progression. *AIDS* **14**:2515–21.

41. Pape JW, Jean SS, Ho JL, *et al.* (1993). Effect of isoniazid prophylaxis on incidence of active tuberculosis and progression of HIV infection. *Lancet* **342**:268–72.

42. Fitzgerald DW, Morse MM, Pape JW, *et al.* (2000). Effect of post-treatment isoniazid on prevention of recurrent tuberculosis in HIV-1-infected individuals: a randomised trial. *Lancet* **356**:1470–4.

43. Joseph P, Severe P, Ferdinand S, *et al.* (2006). Multidrug-resistant tuberculosis at an HIV testing center in Haiti. *AIDS* **20**:415–8.

44. Koenig SP, Leandre F, Farmer PE. (2004). Scaling-up HIV treatment programmes in resource-limited settings: the rural Haiti experience. *AIDS* **18**(Suppl 3):S21–5.

45. The Honorable Mildred Aristide. (2001). *Statement by the First Lady of the Republic of Haiti, the Honorable Mildred Aristide, 26 June 2001. United Nations Special Session on HIV/AIDS. Implications for Poverty Reduction: Impact of HIV/AIDS.* Available at http://www.haiti.org/official_documents/la_presidence/Jba/UNITED_26–06–01.htm (accessed October 2007).

46. Stamm WE, Handsfield HH, Rompalo AM, *et al.* (1988). The association between genital ulcer disease and acquisition of HIV infection in homosexual men. *JAMA* **260**:1429–33.

47. Greenblatt R, Lukehart SA, Plummer FA, *et al.* (1988). Genital ulceration as a risk factor for human immunodeficiency virus infection. *AIDS* **2**:47–50.

48. Keet IP, Lee FK, van Griensven GJ, *et al.*(1990). Herpes simplex virus type 2 and other genital ulcerative infections as a risk factor for HIV-1 acquisition. *Genitourin Med* **66**:330–3.

49. Latif AS, Katzenstein DA, Bassett MT, *et al.* (1989). Genital ulcers and transmission of HIV among couples in Zimbabwe. *AIDS* **3**:519–23.

50. Deschamps MM, Pape JW, Hafner A, *et al.* (1996). Heterosexual transmission of HIV in Haiti. *Ann Intern Med* **125**:324–30.

51. Liautaud B. (1992). Preliminary Data on STDs in Haiti. VIII International Conference on AIDS/ III STD World Congress, 19–24 July 1992, Amsterdam, the Netherlands. [Abstract 04302]

52. Behets FM, Génécé E, Narcisse M, *et al.* (1998). Approaches to control sexually transmitted diseases in Haiti, 1992–95. *Bull World Health Organ* **76**:189–94.

53. Pape J. (1987). Outcome of Offspring of HIV-infected pregnant women in Haiti. In: Shinazi R, Mahmias A, eds. *AIDS in Children, Adolescents, and Heterosexual Adults.* New York: Elsevier Science Publishing. p216–8.

54. Halsey NA, Boulos R, Holt E, *et al.* (1990). Transmission of HIV-1 infections from mothers to infants in Haiti. Impact on childhood mortality and malnutrition. The CDS/JHU AIDS Project Team. *JAMA* **264**: 2088–92.

55. Behforouz HL, Farmer PE, Mukherjee JS. (2004). From directly observed therapy to accompagnateurs: enhancing AIDS treatment outcomes in Haiti and in Boston. *Clin Infect Dis* **38**(Suppl 5):S429–36.

56. Walton DA, Farmer PE, Lambert W, *et al.* (2004). Integrated HIV prevention and care strengthens primary health care: lessons from rural Haiti. *J Public Health Policy* **25**:137–58.

57. Peck R, Fitzgerald DW, Liautaud B, *et al.* (2003). The feasibility, demand, and effect of integrating primary care services with HIV voluntary counseling and testing: evaluation of a 15-year experience in Haiti, 1985–2000. *J Acquir Immune Defic Syndr* **33**:470–5.

58. World Health Organization. (2006). *Antiretroviral Therapy for HIV Infection in Adults and Adolescents in Resource-Limited Settings: Toward Universal Access. Recommendations for a Public Health Approach.* Geneva: WHO.

Chapter 23

Country review: Malawi

Erik J. Schouten*, Simon D. Makombe, Anthony D. Harries and Kelita Kamoto

Background

Malawi is a low-income country in southern Africa and one of the poorest countries in the world. Its gross domestic product (GDP) is a mere US$149 per capita per year, and it ranks 166th out of 177 countries in the Human Development Index. Over three-quarters of the population live on less that US$2 per day [1]. With an HIV prevalence of 14% (95% CI:12–17%), the eighth highest in the world, it is also one of the countries hardest hit by HIV/AIDS [2].

Highly active antiretroviral therapy (HAART) became available in many countries around the world in the second half of the 1990s, but it was not until the scale-up of therapy in 2003–4 that HAART became available in low-income countries. The aim of this chapter is to describe the epidemiological characteristics of HIV infection in Malawi, to present the antiretroviral therapy (ART) scale-up programme, to analyse the reasons why the country was able to achieve a good degree of success and to discuss challenges of the programme.

Epidemiology

The first AIDS diagnosis was made in Malawi in 1985. Retrospective analysis of blood samples collected from 1981 to 1984 and from 1987 to 1989 as part of a community-based study in a district in northern Malawi showed that HIV was introduced into the district in the very early 1980s from many sources, and that immigration and travel were important in the repeated introduction and establishment of the HIV epidemic [3]. From 1982 to 1984, small numbers of different HIV-1 subtypes (A, C and D) were present, and by 1987–9, 152 of 168 sequences (90%) were subtype C [4]. HIV-1 subtype C is now the predominant subtype in Malawi. This was confirmed by a HIV drug resistance study that was carried out in 2007 in which 43 (91%) of 47 successfully sequenced samples were shown to be HIV-1 subtype C viruses, with the remainder being recombinants of subtype C [5].

Like most sub-Saharan countries, Malawi monitors HIV prevalence mainly through antenatal clinic (ANC) sentinel surveillance. The surveillance is conducted every two years using the same methodology in the same sentinel sites, and the system has collected data from 19 sites since 1994, although some sentinel sites started data collection as early as 1990. Data from sentinel surveillance sites indicate that prevalence increased rapidly from the late 1980s to the early 1990s. By the mid-1990s, prevalence had stabilized, and since then it has remained fairly constant. In 2005, the total number of people infected with HIV was estimated to be between 780,000 and 1.12 million. This figure includes 69,000–100,000 children under the age of 15. Every year

* Corresponding author.

another 96,000 people are newly infected with HIV and 86,000 people die of AIDS-related causes [6]. Overall HIV prevalence in Malawi appears to have stabilized, and there has been a general decline in HIV prevalence among ANC attendees aged 15–24 years since 1999.

HIV has not spread equally among the population. HIV prevalence among women is about 30% higher than among men, with women becoming infected earlier in life; the prevalence in women in the 20–24 year age group is three times higher (13.2% versus 3.9%) than in men. In people over 30 years of age, prevalence is similar for both sexes [7] (Figure 23.1). The epidemic also shows a geographical heterogeneity. Prevalence in urban areas is higher than in rural areas (21.6% versus 12.1%) and is higher in the southern region of the country (17.6%) compared with the central (6.5%) and northern regions (8.1%). HIV prevalence in the wealthiest quintile of the population is twice that of the lowest quintile (16% versus 8%). This relationship exists for both women and men, although it is more pronounced in the latter group.

Heterosexual contact is the principal mode of HIV transmission in Malawi, while mother-to-child transmission (MTCT) of HIV accounts for approximately 25% of all new HIV infections [6]. Injection drug use in Malawi is hardly ever reported, and this does not seem to play any significant role in HIV transmission in the country. Homosexuality is illegal, regarded as taboo, and is not addressed in the national response to HIV.

Primary and newly diagnosed chronic infection

Monitoring of HIV drug resistance in individual patients is not possible in Malawi due to resource constraints. However, in both the ART guidelines and the national ART Scale-Up Plan, annual surveillance and monitoring for drug resistance at selected sites is recognized to be an important and vital component of successful national ART delivery. A protocol was developed to monitor HIV viral suppression and the emergence of drug resistance among patients receiving ART and to determine its prevalence in recently infected populations using threshold surveillance methods. Using the World Health Organization (WHO) threshold survey approach to assess drug resistant HIV transmission, a survey was carried out in Lilongwe, the capital of Malawi, in 2006. Transmitted drug resistance among the population surveyed was found to be <5% for all relevant antiretroviral drugs and drug classes. The finding of <5% transmitted

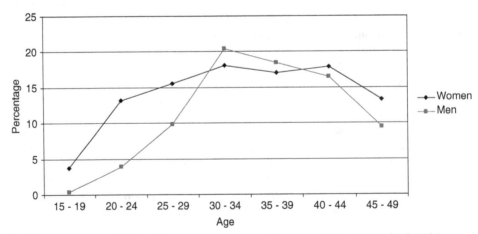

Fig. 23.1 Percentage of HIV-positives among women and men aged 15–49 in Malawi, 2004.
Source: Malawi Demographic and Health Survey 2004.

resistance among people with primary and untreated chronic infection in the capital city, where ART has been available for the longest time, implies that the current first-line ART regimen can be used with confidence [5].

A patient who has tested positive for HIV and is symptomatic or has a past history of pulmonary tuberculosis (TB) will be referred to one of the 104 public sector or 38 private sector ART clinics for further assessment. In the ART clinic, the patient will be evaluated for ART, and those who are assessed at WHO clinical stage 3 or 4, those with a low CD4-lymphocyte count (<250 cells/mm^3), or patients in WHO clinical stage 2 with a total lymphocyte count <1200 cells/mm^3 are eligible for ART. Once opportunistic infections (OIs) are stabilized, patients undergo group counselling, and this is followed a few days later by individual counselling. If the patient has a clear understanding of the implications of ART, treatment is started. Those who are asymptomatic are referred to the general health services for appropriate management and advice [8].

ART strategies

The criteria for choosing the first-line ART regimen include: the need for a standardized regimen across the country; ease of administration (once or twice daily, available as a fixed-dose combination and ingestion not related to food intake); few side effects (especially side effects requiring laboratory monitoring); lack of interaction with rifampicin; previous experience with use; and price. The first-line regimen chosen was a fixed-dose combination of stavudine (d4T)/lamivudine (3TC)/nevirapine (NVP), and this remains the first-line regimen in current use. In the event of adverse reactions that are serious enough to necessitate a change in drug treatment, either d4T is replaced by zidovudine (ZDV) or NVP is replaced by efavirenz (EFV). These are called alternative first-line regimens.

The second-line regimen is used in case of treatment failure, which is defined as a patient having been on ART and adhering to therapy for six months or longer, with either the development of a new WHO clinical stage 4 feature or a CD4 count/percentage that has declined to pre-treatment values or declined to <50% of peak value. These CD4 measurements need to be confirmed one month later. The chosen second-line option for adults is: ZDV/3TC/tenofovir (TDF)/lopinavir (LPV).

Alternative and second-line regimens are not available in all ART sites. Patients in need of an alternative ART regimen are referred to a clinic with experienced staff who will assess them, and in the case of treatment failure, patients are referred to a specialist at one of the four central hospitals in the country. As sites have become more experienced in the use of ART, more sites directly give alternative first-line therapy.

The first-line and alternative first-line regimens for children are identical to the adult regimens and are administered as divided tablets. The second-line regimen consists of: abacavir (ABC)/didanosine (ddI)/LPV. For all patients, adults and children alike, patients are seen two weeks after ART is started, and then followed up initially every four weeks. If they are stable and adherent to therapy by six months, patients can then be followed up every eight weeks.

The national scale-up of the ART programme started in 2004, not long after the launch of the '3 by 5' initiative by the WHO and the Joint United Nations Programme on HIV/AIDS (UNAIDS). The international goal was to start 3 million people in developing countries on ART by the end of 2005 [9]. Although the target was not met, the initiative encouraged many governments to develop bold plans to scale up access to ART. By December 2006, WHO and UNAIDS estimated that more than 2 million people from low- and middle-income countries had been placed on treatment, 1.3 million of whom were in sub-Saharan Africa [10].

In January 2004, approximately 3000 people received ART in nine public health facilities in Malawi. Due to the severe capacity constraints of the Malawi health sector, it was recognized right from the start that ART delivery using a wide range of treatment options would not work, and that the key to rapid and massive scale-up was to keep the principles and practice of ART delivery as simple as possible. The chosen strategy was based on a public health approach [11,12], to scale up as fast as possible and to have the biggest impact on the health of the population by rolling out first-line ART only and providing alternative and second-line therapy in a very limited number of facilities. Standardized diagnosis and case finding were initiated, and no laboratory tests or laboratory monitoring were needed to start ART. Moreover, many of the principles of directly observed treatment (DOTS)—the system used to successfully deliver anti-tuberculosis (TB) treatment to people in some of the poorest countries of the world—were adapted to ART delivery.

A standardized system was developed, following the TB control system of case finding, treatment initiation, registering, recording and reporting of cases and outcomes. All stakeholders such as mission hospitals, universities, private sector, development partners (e.g. the WHO, the United Nations Children's Fund (UNICEF)), and national (e.g. Lighthouse) and international (e.g. Médecins Sans Frontières (MSF)) non-governmental organizations (NGOs) were included in the development of treatment guidelines and scale-up plans, and they bought into the implementation of the standard system. An important policy decision was made that ART was to be free for all patients in the public sector, and heavily subsidized in the private sector.

Every three months, the HIV Unit of the Ministry of Health and its partners conduct supervisory and monitoring visits to all ART sites in the country [13]. The purpose is to ensure that guidelines and standards are being adhered to, to collect data for national reporting, to provide encouragement and support, and to obtain drug stock levels to help with drug procurement.

Malawi's drug supply management system has several distinguishing elements [14]. Antiretroviral drugs are directly delivered to ART sites by the procurement agent every six months using a 'push system', in which the HIV Unit in the Ministry of Health determines the quantity of drugs to be delivered to each ART clinic. Facilities were initially classified on the basis of a number of parameters, including the number of TB patients they were treating, as the TB burden was considered to be a reasonable indicator for HIV burden. Low-burden facilities were given an allocation or 'ceiling' of antiretroviral drugs to recruit 25 new patients per month; medium-burden facilities could recruit 50 new patients per month; and high-burden facilities could recruit 150 new patients per month. Sites were instructed not to recruit any patients over and above this monthly ceiling. These ceilings can be increased if a facility shows it has the capacity to recruit more patients, but only after adequate drug supply is guaranteed. This system has thus far prevented the country from running out of drug supplies. A pre-packed kit system with 'starter packs' and 'continuation packs' was also introduced. A starter pack contains enough drugs to start 25 patients on ART for three months, and a continuation pack contains enough drugs to keep 75 patients on therapy for a similar period of three months. The classification and pre-packing of ART drugs has facilitated quantification and drug ordering. Malawi has also developed special packaging for antiretroviral drugs.

Involvement of the private sector

Health providers in the private sector were eager to join the national scaling up of ART. Within a year of the national programme's launch, the first private sector ART clinics had opened and were following the national system of standardized diagnosis, treatment, recording and reporting. Antiretroviral drugs are provided free of charge to such clinics, and patients pay a nominal fee (US$3.50) for their drug supplies, over and above the usual consultation fee.

The number of people on treatment in the private sector is not more than 5% of the total number of people on ART in Malawi. The main advantage of the private sector being in line with the public sector is that patients on ART in the private sector use a regimen that follows the national protocol, and the Ministry of Health receives quarterly reports from all 38 of the country's private sector treatment sites. Involvement of the private sector at an early stage of the programme's development proved essential for an uncomplicated public-private partnership [15].

Incidence of opportunistic infections

During quarterly supervision, data on the following four HIV-related diseases are collected: TB; Kaposi's sarcoma (KS); cryptococcal meningitis (CM); and oesophageal candidiasis (OC). Of the 13,370 patients that started ART between January and March 2007, 1596 had a history of TB, and 772, 600, and 1547 were diagnosed with KS, CM and OC, respectively [16].

Survival

Early mortality is a problem; approximately 8.5% of patients starting on ART die within the first three months of treatment [16]. One reason for this is that many people start ART late and are already (very) ill; 65% of patients starting ART are in WHO clinical stage 3, and 22% are in stage 4. At the moment, only 17 sites in Malawi have the capacity to provide CD4 testing, and this means that only 13% of patients start ART on the basis of being in WHO clinical stage 1 or 2 with a low CD4-lymphocyte count. Increased access to CD4-lymphocyte counts may help to get patients started earlier on ART, and this may reduce early mortality. A relation between early mortality and low body mass index (BMI) and fever (HIV wasting syndrome) is seen, but more research into the etiology of early mortality is needed. Cotrimoxazole prophylaxis is associated with a significant reduction in mortality for HIV-infected individuals who are not on ART, even in areas with high bacterial resistance to the antibiotic. A study carried out in Malawi showed that cotrimoxazole (CTX) taken concomitantly with ART reduces six-month mortality by 41% [17]. Increasing the current proportion (60%) of people on ART who are also receiving cotrimoxazole preventive therapy (CPT) may further reduce early mortality.

During quarterly supervision of ART sites, data are collected to establish survival analysis. People who move from one clinic to another (transfer out–transfer in) cannot be tracked adequately and are presumed alive. The most recent six-month survival analysis indicated that 81% of patients were alive (73% alive and on ART, and 8% transferred out and presumed alive). The 12-month, 18-month and 24-month survival analyses indicated that 74%, 70% and 70% of patients, respectively, were alive (either on ART, or transferred out and presumed alive).

Antiretroviral therapy has made an important contribution to survival; a study in Blantyre found that in the absence of ART, the 12-month incidence of death in HIV-infected patients with WHO clinical stage 4 and stage 3 was 88% and 62%, respectively [18]. The impact of ART on adult mortality in the community is currently being examined. For example, mortality data have been collected from eight private and parastatal companies in Malawi, where staff have had increased access to ART since 2003. All eight companies have seen a reduced mortality level, with the total mortality dropping from 445 in 2002 to 222 in 2006 (Figure 23.2).

Drug resistance

Before national guidelines and a national system of drug delivery were developed and implemented, patients were being treated with antiretroviral drugs in both the private and the public sectors. In the public sector in 2000, a combination of ZDV and 3TC was used for small numbers of patients (50–100) for about one year before the current regimen of d4T/3TC/NVP

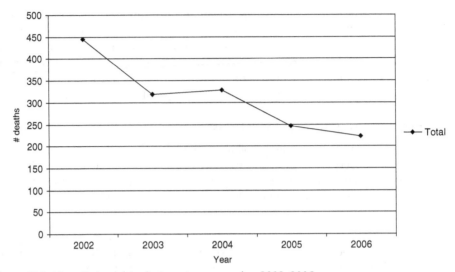

Figure 23.2 Mortality in eight private sector companies, 2002–2006

Source: Proceedings of the meeting and Preliminary Findings of Triangulation of Data on the Malawi National Response to HIV/AIDS: Impact on Prevention, Morbidity, and Mortality. Lilongwe, Malawi, 6–8 June 2007

(or co-formulated Triomune) was introduced. At the same time, monotherapy and dual therapy regimens were being used in the private sector, and such regimens had a high risk of promoting drug resistance. The use of single-dose NVP in prevention of mother-to-child transmission (PMTCT) programmes also potentially increased the risk of drug resistance to the non-nucleoside reverse transcriptase inhibitor (NNRTI) (i.e. NVP) component of Malawi's ART regimen.

Since mid-2004, the country has adopted the national system, and the first-line triple therapy combination is the regimen of choice in all facilities. A proposal and protocol were drafted, first to monitor HIV viral suppression and drug resistance among patients receiving ART, and second to carry out HIV drug resistance threshold surveillance among newly infected individuals. The results of the threshold study, which has been recently completed, showed that all samples were HIV-1 subtype C viruses and that no mutations on the WHO list for mutations associated with transmitted resistance were seen among the genotyped specimens. Therefore, transmitted drug resistance among the surveyed population is classified as <5% for all relevant drugs and drug classes.

Side effects

The major side effects of the first-line regimen (d4T, 3TC, and NVP) are shown in Table 23.1 [8]. According to quarterly monitoring reports, approximately 5% of patients on ART have significant side effects, but it is likely that these data underestimate the magnitude of the problem. Less that 5% of the population on treatment is on one of the alternative first-line regimens, and the first-line regimen may be associated with long-term side effects such as lactic acidosis and lipodystrophy syndrome. As these are often associated with the d4T component, Malawi has been advised by some international experts to change its first-line regimen. Alternatives for d4T (e.g. ZDV) need laboratory monitoring and will more than double the price of antiretroviral drugs (Table 23.2). Because of the very limited laboratory capacity in Malawi and concerns about financial sustainability, Malawi has so far been inclined to continue with a d4T-based regimen.

Table 23.1 Major side effects with d4T/3TC/NVP

Immediate Side Effects
Peripheral neuropathy
Hepatitis
Pancreatitis
Cutaneous hypersensitivity
Long-Term Side Effects
Peripheral neuropathy
Lactic acidosis
Lipodystrophy syndrome

Source: Ministry of Health, Malawi (2006) [8].

HIV and TB

Every year, approximately 27,000 people are diagnosed with TB, and an estimated 70% of these patients are co-infected with HIV. The new TB regimen contains rifampicin throughout the six-month regimen. As rifampicin reduces plasma concentrations of NVP, there has been concern that the combined use of ART and anti-TB treatment may lead to emerging drug resistance. Increasing the dose of NVP is difficult to manage logistically, and this may also lead to increased hepatotoxicity. EFV is a potential alternative for NVP, but as over 60% of Malawian patients are female, and contraception is, in many cases, not guaranteed, this is not a viable option. Evidence is gradually accumulating to indicate that plasma levels of NVP are still within the effective range when ART and rifampicin are combined, and the outcomes of patients on rifampicin and NVP are generally good. As a result, Malawi has decided to implement NVP-based regimens with rifampicin under close monitoring of treatment outcomes. Due to the risk of immune reconstitution disease, ART is started after the initial two-month phase of anti-TB treatment has been completed.

HIV and malaria

HIV infection and malaria are two of the most common and important health problems in sub-Saharan Africa, and there is growing evidence of interactive pathology. In Malawi, where malaria is endemic, a pilot study showed that it is feasible to distribute insecticide-treated bed nets (ITNs) to patients attending ART clinics.

Healthcare delivery

Malawi faces one of the worst human resource crises in the world [19]. The realization by international donors that 'Universal Access for HIV/AIDS' would be impossible without addressing this crisis helped Malawi to obtain substantial funds to implement a six-year Emergency Human Resources Plan. The human resource constraints had a large impact on the design of the ART scale-up plan. It was clear from the beginning that scaling up ART with physicians initiating treatment would not work. Instead, clinical officers and medical assistants were key to initiating ART, while nurses played a major role in following up patients. By 31 March 2007, a total of 69,389 patients, or 1% of the adult population, were on treatment. This success brought up the question of whether other cadres of staff with less training could be used to deliver ART. There are discussions and debates currently in progress about whether nurses can initiate treatment

Table 23.2 Costs of ART per person per year in Malawi

	Costs of ARVs per month (US$) (based on latest costs estimate)	Costs per year (US$) including costs of transport, storage, distribution, wastage	Proportion of people on regimen	Costs in US$
First-line regimen (d4T,3TC,NVP)	7.20	107.64	95.0%	-
Alternative first-line regimen I (ZDV,3TC,NVP)	16.43	245.63	3.0%	-
Alternative first-line regimen II (d4T,3TC,EFV)	26.50	396.18	1.0%	-
Second-line regimen (ZDV,3TC,Tenofovir, Lopinavir/Ritonavir)	70.35	1,051.73	1.0%	-
Average cost of ARVs per person per year				125.61
Costs of drugs for CPT				10.37
Costs of drugs for HIV-related diseases				10.00
Costs of therapeutic feeding for patients on ART per person per year				21.35
Costs for training, IEC, M&E, supervision, OR, health education, infrastructure, etc.				24.35
Staff costs per person per year on ART				27.04
Other service delivery costs (clinic running costs, laboratory support)				10.00
Average total costs of ART programme				228.72

Source: Erik Schouten. Calculation of costs of ART per person per year. Based on data from procurement agency and programmatic data. May 2007

and whether health surveillance assistants (with 10 weeks of training) can be used to follow up patients on treatment. This so-called shifting of tasks to cadres with less training is a core component of the ART scale-up approach and key to the WHO's 'Treat, train and retain' strategy. Scaling up ART with staff who have a minimal amount of training can only be done with a programme that is highly standardized, simplified, and has a strong supervision and monitoring component.

Training of staff

A large number of staff have been trained in ART. Training consists of a five-day module in which the emphasis is on clinical staging, initiation of ART, management of side effects, and monitoring and recording the treatment response. All participants undertake a formal written examination at the end of the module and must obtain a pass mark of 70% or more to be certified in ART delivery. Between 2004 and 2006, 1691 healthcare workers (776 clinicians and 915 nurses) were trained and certified in the public sector, and 400 (164 clinicians and 236 nurses) were similarly trained in the private sector. The ART module has been incorporated into the undergraduate curricula of the medical, health science and nursing training institutions of the country.

ART delivery sites

There are 144 ART sites in the country. In the first instance, 60 central, district and mission hospitals were prepared and started delivering ART, later followed by 46 mainly smaller mission hospitals, rural hospitals and health centres. In the private sector, 38 facilities (hospitals and clinics) were accredited and delivering ART by the end of March 2007.

Patients on ART

Malawi has the fourth highest coverage of ART in all of sub-Saharan Africa [10] and, in April of 2007, reached the milestone of 100,000 people started on ART since the programme began. Even though the numbers of people starting ART are considerable, 50% of those eligible for treatment still do not have access. The capacity of the health sector is a limiting factor in reaching universal access.

Some of the characteristics of patients in the public and private sectors are shown in Table 23.3, and treatment outcomes are shown in Table 23.4. As previously mentioned, patients are grouped together in quarterly cohorts, and this allows, through the routine system, time-bound treatment outcome analysis. For example, all patients registered in a cohort between July and September 2006 could have their outcomes assessed on 31 March 2007, constituting a six-month outcome analysis; it is recognized that, in effect, this means an analysis of patient outcomes

Table 23.3 Characteristics of patients ever started on ART in Malawi up to 31 March 2007

	Public sector	Private Sector	Total
Total number started on ART	95,674	3861	99,535
Number (%) males	38,142 (40)	2007 (52)	40,149 (40)
Number (%) females	57,532 (60)	1854 (48)	59,386 (60)
Number (%) adults	88,337 (92)	3691 (96)	92,028 (92)
Number (%) children (below 15 years)	7337 (8)	170 (4)	7507 (8)
Number (%) on ART due to:			
WHO Clinical Stage 3	62,362 (65)	1672 (43)	64,034 (64)
WHO Clinical Stage 4	21,293 (22)	846 (22)	22,139 (22)
WHO Stage 1 and 2 with low CD4	12,019 (13)	1343 (35)	13,362 (13)
Number (%) on ART due to:			
Active or previous TB	15,126 (16)	317 (8)	15,443 (16)
Referral from PMTCT	1346 (2, of women)	0 (0)	1346 (1)

Source: [16] and .Malawi Business Coalition Against HIV/AIDS. Private sector quarterly supervision report. 15th May 2007. Blantyre, Malawi.

Table 23.4 Treatment outcomes of patients ever started on ART in Malawi up to 31 March 2007

	Public sector	Private Sector	Total
Total number started on ART	95,674	3861	99,535
Number (%) alive and on ART	66,438 (69)	2951 (76)	69,389 (70)
Number (%) dead	11,108 (12)	269 (7)	11,377 (11)
Number (%) lost to follow-up	9483 (10)	158 (4)	9641 (10)
Number (%) stopped treatment	389 (0)	6 (0)	395 (0)
Number (%) transferred out	8252 (9)	477 (12)	8729 (9)
Of those alive and on ART:			
Number (%) on first-line regimen	63,883 (96)	2762 (94)	66,645 (96)
Number (%) on alternative regimen	2349 (3)	172 (6)	2521 (4)
Number (%) on second-line regimen	196 (0)	17 (1)	213 (0)
Of those alive and on ART:			
Number (%) with ambulatory status known	64,682 (97)	2946 (100)	67,628 (97)
Number (%) ambulatory	63,156 (98)	2914 (99)	66,070 (98)
Number (%) with work status known	64,682 (97)	2946 (100)	67,628 (97)
Number (%) able to work	61,527 (95)	2914 (99)	64,441 (95)
Number (%) with side effects known	60,895 (92)	-	-
Number (%) with side effects	2855 (5)	-	-
Number (%) where pill counts were done	48,541 (73)	524 (18)	49,065 (71)
Number (%) with 95% adherence	45,576 (94)	511 (98)	46,087 (94)
Number dying with date/time recorded	11,108	Not known	Not known
Number (%) dying in first month	3526 (32)	-	-
Number (%) dying in second month	2519 (23)	-	-
Number (%) dying in third month	1348 (12)	-	-
Number (%) dying after third month	3715 (33)	-	-

Source: [16] and Malawi Business Coalition Against HIV/AIDS. Private sector quarterly supervision report. 15 May 2007. Blantyre, Malawi.

six to nine months after starting ART. Patients registered 12 months previously, between January and March 2006, could also have their outcomes assessed on 31 March 2007, constituting a 12-month outcome analysis. Recent six-month, 12-month, 18-month and 24-month treatment outcome analyses of different cohorts from sites around the country showed that 73%, 63%, 59% and 56% of patients, respectively, were alive and still on ART at their initial treatment site.

Equity and access to ART

Equity in the health sector response to HIV/AIDS has been a concern from the outset of the programme [20]. Apart from concerns about who does and does not have access to ART, the implementation of a national ART programme may have a negative effect on the implementation of other essential health services. The Ministry of Health and National AIDS Commission have, at national level, recognized the importance of equity in the national scale-up of ART. Through a consultative process, a policy was developed presenting principles for promoting equity in access to ART [21]. The major decisions were that:

- ART would be rolled out throughout the country instead of on a district by district basis;
- ART would be free of charge in the public sector (including mission hospitals) and at heavily subsidized rates in the private sector;
- targeted gender-sensitive health promotion of ART would be made to groups of people considered to be in 'strategic' or vulnerable situations; and
- ART provision would support the provision of essential health services, particularly within the public health sector, and equity monitoring (including disaggregation by sex and age) would be conducted as part of the ART scale-up.

The monitoring of equity has been carried out through ongoing quarterly supervision and monitoring visits by the HIV Unit of the Ministry of Health, and special surveys have been conducted to look into access to ART according to social, economic, demographic and geographic characteristics. This includes identifying groups who are being marginalized in terms of treatment and the barriers that prevent access to treatment in other sectors of the population [21].

Three main categories of patients have been, and still are, relatively underserved. Up until 2005, only 5% of patients were children, and from a small sub-analysis, only very few were under one year of age. This was similar to reports from other African countries [23]. In Malawi, an estimated 10–15% of patients on ART should be children [6], but the small actual number reflects the difficulties faced by clinicians in diagnosing and managing HIV in infants, and in treating children with split-tablet doses. To improve this situation, technical recommendations to simplify the diagnosis of HIV in infants have been developed, and specific paediatric drug formulations are being advocated. The WHO's new, revised paediatric guidelines [24] released in early 2006 have assisted substantially in addressing some of these difficulties. The update of the National ART Guidelines, with a greater focus on paediatric ART, and the increased experience of Malawian clinicians combined with targeted training had boosted the proportion of children on ART from 5% to 10% by the end of March 2007 [16].

Very few HIV-positive pregnant women are referred for ART. Many of these mothers are asymptomatic, and eligibility for ART depends on increased availability of CD4 testing. Potential solutions include more capacity in the country to measure CD4-lymphocyte counts, easier ways of performing the test, and an explicit priority for CD4 testing directed at HIV-positive pregnant women.

Finally, the proportion of TB patients placed on ART is too small. With a national HIV-seroprevalence rate of 70% among TB patients [25] and 27,000 new TB patients being diagnosed and treated every year in the country, approximately 19,000 eligible TB patients annually should be receiving ART. However, there are technical difficulties with placing HIV-infected TB patients on ART, including drug-drug interactions between rifampicin and NNRTIs [26], concerns about immune reconstitution disease, and the fact that, in Malawi, ART is delivered largely from hospital clinics while anti-TB treatment is largely decentralized to health centres [27].

Economics

The costs of the ART programme in Malawi have been calculated. Based on the current regimen (which is the least expensive on the market), a very low proportion of patients on alternative or second-line drugs, and minimal use of laboratory monitoring, the annual cost is estimated at US$229 per person. This includes: the costs of antiretroviral drugs, drugs for HIV-related diseases, and CPT; therapeutic feeding; training; health promotion; supervision; monitoring and evaluation (M&E); operational research (OR); infrastructure development; staff salaries; and costs of laboratory services and salaries (Table 23.2).

If Malawi can maintain the current pace of ART scale-up, starting 45,000 people per year on ART [28], it is expected that approximately 200,000 people will be alive and on treatment by 2015. If the costs do not change, the antiretroviral drugs alone would constitute 30% of the total health budget. Any change in the current first-line ART regimen, e.g. moving away from the use of d4T and replacing it with ZDV, as several international experts have advised, would double the average cost of antiretroviral drugs and increase the total costs of the programme by 60%. Malawi may be reluctant to make these changes, since its economy is too small to support the national scale-up of ART on its own; the programme is largely dependent on foreign donors. Although the G8 countries pledged, at the Gleneagles summit in 2005, to increase overseas development assistance (ODA), and called on UNAIDS, WHO and other international bodies to develop and implement a package for HIV prevention, treatment and care with the aim of attaining, as closely as possible, universal access to treatment for all those who need it by 2010, the funding available through, for example, the Global Fund to fight AIDS, Tuberculosis and Malaria (Global Fund), is far from sufficient to support these promises.

With 75% of the population in Malawi living on less than US$2 per day, and with an average per capita annual income of US$160 [29], it is clear that very few people can afford to pay for ART. The option of charging at least some patients for ART care has been discussed, but experience in the Lighthouse clinic in Lilongwe, one of the first clinics to provide ART in Malawi, showed that paying for ART led to high drop-out rates and poor adherence, which in turn threatened the development of drug resistance [30]. The decision was made, correctly in our view, that ART was to be made available free of charge.

Given the serious questions around financial sustainability and support of the programme, the important question is whether a change in first-line regimen, as mentioned earlier, will result in the saving of more lives. Malawi strongly believes that it should continue scaling up using the first-line d4T, 3TC and NVP regimen only, avoiding a multiplicity of other regimens because of side effects, and, in particular, should be cautious about expanding expensive second-line therapy. There is an important public health consideration to support this view. Because there are many eligible HIV-infected people who are not yet receiving any treatment, and because over 80% of patients do well on the first-line regimen [31], priority should be given to provision of first-line treatment to those not yet receiving ART rather than offering better care to the minority already on ART. This approach is based on principles of equity and should result in an improved overall health gain.

Conclusion

Malawi has shown that in a severely resource-constrained setting, using a simple, structured, inclusive approach to ART delivery, treatment can be delivered to large numbers of patients with good outcomes. A few facilities in the country are supported by NGOs such as MSF and Dignitas International, or through the private, for-profit sector, but in the majority of facilities, the local healthcare personnel are the sole providers of the ART services.

The most important factors that laid the foundations of the Malawi ART programme are:

◆ clear national ART guidelines with a limited number of treatment regimens, in which an emphasis is also placed on the system of registration, monitoring and recording of results [8];

- a desire by all implementing partners to work together with the Ministry of Health and use national standardized systems;
- an intensive training schedule, teaching healthcare workers how to use ART guidelines;
- a structured system of accrediting ART sites before they are permitted to deliver treatment to patients;
- quarterly supervision and monitoring of all ART delivery sites by the HIV Unit of the Ministry of Health and its partners; and
- no stock-outs of antiretroviral drugs. (Their availability has worked well so far through a parallel procurement system).

Challenges

Malawi has developed a five-year scale-up plan to place 245,000 patients on ART by the end of 2010, as the part of the national response to 'Universal Access to HIV/AIDS prevention, care and treatment'. This will be a daunting challenge, and will only succeed if certain issues can be resolved.

First there is a need to tackle the dire human resource shortfall crisis that pervades sub-Saharan Africa [32] and to further engage in task shifting so that healthcare workers with less training can initiate and manage the follow-up of ART [33].

Second, there is an absolute necessity for ongoing financial support, either from the established players such as the Global Fund and the US President's Emergency Plan for AIDS Relief (PEPFAR), or new players such as UNITAID. There is, however, an absolute shortage of funds. The total funding envelope for Round 7 of the Global Fund is US$500 million, while a five-year proposal for HIV treatment and care in Malawi would amount to at least US$200 million.

Third, there will be a need in the next few years to invest in and secure alternative first-line ART regimens to the ones in current use, as HIV drug resistance and long-term side effects, particularly of d4T, become more of a problem. The price of this alternative is an important factor in light of the financial sustainability of the national ART programme.

Fourth, undertaking regular supervision and reliable drug procurement for the increasing case burden will be essential if antiretroviral drug supplies are to remain uninterrupted and standards are to be maintained.

Finally, HIV prevention methods have to be similarly scaled up, otherwise HIV/AIDS caseloads will continue to increase indefinitely.

Future directions

A successful ART programme should adhere to the principles of scaling up, keeping the programme simple and firmly based on public health principles. Mechanisms for task shifting (through an evidence-based, regulatory framework) as well as the role of communities (e.g. expert patients) need to be further developed, in recognition that the proportion of the HIV-infected adult population in Malawi will increase to 3–5% in the coming years.

References

1. United Nations Development Programme. (2006). *Human Development Report 2006. Beyond scarcity: Power, poverty and the global water crisis.* New York: UNDP.
2. UNAIDS. (2006). *Report on the global AIDS epidemic 2006.* Geneva: UNAIDS.

3. Glynn JR, Pönnighaus J, Crampin AC, *et al.* (2001). The development of the HIV epidemic in Karonga District, Malawi. *AIDS* **15**:2025–2029.

4. McGormack GP, Glynn JR, Crampin AC, *et al.* (2002). Early evolution of the human immunodeficiency virus type 1 subtype C epidemic in rural Malawi. *J Virol* **76**:12890–9.

5. Aberle Grasse J, Kamoto K, Wadonda N, *et al.* (2007). HIV Drug Resistance Surveillance in a National ART Program. 2007 HIV/AIDS Implementers' meeting, 16–19 June 2007, Kigali, Rwanda. [Abstract number 358]

6. National AIDS Commission, Malawi. (2005*). HIV and Syphilis Sero-Survey and National HIV Prevalence Estimates Report 2005*. Lilongwe: Government of Malawi.

7. Government of Malawi. (2004). *Demographic and Health Survey 2004*. Lilongwe: Government of Malawi.

8. Ministry of Health, Malawi. (2006). *Treatment of AIDS. Guidelines for the use of antiretroviral therapy in Malawi, 2nd Edition*. Lilongwe: Government of Malawi.

9. World Health Organization, UNAIDS. (2003). *Treating 3 million by 2005: making it happen: the WHO strategy*. Geneva: World Health Organization/ UNAIDS.

10. WHO, UNAIDS, UNICEF. (2007). *Towards Universal Access: scaling up priority HIV/AIDS interventions in the health sector. Progress Report, April 2007*. Geneva and New York: WHO, UNAIDS and UNICEF.

11. Harries AD, Schouten EJ, Libamba E. (2006). Scaling up antiretroviral treatment in resource-poor settings. *Lancet* **367**:1870–1872.

12. Gilks CF, Crowley S, Ekpini R, *et al.* (2006). The WHO public-health approach to antiretroviral treatment against HIV in resource-limited settings. *Lancet* **368**:505–10.

13. Libamba E, Makombe S, Mhango E, *et al.* (2006). Supervision, monitoring and evaluation of nationwide scale-up of antiretroviral therapy in Malawi. *Bull World Health Organ* **84**:320–6.

14. Harries AD, Schouten EJ, Makombe SD, *et al.* (2007). Ensuring uninterrupted supplies of antiretroviral drugs in resource-poor settings: an example from Malawi. *Bull of the World Health Organ* **85**:152–6.

15. Schouten EJ, Chuka S, Libamba E, *et al.* (2006). Private Sector involvement in National Scale up of Antiretroviral therapy (ART) in Malawi. XVI International AIDS Conference, 13 – 18 August 2006, Toronto, Canada. [Abstract THPE0186]

16. HIV Unit, Ministry of Health, Malawi. (2007). *ART in the public sector in the Malawi. Results up to 31st March 2007*. Lilongwe: Government of Malawi.

17. Lowrance D, Makombe S, Harries A, *et al.* (2007). Cotrimoxazole Prophylaxis Reduced the Early Mortality of HIV-infected Patients on ART in Malawi. 14th Conference on Retroviruses and Opportunistic Infections, 25–27 February 2007, Los Angeles, CA, USA. [Abstract 83]

18. Van Oosterhout JJG, Luafer MK, Graham SM, *et al.* (2005). A community-based study of the incidence of trimethoprim-sulfamethoxazole-preventable infections in Malawian adults living with HIV. *J Acquir Immune Defic Syndr* **39**:626–631.

19. Ministry of Health. (2004). *Human Resources in the health sector: toward a solution*. Lilongwe: Government of Malawi.

20. Kemp J, Aitken JM, LeGrand S, Mwale B. (2003). *Equity in Health Sector Responses to HIV/AIDS in Malawi. Equinet Discussion paper 5*. Harare, Zimbabwe: EQUINET.

21. National AIDS Commission, Malawi. (2005). *Policy on equity in access to Antiretroviral Therapy (ART) in Malawi*. Lilongwe: Government of Malawi.

22. Banda T, Hedt B, Aberle-Grasse J, Makwiza I, Schouten, E. (2007). *Universal access to Antiretroviral Therapy – A study to explore factors limiting in reaching universal access to antiretroviral therapy. A proposal developed in collaboration with WHO*. Lilongwe: Government of Malawi.

23. The United Nations Children's Fund (UNICEF). (2005). *The global campaign on children and AIDS: Unite for children. Unite against AIDS*. New York: UNICEF.

24. World Health Organization. (2006). *Antiretroviral therapy of HIV infection in infants and children in resource-limited settings, towards universal access: recommendations for a public health approach*. Geneva: WHO.

25. Kwanjana J, Harries AD, Gausi F, Nyangulu DS, Salaniponi FML. (2001). HIV-seroprevalence in patients with tuberculosis in Malawi. *Malawi Med J* **13**:7–10.

26. Kwara A, Flanigan TP, Carter EJ. (2005). Highly active antiretroviral therapy (HAART) in adults with tuberculosis: current status. *Int J Tuberc Lung Dis* **9**:248–257.

27. Zachariah R, Teck R, Ascurra O, *et al.* (2005). Can we get more HIV-positive tuberculosis patients on antiretroviral treatment in a rural district of Malawi? *Int J Tuberc Lung Dis* **9**:238–247.

28. Harries AD, Schouten EJ, Libamba E. (2006). Scaling up antiretroviral treatment in resource-poor settings. *Lancet* **367**:1870–1872.

29. World Bank Group. (2004). *Country "at a glance" reports: Malawi, Tanzania, Zambia, Mozambique, South Africa*. Washington, DC: World Bank.

30. Phiri SJ, Nkhoma EC, Mhango E, *et al.* (2004). The Lighthouse project: A model of integrated services for HIV/AIDS care in Lilongwe, Malawi. XV International Conference on AIDS, 11–16 July 2004, Bangkok, Thailand. [Abstract B11828]

31. Libamba E, Makombe S, Harries AD, *et al.* (2005). Scaling up antiretroviral therapy in Africa: learning from tuberculosis control programmes – the case of Malawi. *Int J Tuberc Lung Dis* **9**:1062–71.

32. Hongoro C, MacPake B. (2004). How to bridge the gap in human resources for health. *Lancet* **364**:1451–1456.

33. Van Damme W, Kober K, Laga M. (2006). The real challenges for scaling up ART in sub-Saharan Africa. *AIDS* **20**:653–656.

Chapter 24

Country review: Senegal

Papa Salif Sow

Introduction

Senegal is a low-income country in West Africa with 10 million inhabitants. There are 11 administrative regions in the country, and the health system is decentralized, with two university teaching hospitals, 17 regional hospitals, 58 health districts, and 830 health posts. In Senegal, 93% of the population is Muslim and 5% Christian, and male circumcision is universal from birth to age seven. In a 1994 population-based survey in Dakar, the capital of Senegal, less than 5% of the population reported drinking alcohol in the month prior to the survey. Sex work was legalized in 1969, and since then regular screening and treatment for sexually transmitted diseases (STDs) has been offered to female sex workers (FSWs) in the cities where they are found in high concentrations. The number of non-registered FSWs is not known but is estimated to be equal to the number of registered FSWs. A population-based survey in Dakar in the early 1990s showed that the median age at initiation of sexual intercourse was 18 years for both women and men. The median age at first marriage was 19 years for women and 28 years for men, this age difference being associated with high levels of polygamy in keeping with the religious mores of this society [1].

Epidemiology

Senegal is a country with a concentrated HIV epidemic. The prevalence is estimated at 1.5% in the general population, 17–30% in FSWs and 21% in men who have sex with men (MSM). The majority of patients (80%) are infected with HIV-1, 15% with HIV-2, and 5% are dually reactive HIV-1 and HIV-2; the CRF-02 AG strains are more prevalent. There are 80,000 people currently living with HIV in Senegal [2].

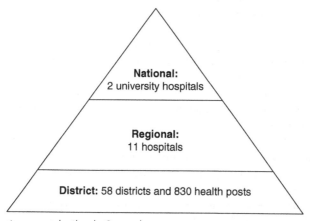

Fig. 24.1 Health system organization in Senegal.

The HIV-2 virus was described for the first time in Senegalese FSWs in 1985, by Senegalese researchers in collaboration with colleagues from France (Lomges, Tours) and from the United States (Harvard AIDS Institute). The first AIDS case was hospitalized and described in 1986 in the Department of Infectious Diseases at Fann Hospital, the university teaching hospital in Dakar. Between 1989 and 1996, the levels of HIV infection estimated in four urban sentinel sites remained stable at around 1.2% in pregnant women and 3% in male STD patients; this low HIV prevalence in the general population in Senegal contrasts with the situation in a number of West African countries [1]. Blood transfusion safety was established at the start of the HIV epidemic and the level of knowledge of preventive practices relating to HIV/AIDS among the general population exceeded 90% in the early 1990s.

From 1991 to 1996, a 30–66% decrease in STD prevalence rates was observed in pregnant women and sex workers in Dakar. In 1997, 33% of men aged 15–49 years in Dakar reported having engaged in sexual activity with people other than their regular partners, and among them, 67% reported condom use. It is impossible to know what course the HIV epidemic in Senegal would have taken in the absence of prevention efforts. While several factors pre-dating the occurrence of AIDS in Senegal laid the groundwork for a positive response, data from a number of sources do reveal how successful the HIV prevention efforts were. Senegal can rightfully claim to have contained the spread of HIV by intervening early and comprehensively to increase knowledge and awareness of HIV/AIDS and to promote safe sexual behaviour.

Response to HIV in Senegal

A strong public response to the HIV/AIDS epidemic was developed by the Senegalese authorities. In terms of the organization of health and health information services, three factors seem to have provided a good grounding for an effective response to the HIV/AIDS epidemic in Senegal. The first was the existing STD screening and treatment programme for registered FSWs, which had been running since 1969. The second was the creation of a national STD control programme established in most health facilities, which started in 1988 and offered care in specialized STD clinics. The programme has since evolved, and the management of STDs is now widely integrated into regular primary health care services, with care providers having been trained, and a system of cost recovery for STD drugs in place to ensure sustainability. The drop in the prevalence of STDs among pregnant women and sex workers in Dakar between 1991 and 1996 is due to the success of this programme. The third factor was the presence of a large number of non-governmental organizations (NGOs) that had already developed a tradition of commitment to health through the promotion of vaccination and control of malaria.

There were four special features of the Senegalese response to the HIV epidemic. The first was the early establishment of a transfusion policy centred on the prevention of transmission of HIV through blood. Compulsory screening of every batch of blood for HIV infection was set up in 1987 in the all 11 regions of Senegal.

The second feature was the use of existing STD screening and treatment services as entry points for information, counselling, condom provision, and promotion of safer behaviours, especially among sex workers.

The third feature of the Senegalese response was the extent of social mobilization in the development of information, education and communication (IEC) campaigns to promote responsible and safe sexual behaviour and to encourage the use of condoms. The existing network of hundreds of NGOs served as the basis for this mobilization. Local communication efforts to promote change in behaviour was essential and took place in the workplace, in schools and universities, stations, on roads, in markets, kiosks, touring cinema buses in outlying regions, and through national days of action. Tens of thousands of IEC materials (brochures, handbooks, videos, posters, etc.) were produced by the National AIDS Prevention Committee (NAPC) and NGOs. By 1992, the Ministry of Education had included sex education with an HIV component in the school curriculum for children aged 12 and over. Teachers were trained and educational brochures were included in the curriculum, and during the course of 1997, over 130,000 school manuals devoted to IEC on HIV/AIDS were distributed in public and private teaching establishments. IEC activities covered the whole of the country, thanks to the media and regional and departmental AIDS control committees.

The fourth feature of the response was the concerted and effective effort to include religious and community leaders and politicians at all levels in HIV prevention activities. Widely publicized national conferences were held by both Muslim and Christian leaders, who lent considerable moral support to the provision of universal information about AIDS and other STDs, as well as to efforts to promote responsible sexual behaviour. Senegal also benefited from major technical and financial contributions from its international partners in AIDS control. Technical or donor agencies, including the World Health Organization (WHO), the European Union, the United States Agency for International Development (USAID) and Coopération Française, regularly conducted reviews of Senegal's national programme. These independent evaluations helped to refocus prevention and control activities on a regular basis.

Prevention

With strong political and community commitment, the NAPC, which was set up in 1986, made an early and extensive response to the epidemic. This response included:

- prevention of transmission through blood by means of systematic HIV screening of all blood used for transfusion;
- prevention of sexual transmission through awareness campaigns for safer sex;
- widespread screening and treatment of STDs;
- promotion of condom use and provision of affordable, good quality condoms; and
- special interventions for groups at high risk of HIV infection, such as FSWs.

A focus on prevention at the beginning of the HIV epidemic was and is advocated as the most cost-effective way of controlling or even stopping the epidemic.

Treatment of opportunistic infections

During the period 1986–96, focus turned to the treatment of opportunistic infections (OIs). There was no national antiretroviral therapy (ART) programme at this time. The most prevalent OIs were tuberculosis (TB), chronic diarrhoea, oesophageal candidiasis and bacteraemia due to *Salmonella typhi murium* and *Streptococcus pneumonia* [3,4]. A great deal of clinical research on OIs was conducted in Senegal in collaboration with France's *Agence Nationale de Recherches sur le SIDA* (ANRS) as well as the University of Washington at Seattle and the Havard AIDS Institute in the United States.

A prospective study of high-grade squamous intraepithelial lesion (HSIL) development among Senegalese women with and without HIV-1 and/or HIV-2 infection and high-risk human papilloma virus (HPV) infection was conducted [5]. Study subjects included 627 women who were assessed every four months for squamous intraepithelial lesion and HPV DNA over a mean follow-up of 2.2 years. During follow-up, 71 (11%) of the women developed HSIL as detected by cytology. HIV-infected women with high-risk HPV types were at the greatest risk for developing HSIL. In multivariable Cox regression modelling, persistent infection (hazard ratio (HR)=47.1; 95% confidence interval (CI) =16.3–136) and transient infection (HR=14.0; 95% CI=3.7–54) with oncogenic HPV types were strongly associated with HSIL risk. In univariate analyses, HIV-positive women infected with HIV-2 were less likely to develop HSIL (HR=0.3; 95% CI=0.1–0.9) than HIV-positive women infected with HIV-1. HIV-positive women with CD4+ cell counts between 200 and 500 cells/mm^3 (HR=2.2, 95% CI=0.8–6.3) or less than 200 cells/mm^3 (HR=5.5; 95% CI=2.0–15.2) were at greater risk for HSIL than HIV-positive women with CD4 counts of more than 500 cells/mm^3. High plasma HIV levels were associated with increased HSIL risk (HR for each order of magnitude increase in the level of HIV plasma RNA =1.4; 95% CI=1.1–1.7). HIV-1 and HIV-2 are associated with increased risk for development of HSIL. This risk appears to be primarily associated with the increased HPV persistence resulting from immunosuppression related to HIV-1 and/or HIV-2 infection.

Another study included 2065 consecutive patients aged 35 years or older presenting to community health clinics in Dakar, who had not been previously screened for cytologic abnormalities or HPV. Cytologic diagnosis and HPV detection were accomplished using a ThinPrep® Pap test and a polymerase chain reaction (PCR)-based reverse-line strip assay, respectively. Odds ratios (OR) and associated 95% confidence intervals were estimated using polynomial logistic regression. Cytologic abnormalities were found in 426 women (20%), including 254 (12%) with atypical squamous cells of undetermined significance, 86 (4%) with low-grade squamous intraepithelial lesions, 66 (3%) with HSIL, and 20 (1%) with invasive cancer. Infection with HPV was detected in 18%. Among women with negative cytologic results, the prevalence of high-risk but not low-risk HPV types increased with age. HPV16 (2.4%) and HPV58 (1.6%) were the most frequently detected HPV types in this population, as well as being those most strongly associated with risk of HSIL/cancer (HPV16: OR=88; 95% CI=39–200; HPV58: OR=51; 95% CI=16–161). These data suggest that in addition to HPV16, HPV58 should be considered in the strategic planning of vaccination against cervical cancer in this geographical region [6].

Antiretroviral therapy (ART)

In August 1998, the government of Senegal launched a national initiative for access to ART, known as the Highly Active Antiretroviral Therapy Initiative (ISAARV), which began as a pilot project at three selected university hospital sites within Dakar over the three-year period 1998–2001 [7]. The inclusion criteria for access to ART included symptomatic and asymptomatic HIV-positive patients with CD4 counts less than 200cells/mm^3. Viral load criteria were not required for starting ART; testing was done once a year or in case of clinical immunologic failure. Haematology, renal and liver evaluations were done at day one, one month later, and every four months subsequently. Patients had free access to HIV serology tests, antiretroviral drugs, drugs for OIs, CD4 count and viral load testing.

For this pilot study, a prospective observational cohort study was established in Dakar in August 1998. Initial treatment consisted of two nucleoside reverse transcriptase inhibitors (NRTIs) and one protease inhibitor (PI). Fifty-eight treatment-naïve patients, most of whom were infected by the HIV-1 CRF02-AG strain, were enrolled. The majority of these patients were at an advanced stage of HIV disease (86.2% had AIDS). Adherence was good in 87.9% of patients, and treatment was effective in most of them. Thus, HIV-1 RNA was undetectable in 79.6%, 71.2%, 51.4% and 59.3% of patients at months 1, 6, 12 and 18, respectively, and the median viral load reduction was 2.5 log$_{10}$ copies/mL. The CD4 cell count rose by a median of 82, 147, and 180 cells/mm^3 at months 6, 12 and 18, respectively. At the same points in time, the cumulative probability of remaining alive or free of new AIDS-defining events was 94.8%, 85.0% and 82.3%, respectively. Most adverse effects (80.8%) were mild or moderate, and there were only two cases of drug resistance. This study shows that highly active antiretroviral therapy (HAART) is feasible and well tolerated in Senegalese patients. Clinical and biological results were comparable to those seen in western cohorts, despite differences in the HIV-1 subtype distribution and an advanced disease stage when the treatment was initiated [8,9]. Contrary to other recent studies in Africa, viral resistance rarely emerged [10].

The next important challenge became the decentralization and scale-up of ART in all 11 regions of the country. To address this, a system of *parrainage*, or mentoring, was established with the goal of enabling local physicians to prescribe ART. The mentor is a Dakar-based physician at a major academic clinical centre who has significant expertise in using antiretroviral drugs and treating HIV-positive patients. There is a separate mentor for each region. Initially, mentors spend four days on site in their respective regions. These meetings are mainly intended for physicians and focus on inclusion criteria and issues of monitoring patients on treatment in particular. Subsequent visits are arranged every three months by the mentor, and in between visits, close telephone or e-mail contact is maintained between local physicians and the mentor to address specific problems pertaining to monitoring and antiretroviral regimens as they arise.

First-line antiretroviral (ARV) regimens combine two NRTIs and a non-nucleoside reverse transcriptase inhibitor (NNRTI), while protease inhibitors are used for HIV-2-infected patients and for second-line treatment. Cotrimoxazole prophylaxis is provided free of charge to all HIV-infected patients with CD4 cell counts less than 350 cells/mm^3, and women are screened for cervical dysplasia. Post-exposure prophylaxis is available for health staff in the public health centres. Antiretroviral regimens for the prevention of mother-to-child transmission (PMTCT) include the combination of zidovudine (ZDV), lamivudine (3TC) and a single dose of nevirapine (NVP), and alternatives to breastfeeding are offered free of charge to all babies born to HIV-infected mothers. A patient education programme using local languages has been developed under the supervision of social workers; the objective of this programme is to strengthen the patient's level of understanding in order to improve adherence.

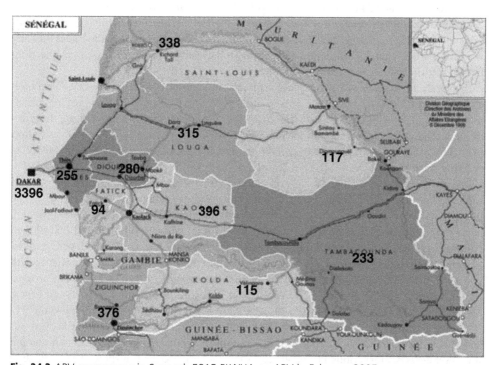

Fig. 24.2 ARV programme in Senegal: 5915 PLWHA on ARV in February 2007.

This mentoring system has had a great impact on scaling up access to ART in Senegal. The number of treatment centres increased from four in 2002 to 55 in February 2007 (16 in Dakar and 39 in other regions), and the number of physicians trained in ART increased from 12 to 125 in the same period. More importantly, the number of patients on ART increased from 980 in 2002 to 5915 in February 2007, which represents 27% coverage of those in need of treatment (see Figure 24.2). Also, there has been a significant reduction in the distances travelled by patients to obtain treatment; since February 2005, there has been access to ART in all 11 Senegalese regions, making it a truly nationwide programme.

After eight years of ART in Senegal (1998–2006), some 5200 HIV patients had been treated with antiretroviral drugs. At baseline, 95% of patients were treatment-naïve and 82% had AIDS. Median age was 37 years, and 54.7% were female. Body mass index was less than 19 kg/m^2 in 38.6% of cases. Median CD4 count was less than 50 $cells/mm^3$ in 24.3% of cases, and between 50 and 199 $cells/mm^3$ in 38.5%, while mean viral load was 5.2 log copies/mL. The majority of the patients (60%) were treated with ZDV/3TC/efavirenz (EFV). Patients' median weight increased from 58 kg at day 0 to 68 kg at 84 months (seven years) on therapy. Antiretroviral efficacy was high, with 60–80% of the patients consistently having viral loads less than 500 copies/mL and the CD4 cell count increased to a median of 225 $cells/mm^3$. Drug resistance occurred in 12.5% of cases, with 33% of the patients changing their ARV regimens after seven years on treatment.

Tuberculosis is the most common OI seen in Senegalese patients receiving ART [11]. This is probably due to the fact that the majority of patients discovered their HIV status very late, after the occurrence of an OI at an advanced stage. The overall incidence of death is 6.3 per 100 person-years (95% CI:5.26–7.7), with most deaths occurring during the first year after initiation of ART; the probability of dying during the first year is 11.7% (95% CI:8.9%–15.3%). However, the death rate then decreases over time, yielding a cumulative probability of dying of 17.4% (95% CI:13.9%–21.5%) and 24.6% (95% CI:20.4%–29.4%) at two and five years, respectively.

Causes of death were mostly due to mycobacterial infections, neuropenic infections and septicaemia. According to Etard et al. [11], data from the Senegalese cohort study underlines the early mortality pattern after ART initiation and highlights the leading role of mycobacterial infections in the cause of death of Senegalese HIV patients.

During the first decade of ART in Senegal, priority was given to the evaluation of clinical trials using simplified antiretroviral regimens in order to improve treatment adherence in patients living in countries with limited resources. In 2000–1, a study was set up to investigate the effectiveness of, as well as adherence and tolerance to, a once-daily ART regimen in Senegalese adults [12]. This study was carried out in collaboration with ANRS and the *Institut de Médecine et d'Épidémiologie Appliquée* (IMEA) in France.

In a prospective, open-label, single-arm study, 40 treatment-naïve HIV-1-infected patients took the following three drugs once a day at bedtime: didanosine (ddI), 3TC and EFV. The primary endpoint was the percentage of patients with plasma HIV-1 RNA below 500 copies/mL at six months; analysis was done on an intention-to-treat basis. Results showed that 85% of patients were at US Centers for Disease Control and Prevention (CDC) stage B or C and the plasma HIV RNA level was 5.4 log_{10} copies/mL at baseline. The percentage of patients with plasma HIV-1 RNA below 500 copies/mL at six months was 95% (95% CI:83–99). The proportion of patients with plasma HIV-1 RNA below 50 copies/mL at months 3, 6, 9, 12 and 15 was 26% (n=39; 95% CI:12–39), 78% (n=40; 95% CI:65–90), 70% (n=40; 95% CI:56–84), 77% (n=39; 95% CI:64–90), and 69% (n=39; 95% CI:55–84), respectively. The CD4 cell count was 164 $cells/mm^3$ at baseline and 299 $cells/mm^3$ at month 15. Permanent treatment discontinuation was never necessary for serious adverse effects. Adherence was excellent, as shown by plasma drug concentrations and according to the results of a questionnaire. Researchers concluded that this once-daily regimen of ddI, 3TC and EFV was safe, easy to take, and demonstrated strong anti-retroviral and immunologic effects in African patients with advanced HIV infection.

In another study, the effectiveness and safety of ART in HIV-1-infected patients in resource-limited African countries was assessed. HIV-1 screening, therapy, counselling, monitoring, training and education were provided free of charge [13]. This was an open-label cohort programme involving 206 treatment-naïve HIV-1-infected patients recruited in four urban clinics in Senegal, Côte d'Ivoire, Uganda and Kenya and treated with ritonavir (RTV)-boosted saquinavir (SQV), 3TC and ZDV. The primary outcome was a plasma viral load (pVL) of 400 copies/mL after 96 weeks of treatment. Secondary analyses included CD4 cell count changes and the occurrence of adverse events. Overall virologic and immunologic responses to ART in resource-limited African settings were found to be as good as in western settings.

In another recent study in collaboration with ANRS and IMEA, the efficacy of a once-daily regimen using tenofovir (TDF), emtricitabine (FTC) and EFV was evaluated. A total of 40 patients were included and followed up during 96 weeks of treatment. The clinical and immuno-virologic results were very good, showing a significant increase in CD4 count and a decrease in viral load. The adherence to this once-daily antiretroviral regimen was excellent [14].

Conclusion

There remain many challenges relative to HIV and ART in Senegal, including insufficient scale-up of the PMTCT programme and weakness in the paediatric component of the Senegalese initiative for access to care and treatment. Access to voluntary counselling and HIV testing needs to be strengthened by increasing the availability of HIV care centres throughout the country. There are also limited antiretroviral drugs available for second-line regimens, particularly RTV-boosted drugs. Support from the Senegalese government, the World Bank, the Global Fund to Fight AIDS, Malaria and Tuberculosis, and from bilateral and multilateral partners, together with the involvement of the private sector, will help to overcome these challenges.

Acknowledgements

The author wishes to expresses his sincere gratitude to the entire Senegalese team and its international partners for their involvement in the Senegalese HIV programme, including care and research, since 1985: Ndèye Coumba Touré-Kane, Cheikh Tidiane Ndour, Ibrahima Ndiaye, Ndèye Fatou Ngom-Guèye, Ndella Diakhaté, Adama Ndir, Mouhamadou Baila Diallo, Pape Mandoumbé Guèye, Khadidiatou Ba Fall, Ibrahima Traoré, Pape Gallo Sow, Khoudia Sow, Safiatou Thiam, Bara Ndiaye, Karim Diop, Djibril Faye, Papa Alassane Diaw, Halimatou Diop-Ndiaye, Abdoulaye Sidibé Wade, Abdoulaye Ly, Abdoulahat Mangane, Phyllis Kanki, Nancy Kiviat, Eric Delaporte, Awa Marie Coll-Seck, Souleymane Mboup and Ibra Ndoye.

References

1. Meda N, Ndoye I, M'Boup S, et al. (1999). Low and stable HIV infection rates in Senegal: natural course of the epidemic or evidence for success in prevention. *AIDS* 13:1397–1405.

2. Toure-Kane C, Montavon C, Faye MA, et al. (2000). Identification of all HIV type 1 group M subtypes in Senegal, a country with low and stable seroprevalence. *AIDS Res Hum Retroviruses* 16:603–9.

3. Ndour M, Sow PS, Coll-Seck AM, et al. (2000). AIDS caused by HIV1 and HIV2 infection: are there clinical differences? Results of AIDS surveillance 1986–97 at Fann Hospital in Dakar, Senegal. *Trop Med Int Health* 5:687–91.

4. Sow PS, Hawes SE, Critchlow CW, et al. (2004). Characteristics and Presenting Complaints of Outpatients with Undiagnosed HIV Infection: Potential Utility in Selecting Subjects for HIV Testing. J Acquir Immune Defic Syndr 37:1520–28.

5. Hawes SE, Critchlow CW, Sow PS, et al. (2006). Incident high-grade squamous intraepithelial lesions in Senegalese women with and without human immunodeficiency virus type 1 (HIV-1) and HIV-2. J Natl Cancer Inst 98:100–9.

6 Xi LF, Papa Toure, Cathy W, et al. (2003). Prevalence of specific types of Human Papillomavirus and Cervical Squamous Intraepithelial lesions in consecutive, previously unscreened West African Women over 35 years of age. Int J Cancer 103(6):803–9.

7. Laurent C, Ngom Gueye NF, Ndour CT, et al. ANRS 1215/1290 Study Group. (2005). Long-term benefits of highly active antiretroviral therapy in Senegalese HIV-1-infected adults. J Acquir Immune Defic Syndr 38:14–7.

8. Desclaux A, Ciss M, Taverne B, et al. (2003).Access to antiretroviral drugs and AIDS management in Senegal. AIDS 17(suppl 3):S95–101.

9. Ndour CT, Batista G, Manga NM, et al. (2006). Efficacy and tolerance of antiretroviral therapy in HIV-2 infected patients in Dakar: preliminary study. Med Mal Infect 36:111–4.

10. Vergne L, Toure Kane C, Laurent C, et al. (2003). Low rate of genotypic HIV-1 drug-resistant strains in the Senegalese Government Initiative of access to antiretroviral therapy. AIDS 17(suppl 3):S31–S38.

11. Etard JF, Ndiaye I, Thierry-Mieg M, et al. (2006). Mortality and causes of death in adults receiving highly active antiretroviral therapy in Senegal: a 7-year cohort study. AIDS 20:1181–9.

12. Landman R, Schiemann R, Thiam S, et al. (2003). Once-a-day highly active antiretroviral therapy in treatment naïve HIV-1 infected adults in Senegal. AIDS 17:1017–1022.

13. Sow PS, Otieno LF, Bissagnene E, et al, on behalf of the Cohort Program to Evaluate Access to Antiretroviral Therapy and Education Project Team. (2007). Implementation of an Antiretroviral Access Program for HIV-1-Infected Individuals in Resource-Limited Settings: Clinical Results from 4 African Countries. J Acquir Immune Defic Syndr 44:262–7.

14. Landman R, Diallo M, Diakhate, et al. (2006). Evaluation of TDF/FTC/EFV Once Daily First-Line Regimen in West Africa. 13th Conference on Retroviruses and Opportunistic Infections (CROI), 5-9 February 2006, Denver, USA. [Poster 543].

Chapter 25

Country review: Zambia

Moses Sinkala and Benjamin H. Chi*

Introduction

A former British colony, Zambia is a landlocked country in southern Africa that gained its independence in 1962 and elected its first president in 1964. The country's economy has been based on a wealth of mineral resources—particularly copper—found in the Copperbelt and North-Western Province. The major decline in worldwide copper prices in the 1970s, however, has led to a dramatic and sustained economic downturn. By 2003, it was estimated that 76% of adult Zambians were living on less than US$1 a day [1], making this one of the most impoverished nations in the world.

Like many of its neighbouring countries, Zambia has been devastated by the HIV epidemic. Nearly 100,000 people, or 1% of Zambia's total population, die each year from AIDS-related causes [2]. While HIV prevention programmes have been in place for more than a decade, treatment for the disease has been out of reach for most HIV-infected Zambians due to issues of availability and cost. In 2004, however, the Zambian government began implementing what would become one of the largest HIV care and treatment programmes in the region. Within three years, the number of individuals starting life-prolonging antiretroviral therapy (ART) increased dramatically, from 5000 to over 75,000 nationwide. In this chapter, we describe the implementation and rapid scale-up of ART services, and report early patient outcomes from a large programmatic cohort. Although the history of ART in Zambia is limited thus far, we believe the country's experience provides unique insight into the potential impact of HIV treatment in settings of high prevalence and low resources.

HIV in Zambia

Indirect evidence suggests that AIDS was present in Zambia as early as the mid-1980s [3]. After a rapid rise in the 1990s [4], HIV prevalence has steadily declined in both urban and rural settings. This trend has been observed in both antenatal-based sentinel surveillance for HIV [5,6] and nationally representative, community-based surveys [7,8]. By 2002, the prevalence among the adult population was estimated at 16% by the community-based Demographic and Health Survey [9]. For the most part, the subtype C HIV that predominates in Zambia has spread through heterosexual transmission. Homosexuality and injection drug use are believed to play only a limited role in HIV transmission [4], though few studies have examined at-risk populations in a systematic fashion.

HIV prevalence has generally remained higher in cities and towns when compared with rural areas. The 2002 Demographic and Health Survey reported prevalence rates of 23% and 11%,

* Corresponding author

respectively [9], a roughly twofold difference that has been observed since the late 1990s [10]. As expected, higher prevalence rates have been found among mobile or at-risk populations. In 2001, researchers observed that nearly 70% of sex workers in the copper-mining town of Ndola were HIV-infected [11]. Prevalence rates among antenatal attendees have ranged between 25% and 30% in most urban centres, including the nation's capital, Lusaka [12,13]. Gender imbalances in HIV prevalence have also been demonstrated within younger age groups. Sexually active women under the age of 25, for example, appear to be up to six times more likely to be infected with HIV when compared with their male counterparts. The reasons behind this phenomenon are unclear, but probably cannot be explained by differences in sexual behaviour (e.g. age of sexual debut, number of reported sexual partners) alone [14].

Although few formal studies have examined this issue, HIV contributes significantly to Zambia's high general mortality rates [9]. The rise from 159 deaths per 1000 individuals in 1985 to 623 deaths per 1000 in 1995 is considered strong indirect evidence that the rising prevalence of HIV over this period played an important role in the country's overall mortality rates [15]. Given the country's high disease prevalence, the population-attributable fraction of HIV mortality is likely to be within the high range (24–74%) described in regional cohorts [16]. In 2000, the Joint United Nations Programme on HIV/AIDS (UNAIDS) estimated that 60% of all 15-year-old boys in Zambia will eventually die of AIDS-related causes [17]. This serves as a stark reminder of the chronic and devastating nature of the disease process.

These mortality trends are also consistent within subpopulations. Despite a high prevalence of risk factors such as malnutrition, HIV infection was associated with a nearly twofold risk of mortality among hospitalized children in Lusaka [18], a finding consistent with regional experiences [19]. From 1993 to 2004, the proportion of AIDS-related maternal deaths at the University Teaching Hospital in Lusaka rose significantly, from 1.4% to 6.5% [20].

Opportunistic infections (OIs) play a significant and direct role in AIDS-related mortality. The incidence of tuberculosis (TB) and HIV co-infection is high across the country [21]. Up to 70% of patients under TB treatment are believed to be HIV-co-infected [22, 23]. When individuals testing HIV-positive are screened for TB, more than a third have laboratory evidence of pulmonary disease [24]. In a study of 230 patients conducted during Zambia's pre-ART era, diagnosis of cryptococcal meningitis was associated with a universal fatality rate at six months following diagnosis, despite aggressive treatment at the country's only tertiary care centre [25]. Other OI-related causes of mortality have included wasting syndrome [26, 27], Kaposi's sarcoma [28], and cervical cancer among women [29]. The impact of OIs on mortality is by no means limited to HIV-infected adults. A necropsy study in 2002 found a high prevalence of AIDS-related pulmonary infections among children who had died of respiratory disease. Among the 180 HIV-infected children in the series, 41% were diagnosed with acute pyogenic pneumonia, 29% with *Pneumocystis carinii* pneumonia, and 18% with pulmonary TB [30].

In many ways, the impact of HIV on human health has been exacerbated by the social and cultural response to the epidemic. Despite the high prevalence in the general adult population, individuals with HIV infection have traditionally faced stigma. Qualitative studies on the topic have painted a picture of social isolation, discrimination, internalized guilt, and despair among those infected by the virus [31]. Fear of these social consequences contributed greatly to the low testing rates for HIV in the 1990s and early 2000s [32]. This reluctance to undergo HIV testing has been documented in many segments of the population, including healthcare providers [33, 34]. With improved strategies for patient confidentiality and patient education [35], testing rates have steadily risen. The increased availability of HIV treatment has undoubtedly had a strong impact on AIDS-related stigma.

As in many African countries [36], the economic impact of HIV in Zambia has been severe. A study of 33 Zambian businesses found that employee mortality increased steadily between 1987 and 1993, from 0.25 deaths to 1.83 deaths per 100 person-years [37]. In another study, up to 20% of the workforce reported taking sick leave within the previous 12 months, with absences ranging from two to six months at a time [38]. Evaluation of the education sector found that the impact of HIV on primary education resulted in an annual cost of US$1.3–3.1 million, or roughly 3% of the Ministry of Education's total annual budget. Nearly three-quarters (71%) of these costs were attributed to teacher absenteeism, while the remainder was due to the replacement of trained educators (22%) and funeral expenses (7%) [39].

HIV has had a deleterious effect on the healthcare sector as well. Although the 'brain drain' of African healthcare providers has received considerable attention [40–42], recent estimates suggest that AIDS-attributable deaths may be having an even greater impact on Zambia's human resource crisis [43]. One study found that up to 3.5% of all healthcare providers die each year, many prematurely (mean age=38 years). From 2000 to 2003, death claimed more nurses and clinical officers (68%) than did resignation (23%) or retirement (9%) [44]. The loss of trained medical personnel at such high proportions annually represents one of the greatest challenges to ART scale-up across Zambia.

The HIV epidemic in Zambia has taken a tremendous toll, both in human health and economic development. Despite these rather sobering statistics, however, some encouraging trends have been evident. Since 1990, community-based surveys have shown significant increases in AIDS knowledge and decreases in reported risk behaviours [45,46]. When viewed alongside the rapid expansion of access to ART across the country—the focus of this chapter—we believe there is great cause for optimism.

ART in Zambia

In 2004, Zambia's Ministry of Health set forth national guidelines for HIV treatment [47], closely following those of the World Health Organization (WHO) [48]. Currently in their second iteration, these guidelines rely heavily on WHO-defined clinical staging of HIV disease and CD4 counts to determine treatment eligibility. Initiation is recommended for individuals with CD4 counts <200 cells/mm^3, WHO stage 4 disease, or WHO stage 3 disease with CD4 counts <350 cells/mm^3. Access to CD4 count technology has become increasingly available across Zambia and is considered part of the country's minimum package for ART expansion.

For adults and adolescents, first-line regimens incorporate non-nucleoside reverse transcriptase inhibitors (NNRTIs) nevirapine (NVP) or efavirenz (EFV), along with two nucleoside reverse transcriptase inhibitors (NRTIs)—lamivudine (3TC) with either stavudine (d4T) or zidovudine (ZDV). Both brand-name and generic formulations of antiretroviral drugs have been approved by the Zambian government. In 2007, both tenofovir (TDF) and emtricitabine (FTC) were incorporated into the first-line options for ART due to their once-daily dosing and improved tolerability compared with other drugs.

Long-term monitoring for ART is based on immunologic (e.g. suboptimal rise or decrease in CD4 counts) and clinical (i.e. increasing WHO stage) evaluation. Criteria for treatment failure have not been standardized nationally. Second-line regimens in Zambia are tailored to the individual patient, but usually incorporate protease inhibitors (PIs) such as lopinavir/ritonavir (LPV/r), along with non first-line NRTIs such as didanosine (ddI) and abacavir (ABC).

Due to issues of cost and technical complexity, neither routine virologic monitoring nor HIV resistance testing are widely available in Zambia. Current investigation has focused on targeted use of these expensive assays for complicated medical cases. The inability to provide this level of monitoring for all individuals on ART is an area of public health concern [49], given the widespread use of short-course monotherapy regimens for prevention of mother-to-child transmission (PMTCT) of HIV (including single-dose NVP [12,50]) and poor regulation of antiretroviral drug use early in the HIV epidemic, particularly in the private sector. Work in the pre-ART era in Zambia found that primary drug resistance was minimal among ART-naïve HIV-infected patients [51]. To date, severe resource limitations have not permitted programmatic follow-up of resistance patterns; however, population-based surveillance has been planned [52].

Provision of ART to children has proven challenging due to the limited diagnostic capability within the first 18 months of life. Virologic methods for early infant diagnosis (i.e. polymerase chain reaction (PCR) assays) have only recently become available in Zambia and remain limited to urban centres. For the majority of programmes in the country, diagnosis of HIV among children younger than 18 months is thus based on confirmed maternal HIV status, CD4 percentage and clinical staging of HIV disease. Children older than 18 months are diagnosed via standard HIV antibody assays using a serial algorithm of rapid tests. Criteria for ART initiation in children are based on WHO guidelines [53]; first-line regimens are similar to those for adults. Depending on the age of the child, parents are either provided with syrup formulations, or they are instructed to dissolve tablets into liquid suspensions at home.

Until recently [54], PMTCT programmes in Zambia relied heavily on single-dose NVP for perinatal HIV prophylaxis. With the expansion of ART services, however, more complex regimens are now considered part of the national standard of care [55]. Women are first screened for treatment eligibility via CD4 screening and clinical staging of disease. Those who meet the criteria for ART initiation are started on a first-line regimen, preferably a ZDV-containing combination. HIV-infected pregnant women who are not treatment-eligible are offered ZDV monotherapy from 32 weeks gestation onward, with a 'boost' of single-dose NVP during labour. Infants are given a single dose of NVP syrup in the first 72 hours of life, followed by a seven-day regimen of ZDV syrup. This modification of the highly efficacious Thai PHPT-2 regimen [56] is currently being implemented across Zambia. The integration of CD4 screening into routine PMTCT is an important programme component and could minimize NVP exposure among women who urgently need ART [57,58].

Expansion of ART access

In 2004, the Ministry of Health initiated a massive effort to expand access to ART across Zambia. Although small provincial programmes had been in place since 2002, the integration of services at the primary care level resulted in an unprecedented number of new enrolments. By the beginning of 2007, over 75,000 individuals had begun long-term HIV treatment, an increase of more than 15 times in under three years. Zambia's ART experience highlights the feasibility of rapid scale-up in the face of severe human and material resource constraints. A number of internal and external factors have contributed to the success, as described below.

Government leadership

The Zambian government has taken on a strong leadership role in the country's response to its HIV epidemic. Recognizing the breadth of the HIV problem in Zambia, the government has set ambitious targets for numbers of people on ART in 2003, both for the World Health Organization's '3 by 5' initiative and for its call for universal access [59]. It has also moved quickly to establish national guidelines for care, to coordinate the implementation of services, and to procure antiretroviral drugs [60]. The government's decision to eliminate patient fees for antiretroviral drugs in the public sector (see below) continues to have a tremendous impact on the success of the national programme.

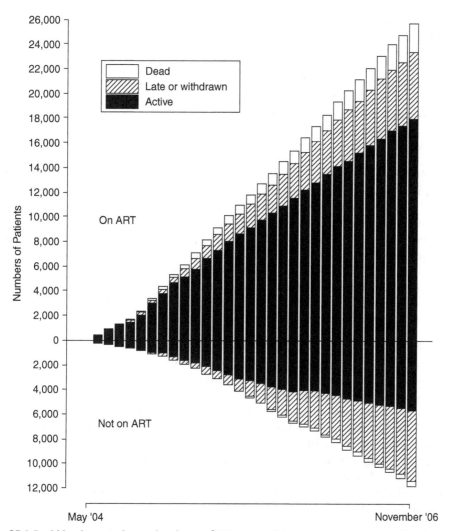

Fig. 25.1 Rapid implementation and scale-up of HIV care and treatment in Lusaka, Zambia, from May 2004 to November 2006.

Source: [62]

Focused efforts in urban settings

The roll-out of services has been most visible in Lusaka, where in less than three years 45,421 new patients had enrolled in long-term HIV care and 25,579 had initiated ART (Figure 25.1) [61,62]. Higher HIV prevalence, greater population density, fewer staff deficits and a more structured district healthcare system all contributed to the rapidity of programme expansion [63]. Although access to ART in rural settings has expanded, the initial prioritization of urban sites was considered necessary in order to reach the largest number of people in need in the shortest amount of time.

Treatment at the primary care level

The decentralized model for programme scale-up provided greater access for ART services across the country. In Lusaka, for example, the 26 primary care clinics of the district's health management team are distributed throughout the entire city and log as many as 3.5 million patient visits per year. The accessibility of these specialized HIV services, as well as referrals from other health-care departments such as TB and antenatal care [23], contributed significantly to rapid scale-up.

Elimination of patient fees

For an individual patient, the financial cost of drugs is a well-known barrier to ART initiation and adherence [64]. In 2004, the Ministry of Health launched a district-wide pilot programme to eliminate user fees for ART in Lusaka; based on the success of this programme, the policy was adopted nationwide by 2005. This has made access to ART equitable across all segments of the population [65,66], allowing many to initiate and continue therapy without concerns over cost.

Community sensitization and mobilization

Despite numerous educational campaigns over the past decade, fear of stigmatization among HIV-infected individuals remains a critical barrier to testing and treatment. Alongside programme scale-up, intensive countrywide efforts have been made to increase community awareness about HIV and ART. Campaigns have utilized a variety of media, including radio shows, television announcements, pamphlets, educational lectures and community dramatic productions. Grass-roots formation of facility-based peer and support groups has led to the empowerment of HIV-infected individuals within their communities [67]. Targeting specific populations, such as schoolchildren and their parents, with educational messages has also been successful in encouraging HIV testing [68].

Development of clinical care protocols and standardized programme monitoring

Given the shortage of physicians in most primary care settings in Zambia [69], programmes have relied heavily on non-physician clinicians—for example, nurses and clinical officers—to provide patient care. In order to ensure quality medical care, standard clinical protocols were adapted from the government's own guidelines for HIV care and treatment [47]. Intensive training workshops and in-clinic mentoring were implemented for staff at all sites, and medical oversight was provided by a core team of physicians and nurses to ensure that care was provided at an acceptable standard [70]. Integral to this programme monitoring has been the implementation of a nation-wide patient-tracking and outcomes-monitoring system designed to capture key information from individual patient visits [71]. From this database, each site is evaluated according to a standard set of programme indicators, allowing for targeted training in site-specific problem areas.

Previous experience with rapid scale-up of HIV services

The Zambian government's successful implementation of services for voluntary counselling and testing (VCT) and PMTCT provided an important foundation for the later expansion of ART services. Through partnerships between the Ministry of Health and local non-governmental organizations (NGOs), such as the Kara Counselling and Training Trust, VCT was introduced in the country as early as 1992 [72]. Also, following the introduction of single-dose NVP regimens for infant HIV prophylaxis in 2001, PMTCT programmes expanded rapidly across Zambia [12, 73, 74]. Community education, clinic-level operations and the cohort of HIV-infected individuals identified through these national programmes have been integral to the rapid nature of ART services scale-up.

International donors and partners

Another critical component of the rapid scale-up of ART services was the availability of international funding through the US President's Emergency Plan for AIDS Relief (PEPFAR), the World Bank and the Global Fund to Fight AIDS, Tuberculosis and Malaria (Global Fund). Since 2002, Zambia has been the recipient of over half a billion US dollars for countrywide HIV prevention and treatment initiatives [75,76]. Alongside these donors have been numerous collaborating partners at the central and field levels. Development agencies and NGOs have played a key role in rapid programme scale-up in Zambia by helping the national programme to improve clinic logistics, laboratory capacity, staff training, medical oversight, community outreach, supply and drug forecasting, and national and international reporting.

Effects of ART

Despite the rapidity of programme growth in Zambia, patient outcomes have generally been favourable. In Lusaka, where early implementation of the national data system has permitted outcomes evaluation, the survival benefits of initiating ART have been demonstrated. In Figure 25.2, mortality among individuals who initiated ART in Lusaka was compared to a contemporaneous population that was screened and qualified for, but did not start, ART. Patients in the latter group comprised individuals who refused to initiate ART for a variety of reasons and those who were

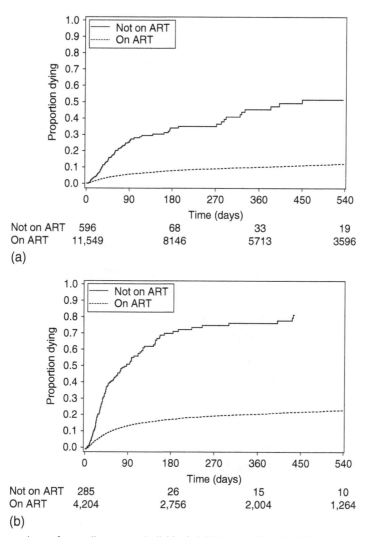

(a)

Not on ART	596	68	33	19
On ART	11,549	8146	5713	3596

(b)

Not on ART	285	26	15	10
On ART	4,204	2,756	2,004	1,264

Fig. 25.2 Comparison of mortality among individuals initiating and not initiating antiretroviral therapy at baseline CD4 cell counts of: (a) 50 and 200 cells/mm³, and (b) under 50 cells/mm³.

Source: [62]

lost to follow-up; survival data were obtained via a district-wide programme to follow up patients with missed clinic visits. Without ART, mortality increased dramatically among these individuals with CD4 counts between 50–200 cells/mm^3 and those with CD4 counts of less than 50 cells/mm^3. The dramatic difference in mortality between these two groups demonstrates the significant improvement in survival associated with ART in this Zambian population.

The initial cohort of patients enrolling in the Lusaka programme represented a relatively sick population. Among the first 21,755 patients presenting for ART eligibility, mean CD4 count was 197 cells/mm^3 (standard deviation (SD)=182 cells/mm^3); 63% had a baseline CD4 count less than 200 cells/mm^3, and 18% had a baseline value of less than 50 cells/mm^3. Of this cohort, 10% met clinical criteria for WHO stage 4 (i.e. clinical AIDS), while another 53% were classified as WHO stage 3. Nearly three-quarters of these patients were initiated on ART based on the Zambian national guidelines [61].

First-line antiretroviral regimens appeared to be reasonably well-tolerated; however, a significant proportion (10%) did require single-drug substitutions due to severe side effects. Among the NRTIs, ZDV was more likely to be substituted compared with d4T (27.1 versus 13.0 substitutions per 100 patient-years). NVP was substituted at a rate of 12 per 100 patient-years. Unfortunately, neither the reasons for drug switching nor their severity were available for analysis [61].

Adherence to antiretroviral regimens has been difficult to measure in the Zambian setting due to the high volume of patients and the limited number of healthcare providers. Thus far, the average number of days a patient is late per month for pharmacy refills has been used as a crude marker for adherence [61]. Although this measure has some limitations, it is easily calculated and has been strongly correlated with patient outcomes in a number of studies [78–81]. In common with other patient populations in the region [82], patients adhere to ART in Zambia at rates comparable to those of developed countries. Nearly 40% of individuals on ART have never missed drug refills; an additional 30% were less than two days late on average per month (Figure 25.3). Not surprisingly, individuals with the poorest adherence (>90th percentile) had nearly

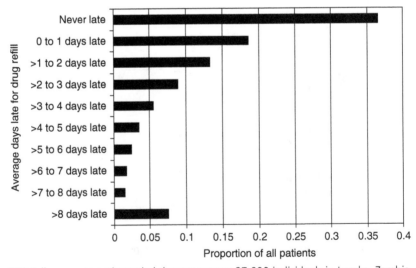

Figure 25.3 Adherence to antiretroviral therapy among 27,000 individuals in Lusaka, Zambia, using timeliness of pharmacy visits as surrogate marker.

Source: [62]

three times greater risk for mortality and a twofold greater risk for clinical treatment failure [62]. In follow-up visits of 271 late patients, common reasons for missed appointments included illness (23%), travelling away from home (16%) and work or personal business (13%). Other important reasons included uncertainty about continuing ART (7%) and negative influence from friends and family (7%) [83].

CD4 response among adults initiating ART in Lusaka has been similar to that seen in North America and Europe [61,84,85]. At six months, the mean increase in CD4 count is 155 cells/mm^3 (SD=182 cells/mm^3); at 12 months, the mean increase is 175 cells/mm^3 (SD=174 cells/mm^3). Patient survival after the first three months of ART initiation is similar to that observed in the United States (5.0 versus 4.3 per 100 person-years); however, mortality appears to be particularly high in the first 90 days (26 per 100 person-years). A variety of causes have been proposed, including immune reconstitution inflammatory syndrome, metabolic disorders and endocrine dysfunction; however, due to limitations in diagnostic tests locally, these etiologies remain poorly understood. In multivariable analysis, strong predictors for death include increasing WHO stage, decreasing CD4 counts, low baseline body mass index, low baseline haemoglobin and poor regimen adherence [61].

Lessons learned and future challenges

From a public health perspective, the Zambian experience provides insight into the feasibility of large-scale programmes in areas of high HIV prevalence and severe resource constraints. In the setting of a structured healthcare system, the scale-up of ART services through primary care centres is possible and allows direct access to large numbers of patients in urgent need of care. With sufficient training, medical oversight and clinical care protocols, non-physician clinicians can play integral roles in patient care [70]. Anecdotally, the availability of ART has led to increased rates of HIV testing and reduced stigma regarding the disease. The number of AIDS-related co-morbidities observed in hospital settings has also dropped dramatically [86]. Despite these positive developments, however, a significant proportion of patients that start ART do not return for clinic appointments, even when efforts are made to follow up those with missed visits [83].

The majority of HIV-infected individuals enrolling in long-term care thus far have presented in late stages of HIV disease. Strategies are needed to effectively identify patients earlier in their disease course via HIV testing and active referral from other clinical care sites (e.g. antenatal care, outpatient care, TB care) [23]. Approaches focusing on couples counselling and increased male involvement hold a great deal of promise [87,88]. Greater programmatic emphasis should also be placed on paediatric HIV care now that virologic tests for early infant HIV diagnosis are available in parts of the country. Preventive care and disease screening could lead to improved long-term health outcomes. Early enrolment would also facilitate the timely initiation of ART before the onset of acute AIDS-defining conditions.

As global initiatives for HIV shift from urgent scale-up to a sustained health response [89], the focus of healthcare services in Zambia must shift as well. While the primary goal of rapid scale-up—averting AIDS-related deaths—remains extremely relevant, greater attention must be paid to quality of life for those living chronically with the disease. Long-term clinical monitoring for side effects and improved diagnostic capacity for opportunistic infections are important, but will only have an impact if healthcare providers and patients can effectively alter health behaviours towards chronic (versus acute) medical care.

Evaluating the long-term response to ART remains a challenge in Zambia. Clinical and immunologic monitoring have provided a basis for detecting treatment failure, but current algorithms perform poorly in field settings. The role of virologic and resistance testing in determining treatment failure must be defined. Although routine deployment would be prohibitively expensive in this setting, selective use within strict treatment failure algorithms could provide a cost-effective alternative with considerable individual and public health benefits.

Efforts to address the human resource crisis must continue [90]. In settings where the number of physicians is limited, training of non-physician clinicians must be initiated. In Lusaka, development of a 'triaging' programme for nurses, designed to provide basic skills in clinical examination and laboratory interpretation, is an example of the task-shifting strategies that are critically needed if ART service roll-out is to continue nationwide [70]. Collaboration with traditional healers for comprehensive HIV care is another promising response to health provider shortages [91], particularly given the large number of practitioners and the widespread use of these traditional medicines among patients [92]. Initiatives specifically designed for healthcare workers are also needed to address staff burnout over time and to promote HIV testing, care and treatment among providers themselves.

Conclusion

Despite having one of the world's highest HIV burdens, numerous factors have delayed ART scale-up in Zambia over much of the last 20 years. These have included the high cost of antiretroviral drugs, the limited availability of specialized laboratory tests and the severe resource constraints of the public health sector. In the past five years, however, numerous external and internal developments have set the stage for an unprecedented public health response to the HIV epidemic. Unlike many high- and medium-income countries, the history of ART in Zambia is just beginning.

While early patient outcomes have been favourable, the true success of ART thus far exists at the public health level; the effective implementation of comprehensive, resource-appropriate ART services has greatly facilitated the rapid roll-out of services. As the national ART programme slowly shifts from urgent scale-up to sustained health response, however, new strategies will be needed to address the complexities of long-term care, such as treatment response and adverse effects. Policy makers will also need to maintain an equitable distribution of funding between HIV and non HIV health services, while ensuring that growing ART programmes remain sustainable with minimal donor commitment. Lastly, alongside treatment, intensive efforts in HIV prevention must continue through community education, service implementation, and vaccine and microbicide development. Without these efforts, the gains made by programmes in Zambia will be overwhelmed by the growing numbers of men, women and children who become newly HIV-infected and eventually require ART themselves.

Acknowledgements

The authors wish to express their thanks to Stewart Reid and Jeffrey Stringer for their insightful comments and thoughtful editing of this chapter.

References

1. United Nations Statistics Division. *Millennium Development Goal Indicators.* Available at http://mdgs.un.org/unsd/mdg/Data.aspx (accessed on March 27, 2007).
2. UNAIDS. (2006). *Report on the global AIDS epidemic.* Geneva: World Health Organization.
3. Iliffe J. (2006). *The African AIDS epidemic: a history.* Oxford: James Curry Ltd.
4. Nyaywa S, Chirwa B, Van Praag E. (1990). Zambia's early response to AIDS. *Progress reports on health & development in Southern Africa,* Fall-Winter 1990:10–12.

5. Fylkesnes K, Musonda RM, Sichone M, Ndhlovu Z, Tembo F, Monze M. (2001). Declining HIV prevalence and risk behaviours in Zambia: evidence from surveillance and population-based surveys. AIDS 15:907–16.

6. Sandoy IF, Kvale G, Michelo C, Fylkesnes K. (2006). Antenatal clinic-based HIV prevalence in Zambia: declining trends but sharp local contrasts in young women. *Trop Med Int Health* 11:917–28.

7. Michelo C, Sandoy IF, Dzekedzeke K, Siziya S, Fylkesnes K. (2006). Steep HIV prevalence declines among young people in selected Zambian communities: population-based observations (1995–2003). *BMC Public Health* 6:279.

8. Michelo C, Sandoy IF, Fylkesnes K. (2006). Marked HIV prevalence declines in higher educated young people: evidence from population-based surveys (1995–2003) in Zambia. AIDS 20:1031–8.

9. Central Statistical Office Zambia, Central Board of Health Zambia, ORC Macro. (2003). *Zambia Demographic and Health Survey 2001–2002*. Calverton, Maryland, USA: Central Statistical Office, Central Board of Health, ORC Macro.

10. Fylkesnes K, Musonda RM, Kasumba K, *et al.* (1997). The HIV epidemic in Zambia: socio-demographic prevalence patterns and indications of trends among childbearing women. AIDS 11:339–45.

11. Morison L, Weiss HA, Buve A, *et al.* (2001). Commercial sex and the spread of HIV in four cities in sub-Saharan Africa. AIDS 15 (Suppl 4):S61–9.

12. Stringer EM, Sinkala M, Stringer JS, *et al.* (2003). Prevention of mother-to-child transmission of HIV in Africa: successes and challenges in scaling up a nevirapine-based program in Lusaka, Zambia. AIDS 17:1377–82.

13. Stringer JS, Sinkala M, Maclean CC, *et al.* (2005). Effectiveness of a city-wide program to prevent mother-to-child HIV transmission in Lusaka, Zambia. AIDS 19:1309–15.

14. Glynn JR, Carael M, Auvert B, *et al.* (2001). Why do young women have a much higher prevalence of HIV than young men? A study in Kisumu, Kenya and Ndola, Zambia. AIDS 15 (Suppl 4):S51–60.

15. Blacker J. (2004). The impact of AIDS on adult mortality: evidence from national and regional statistics. AIDS 18(Suppl 2):S19–26.

16. Porter K, Zaba B. (2004). The empirical evidence for the impact of HIV on adult mortality in the developing world: data from serological studies. AIDS 18(Suppl 2):S9-S17.

17. Joint United Nations Programme on HIV/AIDS. (2000). *Report on the global HIV/AIDS epidemic.* Geneva: UNAIDS.

18. Chintu C, Luo C, Bhat G, *et al.* (1995). Impact of the human immunodeficiency virus type-1 on common pediatric illnesses in Zambia. *J Trop Pediatr* 41:348–53.

19. Newell ML, Coovadia H, Cortina-Borja M, Rollins N, Gaillard P, Dabis F. (2004). Mortality of infected and uninfected infants born to HIV-infected mothers in Africa: a pooled analysis. *Lancet* 364:1236–43.

20. Mazimba C, Collins W, Kaseba CM, Chi B. (2005). HIV-related maternal mortality in Lusaka, Zambia. 3rd IAS Conference on HIV Pathogenesis and Treatment, 2005, Rio de Janeiro, Brazil. [Abstract MoPe11.6C19]

21. Mwaba P, Maboshe M, Chintu C, *et al.* (2003). The relentless spread of tuberculosis in Zambia – trends over the past 37 years (1964–2000). *S Afr Med J* 93:149–52.

22. Ayles H, Ginwalla R. (2003). The Zambian ProTEST Experience. "Lessons Learnt" Workshop on the Six ProTEST Pilot Projects in Malawi, South Africa, and Zambia, 2003. Durban, South Africa. Slides available at http://www.hiv.gov.gy/edocs/protest_zambia.ppt

23. Chi BH, Fusco H, Sinkala M, Goldenberg RL, Stringer JS. (2005). Cost and Enrollment Implications of Targeting Different Source Population for an HIV Treatment Program. *J Acquir Immune Defic Syndr* 40:350–5.

24. Jham M, Levy J, Kancheya N, *et al.* (2006). Screening for tuberculosis (TB) in HIV voluntary counseling and testing (VCT) services in Lusaka, Zambia. XVI International AIDS Conference, 2006, Toronto, Canada. [Abstract MoKc203]

25. Mwaba P, Mwansa J, Chintu C, *et al.* (2001). Clinical presentation, natural history, and cumulative death rates of 230 adults with primary cryptococcal meningitis in Zambian AIDS patients treated under local conditions. *Postgrad Med J* **77**:769–73.

26. Kelly P, Zulu I, Amadi B, *et al.* (2002). Morbidity and nutritional impairment in relation to CD4 count in a Zambian population with high HIV prevalence. *Acta Tropica* **83**:151–8.

27. Kelly P, Davies SE, Mandanda B, *et al.* (1997). Enteropathy in Zambians with HIV-related diarrhoea: regression modelling of potential determinants of mucosal damage. *Gut* **41**:811–6.

28. Olsen SJ, Chang Y, Moore PS, Biggar RJ, Melbye M. (1998). Increasing Kaposi's sarcoma-associated herpesvirus seroprevalence with age in a highly Kaposi's sarcoma endemic region, Zambia in 1985. *AIDS* **12**:1921–5.

29. Parham GP, Sahasrabuddhe VV, Mwanahamuntu MH, *et al.* (2006). Prevalence and predictors of squamous intraepithelial lesions of the cervix in HIV-infected women in Lusaka, Zambia. *Gynecol Oncol* **103**:1017–22.

30. Chintu C, Mudenda V, Lucas S, *et al.* (2002). Lung diseases at necropsy in African children dying from respiratory illnesses: a descriptive necropsy study. *Lancet* **360**:985–90.

31. Nyblade L, Pande R, Mathur S, *et al.* (2003). *Disentangling HIV and AIDS stigma in Ethiopia, Tanzania, and Zambia.* Washington D.C.: International Center for Research on Women. Available at http://www.icrw.org/docs/stigmareport093003.pdf (accessed April 12, 2007).

32. Fylkesnes K, Haworth A, Rosensvard C, Kwapa PM. (1999). HIV counselling and testing: overemphasizing high acceptance rates a threat to confidentiality and the right not to know. *AIDS* **13**:2469–74.

33. Thierman S, Chi BH, Levy JW, Sinkala M, Goldenberg RL, Stringer JS. (2006). Individual-level predictors for HIV testing among antenatal attendees in Lusaka, Zambia. *Am J Med Sci* **332**:13–7.

34. Chi BH, Chansa K, Gardner MO, *et al.* (2004). Perceptions toward HIV, HIV screening, and the use of antiretroviral medications: a survey of maternity-based health care providers in Zambia. *Int J STD AIDS* **15**:685–90.

35. Fylkesnes K, Siziya S. (2004). A randomized trial on acceptability of voluntary HIV counselling and testing. *Trop Med Int Health* **9**:566–72.

36. (2000). *AIDS update: impact on African labour force to be "very severe".* London: WorldWork. **33**:7,16.

37. Baggaley R, Godfrey-Faussett P, Msiska R, *et al.* (1994). Impact of HIV infection on Zambian businesses. *BMJ* **309**:1549–50.

38. Guinness L, Walker D, Ndubani P, Jama J, Kelly P. (2003). Surviving the impact of HIV-related illness in the Zambian business sector. *AIDS Patient Care STDS* **17**:353–63.

39. Grassly NC, Desai K, Pegurri E, *et al.* (2003). The economic impact of HIV/AIDS on the education sector in Zambia. *AIDS* **17**:1039–44.

40. Kober K, Van Damme W. (2004). Scaling up access to antiretroviral treatment in southern Africa: who will do the job? *Lancet* **364**:103–7.

41. Pang T, Lansang MA, Haines A. (2002). Brain drain and health professionals. *BMJ* **324**:499–500.

42. Stilwell B, Diallo K, Zurn P, Vujicic M, Adams O, Dal Poz M. (2004). Migration of health-care workers from developing countries: strategic approaches to its management. *Bull World Health Organ* **82**:595–600.

43. Feeley F. (2006). Fight AIDS as well as the brain drain. *Lancet* **368**:435–6.

44. Feeley R, Rosen S, Fox M, Macwan'gi M, Mazimba A. (2004). *Cost of AIDS among public healthcare professionals.* Lusaka, Zambia: Central Board of Health, Zambia. Available at http://www.bu.edu/dbin/sph/research_centers/documents/ImpactofAIDSonZambiahealthsector June2004.pdf (accessed on 30 March 2007).

45. Bloom SS, Banda C, Songolo G, Mulendema S, Cunningham AE, Boerma JT. (2000). Looking for change in response to the AIDS epidemic: trends in AIDS knowledge and sexual behavior in Zambia, 1990 through 1998. *J Acquir Immune Defic Syndr* **25**:77–85.

46. Agha S. (2002). Declines in casual sex in Lusaka, Zambia: 1996–1999. *AIDS* **16**:291–3.

47. Zambian National AIDS Council. (2004). *National Guidelines for Management and Care of Patients with HIV/AIDS*. Lusaka, Zambia: Printech Press.

48. World Health Organization. (2006). *Antiretroviral therapy for HIV infection in adults and adolescents in resource-limited settings: towards universal access*. Geneva: WHO.

49. Zulu I, Schuman P, Musonda R, *et al.* (2004). Priorities for antiretroviral therapy research in sub-Saharan Africa: a 2002 consensus conference in Zambia. *J Acquir Immune Defic Syndr* **36**:831–4.

50. Eshleman SH, Mracna M, Guay LA, *et al.* (2001). Selection and fading of resistance mutations in women and infants receiving nevirapine to prevent HIV-1 vertical transmission (HIV-NET 012). *AIDS* **15**:1951–7.

51. Handema R, Terunuma H, Kasolo F, *et al.* (2003). Prevalence of drug-resistance-associated mutations in antiretroviral drug-naive Zambians infected with subtype C HIV-1. *AIDS Res Hum Retroviruses* **19**:151–60.

52. Lazzari S, de Felici A, Sobel H, Bertagnolio S. (2004). HIV drug resistance surveillance: summary of an April 2003 WHO consultation. *AIDS* **18**(Suppl 3):S49–53.

53. World Health Organization. (2006). *Antiretroviral therapy of HIV infection in infants and children in resource-limited settings: towards universal access*. Geneva: WHO.

54. Chi BH, Chintu N, Lee A, Stringer EM, Sinkala M, Stringer JS. (2007). Expanded services for the prevention of mother-to-child HIV transmission: field acceptability of a pilot program in Lusaka, Zambia. *J Acquir Immune Defic Syndr* **45**:125–7.

55. Zambian National AIDS Council. (2004). *Zambian national protocol guidelines: integrated PMTCT of HIV/AIDS*. Lusaka, Zambia: Printech Press.

56. Lallemant M, Jourdain G, Le Coeur S, *et al.* (2004). Single-dose perinatal nevirapine plus standard zidovudine to prevent mother-to-child transmission of HIV-1 in Thailand. *N Engl J Med* **351**:217–28.

57. Lockman S, Shapiro RL, Smeaton LM, *et al.* (2007). Response to antiretroviral therapy after a single, peripartum dose of nevirapine. *N Engl J Med* **356**:135–47.

58. Chi BH, Sinkala M, Stringer EM, *et al.* (2007). Early clinical and immune response to NNRTI-based antiretroviral therapy among women with prior exposure to single-dose nevirapine. *AIDS* **21**:957–64.

59. WHO/UNAIDS. (2006). *Progress on global access to HIV antiretroviral therapy: a report on "3 by 5" and beyond*. Geneva: World Health Organization.

60. WHO/UNAIDS. (2004). *"3 by 5" Progress Report: December 2004*. Geneva: World Health Organization.

61. Stringer JS, Zulu I, Levy J, *et al.* (2006). Rapid scale-up of antiretroviral therapy at primary care sites in Zambia: feasibility and early outcomes. *JAMA* **296**:782–93.

62. Sinkala M, Levy J, Zulu I, Mwango A, *et al.* (2006). Rapid scale-up of antiretroviral services in Zambia: 1-year clinical and immunological outcomes. 13th Conference on Retroviruses and Opportunistic Infections, February 5–8, 2006, Denver, USA. [Abstract 64]

63. Ministry of Health Zambia, Central Statistical Office Zambia, ORC Macro. (2005). *Zambia HIV/AIDS Service Provision Assessment Survey*. Calverton, Maryland, USA: Ministry of Health, Central Statistical Office, ORC Macro.

64. Bisson GP, Frank I, Gross R, *et al.* (2006). Out-of-pocket costs of HAART limit HIV treatment responses in Botswana's private sector. *AIDS* **20**:1333–6.

65. Bennett S, Chanfreau C. (2005). Approaches to rationing antiretroviral treatment: ethical and equity implications. *Bull World Health Organ* **83**:541–7.

66. Rosen S, Sanne I, Collier A, Simon JL. (2005). Rationing antiretroviral therapy for HIV/AIDS in Africa: choices and consequences. *PLoS Med* **2**:e303.

67. Mukuka I, Spadoni S, Chirwa S, *et al.* (2006). Clinic-based treatment support groups provide education, family support, empowerment, and HIV/AIDS awareness in communities in Lusaka, Zambia. XVI International AIDS Conference, 2006, Toronto, Canada. [Abstract MoPE0936]

68. Banda S, Sakala S, Banda E, *et al.* (2006). Voluntary HIV counseling and testing (VCT): is it feasible in schools? XVI International AIDS Conference, 2006, Toronto, Canada. [Abstract WePE0448]

69. Zambian Ministry of Health. (2005). *Human resources for health strategic plan (2007 – 2010)*. Lusaka, Zambia: Printech Press.

70. Morris M, Bolton C, Mwanza J, *et al.* (2006). Ensuring quality patient care during rapid scale-up of antiretroviral (ARV) therapy in Zambia. XVI International AIDS Conference, 2006, Toronto, Canada. [Abstract ThPE0193]

71. Fusco H, Hubschman T, Mweeta V, *et al.* (2005). Electronic patient tracking supports rapid expansion of HIV care and treatment in resource-constrained settings. 3rd IAS Conference on HIV Pathogenesis and Treatment, 2005, Rio de Janeiro, Brazil. [Abstract MoPe11.2C37]

72. Baggaley R, Kelly M, Weinreich S, *et al.* (1998). HIV counselling and testing in Zambia: the Kara Counselling experience. *SAfAIDS News* 6:2–8.

73. Guay LA, Musoke P, Fleming T, *et al.* (1999). Intrapartum and neonatal single-dose nevirapine compared with zidovudine for prevention of mother-to-child transmission of HIV-1 in Kampala, Uganda: HIVNET 012 randomised trial. *Lancet* 354:795–802.

74. Sinkala M, McFarlane Y, Nguni C, *et al.* (2005). Scale-up of PMTCT services in Zambia. President's Emergency Plan for AIDS Relief 2nd Annual Meeting, Supporting National Stategies: Building on Success, 23–27 May 2005, Addis Ababa, Ethiopia.

75. U.S. President's Emergency Plan for AIDS Relief. *Country profile: Zambia.* Available at http://www.pepfar.gov/press/75974.htm (accessed on 11 January 2007).

76. The Global Fund for AIDS Tuberculosis and Malaria. *Zambia and the Global Fund: portfolio of grants.* Available at http://www.theglobalfund.org/Programs/Portfolio.aspx?countryID=ZAM &lang= (accessed on 11 January 2007).

77. World Bank. *Country information: Zambia.* Washington D.C.: World Bank. Available at http://web.worldbank.org/WBSITE/EXTERNAL/COUNTRIES/AFRICAEXT/EXTAFRHEANUTPOP/ EXTAFRREGTOPHIVAIDS/0,,contentMDK:20450536~pagePK:34004173~piPK:34003707~theSite PK:717148,00.html (accessed on 11 January 2007).

78. Berg MB, Safren SA, Mimiaga MJ, Grasso C, Boswell S, Mayer KH. (2005). Nonadherence to medical appointments is associated with increased plasma HIV RNA and decreased CD4 cell counts in a community-based HIV primary care clinic. *AIDS Care* 17:902–7.

79. Rastegar DA, Fingerhood MI, Jasinski DR. (2003). Highly active antiretroviral therapy outcomes in a primary care clinic. *AIDS Care* 15:231–7.

80. Lucas GM, Chaisson RE, Moore RD. (1999). Highly active antiretroviral therapy in a large urban clinic: risk factors for virologic failure and adverse drug reactions. *Ann Intern Med* 131:81–7.

81. Nachega JB, Hislop M, Dowdy DW, *et al.* (2006). Adherence to Highly Active Antiretroviral Therapy Assessed by Pharmacy Claims Predicts Survival in HIV-Infected South African Adults. *J Acquir Immune Defic Syndr* 43:78–84.

82. Mills EJ, Nachega JB, Buchan I, *et al.* (2006). Adherence to antiretroviral therapy in sub-Saharan Africa and North America: a meta-analysis. *JAMA* 296:679–90.

83. Krebs D, Chi B, Mulenga Y, Cantrell RA, Levy J. (2006). A community-based contact tracing program for patients enrolled in a district-wide program for antiretroviral therapy (ART). XVI International AIDS Conference, 2006, Toronto, Canada. [Abstract TuPE0143]

84. Mocroft A, Madge S, Johnson AM, *et al.* (1999). A comparison of exposure groups in the EuroSIDA study: starting highly active antiretroviral therapy (HAART), response to HAART, and survival. *J Acquir Immune Defic Syndr* 22:369–78.

85. Kitchen CM, Kitchen SG, Dubin JA, Gottlieb MS. (2001). Initial virological and immunologic response to highly active antiretroviral therapy predicts long-term clinical outcome. *Clin Infect Dis* 33:466–72.

86. Mwaba P, Zulu I, Kafula T, *et al.* (2004). The GRZ ARV Pilot Program: The UTH Experience. *Zambian Medical Journal* **6:**118–20.

87. Bulterys M. (2007). PMTCT of HIV in resource-poor settings: why are we doing so badly?. 14th Conference on Retroviruses and Opportunistic Infections, 2007, Los Angeles, CA, USA. [Abstract 11]

88. Farquhar C, Kiarie JN, Richardson BA, *et al.* (2004). Antenatal couple counseling increases uptake of interventions to prevent HIV-1 transmission. *J Acquir Immune Defic Syndr* **37:**1620–6.

89. World Health Organization. (2006). *Progress on global access to HIV antiretroviral therapy: a report on "3 by 5" and beyond.* Geneva: WHO.

90. Reid S. (2006). Human resource: a critical factor for the success of ART scale-up in resource-limited settings. 37th Union World Conference on Lung Health, 31 October–4 November 2006, Paris, France.

91. Burnett A, Baggaley R, Ndovi-MacMillan M, Sulwe J, Hang'omba B, Bennett J.(1999). Caring for people with HIV in Zambia: are traditional healers and formal health workers willing to work together? *AIDS Care* **11:**481–91.

92. Banda Y, Chapman V, Goldenberg RL, *et al.* (2007). Use of traditional medicine among pregnant women in Lusaka, Zambia. *J Altern Complement Med* **13:**123–7.

Part 5

Future challenges in the next decade of HAART

Chapter 26

The clinical challenges of lifetime HAART

Roger Paredes*, Renslow Sherer and
Bonaventura Clotet

Introduction

HIV is a transmissible viral disease with a zoonotic origin that, to date, cannot be cured nor be prevented with an effective vaccine. Without adequate treatment, HIV infection typically progresses within a few years to severe immunodeficiency and death. Lack of awareness of HIV-positive serostatus delays the initiation of adequate treatment and defers the establishment of secondary preventive measures, increasing the risk of clinical complications and HIV transmission [1].

The advent of highly active antiretroviral therapy (HAART) in the past decade has transformed the clinical picture of HIV infection in countries that can afford the therapy's cost. The global impact of HIV/AIDS is still appalling due to economic and social inequalities, particularly for women and children living in resource-poor areas of the world [2,3].

HIV-1 infection has a more benign course when optimal therapy can be continuously provided. In resource-rich countries, the incidence of AIDS-defining conditions has been greatly reduced since the widespread use of HAART began [4–6]; the life expectancy of HIV-infected individuals is now approaching that of other common chronic diseases. Indeed, most HIV-1-infected patients have autonomy and physical and cognitive functioning similar to their non HIV-infected peers [7], with significant declines in depression scores and an improvement in several neurocognitive domains being observed over time [8].

Despite these remarkable improvements, antiretroviral therapy (ART) falls short of achieving some key objectives. The first, and most important, is that HAART is unable to clear HIV infection or to persistently diminish viral virulence. HIV exhibits five characteristics no known human pathogen has combined before, which prevent its eradication:

- HIV infects CD4+ T-lymphocytes and macrophages and subverts the immune system by inducing immune activation and utilizing its milieu towards its own replicative advantage [9–14];
- HIV irreversibly integrates its DNA into the host's genome [15–22];
- HIV has a quasispecies distribution that permits rapid fitness adaptation to varying environments [23–27];
- HIV infects latent cellular viral reservoirs and is compartmentalized in anatomical sanctuaries with different replication kinetics [28–37]; and
- HIV is prone to rapid antigen variation and epitope masking using the host's autologous glycoproteins [38–39].

* Corresponding author.

Cumulative evidence demonstrates that, regardless of the clinical context and schedule chosen, ART interruption is followed by immediate bursts in viral replication, decreases in CD4 counts, and the recovery of the pre-treatment risk of clinical progression and death [40–43]. Therefore, currently available ART has to be administered indefinitely and in a continuous manner.

Long-term ART, however, is associated with difficulties in adherence, emotional exhaustion, cumulative toxicity and the development of HIV drug resistance. Many subjects who started therapy under suboptimal regimens or sequentially added new drugs to their regimens are nowadays infected with multi-drug resistant (MDR)-HIV and lack optimal treatment options. Likewise, prolonged ART can induce changes in body fat distribution, metabolic alterations and other long-term toxicities. Changes in corporal appearance have a strong impact on the patient's psychological and social spheres. Often, they complicate treatment adherence and may contribute to the stigmatization of HIV-infected patients. Metabolic abnormalities are difficult to treat and are likely to contribute to an increased risk of myocardial infarction and other cardiovascular complications.

With the control of AIDS-defining diseases and prolonged survival, non AIDS-defining illnesses are increasingly being reported as causes of morbidity and mortality in HIV-infected subjects [5]. In a recent analysis of mortality trends and causes of death in the HIV Outpatient Study (HOPS) cohort, the proportion of deaths attributable to non AIDS diseases increased from 13.1% in 1996 to 42.5% in 2004, and prominently included hepatic, cardiovascular and pulmonary diseases, as well as non AIDS-related malignancies [5].

In regions where HIV and hepatitis C virus (HCV) epidemics overlap, the most frequent non AIDS-related causes of death and hospital admission for HIV-infected subjects are complications derived from chronic HCV infection [44–47]. In the HOPS cohort, liver disease was the only reported cause of death for which absolute rates increased over time [5].

HAART has also modified the epidemiology of cancer in HIV-infected individuals. Common neoplasms in HIV-negative subjects, such as lung, prostate or colon cancers, are increasingly being reported in HIV-infected patients. Lung cancer was the second most frequent cause of death in HIV-infected patients older than 55 years living in New York City between 1999 and 2004, after coronary heart disease [48]. As HIV-infected individuals age, more are developing diseases that are common in geriatric patients, including Alzheimer's disease [49–53]. HIV caregivers need to be aware of this changing epidemiology and manage growing non AIDS-defining co-morbidities appropriately.

Whereas a pharmacologic cure for HIV seems beyond reach in the short term, it is possible to develop better treatment strategies addressing and preventing MDR-HIV, fat redistribution syndrome, metabolic alterations, short-term toxicities and patient adherence. Equally important challenges are to improve HIV surveillance, detection and prevention programmes, reinforce sexual education, reduce social inequalities and increase the commitment of our societies to tackle HIV infections in less favoured populations.

In this chapter we summarize the principal challenges of ART in both resource-rich and developing world settings as of the end of year 2006 and discuss the options available to address them.

The HAART paradigm

Defining 'HAART'

The term 'highly active antiretroviral therapy' (or HAART) was first coined between 1995 and 1996 to define antiretroviral drug combinations including two nucleoside reverse transcriptase inhibitors (NRTIs) and one protease inhibitor (PI) [54]. Between 1996 and 1999, combinations of two NRTIs plus one non-nucleoside reverse transcriptase inhibitor (NNRTI) also demonstrated high antiviral and immune-boosting activity [55–57]. Initial studies suggested that triple-NRTI regimens were as active as PI- or NNRTI-based combinations [58]. However, the ACTG 5095 study demonstrated the antiviral inferiority of triple-NRTI regimens relative to modern PI- or NNRTI-based HAART in treatment-naïve individuals. At present, triple-NRTI combinations are not recommended to treat HIV infection [60,61]. The only possible exception is the combination of abacavir (ABC)/ zidovudine (ZDV)/ lamivudine (3TC) or tenofovir (TDF), always as an alternative approach to limit toxicity or major drug interactions—for example, when concomitant administration of tuberculostatics or certain immunosuppressants is required—when other treatment options are not suitable. New antiretroviral drug classes inhibiting viral entry and integration hold promise for broadening the definition of HAART in the near future.

When to start therapy

In spite of the major advances in ART that have occurred in the last decade, the optimal time for initiating treatment is still uncertain. Based on the inherent difficulty with designing and executing such studies, it is unlikely that a well-powered, randomized, controlled trial will be conducted to answer this question.

Early expectations for HIV-1 eradication, together with inadequate understanding of viral reservoir dynamics and long-term antiretroviral toxicity, led to the 'hit hard, hit early' doctrine of 1995 [62–64]. This approach postulated the initiation of HAART as soon as HIV-1 infection was diagnosed in order to preserve and improve the immune status of HIV-1-infected subjects and, eventually, eradicate HIV-1 infection.

By 1998, it was already clear that HIV-1 infection could not be eradicated with the available treatment armamentarium [9,35–37,65]; on the contrary, patients and caregivers were witnessing a striking increase of primary and secondary antiretroviral resistance [66–76], metabolic toxicities and fat redistribution syndrome [77–84]. When several studies suggested that subjects starting HAART in later stages of HIV infection could achieve immunologic recovery similar to those starting with higher CD4 counts, treatment guidelines shifted to a 'delayed initiation of therapy' paradigm—i.e. 'hit hard, but only when necessary' [85]. The threshold for therapy initiation was set at a CD4 count of 200 cells/mm³. The goal was to preserve the clinical benefit of HAART in terms of survival and morbidity while minimizing management-related complications.

Starting therapy below a CD4 count of 200 cells/mm³, however, proved to be too hazardous; there was a higher risk for AIDS-defining events, treatment-derived toxicities, neurocognitive impairment and impaired immune reconstitution when compared with starting therapy at CD4 counts between 200–350 cells/mm³ [86]. As new, more potent, convenient and less toxic antiretroviral drugs with alternative resistance profiles were developed, it became less necessary to delay therapy until CD4 counts were so low.

The pendulum is now swinging towards a 'not-so-delayed initiation of therapy' paradigm. As of late 2006, treatment guidelines recommend the initiation of ART in HIV-1-infected individuals that develop symptoms of HIV-infection or have CD4 counts between 200–350 cells/mm³. Within this CD4 count interval, plasma HIV-1 RNA levels >100,000 copies/mL or rapidly deteriorating CD4 counts favour earlier rather than later therapy initiation [60].

Components of HAART: the 'third' drug

At present, both PI- and NNRTI-based regimens are suitable options for first-line regimens, although some prefer to reserve PI-based regimens for subjects in more advanced stages of HIV-1 infection and with lower CD4 counts. In general, NNRTI-based regimens are more frequently prescribed as first-line therapy for the following reasons:

- Efavirenz (EFV)-based HAART regimens are at least as potent as PI-based regimens in antiretroviral-naïve subjects. A growing number of studies comparing EFV to PIs have provided no solid evidence that first-line nevirapine (NVP)-based regimens are less effective than those including EFV;

- NNRTI-based regimens tend to be better tolerated and less associated with metabolic abnormalities than most PI regimens, with the exception of those based on atazanavir (ATV);

- EFV-based HAART combinations require fewer pills. A combination of TDF/emtricitabine (FTC)/EFV is the only full-potency HAART regimen that is co-formulated in a single, once-daily pill (marketed as Atripla®);

- Whereas early PI failure can potentially be rescued with another PI, sequential NNRTI therapy is usually not possible because NNRTIs have a low genetic barrier, and resistance mutations often generate extensive cross-class resistance. The new-generation NNRTI, etravirine (or TMC-125), retains antiviral efficacy against viruses with the K103N mutation. The efficacy of this drug, however, decreases as other NNRTI mutations (e.g. L100I, Y181C, G190S/A and others) accumulate [87,88]. On the contrary, high-level PI resistance requires the accumulation of multiple resistance mutations. Early PI failure is often associated with the emergence of specific resistance mutations for that PI, but not for others. In fact, certain PI resistance mutations (e.g. I50L, L76V, N88S) may increase viral susceptibility to other PIs. While continued viral replication under PI-selective pressure leads to the accumulation of minor resistance mutations and cross-PI-resistance, early detection of virologic failure in PI-based regimens usually allows for subsequent treatment with other PIs. Moreover, new-generation PIs such as tipranavir (TPV) and darunavir (DRV) retain antiviral activity in the presence of multiple PI resistance mutations, making them particularly suitable for treating subjects infected with MDR-HIV-1 [89,90].

Among PI regimens, neither ATV- nor ritonavir (RTV)-boosted fosamprenavir (fAPV)-based regimens have been shown to be inferior to therapy with lopinavir (LPV), which is co-formulated with a boosting dose of RTV, in treatment-naïve subjects. Atazanavir is usually preferred as the starting PI when priority is given to improving tolerability and preventing lipid metabolic toxicity. LPV- or RTV-boosted fAPV-containing regimens, in contrast, are usually preferred for patients with low CD4 counts or who present with severe clinical complications.

Due to their impressive antiviral potency, viral target specificity, alternative resistance profile and seemingly low incidence of adverse events, integrase inhibitor-based regimens, including the first in its class to receive US Food and Drug Administration (FDA) approval, raltegravir (RAL), are seen as potentially ideal candidates for first-line therapy [91]. Although initial studies suggest that cross-family resistance is likely, new integrase inhibitors with different resistance profiles are already in the pipeline, suggesting that sequential integrase inhibitor-based therapy may be possible in the future.

It is less certain whether chemokine (C-C motif) receptor 5 (CCR5) antagonists, including the recently FDA-approved maraviroc (MRV), will become regular components of first-line therapy or if, instead, they will remain mainly confined to salvage therapy. In head-to-head comparisons in drug-naïve subjects, regimens based on MRV or vicriviroc (VCV) were less likely to achieve viral suppression below 50 copies/mL than EFV-based combinations. Interestingly, virologic response to MRV seemed to vary between different HIV-1 subtypes. In addition, treatment with CCR5 antagonists requires prior viral tropism testing, which is expensive and not widely available. Mechanisms of resistance to CCR5 inhibitors are not completely understood, and the clinical implications of drug-induced viral tropism shifts need to be further explored. In addition, some uncertainty remains regarding the long-term safety, risk for malignancies, and immune dysregulation associated with CCR5 antagonist treatment. Further follow-up will probably be required before additional CCR5 antagonists become widely available for treatment-naïve subjects.

On the other hand, when combined with an optimized background treatment (OBT), both MRV and VCV have demonstrated remarkable improvements in virologic and immunologic parameters in treatment-experienced subjects compared to placebo, particularly when two or more active regimens including the fusion inhibitor enfuvirtide (ENF) were incorporated in the OBT. Overall, about 12% of subjects receiving CCR5 antagonist therapy experienced on-treatment tropism shifts.

The dual-NRTI backbone

Relatively few NRTI backbones are, in practice, available to treat HIV-1 infection. Certain NRTI combinations have been withdrawn from the treatment frontline in resource-rich settings due to excessive toxicity or pharmacokinetic interactions. Stavudine (d4T) and didanosine (ddI) are associated with an increased risk for mitochondrial toxicity, metabolic disturbances and fat redistribution syndrome, particularly when given in combination. Treatment with TDF/ddI is associated with CD4 count declines and excess risk for pancreatitis and other ddI-derived toxicity. The combination of ZDV and ddI is associated with an excess of anaemia, pancreatitis and other toxicities. On the other hand, co-formulated dual-NRTIs (TDF/FTC (marketed as Truvada®), ABC/3TC (marketed as Epzicom®) and ZDV/3TC (marketed as Combivir®)) increase treatment convenience and facilitate adherence. Regimens including FTC or 3TC even retain residual antiviral activity in the presence of the M184V mutation. Moreover, virologic failure to HAART regimens including potent 'third drugs' (e.g. RTV-boosted PIs) is often associated with limited resistance to NRTIs, which sometimes enables maintaining the dual-NRTI backbone in subsequent treatment lines.

The preferred dual-NRTI combinations are co-formulated TDF/FTC or co-formulated ZDV/3TC. Alternative dual-NRTI options include co-formulated ABC/3TC and ddI plus 3TC or FTC. New NRTI combinations are needed to enable a more rational use of 'third drug' options.

The future of HAART

According to economist John Kenneth Galbraith, 'there are two kinds of forecasters: those who don't know, and those who don't know they don't know' [92]. Of course, we don't know how HIV infection will be treated in the future. New drugs inhibiting multiple viral and cell targets are currently being incorporated into the treatment armamentarium, and many more are in the pipeline. It is clear, however, that any future treatment sequence will depend on the following parameters: antiviral potency; toxicity profile; resistance profile (genetic barrier and cross-class resistance); dosing convenience; food- or drug-drug interactions; and cost. Based on what we know at present, a future HAART sequence may look as depicted in Figure 26.1.

Options for first-line therapy in subjects infected with a wild-type HIV could include NNRTI-, PI-, or integrase inhibitor-based regimens (e.g RAL or elvitegravir (ELV)). It is uncertain whether CCR5 antagonist-based therapy would be suitable for first-line therapy or if, instead, it would remain preferably confined to the treatment of MDR-HIV-1 infection.

Second-line therapy for subjects with first-line integrase inhibitor failure could include: treatment with an RTV-boosted PI (LPV, RTV-boosted ATV (ATV/r), RTV-boosted fAPV (fAPV/r)); an NNRTI (EFV or NVP); or an RTV-boosted PI plus an NNRTI. Alternatively, an integrase inhibitor with a different resistance to RAL or ELV and a different resistance profile (e.g. MK-2048) could be combined with either an NNRTI (EFV or NVP) or an RTV-boosted PI (ATV/r, fAPV/r, or LPV).

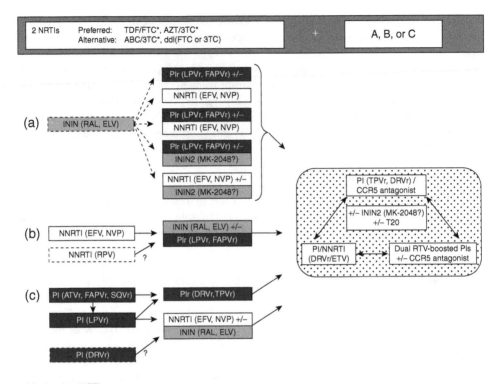

* Co-formulated NRTIs

Fig. 26.1 Hypothetical future HIV-1 treatment.

Notes (1): HIV-1 infected subjects would probably be treated with two NRTIs, preferably in a single pill, plus treatment options included in arms A, B, or C. Dashed boxes and arrows indicate new ININs, NNRTIs, and ritonavir-boosted PIs being tested as first-line therapy as of late 2006. Question marks indicate higher uncertainty that TPV or DRVr will become regular components of first-line therapy than, for example, RAL or ELV. Continous boxes and arrows indicate well-established therapy indications and switches as of late 2006. The oval on right includes different valid salvage therapy options, which should be chosen depending on prior resistance testing and patient's clinical history, if they have not been used before. An ININ2 and/or T20 could be added to any of the three main salvege regimens if they have not been used before.

Notes (2): ININ=integrase inhibitors; ININ2=ININ with alternative resistance profile to raltegravir or elvitegravir; NNRTI=non-nucleoside reverse transcriptase inhibitor; PI=protease inhibitor; RAL=raltegravir.

For patients in whom first-line NNRTI-based regimens have failed, second-line therapy could include an integrase inhibitor plus an RTV-boosted PI. Due to its low genetic barrier, the integrase inhibitor should probably be administered alongside another potent drug. Treatment with the integrase inhibitor plus a RTV-boosted PI would seem preferable to treatment with the PI alone because it could potentially lead to deeper suppression of residual replication and help deplete the viral reservoir in the long term.

Patients exhibiting early failure to first-line ATV- or fAPV/r-based therapy could theoretically be treated with LPV-based regimens if minor PI resistance mutations had not accumulated. Alternatively, subjects could start directly with a LPV-based regimen. Ongoing head-to-head comparisons of RTV-boosted DRV (DRV/r) or RTV-boosted TPV (TPV/r) with LPV in treatment-naïve subjects will help clarify the role of DRV/r- or TPV/r-based regimens as first-line therapy.

Second-line therapy after PI failure could include an NNRTI (EFV, NVP) plus an integrase inhibitor (RAL, ELV). Given that both drug classes display high antiviral potency but low genetic barriers, the inclusion of at least a third active compound in the regimen (an NRTI, a nucleotide reverse transcriptase inhibitor (NtRTI) such as TDF, or a PI) should probably be warranted.

Antiviral combinations most suitable for treating MDR-HIV-1 would be defined according to treatment history, adverse events and viral resistance profiles. Among the three options available, most subjects would probably start with a new generation PI (TPV/r or DRV/r) combined with a new generation NNRTI (etravirine) and/or a CCR5 antagonist (MRV or VCV). Alternatively, highly treatment-experienced subjects could be treated with double RTV-boosted PIs. Enfuvirtide and new integrase inhibitors with complementary resistance profiles (MK-2048) could be added to the aforementioned regimens if they had not been administered before.

Long-term adherence to ART

Long-term adherence to ART is the cornerstone for virologic success. Extensive research has been devoted to determining factors related to better treatment adherence as well as to designing clinical interventions able to improve it [93,94].

Of particular interest has been the analysis of medication characteristics that may facilitate treatment adherence [95]. Newer, simplified antiretroviral regimens fit better with patients' daily activities and achieve equal or superior antiviral efficacy than former, more complex approaches. Early HAART lines may include co-formulated drugs in a single tablet, administered once a day. Once-daily regimens increase patients' satisfaction with their therapy and may also improve practical aspects related to quality of life [95]. Twice-daily regimens, however, are also a good option for many patients. In a recent systematic review of HAART regimens tested in clinical trials, pill count was not a significant predictor of HIV-1 RNA suppression <50 copies/mL [96]. In general, NNRTI and RTV-boosted PI regimens require lower levels of adherence to achieve viral suppression <50 copies/mL than do non-boosted PIs. No solid evidence is available suggesting that NNRTIs are more or less forgiving than RTV-boosted PIs, however. Clinicians must seek to minimize ART toxicity and ensure adequate plasma drug levels.

It is important to note that clinical interventions are of equal importance to behavioural interventions in promoting adherence to HAART. Besides treatment simplicity, tolerability and favourable pharmacokinetic profile, patients' health beliefs, social environment, relationship with the healthcare team, and spiritual and religious beliefs are other essential factors for a proper treatment adherence [97–109]. Healthcare providers should discuss the suitability of starting treatment with their patients, addressing the advantages and disadvantages of the different options available. In addition to collecting objective health data, caregivers should also understand patients' perspectives and expectations regarding their own health [110]. Treatment initiation should preferably be postponed until the patient is committed to improving his or her own health status.

When possible, antiretroviral regimens should suit patients' lifestyle needs. If equally potent regimens are available, treatment simplicity and convenience should be prioritized. Patients should be informed about the tolerability of the regimen, including potential side effects. They should be trained to respond appropriately in the event of toxicity and have a clear referral system to specialized care in order to minimize the impact of adverse drug events [100]. A clear understanding of the risks and benefits of ART might help reduce unjustified fears of medication and lead to improved treatment adherence.

Adequate levels of adherence might not be difficult to achieve during the early stages of therapy, particularly considering the elevated patient motivation, the emotional distress associated with the recent diagnosis, the perceived threat to the patient's own health, and the simplicity, convenience and limited toxicity of modern first-line antiretroviral regimens. However, adherence may progressively decrease thereafter due to a gradual relaxation of these attitudes, a decrease in motivation and a perceived lowering of, or distancing from, the illness threat. As observed in other chronic conditions, prolonged asymptomatic periods during a disease can complicate long-term adherence. Therefore, adherence interventions should continually be provided throughout ART and should be integrated into routine patient care.

Self-reported adherence correlates well with other objective methods like therapeutic drug monitoring and may be a good indicator of patients' behaviour in the clinical setting [111]. However, the reliability of this approach depends on the quality of communication between the clinician and the patient. A positive relationship between patient and healthcare provider, including empathy, mutual respect and engagement, is associated with better adherence and health outcomes and should always be promoted [112].

Non-adherent behaviours in long-term experienced patients tend to be associated with emotional and social problems rather than with practical aspects of medication management [113]. Psychological factors are strongly related to adherence and may also contribute to HIV progression [114]. Multidisciplinary teams of specialized professionals—physicians, nurse practitioners, psychologists, dieticians, and social workers—providing comprehensive healthcare might provide more effective patient care and help overcome problems related to long-term adherence.

The assessment and management of adherence should be integrated with other health-promoting and behaviour-modifying activities such as modification of sexual risk behaviour, cessation of toxic habits, promotion of regular exercise and a healthy diet, etc. Adherence interventions should be comprehensive and should encourage patients to take their medication properly, as well as to live healthier lives.

Antiretroviral toxicity

Adverse events can be a direct cause of suboptimal treatment adherence and unplanned interruptions of therapy. Unexpected toxicities can lead to a patient's distrust in his or her medication, caregivers or treatment plan. In some HIV-infected individuals with solid indications for starting therapy, the fear of suffering long-term toxicity (particularly body fat redistribution) may lead to hazardous voluntary delays in initiation of treatment. Several factors predisposing to antiretroviral toxicity have been identified. NVP-derived hepatotoxicity is more frequent during pregnancy in women with CD4 counts above 250 cells/mm^3 [115,116] and in patients co-infected with HIV and hepatitis B virus (HBV) or HCV [117]. EFV-related central nervous system (CNS) symptoms are more frequent in patients with psychiatric conditions, in certain ethnic groups [118], and in patients homozygous for the CYP2B6*6 allele [119]. Abacavir-associated hypersensitivity is significantly more incident in individuals with the HLA-B*5701 haplotype [120–122].

Short-term toxicity occurs within the first weeks of therapy. Often, the clinical picture includes an acute presentation of mild symptoms or analytical disturbances, which remit or significantly improve in few weeks and rarely require the discontinuation of therapy. Occasionally, short-term toxicity can be severe and even life-threatening (e.g. NNRTI-associated Stevens-Johnson's syndrome or ABC-related anaphylaxis), requiring immediate treatment interruption and, sometimes, life support measures. In the particular case of ABC-related hypersensitivity, short-term toxicity precludes a patient's re-exposure to the drug.

Long-term toxicity has a subacute or chronic onset. Symptoms and signs start gradually and, if they are not pre-emptively pursued, may remain unrecognized during long time periods (months or even years). Long-term toxicity is usually cumulative and difficult to manage with pharmacologic interventions, even if therapy is interrupted. Although different antiretrovirals are associated with different incidence, severity and rapidity of onset of symptoms and signs, all anti-HIV drugs may contribute to some extent to most long-term toxicities. Often, the patho-geneses of long-term toxicities are not fully understood, and factors like duration of HIV infec-tion, immune deterioration, aging or other co-morbidities may play an important pathogenic role. Long-term toxicity may have a profound impact on patients' physical, psychological and social spheres. It may also compromise treatment adherence and the efficacy of antiretroviral regimens, leading to ART failure.

Fat redistribution syndrome (FRS)

Fat redistribution syndrome is probably the most challenging long-term antiretroviral toxicity. All antiretrovirals may contribute to the syndrome, but NRTIs are more frequently associated with peripheral lipoatrophy, and PIs tend to produce abnormal central fat accumulation or combined syndromes [79]. Therapy with NNRTIs is less clearly related to FRS, although they may con-tribute to concomitant lipid abnormalities.

The routine follow-up of HIV-infected patients should include serial measurements of body fat composition using Dual Energy X-Ray Absortiometry (DEXA) or computerized tomography (CT), including at least one measurement before starting therapy [122]. Patient self-reporting and physician examination, however, correlate well with objective measurements. Therefore, standardized questionnaires and clinical assessments are also adequate tools for diagnosing and monitoring the syndrome if objective measurements are not available.

The current consensus is that lipoatrophy and fat accumulation are different clinical entities with different pathogenesis and different clinical management [123]. Different NRTIs induce various degrees of 'mitochondrial toxicity' by interfering with the mitochondrial gamma-DNA polymerase and other critical enzymes in different metabolic pathways, ultimately altering the cellular oxidative and lipid metabolisms [84,124,125]. Stavudine (d4T), ZDV, and ddI—and particularly d4T and ddI combined—are strongly associated with the development of lipoatrophy. 3TC produces less lipoatrophy than the previously mentioned drugs. ABC and TDF could delay or even improve lipoatrophy in some patients [123,125,126].

To prevent the development of lipoatrophy and other toxicities, current guidelines recommend delaying the initiation of ART until CD4 counts fall between 200–350 cells/mm³ and avoiding treatment with d4T or ddI as long as alternative regimens are available [127]. In the presence of lipoatrophy, different studies suggest that a change of ZDV or d4T to either ABC or an NRTI-sparing regimen [128–131] may be the best option currently available. However, fat alterations may improve very slowly and to a moderate degree. Early studies demonstrated the lack of effect on abnormal body changes of switching the PI component for NNRTIs [132]. Other treatments, such as peroxisome proliferator-activated receptor (PPAR)-gamma inhibitors, have exhibited minimal or no improvements in lipoatrophy, although they might help slow down the progres-sion of fat loss [133,134]. Finally, in cases of moderate or severe lipoatrophy affecting the face, reconstructive procedures with facial fillers, including Sculptra™ (poly-L-lactic acid, the only FDA-approved product for lipoatrophy), Silikon® 1000 (polydimethylsiloxane), Bio-Alcamid™ (poly-Alkyl-Imide) and PMMA (polymethyl-methacrylate) may be indicated [135–137].

Autologous fat transfer may be indicated in individuals with enough residual subcutaneous fat in the abdomen or in the dorso-cervical region [138–142]. In a prospective comparison of autol-ogous fat transfer, injections of reabsorbable polylactic acid, and non-reabsorbable polyacry-lamide hydrogel filler materials for the treatment of HIV-related facial lipoatrophy, all three procedures achieved comparable results after 24 weeks and were highly effective in improving the aesthetic satisfaction of the patients [138]. Autologous fat transplantation procedures, though, require surgical procedures and may not be as durable as facial fillings. Infrequently, autologous fat transplantation may be associated with disfiguring facial lipohypertrophy at the graft site together with recurrent fat accumulation at the tissue harvest site, particularly if fat is obtained from the dorso-cervical fat pad [139].

To date, there is no satisfactory pharmacologic treatment for fat accumulation [123]. Growth hormone is associated with dose-dependent improvements in patients with HIV-associated visceral fat accumulation [143,144], but also with predictable and dose-dependent side effects. The optimal dose and duration of treatment with growth hormone has not been established. Although initial studies suggested that rosiglitazone and metformin could improve fat accumulation [145], recent randomized controlled trials did not observe significant visceral fat reductions after treatment with metformin and rosiglitazone in combination or alone [146–148]. Indeed, a modest increase in limb fat was noted among the rosiglitazone-treated patients in one study [149]. Testosterone replacement in obese men with low serum testosterone and a waist:hip ratio above 0.95 led to the unexpected loss of limb fat, whereas no effect was observed on central fat deposits [150].

While surgical resection of localized fat deposits (e.g. the dorso-cervical fat pad) may be a temporary solution for some patients, fat accumulation occurs in and around viscerae and occupies the interstitial space of several tissues like the muscles of the dorso-cervical area. Therefore, fat deposits are not easy to remove by surgical procedures, and abnormal deposits often recur after their excision. Unfortunately, PI-sparing options are only available for patients without prior NNRTI exposure. A switch to more novel PIs with better metabolic profile, such as RTV-boosted ATV, might be an option worth exploring in some cases [151,152]. Due to their viral target specificity, it is expected that new integrase inhibitors may have a favourable impact on lipid metabolism, but it is too early to draw any conclusions on this issue.

Metabolic complications

Long-term ART is often complicated with hypercholesterolaemia, hypertriglyceridaemia and insulin resistance. Increase in plasma lipid concentrations may affect up to 70–80% of HIV-positive subjects treated with a PI-containing regimen and is frequently associated with fat redistribution syndrome [153]. According to data from the Swiss HIV Cohort [154], increasing exposure to either PI- or NNRTI-based therapy increases non-high density lipoprotein (HDL) cholesterol levels; increasing exposure to NNRTI-based therapy is associated with increases in HDL cholesterol levels and decreases in triglyceride levels. In contrast, PI-based therapy is associated with increased triglyceride levels.

High blood pressure (HTA) has also been frequently reported in HIV-infected patients. Some authors have linked HTA with lipid and glucose abnormalities as part of a wider metabolic syndrome, but there is no consensus on this issue. High blood pressure is likely to be mediated by increases in body mass index (BMI), and some PIs (e.g. LPV) may be more likely to cause HTA than others (e.g. ATV) [155,156].

Bone density abnormalities are also frequently seen, but the pathogenesis probably combines the direct effects of ART with other factors such as HIV infection itself, aging, gender, ethnic origin, alcohol consumption, menstrual irregularities, smoking and other co-morbidities [82,83,157–166].

As with fat redistribution syndrome, all marketed antiretroviral drugs can produce metabolic alterations. All PIs can alter the lipid metabolism, especially if they are boosted with RTV. ATV, however, has a much more favourable impact on lipid and glucose metabolism than the other PIs, even when it is co-administered with RTV [151,152,167–169]. Atazanavir is also less likely to cause HTA than LPV [155]. Whereas therapies with different non RTV-boosted PIs are associated with different lipid profiles [154], it is uncertain whether all RTV-boosted PIs other than ATV/r have comparable effects on lipid metabolism. In the recent KLEAN Study, both fAPV/r and LPV, each in a TDF/FTC background, were associated with similar incidence of grade 3–4 hypercholesterolaemia, hypertriglyceridaemia and glucose alterations. However, LPV-based treatment was associated with fewer lipid disturbances than therapy including RTV-boosted indinavir (IDV) in previous studies. Despite the beneficial profile of ATV on lipid and glucose metabolism and HTA, this drug interferes with the liver microsomal enzyme system, probably through direct inhibition of UGT1A1-mediated bilirubin glucuronidation [170], inducing reversible increases of unconjugated bilirubin. Long-term metabolic toxicity is less evident for ATV than for the remaining PIs.

Overall, NNRTI therapy is associated with a more favourable lipid profile than PI-based therapy [154], although it also alters the lipid metabolism. Nevirapine, however, is associated with a better lipid profile than EFV. A prospective non-randomized study comparing first-line therapies including EFV or LPV reported a similar risk for total and low-density lipoprotein (LDL) cholesterol increases in both arms, but a higher risk for hypertriglyceridaemia in the LPV group [171]. In a retrospective review of prospectively collected samples from 1065 treatment-naïve HIV-infected patients starting HAART in 2000, there was a slight difference between NVP- and EFV-containing regimens in triglyceride levels, which tended to increase with increasing exposure to EFV and to decrease with increasing exposure to NVP [154]. In a prospective analysis of lipids and lipoproteins of the 2NN study comparing patients allocated to NVP or EFV in combination with d4T and 3TC, NVP-containing regimens were associated with significantly higher HDL cholesterol increases and significantly smaller increases in total cholesterol, non HDL-cholesterol, LDL-cholesterol and triglycerides than EFV-containing regimens [172]. Data from the Fat Redistribution and Metabolic Change in HIV Infection study (FRAMS) and the Atlantic Study confirm that first-line NVP treatment is associated with a favourable lipoprotein profile, i.e. an increase in HDL-cholesterol and apoA1 plasma levels [173].

Several studies have demonstrated improvements in the lipid metabolism of patients who switched from a PI-based regimen to an NVP-based regimen [77,174,175]. In one study, the replacement of the PI by NVP improved the lipid profile both by reducing the number and lipid content of atherogenic LDL particles and by increasing the protective HDL fraction [77]. Total triglyceride levels remained unchanged, but there was a reduction in the VLDL-1 fraction that contributed to the reduction of LDL particles. The benefit of EFV substitution for PI therapy on the lipid profile is less clear. Some studies have detected reductions in triglyceride levels and fasting insulin resistance index [176], while others have not [81,177]. Indeed, a switch from EFV to NVP in patients with virologically controlled HIV infection but suffering adverse effects led to improvements in dyslipidaemia, including decreases in total and LDL cholesterol and triglyceride levels, and increases in HDL cholesterol [178].

Long-term NRTI therapy with d4T, ddI, ZDV or 3TC is also associated with altered lipid parameters, while ABC and TDF present a more benign lipid profile. All current guidelines recommend prioritizing regimens other than d4T and ddI in order to minimize the development of lipid and glucose metabolism disturbances. Switch of PIs, d4T or ddI to ABC or TDF has consistently improved the lipid and glucose profile in different studies.

Treatment of HIV dyslipidaemia should include lifestyle modifications such as a low-fat diet, increased exercise, reduced alcohol consumption and smoking cessation. In many patients, however, these changes alone will not correct lipid levels [179]. Potentially effective strategies in some patients include changing the PI component of ART to another PI or non-PI and/or lipid-lowering drugs. The choice of hypolipidaemic drugs is problematic because of potential pharmacologic interactions with antiretroviral drugs and other antimicrobial agents associated with an increased risk of toxicity and intolerance. Statins are considered the first-line therapy for the PI-related hypercholesterolaemia, while fibrates are recommended when predominant hypertriglyceridaemia is of concern [153]. In any case, the need to maintain viral suppression must be balanced with the need to treat abnormal lipid levels.

Genetic predisposition to metabolic complications

The completion of the human genome sequence has generated unprecedented possibilities to study the genetic correlates of human diseases [180]. Not surprisingly, the patent need to minimize antiretroviral toxicity has fostered extensive research on genetic susceptibility to HIV and ART effects. A growing number of genetic polymorphisms are being correlated with toxicity susceptibility profiles. For example, Rotger *et al.* [181] found that, regardless of diverse ethnicities, individuals with extremely high EFV plasma concentrations consistently presented two copies of CYP2B6 loss-of-function alleles. In an exploratory pharmacogenetic analysis of the ACTG 384 Study [119], a single nucleotide polymorphism in the resistin gene was significantly associated with risk of developing adverse metabolic changes on HAART. It is important to note that, in most cases, such polymorphisms need to be validated in prospective cohorts. In addition, the mechanisms by which they modify the host's susceptibility are often unknown. This is a rapidly evolving field that is likely to produce very interesting data in forthcoming years. However, clinical interpretations need to be cautious until further research is completed and more robust concepts are settled.

Cardiovascular disease

HIV-infected patients receiving ART are at increased risk of suffering acute myocardial infarction at a rate directly proportional to the duration of treatment [182]. In a recent retrospective analysis of the causes of death of HIV-infected individuals in New York City between 1999 and 2004 [48], 76% of non HIV-related deaths were attributed to substance abuse, cardiovascular disease (CVD), and age-appropriate malignant conditions. Coronary heart disease was the leading cause of non HIV-related deaths in people 55 years of age or older, followed by lung cancer.

Smoking constitutes the single most significant contribution to increased risk of CVD in HIV-positive patients, particularly men, independent of other risk factors [183]. Lipid and glucose metabolism abnormalities coupled with HTA, older age, male sex, prior history of CVD, obesity, and possibly the direct effect of some antiretroviral drugs, contribute to the increased risk for cardiovascular complications [184]. Long-term ART has been associated with endothelial dysfunction, reduced flow-mediated dilation and progressively increased carotid intima-media thickness.

In the prospective Data Collection on Adverse events of Anti-HIV Drugs (D:A:D) Study [182], the incidence of a first myocardial infarction was 3.5 per 1000 person-years (126 out of 23,468 participants), a quarter of which were fatal. There were an additional 77 events related to ischaemia, including coronary-artery angioplasty or bypass surgery, ischaemic stroke and carotid endarterectomy. The incidence of myocardial infarction or of any ischaemic vascular event increased directly with longer exposure to ART (relative risk=1.26; 95% confidence interval (CI):1.12–1.41 per additional year of exposure; p<0.001). However, while the risk of myocardial infarction in relation to the duration of ART remained significant, it was relatively reduced in analyses that adjusted for increased cholesterol levels, suggesting that metabolic abnormalities induced by ART contributed to the increased morbidity observed.

Follow-up data from the same study indicated that increased PI exposure was associated with an increased risk of myocardial infarction, which was partly explained by dyslipidaemia [185]. Conversely, although there were fewer years of experience, there was no evidence that increased NNRTI exposure was associated with risk of myocardial infarction.

Among the other, less frequent cardiovascular complications seen during prolonged HIV therapy, one anecdotal report described a case of QT prolongation and Torsade de Pointes in a subject who initiated EFV [186]. The incidence of HIV-associated pulmonary hypertension (0.21%) does not seem to have decreased during the HAART era, according to two recent studies, and has to be included in the differential diagnosis of dyspnoea in HIV-infected individuals.

Hyperlactataemia and metabolic acidosis

The most threatening long-term toxicity of NRTI therapy is lactic acidosis [187]. There is a continuum of severity in the clinical presentation of hyperlactataemia syndromes, ranging from asymptomatic hyperlactataemia to severe metabolic acidosis with steatohepatitis, multiple organ failure, and death. Different NRTI combinations exhibit additive or synergistic long-term mitochondrial toxicity *in vitro* [188].

Subclinical hyperlactataemia, with serum lactate levels between 2.0 and 5.0 mmol/L and no acid/base abnormalities, is frequent among HIV-infected patients receiving NRTIs (especially with d4T, ZDV, and ddI). The clinical course of this entity is usually benign and has an excellent prognosis. The management of asymptomatic hyperlactataemia should be conservative at first, but watchful. Elevated lactate levels should be confirmed at least in a second determination and closely monitored thereafter, together with acid/base equilibrium and liver enzymes. Frequently, lactate levels will remain stable or improve without the need to withdraw the NRTIs. However, if they remain high or approach 5 mmol/L, it is prudent to replace the culprit NRTIs with ABC, TDF, 3TC or FTC, or change to an NRTI-sparing regimen.

Symptomatic hyperlactataemia, which includes vomiting, nausea, abdominal discomfort and bloating, is frequent when lactate levels reach 5.0 mmol/L, although symptoms can develop with lower lactate levels. It is associated with mild liver abnormalities but no acid/base alterations. Prognosis is relatively good if NRTIs are immediately interrupted, which is mandatory whenever symptoms are present. When symptoms remit and there are no analytical abnormalities, patients can start therapy with TDF, ABC, 3TC, FTC, or with an NRTI-sparing regimen.

Lactic acidosis is a severe disease with an extraordinarily bad prognosis and a lethality index of >50%. This entity often has a gradual onset of relatively unspecific symptoms, which may delay its diagnosis. It is frequently associated with severe liver damage and extrahepatic organ failure (pancreatitis, respiratory insufficiency, heart failure, metabolic coma, etc.) and requires immediate and aggressive management. Immediate interruption of ART and vigorous intravenous hydration to prevent cardiovascular collapse and assist hepatic and renal clearance of lactate are mandatory. Intensive haemodynamic monitoring is advisable. In case of multiple organ failure, intensive organ substitution therapy may be required. The role of intravenous sodium bicarbonate is more controversial, because it may stimulate respiratory acidosis in cases complicated with encephalopathy or coma. The effectiveness of antioxidants and cofactors of the respiratory chain (e.g. riboflavin, L-carnitin, coenzyme Q, vitamin C) is uncertain, but some advocate their use based on retrospective data and the lack of significant adverse effects. However, dosing and schedules have not been properly defined for these agents. In summary, the principal clinical challenges in hyperlactataemia syndromes are their early diagnosis, and whether and when to interrupt NRTIs. Given the current availability of NRTIs with more favourable mitochondrial toxicity profiles, it does not seem reasonable to delay an NRTI switch if hyperlactataemia is consistently detected.

Renal toxicity

TDF-associated nephrotoxicity, including renal insufficiency and Fanconi's syndrome, has been reported infrequently, but the incidence, risk factors and time to resolution remain uncertain [189–200]. Small reductions from baseline in creatinine clearance, or increases in serum creatinine, have been reported for TDF-treated patients in some [194,196,200], but not other, studies [195,201]. The clinical presentation of TDF-related nephrotoxicity corresponds to proximal renal tubular damage with hypophosphataemia, normoglycaemic glycosuria, proteinuria, and decrease of creatinine clearance [197]. It is more frequent in subjects with already altered renal clearance, other nephropathies, and diabetes. In addition, TDF-induced renal tubulopathy has been associated with certain haplotypes of the ATP-binding cassette gene C2 gene (ABCC2) encoding the multi-drug resistance 2 (MDR2) protein, which mediates the cellular efflux into the urine at the apical membrane [202].

Long-term assessments of renal function in subjects without previous renal dysfunction starting TDF therapy detected statistically, but not clinically significant, decreases in glomerular filtration rate compared to alternative NRTIs [194], or no differences in the renal safety profile between TDF and d4T, each administered in combination with EFV and 3TC [190]. Dose adjustment and monitoring of renal function is warranted if TDF needs to be administered in subjects with mild renal dysfunction. Alternative NRTI compounds might be preferable in subjects with moderate to severe renal impairment.

HIV drug resistance

HIV drug resistance is an essential survival strategy for HIV that stems from its vast capacity to diversify and escape from adverse environmental conditions [203,204]. The substrate for HIV diversity comprises:

- a high viral turnover of virus-producing cells [26,205];
- an error-prone reverse transcriptase, which introduces, on average, one mutation per new virion produced [206,207];
- a high rate of homologous recombination events due to saltatory reverse transcription between the two strands of the diploid HIV genome [208–213];
- the archival nature of 'memory' mutants in the virus reservoir [31,32,35,37,214–218];
- the compartmentalization of viral replication in anatomical sanctuaries [29,33,36]; and
- the effects of genetic drift and selective pressure (immune or pharmacologic) on the evolution of the HIV quasi-species [26,203,219,220].

As a consequence, all variants with single non-deleterious resistance mutations, some with two resistance mutations, and very few with three resistance mutations are likely to exist prior to ART exposure.

Antiretroviral therapy tackles these adaptive mechanisms by taking advantage of two aspects. First, the pre-existence of viral variants resistant to three drugs is highly unlikely, and second, the rate of viral evolution is highly dependent on the viral replication rate. Although viral replication cannot be completely interrupted, HAART can potentially suppress viral load below 50 copies/mL for several years in treatment-naïve patients. However, due to the aforementioned factors, as well as suboptimal adherence, pharmacokinetic or pharmacodynamic problems, pre-existing resistance mutations and the persistence of low-level residual viral replication, resistance will eventually evolve and cause virologic failure [76,221–227]. Given the similarities in molecular structure within compounds of the same antiretroviral family and their interaction with similar target sites, the emergence of resistance to one drug will often extend to the other drugs of the same family to some degree. The presence of active replication under selective antiretroviral pressure will promote the accumulation of additional resistance mutations, further increasing the degree of cross-family resistance [228,229].

Recent findings from the HAART Observational Medical Evaluation and Research (HOMER) cohort indicate that the emergence of antiretroviral resistance among patients starting first-line HAART is associated with a nearly twofold increase in risk of death [230]. Interestingly, the emergence of resistance to NNRTIs was associated with a greater risk of subsequent death (a threefold increase) than the emergence of resistance to any other class of drug. To delay the evolution of HIV drug resistance, it is essential to suppress viral replication profoundly and durably, and to manage viral replication rebounds aggressively.

While most new-generation PIs are associated with specific major resistance mutations, different PIs share many minor resistance mutations [228,229]. Therefore, the early detection of PI failure with few minor PI resistance mutations could enable salvage therapy with another PI. An aggressive approach to treatment failure is warranted in order to avoid persistent replication under a failing PI and to limit accumulation of minor PI resistance mutations.

NNRTIs, in contrast, have a low genetic barrier [228,229]. The emergence of single mutations (e.g. K103N, G190A/S) generates high-level resistance to all members of this family. Until recently, this made sequential treatment with NNRTIs virtually unfeasible. The new NNRTI etravirine, however, retains antiviral efficacy against viruses with the K103N mutation, although susceptibility to etravirine is lost with the accumulation of NNRTI-resistant mutations. It is important to limit the development of NNRTI resistance by maximizing the antiviral potency and resistance barrier of the accompanying drugs (i.e. the NRTI backbone) and by reinforcing treatment adherence. Early treatment switch after NNRTI failure is needed to forestall the accumulation of NRTI and NNRTI resistance mutations and to facilitate a potential rescue with etravirine. Unlike PI or NRTI-resistance mutations, NNRTI resistance mutations have a minimal impact on HIV's replication capacity [231]. Hence, NNRTI maintenance is of little utility to impair viral virulence.

At least four main resistance pathways can be identified in the NRTI family:

- The first involves resistance to 3TC and its related compound FTC. M184V or M184I mutations, situated in the conserved YMMD motif in the reverse transcriptase (RT)'s active site, confer >1000-fold resistance to both drugs [232–234]. M184V/I mutations are less frequent in FTC- than in 3TC-containing regimens, and also decrease the susceptibility to ABC and ddI. M184V hypersensitizes HIV-1 to ZDV and TDF and acts in synergy with these drugs by altering RT's processivity and causing multiple other effects [235–248]. Notably, M184V impairs the replication capacity of mutant viruses in the presence of 3TC, relative to wild-type viruses in the absence of therapy.

- A second resistance pathway comprises the stepwise accumulation of thymidine-analogue resistance mutations (TAMs) at positions 41, 67, 70, 210, 215 and 219, which confer resistance to ZDV and d4T, and partially contribute to ABC and ddI resistance [228,229]. There are two TAM pathways: TAM1 (41L, 210W, 215Y) and TAM2 (67N, 70R and 219E/Q), which tend to be mutually excluding, particularly during early TAM accumulation. In general, significant decreases in NRTI susceptibility require the stepwise accumulation of several resistance mutations [222,225–227,231,249–254].

- The third pathway includes the K65R and L74V mutations plus several accessory mutations (T69N/S/A, V75T) situated in a loop between the β2 and β3 strands in the 'fingers' region of the RT [255]. Mutation K65R is the signature mutation for TDF, although it also confers intermediate levels of resistance to ddI, ABC, 3TC and FTC, and low-level resistance to d4T [69,255–263]. K65R hypersensitizes HIV-1 to ZDV and does not develop in patients receiving ZDV-containing regimens [259]. L74V occurs frequently during ddI and ABC monotherapy [264] and is ddI's signature mutation, one sufficient to cause failure in patients receiving ddI monotherapy. ABC failure, in contrast, requires the accumulation of additional mutations [265]. Furthermore, L74V hypersensitizes HIV-1 to ZDV and, less clearly, to d4T and TDF. Mutations at position 69 are the most commonly detected in HIV-1 genotypes, other than TAMs and M184V, and have been shown to contribute to resistance to every NRTI. V75T confers resistance to d4T, ddI, and zalcitabine (ddC), and generally occurs in the context of multi-nucleoside resistance.

- A fourth and infrequently detected resistance pathway includes multi-nucleoside resistance driven by the Q151M mutation and/or 69 insertions [68,228,229,266]. Insertions in position 69 occur only in 2% of heavily pre-treated patients and confer high-level resistance to TDF and other NRTIs. Q151M is a two base-pair change in a conserved reverse transcriptase region that is close to the first nucleotide of the single-stranded nucleotide template. Q151M alone causes intermediate levels of resistance to ZDV, ddI, d4T and ABC, and is nearly always followed by mutations at positions 62, 75, 77 and 116. Isolates with V75I, F77L, F116Y and Q151M have high-level resistance to each of these NRTIs and low-level resistance to 3TC and TDF.

The clinical relevance of these four resistance profiles regarding long-term ART in resource-rich countries is related to the availability of co-formulated NRTIs. Single-pill co-formulated NRTIs are the NRTI treatment of choice in economically developed countries due to their demonstrated efficacy, simplicity, convenience and favourable adherence profile [60]. ZDV- and TDF-based fixed-dose combinations have complementary resistance patterns, so one can be used as the second line of the other. Despite the lack of clinical trials directly assessing the order in which these regimens should be used, given that TDF- and FTC-associated mutations hypersensitize HIV-1 to ZDV, it seems reasonable to use TDF/FTC regimens as first-line NRTI therapy. Third and further lines of NRTI treatment should be designed according to phenotypic and genotypic resistance analyses.

Multi-drug resistant HIV

Multi-drug resistant HIV infection is an extraordinarily challenging complication of long-term ART. In a US survey [66], 75%, 50% and 13% of viraemic patients receiving HAART had viruses resistant to at least one, two and three classes of antiretroviral drugs, respectively. Exposure to suboptimal therapy is the main risk factor for MDR-HIV. Advanced HIV disease, higher HIV-1 RNA levels and lower CD4 counts are also associated with this condition. Most patients currently exhibiting MDR-HIV started therapy in the pre-HAART era, or showed particularly erratic adherence.

To prevent the development of MDR-HIV, it is critical to maximize the success of the first lines of therapy and to plan subsequent treatment lines proactively. Unless there is an imperative medical reason—which is infrequently the case—ART should not be initiated until the patient has a full understanding of its benefits and problems and he or she is committed to adhere to and face lifelong therapy. Maximum antiviral potency should be sought but should also be balanced with convenience, tolerability and potential pharmacokinetic interactions, and should always preserve future treatment options.

The main treatment strategy in the presence of MDR-HIV is the optimization of the antiretroviral background—preferably based on phenotypic resistance information—and the addition of new drugs with preserved antiviral activity, if available. The main clinical goal of the management of MDR-HIV is to preserve CD4 counts and avoid clinical complications [228,229]; however, a significant proportion of subjects treated with the new antiretroviral drugs and classes will be able to suppress HIV-1 RNA levels to <50 copies/mL. Given the scarcity of adequate treatment alternatives and the presence of MDR-HIV, it seems reasonable to consider the following management principles:

◆ If two active drugs are available, they should be administered with an antiretroviral background optimized according to (preferably phenotypic) resistance information. This is the only scenario where viral suppression <50 copies/mL is, at least transiently, achievable in a considerable proportion of patients and should thus be a goal of therapy. Initial results from clinical trials including new PIs (DRV), NNRTIs (etravirine), integrase inhibitors (RAL, ELV), and CCR5 antagonists (MRV, VCV) forecast an upsurge of highly effective new treatment options for subjects currently infected with MDR-HIV. Genotype-based optimization of already available regimens has a limited impact on subsequent HIV-1 RNA reductions in patients with MDR-HIV.

- If only one active drug is available, the patient is clinically stable, and his/her immune status is relatively preserved, it may be preferable to delay the administration of this drug until a second active drug becomes available. Virtual monotherapy (i.e. the addition of only one active drug to a resistant background) is deemed to lead to early treatment failure [267] and rapid abolition of the activity of the new compound due to the development of resistance. Indeed, virtual monotherapy probably will not have a clinical impact in terms of prolonged survival or preservation of immune responses.

- If the patient's clinical context is severe, and/or a 'watchful waiting' or a 'minimal intervention' strategy is considered too hazardous, a salvage regimen should be administered without delay. This treatment should be optimized according to phenotypic resistance information, toxicity profile and patient's tolerability and acceptance, and should include as many drugs as necessary in the clinician's judgement. Dual-boosted PI-based regimens such as LPV/ATV/r or LPV/ saquinavir(SQV)/r may be useful in this context [268,269].

- If MDR-HIV is associated with relatively stable CD4 counts and the patient's clinical status is maintained, alternative treatment strategies directed to impair viral fitness might be considered, preferably in the context of closely monitored clinical studies. It is important to note that none of these strategies has been properly validated in clinical trials. Anecdotal reports suggest that the interruption of some components of HAART (PIs or NRTIs) may delay the emergence of more fit, and therefore more virulent, wild-type viruses [270]. A simple and safe strategy to partially constrain viral fitness is to maintain 3TC therapy even in subjects with the M184V mutation [271,272]. Nevertheless, the utility of this strategy has not been confirmed in clinical studies so far.

- Complete HAART interruption should never be attempted in subjects with MDR-HIV, because this strategy is associated with rapid clinical progression and a significant increase in death rates [41,42].

Non AIDS-defining conditions

As a consequence of the success of long-term HAART on prolonging life expectancy and reducing 'classical' complications, a number of non AIDS-defining conditions that were rarely seen in the early years of the HIV pandemic are increasingly being reported in HIV-infected patients. An adequate management of non AIDS-defining conditions is essential for the long-term management of HIV infection.

Cancer

HIV-infected individuals are at a higher risk for cancer than the general population. Because HIV infection induces immune deregulation, usual cancer risk factors (e.g. smoking, alcohol consumption, viral co-infections) are found in excess among HIV-positive individuals, and the aging of HIV-infected individuals increases their likelihood of developing cancers afflicting the general population [273–275]. The advent of HAART a decade ago contributed to a reduction in incidence of, and an amelioration in the prognosis for, some neoplasms, but had little effect on others [275–277]. In the face of this changing epidemiology, it is important to note that:

- the risk for AIDS-defining cancers has not continued to decline during the HAART era;
- despite reductions in their incidence over the last two decades, Kaposi's sarcoma (KS) and non-Hodgkin's lymphoma (NHL) still account for more than 60% of neoplasms seen in Western HIV-infected patients at present; and

♦ the incidence of most non AIDS-defining neoplasms has remained constant over time [275,278].

ART has increasingly and progressively lowered the incidence of, and improved the prognosis for, herpes virus-related malignancies such as KS and NHL. While HAART is likely to have led to the sharp decrease in the incidence of KS and NHL in 1996, the incidence of these diseases had already started to decrease in the early 1990s, probably because of the growing use of single and dual antiretroviral drug regimens [275]. Although PIs have specific anti-oncogenic effects unrelated to their antiviral activity (i.e. inhibition of cell proliferation and induction of apoptosis in cultured cancer cells, blockade of endothelial- and tumour-cell invasion, *in vivo* antiangiogenic effects, tumour growth inhibition and direct anti-inflammatory effects) [279], NNRTI-based HAART is as protective for systemic NHL and KS as PI-based HAART, and these are significantly more protective than either NRTIs alone or a total absence of antiretroviral drugs [277,280].

Kaposi's sarcoma remains the most common AIDS-associated cancer in Western countries and is an important cause of morbidity and mortality worldwide, particularly in sub-Saharan Africa [276,277]. Several mechanisms by which HAART might reduce or prevent KS have been proposed [277], including:

♦ immune reconstitution against Kaposi's sarcoma-associated herpes virus (KSHV) and cytotoxic T-lymphocyte (CTL)-mediated killing of KSHV-infected spindle cells;

♦ reduction of circulating levels of HIV-1 Tat and other inflammatory cytokines;

♦ direct anti-spindle cell and/or anti-angiogenic effect of protease inhibitors; and

♦ potential inhibition of KSHV replication by HAART.

AIDS-related NHL often has an extranodal presentation, involves the bone marrow, and has an aggressive clinical course and poor prognosis [276]. HAART reduces the incidence and improves the response rate and survival, in part by restoring CTL responses and reducing chronic antigen stimulation. Regarding NHL subtypes, major reductions have been observed in cerebral lymphoma, immunoblastic lymphoma and Burkitt's lymphoma since the advent of HAART [278]. The clinical presentation of AIDS-related NHL is not altered by HAART, except that CD4 counts at NHL diagnosis tend to be higher than in patients not receiving treatment [281]. Response rates and survival duration statistics are approaching those seen in the general population with advanced-stage, high-grade NHL [276]. Moreover, the prognostic factors of AIDS-related lymphoma closely resemble those for the general population [282], with CD4 count being an additional independent prognostic factor [276]. In contrast to cancers related to herpes viruses, the incidence or clinical presentation of other AIDS-related cancers has not substantially changed since the beginning of the HIV epidemic [274,275,278].

The increased incidence of human papillomavirus (HPV)-related neoplasms (cervical intraepithelial neoplasia and cervical cancer in women, and squamous intraepithelial lesions and cancer of the anus in HIV-infected women and men) might only reflect the higher prevalence of HPV infections in this population, as there are shared risk factors for both infections [276,277]. In a recent survey of HIV-infected males (including men who have sex with men (MSM) and heterosexuals) in a Spanish tertiary hospital, the prevalence of high-risk HPV types in the anus, penis and mouth was 78%, 36% and 30%, respectively, without evidence of pathology in these areas [283]. Oncogenic genotypes (HPV16, 18 and others) alter the tumour microenvironment and disrupt cell differentiation. Chronic inflammation due to repeated sexually transmitted diseases (STDs) probably promotes the proliferation of HPV-infected cells, but no direct effects of HIV-1 infection have been consistently described.

The lack of impact of HAART on HPV-related cancer incidence has been confirmed in several large cohorts [274,275,278,284]. Similarly, the impact of HAART on the clinical presentation of pre-invasive lesions (cervical intraepithelial neoplasia (CIN)) has been modest at best [285–287]. The incidence and clinical presentation of, and prognosis for, other HPV-related neoplasms (vulval/vaginal cancer, skin cancer, conjunctival cancer, penile intraepithelial and invasive neo-plasia and, probably, oral, tonsillar, laryngeal and oesophageal carcinoma) have remained unal-tered in the HAART era, although some of these cancers are relatively more frequent in HIV-infected subjects than in linked HIV-negative peers.

Lung cancer is the most common non AIDS-related cancer in the United States [275] and is the second most frequent cause of death among HIV-infected individuals aged 55 or older in New York City [48]. Most of the significant excess of lung cancer in HIV individuals is probably related with an increased prevalence of smoking, but it remains unclear whether other factors are also involved. According to Lavole *et al.* [288], lung cancer is usually diagnosed in asymptomatic 45-year-old patients with mild or moderate immunosuppression. In 75–90% of cases, lung can-cer is locally advanced or is already metastatic at diagnosis (stages III-IV), and adenocarcinoma is the most frequent histological type. The prognosis for lung cancer is poorer in HIV-infected patients than in the general population. However, data on the efficacy and toxicity of chemotherapy in this setting are rare and rather imprecise. Surgery remains the standard treatment for localized disease in patients with adequate functional status and general health, regardless of their immune status.

Although Hodgkin's lymphoma (HL) is not considered an AIDS-defining cancer, it is 10–35 times more frequent in HIV-infected patients than in HIV-negative individuals and is virtually always associated with Epstein-Barr Virus (EBV) infection. HIV-infected subjects with HL are more likely than their HIV-negative counterparts to present with stage B symptoms (asthenia, anorexi and night sweats), advanced disease stage, extranodal disease and bone marrow involve-ment. Treatment with HAART concomitantly with dose-intense chemotherapeutic regimens dramatically improves the outcome and response of this disease [289]. In a study analyzing the outcome of patients with HIV-associated HL with respect to the use and efficacy of HAART and other prognostic factors, median survival time in patients without HAART response was 18.6 months, whereas the median survival time in patients with HAART response was not reached (89% overall survival (OS), at 24 months) [290]. Despite the benefits of HAART on the outcome of HL, several studies have described a steady increase in the incidence of this disease over time [274,275,284], for which there is no clear explanation.

The third, fourth and fifth most frequent cancers in HIV-infected subjects are anal, colon and prostate cancers. Anal cancer is overrepresented in HIV-infected individuals (19.6 times more frequent than in the general population) and is linked to HPV infections in the anal mucosa. In contrast, colon cancer is as frequent in HIV-infected subjects as in the general population, and prostate cancer occurs twice as frequently in HIV-negative subjects.

In summary, HIV-infected subjects remain at high risk for cancer even in the HAART era. Aggressive risk reduction strategies including smoking cessation and periodical screening for sex-ually transmitted diseases and pre-neoplasic lesions are warranted in the long-term management of HIV-infected subjects.

HBV and HCV

Worldwide, 12 million people are co-infected with HIV and HCV, 4 million are co-infected with HIV and HBV, and half a million are co-infected with all three viruses. More than 75% of indi-viduals who acquired HIV infection through injection drug use or transfusion of contaminated blood products are also infected with HCV. The prevalence of HCV infection among HIV-positive individuals is over 50% in countries where parenteral transmission is (or was) the main HIV transmission route (e.g. Spain, other countries in the Mediterranean basin, and the Russian

Federation) [291]. In areas where the HIV epidemic was driven by other modes of transmission, less than 10% of HIV-infected patients are also HCV-positive [292]. In Spain, 94% of HIV-infected prisoners are co-infected with HCV [293].

In countries with high prevalence of HBV or HCV/HIV co-infection, liver disease is a major cause of hospital admission, severe morbidity and mortality among HIV-infected individuals. Liver-related deaths were the first cause of non AIDS-related deaths in the D:A:D trial [44], representing 15.5% of all deaths observed. Sixty-six per cent of patients who died had HCV infection, 16.9% were HBV-positive, and 7.1% had dual viral hepatic co-infections. There was a strong association between immunodeficiency and risk of liver-related death. Similarly, in the year 2000, complications derived from viral hepatitis were the first cause of non AIDS-related deaths among HIV-infected subjects in French hospitals [294].

It is important to note that in HIV-infected subjects, the natural history of HBV or HCV chronic infection is much faster, the response to therapy is poorer, and the incidence of adverse events is higher. Those co-infected with HIV-HBV and HIV-HCV and receiving ART have a three- to fourfold higher risk of liver-related serious adverse events or deaths compared with HIV-monoinfected patients [295–298], with risk associated with level of immunodeficiency [22,299]. In the D:A:D study, the risk of liver-related death is increased by 12 times for patients whose latest CD4 count is less than 50 cells/mm^3 compared with patients with a latest CD4 count of more than 500 cells/mm^3 [44]. In addition, initiation of HAART in HIV-HBV co-infected individuals with low CD4 counts may be associated with hepatitis flares during immunologic recovery. Initiation of certain antiretroviral drugs (e.g. NVP, TPV and other PIs), or the interruption of antiretroviral drugs with anti-HBV activity (i.e. 3TC, FTC, TDF), may also cause liver enzyme flares.

End-stage liver disease due to HBV or HCV infection in HIV-infected subjects has an extremely poor prognosis [47]. In a prospective follow-up of all consecutive patients with HCV-related cirrhosis who presented with the first hepatic decompensation in tertiary hospitals of Andalucía, Spain, from January 1997 to June 2004, the median survival after the first hepatic decompensation was 13 months. Independent predictors of survival were Child score [hazard ratio (HR)=1.2; 95% CI:1.08–1.37; p=0.001], CD4 count at decompensation lower than 100 cells/mm^3 (HR=2.48; 95% CI:1.52–4.06; p<0.001), and hepatic encephalopathy as the first hepatic decompensation (HR=2.45; 95% CI:1.41–4.27; p=0.001). Subjects who received HAART had a lower risk of liver-related mortality.

Whereas HCV infection can be eradicated in HIV-infected patients (although HIV-HCV co-infected individuals achieve worse outcomes than those infected solely with HCV), HBV infection requires prolonged antiviral treatment. Early detection and aggressive treatment of viral hepatitis co-infections is crucial for the long-term well-being of HIV-infected individuals. Subjects with end-stage liver disease have an extraordinarily bad prognosis and few may benefit from liver transplantation.

Cognitive disorders and other geriatric syndromes

The number of HIV-infected individuals aged 65 or over has increased tenfold over the past decade [300]. In 2005, 28% of AIDS cases in the United States were over 50 years of age. The US Senate Special Committee on Aging predicted that 50% of nationally prevalent AIDS cases would be over 50 years of age by 2015 [301]. Older HIV-positive individuals have inferior immunologic recovery and accelerated clinical progression. In addition, they experience more co-morbidities necessitating medical interventions, more antiretroviral drug-related adverse events, and have higher mortality. As they age, HIV-infected patients are increasingly more likely to develop the geriatric syndromes that affect the general population.

Of particular importance is cognitive impairment, which includes HIV-associated dementia (HAD) and minor cognitive motor disorder (MCMD) as well as other overlapping diseases like Alzheimer's or Parkinson's diseases [reviewed in 49]. Before the advent of HAART, at least a third of individuals with AIDS had some degree of HIV-associated cognitive deterioration, frequently associated with low CD4 counts. Classic subcortical symptoms of HIV-related dementia (slowed response times, slowness in psychomotor speed, cognitive rigidity, emotional lability, and apathy) were the usual clinical presentation. In comparison, the widespread use of HAART significantly reduced the incidence HIV-associated dementia. At present, cognitive impairment is less incident but just as prevalent as in the pre-HAART era. Cortical symptoms (aphasia, apraxia, agnosia) are more frequently seen, and they present in subjects with higher CD4 counts (also above 200 cells/mm^3). Cognitive deficits can present a fluctuating course because of fluctuations in CNS inflammation.

The relative hazard ratio for dementia in the HAART era is 1.6 per decade of life at AIDS onset [301]. Whether there is a synergistic or an additive relationship between aging and HIV infection on neuropsychological performance remains to be clarified. Neuropathological findings typical from other age-related neurodegenerative diseases such as Alzheimer's disease (increased beta-amyloid deposition, increased extracellular amyloid plaques, and decreased cerebrospinal fluid (CSF) beta-amyloid levels) [218,303–305] and Parkinson's disease [306–310] are increasingly being observed in HIV-infected patients. Therefore, it is possible that different cognitive diseases frequently overlap in older HIV-positive patients. On the other hand, HIV-derived products like the Tat protein, which inhibits neprilysin, an enzyme responsible for amyloid degradation, may mimic the neuropathological findings of age-related dementias [303,311–314].

Among other geriatric syndromes, older HIV-infected patients are at higher risk of bone fractures and falls due to decreased bone mineralization, as well as other metabolic disorders (e.g. diabetes mellitus), malignancies and renal, hepatic, or cardiac dysfunctions. It has been suggested that monoclonal gammopathy of unknown significance (MGUS) may appear earlier in HIV-infected patients, this being more strongly associated with other viral infections such as HBV, HCV or KSHV than is typically seen in an HIV-uninfected cohort [315]. HAART might be beneficial for MGUS, although prospective robust studies are lacking.

It is important to note that HIV diagnosis in older patients is frequently delayed due to stereotyping and false assumptions—for example, that they do not engage in sexual intercourse or that their risk for contracting HIV infection is lower. Another factor is the tendency of older patients to delay seeking medical help due to fear of stigmatization or to different forms of social pressure. Consequently, HIV infection in older patients is frequently diagnosed at late stages of the disease, often when severe complications have already occurred. Information campaigns targeting older patients and their physicians are required, both to prevent HIV transmission and to diagnose and treat HIV infection in a timely manner.

Lifetime HAART in the developing world

The astounding reality of lifetime HAART in the developing world is that it is *achievable*. The estimated annual cost of US$30 billion for care and prevention of HIV, tuberculosis (TB) and malaria equals the amount spent by the United States in Iraq in only six weeks. As eloquently argued by US economist Jeffrey Sachs and others, there are sufficient global health resources now to achieve the Millennium Development Goals for HIV, TB and malaria if only the necessary political will and leadership are present [316]. Compared to this imperative, the challenges of lifetime HAART in the clinics of the developing world are minor, manageable problems.

Lifetime HAART in the developing world presents unique challenges, in addition to those that are familiar in the developed world (Table 26.1), and this is the focus of this section. Sustainable access to prevention, care and treatment is the highest priority and the greatest challenge in both settings, as shown by the estimated 100,000 people living with HIV in the United States who lack treatment [317], though the problem of access is several degrees of magnitude greater in the developing world.

The clinical challenges

The daunting challenges of lifetime HAART in the developed world, such as prolonged treatment adherence, long-term toxicities, drug resistance, persisting unwillingness to engage MSM, co-morbidities such as HBV and HCV infection, and rising mortality from non-HIV health problems like heart disease, injection drug use, renal disease and cancer are discussed in detail in other chapters. It will have to suffice here to note that each of these issues is also of paramount importance to the future of HIV in the developing world, and an important dimension of strategies for their successful management in the North will be their potential applicability to the same problems in developing countries. One issue that merits mention is the ubiquity of thymidine analogues, and d4T in particular, in first-line regimens in the developing world. The inevitable rise in peripheral neuropathy and peripheral lipoatrophy is already being described, and rapid access to second-line drugs that lack these toxicities is a growing priority.

First among the unique obstacles facing people living with HIV and their physicians in the developing world are HIV stigma and discrimination. An elderly woman in China with AIDS stated in 1995 that she would rather die than take an HIV test because of the shame that the diagnosis would bring upon her and her family. This common scenario is repeated too often, to this day, around the world. An environment of tolerance in which to take an HIV test and live with an HIV diagnosis is of paramount importance to effective national and local HIV treatment and prevention programmes. Similarly, health professionals bear the responsibility of ensuring compassionate and non-judgemental care from health workers. The emerging HIV centres of excellence are essential for the nurturing of tolerance and acceptance of HIV testing, treatment and support.

Access to simple, basic information for HIV prevention and HIV testing is another important challenge for lifetime HAART. It is estimated that only 20% of the world's population has

Table 26.1 Clinical challenges of lifetime HAART in the developing world

Comparable to developed world	Unique to developing world
Access and sustainability	Access and sustainability
HIV prevention and expansion of VCT	HIV prevention and expansion of VCT
Adherence	High early mortality
Drug resistance	Diagnosis and treatment of OIs, TB
ART toxicities	Access to second-line drugs
Integration of treatment and prevention	Access to viral load, resistance tests
Hepatitis B/C co-infection	Clade variation
Non-HIV causes of mortality	Human resource crisis, training
	Health system infrastructure
	Laboratory testing and support
	Access to rural areas, IDUs, children, and pregnant women
	Stigma reduction and anti-discrimination

access to needed HIV prevention information and voluntary counselling and testing (VCT) [318]. There is clear evidence from South Africa and Thailand that more people seek VCT when it is more accessible and convenient, and when care and treatment are available to people who test HIV-positive.

Unfortunately, the evolution of care and treatment for women and children in the developing world has mirrored the inequities in the North, and it is still the case that fewer than a quarter of pregnant women and children in need of ART have access to it [318]. Several programmatic obstacles must be overcome to address this problem, including access to paediatric formulations, rapid HIV testing for all pregnant women, training for clinicians in paediatric care and paediatric dosing of ART, DNA testing for infants born to HIV-positive women, and reproductive counselling, including breastfeeding counselling, for HIV-positive women.

Although 10% of HIV in the world is acquired through injection drug use, less than 1% of people living with HIV who are on ART in the world are IDUs [4]. This problem is most acute in the Russian Federation, Eastern Europe, Central Asia, China and South-East Asia. It is nearly impossible for a single clinician to effectively manage HIV infection in an injection drug user (IDU) without a supportive local and national environment that includes harm reduction, counselling and treatment for chemical dependency, and non-judgemental care for the individual and his or her family. Stigma reduction efforts in countries with high rates of injection drug use must include improved tolerance towards drug use and support for harm reduction strategies, as well as HIV stigma reduction efforts.

Although morbidity and mortality from non-HIV conditions are rising in the developing world, the main causes of death continue to be opportunistic infection (OI)-related, and TB is the most common among them. While first-year mortality on ART in the developed world is 2–3%, it is 5–15% in the developing world. Among the many reasons for the greater mortality in the developing world are: the higher prevalence of diseases such as TB, malaria and infectious diarrhoea; the greater prevalence of malnutrition and anaemia; and limitations in the individual healthcare systems.

It is likely that a higher incidence of immune reconstitution disease also contributes to the greater mortality; the average CD4 count at which ART is started is below 100 cells/mm^3 in many sub-Saharan countries, and immune reconstitution inflammatory syndrome (IRIS) is more common when ART is started at CD4 counts below 100 cells/mm^3 [319]. Earlier diagnosis of HIV is one key strategy to reducing this early mortality. Others include greater access to primary and preventive healthcare, improved nutrition and maternal-child health, and better TB detection and treatment.

One of the major obstacles to the optimum diagnosis and treatment of HIV-related OIs has been the severe limitation in clinical laboratories supporting HIV clinical care, and this is also an urgent challenge for the future of lifetime HAART in the developing world. For example, over 90% of people with TB in the world are diagnosed by sputum smear microscopy alone, and the capability for culture and TB drug sensitivities is lacking [320]. Microscopy at best only diagnoses 60% of people living with TB, and in high HIV prevalence areas, the diagnostic yield of microscopy for TB is further reduced to 40% or less. Similarly, in many countries of the developing world, only a single central reference laboratory has the capabilities of a modern HIV laboratory that one would find, say, in the United States, and the vast majority of rural residents with HIV lack access to modern laboratory procedures and equipment.

Inadequate laboratory support also has a great impact on ART management. In the absence of viral load testing, clinicians must manage patients with inadequate tools such as CD4 counts and clinical manifestations of the disease. Management of ART without viral loads has been shown to lead to management errors that include premature discontinuation, prolonged exposure to toxicities from inactive drugs and high-level HIV drug resistance. Optimal management of ART will require rapid scale-up of inexpensive viral load testing using dried blood spot technology in order for the precious resource of ART to be used more effectively.

With the rise in treatment failure due to clinical or immunologic failure and toxicity, access to second-line treatments is an enormous challenge to lifetime HAART in the developing world. At present, access to one or more boosted PIs and second-line NRTIs is the first priority, but in future, access to other new classes and drugs will also be needed.

The greater diversity of HIV clades is another potential challenge for lifetime HAART in the developing world. Fortunately, the impact of non-B clades on the activity of ART has been minimal to date [321]. Minor differences in drug resistance patterns have been described, as well as some differences in transmissibility and CNS manifestations, but none of these differences has substantially altered the enormous impact of ART on morbidity and mortality [322].

Sustaining care and treatment in the developing world

The most daunting challenge of lifetime HAART in the developing world is the implementation of effective health policies and systems of care and prevention that are durable and sustainable. The critical issues to be addressed are shown in Table 26.2, and they are also discussed in detail elsewhere in this book. The first priority is access to care and prevention, with increasing attention to the integration of prevention and care services in recognition of their mutual interdependence. A similarly increasing priority must be placed on the coordination and integration of parallel health services that affect the same populations, in order to maximize scarce health resources and to take advantage of economies of scale, such as coordination of HIV and TB care and diagnostic services, or coordination and integration of services for women, children and orphans with HIV, prevention of mother-to-child transmission (PMTCT)-plus, and maternal-child health.

Accordingly, two parallel activities are invaluable to support this process. In order to build the capacity of health systems to meet the clinical challenges of HAART in the developing world, aggressive health worker training and mentoring, and careful nurturing of the many developing centres of clinical excellence that now can be found throughout the developing world, are essential to meet the needs of the expanding epidemic. Task-shifting of responsibilities from doctors to nurses, and from nurses to community health workers, has been shown to expand capacity and address the human resource crisis in health and prevention services. It should be expanded carefully, with ongoing attention to the need for health professional oversight and to ongoing quality monitoring.

The second essential component is the inclusion of people living with HIV and their communities in policy, decision-making, and service implementation. As we have learned in the North, the active participation and leadership of people with HIV and their communities leads to greater acceptance of AIDS in the community and stigma reduction, while addressing the obvious need for the voices of affected people to be heard and included in the decisions that affect their lives.

Table 26.2 Challenges to sustaining care and treatment in the developing world

Access to care and treatment
Coordination and integration of services (e.g. prevention and care; HIV and TB care)
Provision of comprehensive services
Building capacity of health systems and task shifting
Health worker training and mentoring
Engagement and participation of people living with HIV
Commitment to monitoring and evaluation

To summarize, the greatest challenge to lifetime HAART in the developing world is sustainable access to HIV prevention, care and treatment for all in need. For the first time in history, it is possible for this challenge to be met. In comparison to this challenge, the clinical problems in developing world clinics, though serious, are minor and manageable. It will be critical for the lessons learned in the developed world regarding HIV drug resistance, treatment toxicity and OI management to be applied in the developing world. In addition, the many unique challenges to lifetime HAART in the developing world will require firm resolution on the part of local and national clinicians, health authorities, civil society and people living with HIV, using the tools of a decade of experience with ART and the best practices in prevention and care that have emerged.

The global HIV treatment community has changed radically in the past decade. Most nations of the world have HIV centres of excellence in which knowledgeable clinicians and public health workers are following the best international practices of HIV prevention, care and treatment while training other health workers to expand the network of effective prevention and treatment centres. These centres, along with the clinicians, public health workers, the larger HIV community of stakeholders, and their national leaders and advocates, hold the promise for the future of HIV prevention and care in the developing world. It is now the responsibility of the developing world to further support and foster these centres and the expansion of services to new areas and people living with HIV in a sustainable and cost-effective manner.

Concluding remarks

HAART has achieved formidable successes. In less than a decade, it transformed the clinical presentation and natural history of HIV/AIDS. No other infectious disease has accumulated more knowledge at a faster pace than HIV infection. With no other disease have treatment options evolved further in so little time. However, the unprecedented complexity of HIV infection, the fact that HIV thrives by targeting the immune components specifically designed to eradicate it, and the fact that this disease erupted in human immune systems that were unprepared for counterbalancing its effects, all currently put HIV eradication beyond our reach. Moreover, current ART does not modify the virulence of HIV. Therapy interruption allows HIV to regain full virulence, with associated major declines in CD4 counts and increased risk for clinical progression and death.

We have seen in this chapter that long-term ART involves problems of adherence, resistance and toxicity as well as cost. We have also shown how the successes of HAART have modified the clinical presentation of cancers in HIV-infected individuals and how the aging of HIV-positive patients is gradually increasing the development of geriatric syndromes that were rarely seen just a few years ago. We have also shown that early detection and aggressive management of hepatitis co-infections are needed in order to avoid the severe complications and elevated mortality of end-stage liver disease.

Certainly, the next decade will witness major advances in HIV treatment, with more potent, convenient, and less toxic drugs that have different resistance profiles. Major progress in the development of an effective vaccine can also be expected, particularly as a strategy to slow AIDS progression. Hopefully, the benefits of HAART will extend to all human beings, regardless of nationality, gender or income status.

References

1. Chadborn TR, Delpech VC, Sabin CA, Sinka K, Evans BG. (2006). The late diagnosis and consequent short-term mortality of HIV-infected heterosexuals (England and Wales, 2000–2004). *AIDS* **20**:2371–9.

2. Santos Corraliza E, Fuertes Martin A. (2006). Side effects of antiretroviral therapy. Fisiopathology, clinical manifestations and treatment. *An Med Interna* **23**:338–44.

3. UNAIDS. (2006). *Report on the global AIDS epidemic 2006*. Geneva: UNAIDS. Available at www.unaids.org

4. Mocroft A, Ledergerber B, Katlama C, *et al.* (2003). Decline in the AIDS and death rates in the EuroSIDA study: an observational study. *Lancet* **362**:22–9.

5. Palella FJ Jr, Baker RK, Moorman AC, *et al.* (2006). Mortality in the highly active antiretroviral therapy era: changing causes of death and disease in the HIV outpatient study. *J Acquir Immune Defic Syndr* **43**:27–34.

6. Palella FJ Jr, Delaney KM, Moorman AC, *et al.* (1998). Declining morbidity and mortality among patients with advanced human immunodeficiency virus infection. HIV Outpatient Study Investigators. *N Engl J Med* **338**:853–60.

7. Parsons TD, Braaten AJ, Hall CD, Robertson KR. (2006). Better quality of life with neuropsychological improvement on HAART. *Health Qual Life Outcomes* **4**:11.

8. Gibbie T, Mijch A, Ellen S, *et al.* (2006). Depression and neurocognitive performance in individuals with HIV/AIDS: 2-year follow-up. *HIV Med* **7**:112–21.

9. Ostrowski MA, Krakauer DC, Li Y, *et al.* (1998). Effect of immune activation on the dynamics of human immunodeficiency virus replication and on the distribution of viral quasispecies. *J Virol* **72**:7772–84.

10. Cohen OJ, Kinter A, Fauci AS. (1997). Host factors in the pathogenesis of HIV disease. *Immunol Rev* **159**:31–48.

11. Pantaleo G, Fauci AS. (1996). Immunopathogenesis of HIV infection. *Annu Rev Microbiol* **50**:825–54.

12. Fauci AS. (1996). Host factors and the pathogenesis of HIV-induced disease. *Nature* **384**:529–34.

13. Fauci AS. (1996). Host factors in the pathogenesis of HIV disease. *Antibiot Chemother* **48**:4–12.

14. Rosenberg ZF, Fauci AS. (1990). Immunopathogenic mechanisms of HIV infection: cytokine induction of HIV expression. *Immunol Today* **11**:176–80.

15. Van Maele B, Busschots K, Vandekerckhove L, Christ F, Debyser Z. (2006). Cellular co-factors of HIV-1 integration. *Trends Biochem Sci* **31**:98–105.

16. Lewinski MK, Yamashita M, Emerman M, *et al.* (2006). Retroviral DNA integration: viral and cellular determinants of target-site selection. *PLoS Pathog* **2**(6):e60.

17. Chiu TK, Davies DR. (2004). Structure and function of HIV-1 integrase. *Curr Top Med Chem* **4**:965–77.

18. Brin E, Yi J, Skalka AM, Leis J. (2000). Modeling the late steps in HIV-1 retroviral integrase-catalyzed DNA integration. *J Biol Chem* **275**:39287–95.

19. Hindmarsh P, Leis J. (1999). Retroviral DNA integration. *Microbiol Mol Biol Rev* **63**:836–43.

20. Asante-Appiah E, Skalka AM. (1997). Molecular mechanisms in retrovirus DNA integration. *Antiviral Res* **36**:139–56.

21. Vink C, Plasterk RH. (1993). The human immunodeficiency virus integrase protein. *Trends Genet* **9**:433–8.

22. Sakai H, Kawamura M, Sakuragi J, *et al.* (1993). Integration is essential for efficient gene expression of human immunodeficiency virus type 1. *J Virol* **67**:1169–74.

23. Cristina J. (2005). Genetic diversity and evolution of hepatitis C virus in the Latin American region. *J Clin Virol* **34** (Suppl 2):S1–7.

24. Gonzalez-Lopez C, Gomez-Mariano G, Escarmis C, Domingo E. (2005). Invariant aphthovirus consensus nucleotide sequence in the transition to error catastrophe. *Infect Genet Evol* **5**:366–74.

25. Jerzak G, Bernard KA, Kramer LD, Ebel GD. (2005). Genetic variation in West Nile virus from naturally infected mosquitoes and birds suggests quasispecies structure and strong purifying selection. *J Gen Virol* **86**:2175–83.

26. Coffin JM. (1995). HIV population dynamics in vivo: implications for genetic variation, pathogenesis, and therapy. *Science* **267**:483–9.

27. Smith DB, McAllister J, Casino C, Simmonds P. (1997). Virus 'quasispecies': making a mountain out of a molehill? *J Gen Virol* **78**:1511–9.

28. Chun T-W, Nickle DC, Justement JS, *et al.* (2005). HIV-infected individuals receiving effective antiviral therapy for extended periods of time continually replenish their viral reservoir. *J Clin Invest* **115**:3250–5.

29. Nunnari G, Sullivan J, Xu Y, *et al.* (2005). HIV type 1 cervicovaginal reservoirs in the era of HAART. *AIDS Res Hum Retroviruses* **21**:714–8.

30. Chun TW, Nickle DC, Justement JS, *et al.* (2005). HIV-infected individuals receiving effective antiviral therapy for extended periods of time continually replenish their viral reservoir. *J Clin Invest* **115**:3250–5.

31. Siliciano JD, Siliciano RF. (2004). A long-term latent reservoir for HIV-1: discovery and clinical implications. *J Antimicrob Chemother* **54**:6–9.

32. Siliciano JD, Kajdas J, Finzi D, *et al.* (2003). Long-term follow-up studies confirm the stability of the latent reservoir for HIV-1 in resting CD4+ T cells. *Nat Med* **9**:727–8.

33. Lambotte O, Deiva K, Tardieu M. (2003). HIV-1 persistence, viral reservoir, and the central nervous system in the HAART era. *Brain Pathol* **13**:95–103.

34. Finzi D, Blankson J, Siliciano JD, *et al.* (1999). Latent infection of CD4+ T cells provides a mechanism for lifelong persistence of HIV-1, even in patients on effective combination therapy. *Nat Med* **5**:512–7.

35. Siliciano RF. (1998). A reservoir for HIV in patients on combination antiretroviral therapy. *Hopkins HIV Rep* **10**:1, 5–6, 11.

36. Schrager LK, D'Souza MP. (1998). Cellular and anatomical reservoirs of HIV-1 in patients receiving potent antiretroviral combination therapy. *JAMA* **280**:67–71.

37. Finzi D, Hermankova M, Pierson T, *et al.* (1997). Identification of a reservoir for HIV-1 in patients on highly active antiretroviral therapy. *Science* **278**:1295–300.

38. Richman DD, Wrin T, Little SJ, Petropoulos CJ. (2003). Rapid evolution of the neutralizing antibody response to HIV type 1 infection. *Proc Natl Acad Sci USA* **100**:4144–9.

39. Frost SD, Liu Y, Pond SL, *et al.* (2005). Characterization of human immunodeficiency virus type 1 (HIV-1) envelope variation and neutralizing antibody responses during transmission of HIV-1 subtype B. *J Virol* **79**:6523–7.

40. El-Sadr WM, Lundgren JD, Neaton JD, *et al.* (2006). CD4+ count-guided interruption of antiretroviral treatment. *N Engl J Med* **355**:2283–96.

41. Lawrence J, Mayers DL, Hullsiek KH, *et al.* (2003). Structured treatment interruption in patients with multidrug-resistant human immunodeficiency virus. *N Engl J Med* **349**:837–46.

42. Ruiz L, Ribera E, Bonjoch A, *et al.* (2003). Role of structured treatment interruption before a 5-drug salvage antiretroviral regimen: the Retrogene Study. *J Infect Dis* **188**:977–85.

43. Ruiz L, Paredes R, Gómez G, *et al.* (2007). Antiretroviral therapy interruption guided by CD4 cell counts and plasma HIV-1 RNA levels in chronically HIV-1-infected patients. *AIDS* **21**:169–78.

44. Weber R, Sabin CA, Friis-Moller N, *et al.* (2006). Liver-related deaths in persons infected with the human immunodeficiency virus: the D:A:D study. *Arch Intern Med* **166**:1632–41.

45. Soriano V, Barreiro P, Nunez M. (2006). Management of chronic hepatitis B and C in HIV-coinfected patients. *J Antimicrob Chemother* **57**:815–8.

46. Rockstroh JK. (2006). Management of hepatitis C/HIV coinfection. *Curr Opin Infect Dis* **19**:8–13.

47. Merchante N, Giron-Gonzalez JA, Gonzalez-Serrano M, *et al.* (2006). Survival and prognostic factors of HIV-infected patients with HCV-related end-stage liver disease. *AIDS* **20**:49–57.

48. Sackoff JE, Hanna DB, Pfeiffer MR, Torian LV. (2006). Causes of death among persons with AIDS in the era of highly active antiretroviral therapy: New York City. *Ann Intern Med* **145**:397–406.

49. Valcour V, Paul R. (2006). HIV infection and dementia in older adults. *Clin Infect Dis* **42**:1449–54.

50. Ghafouri M, Amini S, Khalili K, Sawaya BE. (2006). HIV-1 associated dementia: symptoms and causes. *Retrovirology* **3**:28.

51. Anthony IC, Ramage SN, Carnie FW, Simmonds P, Bell JE. (2006). Accelerated Tau deposition in the brains of individuals infected with human immunodeficiency virus-1 before and after the advent of highly active anti-retroviral therapy. *Acta Neuropathol (Berl)* **111**:529–38.

52. Fischer-Smith T, Rappaport J. (2005). Evolving paradigms in the pathogenesis of HIV-1-associated dementia. *Expert Rev Mol Med* **7**:1–26.

53. Goodkin K, Wilkie FL, Concha M, *et al*. (2001). Aging and neuro-AIDS conditions and the changing spectrum of HIV-1-associated morbidity and mortality. *J Clin Epidemiol* **54** (Suppl 1):S35–43.

54. Gilden D. (1996). When HAART is not enough. *GMHC Treat Issues* **10**(10):1–6.

55. Staszewski S, Morales-Ramirez J, Tashima KT, *et al*. Efavirenz plus zidovudine and lamivudine, efavirenz plus indinavir, and indinavir plus zidovudine and lamivudine in the treatment of HIV-1 infection in adults. Study 006 Team. *N Engl J Med* **341**:1865–73.

56. Montaner JS, Reiss P, Cooper D, *et al*. (1998) A randomized, double-blind trial comparing combinations of nevirapine, didanosine, and zidovudine for HIV-infected patients: the INCAS Trial. Italy, The Netherlands, Canada and Australia Study. *JAMA* **279**:930–7.

57. D'Aquila RT, Hughes MD, Johnson VA, *et al*. (1996). Nevirapine, zidovudine, and didanosine compared with zidovudine and didanosine in patients with HIV-1 infection. A randomized, double-blind, placebo-controlled trial. National Institute of Allergy and Infectious Diseases AIDS Clinical Trials Group Protocol 241 Investigators. *Ann Intern Med* **124**:1019–30.

58. Staszewski S, Keiser P, Montaner J, *et al*. (2001). Abacavir-lamivudine-zidovudine vs indinavir-lamivudine-zidovudine in antiretroviral-naive HIV-infected adults: A randomized equivalence trial. *JAMA* **285**:1155–63.

59. Gulick RM, Ribaudo HJ, Shikuma CM, *et al*. (2004). Triple-nucleoside regimens versus efavirenz-containing regimens for the initial treatment of HIV-1 infection. *N Engl J Med* **350**:1850–61.

60. Hammer SM, Saag MS, Schechter M, *et al*. (2006). Treatment for adult HIV infection: 2006 recommendations of the International AIDS Society–USA panel. *Top HIV Med* **14**:827–43.

61. DHHS. (2006). *DHHS Panel on Antiretroviral Guidelines for Adults and Adolescents: Guidelines for the use of antiretroviral agents in HIV-1-infected adults and adolescents. October 10, 2006.* Available at http://www.aidsinfo.nih.gov

62. Bryan CS. (1996). Hit early, hit hard: new strategies for HIV. *J S C Med Assoc* **92**:361–3.

63. Lange J. (1995). Combination antiretroviral therapy. Back to the future. *Drugs* **49**(Suppl 1): 32–7; discussion 8–40.

64. Ho DD. (1995). Time to hit HIV, early and hard. *N Engl J Med* **333**:450–1.

65. Izopet J, Salama G, Pasquier C, *et al*. (1998). Decay of HIV-1 DNA in patients receiving suppressive antiretroviral therapy. *J Acquir Immune Defic Syndr Hum Retrovirol* **19**:478–83.

66. Richman DD, Morton SC, Wrin T, *et al*. (2004). The prevalence of antiretroviral drug resistance in the United States. *AIDS* **18**:1393–401.

67. Ait-Khaled M, Rakik A, Griffin P, *et al*. (2003). HIV-1 reverse transcriptase and protease resistance mutations selected during 16–72 weeks of therapy in isolates from antiretroviral therapy-experienced patients receiving abacavir/efavirenz/amprenavir in the CNA2007 study. *Antivir Ther* **8**:111–20.

68. Naugler WE, Yong FH, Carey VJ, Dragavon JA, Coombs RW, Frenkel LM. (2002). T69D/N pol mutation, human immunodeficiency virus type 1 RNA levels, and syncytium-inducing phenotype are associated with CD4 cell depletion during didanosine therapy. *J Infect Dis* **185**:448–55.

69. Miller MD, Margot NA, Lamy PD, *et al*. (2002). Adefovir and tenofovir susceptibilities of HIV-1 after 24 to 48 weeks of adefovir dipivoxil therapy: genotypic and phenotypic analyses of study GS-96-408. *J Acquir Immune Defic Syndr* **27**:450–8.

70. Dronda F, Casado JL, Moreno S, *et al*. (2001). Phenotypic cross-resistance to nelfinavir: the role of prior antiretroviral therapy and the number of mutations in the protease gene. *AIDS Res Hum Retroviruses* **17**:211–5.

71. Hertogs K, Bloor S, Kemp SD, et al. (2000). Phenotypic and genotypic analysis of clinical HIV-1 isolates reveals extensive protease inhibitor cross-resistance: a survey of over 6000 samples. *AIDS* **14**:1203–10.

72. Havlir DV, Hellmann NS, Petropoulos CJ, et al. (2000). Drug susceptibility in HIV infection after viral rebound in patients receiving indinavir-containing regimens. *JAMA* **283**:229–34.

73. Harrigan PR, Hertogs K, Verbiest W, et al. (1999). Baseline HIV drug resistance profile predicts response to ritonavir-saquinavir protease inhibitor therapy in a community setting. *AIDS* **13**:1863–71.

74. Patick AK, Duran M, Cao Y, et al. (1998). Genotypic and phenotypic characterization of human immunodeficiency virus type 1 variants isolated from patients treated with the protease inhibitor nelfinavir. *Antimicrob Agents Chemother* **42**:2637–44.

75. Nijhuis M, Schuurman R, de Jong D, et al. (1997). Lamivudine-resistant human immunodeficiency virus type 1 variants (184V) require multiple amino acid changes to become co-resistant to zidovudine in vivo. *J Infect Dis* **176**:398–405.

76. Kuritzkes DR, Quinn JB, Benoit SL, et al. (1996). Drug resistance and virologic response in NUCA 3001, a randomized trial of lamivudine (3TC) versus zidovudine (ZDV) versus ZDV plus 3TC in previously untreated patients. *AIDS* **10**:975–81.

77. Negredo E, Ribalta J, Paredes R, et al. (2002). Reversal of atherogenic lipoprotein profile in HIV-1 infected patients with lipodystrophy after replacing protease inhibitors by nevirapine. *AIDS* **16**:1383–9.

78. Hirsch HH, Battegay M. (2002). Lipodystrophy syndrome by HAART in HIV-infected patients: manifestation, mechanisms and management. *Infection* **30**:293–8.

79. Galli M, Cozzi-Lepri A, Ridolfo AL, et al. (2002). Incidence of adipose tissue alterations in first-line antiretroviral therapy: the LipoICoNa Study. *Arch Intern Med* **162**:2621–8.

80. Fellay J, Boubaker K, Ledergerber B, et al. (2001). Prevalence of adverse events associated with potent antiretroviral treatment: Swiss HIV Cohort Study. *Lancet* **358**:1322–7.

81. Doser N, Sudre P, Telenti A, et al. (2001). Persistent dyslipidemia in HIV-infected individuals switched from a protease inhibitor-containing to an efavirenz-containing regimen. *J Acquir Immune Defic Syndr* **26**:389–90.

82. Tebas P, Powderly WG, Claxton S, et al. (2000). Accelerated bone mineral loss in HIV-infected patients receiving potent antiretroviral therapy. *AIDS* **14**:F63–7.

83. Sighinolfi L, Carradori S, Ghinelli F. (2000). Avascular necrosis of the femoral head: a side effect of highly active antiretroviral therapy (HAART) in HIV patients? *Infection* **28**:254–5.

84. Carr A, Samaras K, Chisholm DJ, Cooper DA. (1998). Pathogenesis of HIV-1-protease inhibitor-associated peripheral lipodystrophy, hyperlipidaemia, and insulin resistance. *Lancet* **351**:1881–3.

85. Harrington M, Carpenter CC. (2000). Hit HIV-1 hard, but only when necessary. *Lancet* **355**:2147–52.

86. Palella FJ Jr, Deloria-Knoll M, Chmiel JS, et al. (2003). Survival benefit of initiating antiretroviral therapy in HIV-infected persons in different CD4+ cell strata. *Ann Intern Med* **138**:620–6.

87. Madruga JV, Cahn P, Grinsztejn B, et al. (2007). Efficacy and safety of TMC125 (etravirine) in treatment-experienced HIV-1-infected patients in DUET-1: 24-week results from a randomised, double-blind, placebo-controlled trial. *Lancet* **370**:29–38.

88. Lazzarin A, Campbell T, Clotet B, et al. (2007). Efficacy and safety of TMC125 (etravirine) in treatment-experienced HIV-1-infected patients in DUET-2: 24-week results from a randomised, double-blind, placebo-controlled trial. *Lancet* **370**:39–48.

89. Madruga JV, Berger D, McMurchie M, et al. (2007). Efficacy and safety of darunavir-ritonavir compared with that of lopinavir-ritonavir at 48 weeks in treatment-experienced, HIV-infected patients in TITAN: a randomised controlled phase III trial. *Lancet* **370**:49–58.

90. Clotet B, Bellos N, Molina JM, et al. (2007). Efficacy and safety of darunavir-ritonavir at week 48 in treatment-experienced patients with HIV-1 infection in POWER 1 and 2: a pooled subgroup analysis of data from two randomised trials. *Lancet* **369**:1169–78.

91. Grinsztejn B, Nguyen BY, Katlama C, *et al*. Safety and efficacy of the HIV-1 integrase inhibitor raltegravir (MK-0518) in treatment-experienced patients with multidrug-resistant virus: a phase II randomised controlled trial. *Lancet* **369**:1261–9.

92. *Wall Street Journal*, 22 January 1997. pC1.

93. Carrieri MP, Leport C, Protopopescu C, *et al*. (2006). Factors associated with nonadherence to highly active antiretroviral therapy: a 5-year follow-up analysis with correction for the bias induced by missing data in the treatment maintenance phase. *J Acquir Immune Defic Syndr* **41**:477–85.

94. Rueda S, Park-Wyllie LY, Bayoumi AM, *et al*. (2006). Patient support and education for promoting adherence to highly active antiretroviral therapy for HIV/AIDS. *Cochrane Database Syst Rev* **3**:CD001442.

95. Stone VE, Jordan J, Tolson J, Miller R, Pilon T. (2004). Perspectives on adherence and simplicity for HIV-infected patients on antiretroviral therapy: self-report of the relative importance of multiple attributes of highly active antiretroviral therapy (HAART) regimens in predicting adherence. *J Acquir Immune Defic Syndr* **36**:808–16.

96. Bartlett JA, Fath MJ, Demasi R, *et al*. (2006). An updated systematic overview of triple combination therapy in antiretroviral-naive HIV-infected adults. *AIDS* **20**:2051–64.

97. Altice FL, Mostashari F, Friedland GH. (2001). Trust and the acceptance of and adherence to antiretroviral therapy. *J Acquir Immune Defic Syndr* **28**:47–58.

98. Cheever LW, Wu AW. (1999). Medication Adherence Among HIV-Infected Patients: Understanding the Complex Behavior of Patients Taking This Complex Therapy. *Curr Infect Dis Rep* **1**:401–7.

99. Gebo KA, Keruly J, Moore RD. (2003). Association of social stress, illicit drug use, and health beliefs with nonadherence to antiretroviral therapy. *J Gen Intern Med* **18**:104–11.

100. Gellaitry G, Cooper V, Davis C, Fisher M, Date HL, Horne R. (2005). Patients' perception of information about HAART: impact on treatment decisions. *AIDS Care* **17**:367–76.

101. Holmes WC, Pace JL. (2002). HIV-seropositive individuals' optimistic beliefs about prognosis and relation to medication and safe sex adherence. *J Gen Intern Med* **17**:677–83.

102. Horne R, Buick D, Fisher M, Leake H, Cooper V, Weinman J. (2004). Doubts about necessity and concerns about adverse effects: identifying the types of beliefs that are associated with non-adherence to HAART. *Int J STD AIDS* **15**:38–44.

103. Kemppainen JK, Levine RE, Mistal M, Schmidgall D. (2001). HAART adherence in culturally diverse patients with HIV/AIDS: a study of male patients from a Veteran's Administration Hospital in northern California. *AIDS Patient Care STDS* **15**:117–27.

104. Nachega JB, Lehman DA, Hlatshwayo D, Mothopeng R, Chaisson RE, Karstaedt AS. (2005). HIV/AIDS and antiretroviral treatment knowledge, attitudes, beliefs, and practices in HIV-infected adults in Soweto, South Africa. *J Acquir Immune Defic Syndr* **38**:196–201.

105. Parsons SK, Cruise PL, Davenport WM, Jones V. (2006). Religious beliefs, practices and treatment adherence among individuals with HIV in the southern United States. *AIDS Patient Care STDS* **20**:97–111.

106. Reynolds NR, Testa MA, Marc LG, *et al*. (2004). Factors influencing medication adherence beliefs and self-efficacy in persons naive to antiretroviral therapy: a multicenter, cross-sectional study. *AIDS Behav* **8**:141–50.

107. Roberts KJ. (2000). Physician beliefs about antiretroviral adherence communication. *AIDS Patient Care STDS* **14**:477–84.

108. Roberts KJ. (2000). Barriers to and facilitators of HIV-positive patients' adherence to antiretroviral treatment regimens. *AIDS Patient Care STDS* **14**:155–68.

109. Roberts KJ, Mann T. (2000). Barriers to antiretroviral medication adherence in HIV-infected women. *AIDS Care* **12**:377–86.

110. Locadia M, van Grieken RA, Prins JM, de Vries HJ, Sprangers MA, Nieuwkerk PT. (2006). Patients' preferences regarding the timing of highly active antiretroviral therapy initiation for chronic asymptomatic HIV-1 infection. *Antivir Ther* **11**:335–41.

111. Yasuda JM, Miller C, Currier JS, *et al.* (2004). The correlation between plasma concentrations of protease inhibitors, medication adherence and virological outcome in HIV-infected patients. *Antivir Ther* **9**:753–61.

112. Beach MC, Keruly J, Moore RD. (2006). Is the quality of the patient-provider relationship associated with better adherence and health outcomes for patients with HIV? *J Gen Intern Med* **21**:661–5.

113. Boarts JM, Sledjeski EM, Bogart LM, Delahanty DL. (2006). The differential impact of PTSD and depression on HIV disease markers and adherence to HAART in people living with HIV. *AIDS Behav* **10**:253–61.

114. Ironson G, O'Cleirigh C, Fletcher MA, *et al.* (2005). Psychosocial factors predict CD4 and viral load change in men and women with human immunodeficiency virus in the era of highly active antiretroviral treatment. *Psychosom Med* **67**:1013–21.

115. Taiwo BO. (2006). Nevirapine toxicity. *Int J STD AIDS* **17**:364–9; quiz 70.

116. Hitti J, Frenkel LM, Stek AM, *et al.* (2004). Maternal toxicity with continuous nevirapine in pregnancy: results from PACTG 1022. *J Acquir Immune Defic Syndr* **36**:772–6.

117. Law WP, Dore GJ, Duncombe CJ, *et al.* (2003). Risk of severe hepatotoxicity associated with antiretroviral therapy in the HIV-NAT Cohort, Thailand, 1996–2001. *AIDS* **17**:2191–9.

118. Rotger M, Csajka C, Telenti A. (2006). Genetic, ethnic, and gender differences in the pharmacokinetics of antiretroviral agents. *Curr HIV/AIDS Rep* **3**:118–25.

119. Motsinger AA, Ritchie MD, Shafer RW, *et al.* (2006). Multilocus genetic interactions and response to efavirenz-containing regimens: an adult AIDS clinical trials group study. *Pharmacogenet Genomics* **16**:837–45.

120. Martin AM, Nolan D, Mallal S. (2005). HLA-B*5701 typing by sequence-specific amplification: validation and comparison with sequence-based typing. *Tissue Antigens* **65**:571–4.

121. Martin AM, Nolan D, Gaudieri S, *et al.* (2004). Predisposition to abacavir hypersensitivity conferred by HLA-B*5701 and a haplotypic Hsp70-Hom variant. *Proc Natl Acad Sci USA* **101**:4180–5.

122. Mallal S, Nolan D, Witt C, *et al.* (2002). Association between presence of HLA-B*5701, HLA-DR7, and HLA-DQ3 and hypersensitivity to HIV-1 reverse-transcriptase inhibitor abacavir. *Lancet* **359**:727–32.

123. Grinspoon S, Carr A. (2005). Cardiovascular risk and body-fat abnormalities in HIV-infected adults. *N Engl J Med* **352**:48–62.

124. Milinkovic A, Martinez E. (2005). Current perspectives on HIV-associated lipodystrophy syndrome. *J Antimicrob Chemother* **56**:6–9.

125. Kotler DP. (2003). HIV lipodystrophy etiology and pathogenesis. Body composition and metabolic alterations: etiology and pathogenesis. *AIDS Read* **13**(4 Suppl):S5–9.

126. Grinspoon SK. (2005). Metabolic syndrome and cardiovascular disease in patients with human immunodeficiency virus. *Am J Med* **118** (Suppl 2):23S–8S.

127. Hammer SM, Saag MS, Schechter M, *et al.* (2006). Treatment for adult HIV infection: 2006 recommendations of the International AIDS Society-USA panel. *JAMA* **296**:827–43.

128. Negredo E, Molto J, Burger D, *et al.* (2005). Lopinavir/ritonavir plus nevirapine as a nucleoside-sparing approach in antiretroviral-experienced patients (NEKA study). *J Acquir Immune Defic Syndr* **38**:47–52.

129. Maggiolo F, Ripamonti D, Suter F. (2005). Switch strategies in patients on effective HAART. *J Antimicrob Chemother* **55**:821–3.

130. Carr A, Workman C, Smith DE, *et al.* (2002). Abacavir substitution for nucleoside analogs in patients with HIV lipoatrophy: a randomized trial. *JAMA* **288**:207–15.

131. Nolan D, Mallal S. (2003). Thymidine analogue-sparing highly active antiretroviral therapy (HAART). *J HIV Ther* **8**:2–6.

132. Ruiz L, Negredo E, Domingo P, *et al.* (2001). Antiretroviral treatment simplification with nevirapine in protease inhibitor-experienced patients with HIV-associated lipodystrophy: 1-year prospective follow-up of a multicenter, randomized, controlled study. *J Acquir Immune Defic Syndr* **27**:229–36.

133. Gavrila A, Hsu W, Tsiodras S, *et al.* (2005). Improvement in highly active antiretroviral therapy-induced metabolic syndrome by treatment with pioglitazone but not with fenofibrate: a 2 x 2 factorial, randomized, double-blinded, placebo-controlled trial. *Clin Infect Dis* **40**:745–9.

134. Calmy A, Hirschel B, Hans D, Karsegard VL, Meier CA. (2003). Glitazones in lipodystrophy syndrome induced by highly active antiretroviral therapy. *AIDS* **17**:770–2.

135. Mori A, Lo Russo G, Agostini T, Pattarino J, Vichi F, Dini M. (2006). Treatment of human immunodeficiency virus-associated facial lipoatrophy with lipofilling and submalar silicone implants. *J Plast Reconstr Aesthet Surg* **59**:1209–16.

136. Mest DR, Humble G. (2006). Safety and efficacy of poly-L-lactic acid injections in persons with HIV-associated lipoatrophy: the US experience. *Dermatol Surg* **32**:1336–45.

137. Engelhard P. (2006). Correction options for lipoatrophy in HIV-infected patients. *AIDS Patient Care STDS* **20**:151–60.

138. Guaraldi G, Orlando G, De Fazio D, *et al.* (2005). Comparison of three different interventions for the correction of HIV-associated facial lipoatrophy: a prospective study. *Antivir Ther* **10**:753–9.

139. Guaraldi G, De Fazio D, Orlando G, *et al.* (2005). Facial lipohypertrophy in HIV-infected subjects who underwent autologous fat tissue transplantation. *Clin Infect Dis* **40**(2):e13–5.

140. Burnouf M, Buffet M, Schwarzinger M, *et al.* (2005). Evaluation of Coleman lipostructure for treatment of facial lipoatrophy in patients with human immunodeficiency virus and parameters associated with the efficiency of this technique. *Arch Dermatol* **141**:1220–4.

141. Serra-Renom JM, Fontdevila J. (2004). Treatment of facial fat atrophy related to treatment with protease inhibitors by autologous fat injection in patients with human immunodeficiency virus infection. *Plast Reconstr Surg* **114**(2):551–5; discussion 6–7.

142. Talmor M, Hoffman LA, LaTrenta GS. (2002). Facial atrophy in HIV-related fat redistribution syndrome: anatomic evaluation and surgical reconstruction. *Ann Plast Surg* **49**(1):11–7; discussion 117–8.

143. Burgess E, Wanke C. (2005). Use of recombinant human growth hormone in HIV-associated lipodystrophy. *Curr Opin Infect Dis* **18**:17–24.

144. Luzi L, Meneghini E, Oggionni S, Tambussi G, Piceni-Sereni L, Lazzarin A. (2005). GH treatment reduces trunkal adiposity in HIV-infected patients with lipodystrophy: a randomized placebo-controlled study. *Eur J Endocrinol* **153**:781–9.

145. Grinspoon S. (2003). Mechanisms and strategies for insulin resistance in acquired immune deficiency syndrome. *Clin Infect Dis* **37**(Suppl 2):S85–90.

146. Sutinen J, Kannisto K, Korsheninnikova E, *et al.* (2004). Effects of rosiglitazone on gene expression in subcutaneous adipose tissue in highly active antiretroviral therapy-associated lipodystrophy. *Am J Physiol Endocrinol Metab* **286**(6):E941–9.

147. Sutinen J, Hakkinen AM, Westerbacka J, *et al.* (2003). Rosiglitazone in the treatment of HAART-associated lipodystrophy – a randomized double-blind placebo-controlled study. *Antivir Ther* **8**:199–207.

148. Wohl DA. (2004). Diagnosis and management of body morphology changes and lipid abnormalities associated with HIV Infection and its therapies. *Top HIV Med* **12**:89–93.

149. Mulligan K, Yang Y, Koletar S, *et al.* (2006). Effects of Metformin and Rosiglitazone on Body Composition in HIV-infected Patients with Hyperinsulinemia and Elevated Waist/Hip Ratio: A Randomized, Placebo-controlled Trial. 13th Conference on Retroviruses and Opportunistic Infections (CROI), 5–8 February, 2006, Denver, CO, USA. [Abstract 147]

150. Shikuma C, Parker R, Sattler F, *et al.* Effects of Physiologic Testosterone Supplementation on Fat Mass and Distribution in HIV-infected Men with Abdominal Obesity: ACTG 5079. 13th Conference on Retroviruses and Opportunistic Infections (CROI), 5–8 February 2006, Denver, CO, USA. [Abstract 149]

151. Jemsek JG, Arathoon E, Arlotti M, *et al.* (2006). Body fat and other metabolic effects of atazanavir and efavirenz, each administered in combination with zidovudine plus lamivudine, in antiretroviral-naive HIV-infected patients. *Clin Infect Dis* **42**:273–80.

152. Haerter G, Manfras BJ, Mueller M, Kern P, Trein A. (2004). Regression of lipodystrophy in HIV-infected patients under therapy with the new protease inhibitor atazanavir. *AIDS* **18**:952–5.

153. Calza L, Manfredi R, Chiodo F. (2003). Hyperlipidaemia in patients with HIV-1 infection receiving highly active antiretroviral therapy: epidemiology, pathogenesis, clinical course and management. *Int J Antimicrob Agents* **22**:89–99.

154. Young J, Weber R, Rickenbach M, *et al.* (2005). Lipid profiles for antiretroviral-naive patients starting PI- and NNRTI-based therapy in the Swiss HIV cohort study. *Antivir Ther* **10**:585–91.

155. Crane HM, Van Rompaey SE, Kitahata MM. (2006). Antiretroviral medications associated with elevated blood pressure among patients receiving highly active antiretroviral therapy. *AIDS* **20**:1019–26.

156. Thiebaut R, El-Sadr WM, Friis-Moller N, *et al.* (2005). Predictors of hypertension and changes of blood pressure in HIV-infected patients. *Antivir Ther* **10**:811–23.

157. Pan G, Yang Z, Ballinger SW, McDonald JM. (2006). Pathogenesis of osteopenia/osteoporosis induced by highly active anti-retroviral therapy for AIDS. *Ann N Y Acad Sci* **1068**:297–308.

158. Curtis JR, Smith B, Weaver M, *et al.* (2006). Ethnic variations in the prevalence of metabolic bone disease among HIV-positive patients with lipodystrophy. *AIDS Res Hum Retroviruse* **22**:125–31.

159. Bongiovanni M, Fausto A, Cicconi P, *et al.* (2005). Osteoporosis in HIV-infected subjects: a combined effect of highly active antiretroviral therapy and HIV itself? *J Acquir Immune Defic Syndr* **40**:503–4.

160. Martin K, Lawson-Ayayi S, Miremont-Salame G, *et al.* (2004). Symptomatic bone disorders in HIV-infected patients: incidence in the Aquitaine cohort (1999–2002). *HIV Med* **5**:421–6.

161. Brown TT, Ruppe MD, Kassner R, *et al.* (2004). Reduced bone mineral density in human immunodeficiency virus-infected patients and its association with increased central adiposity and postload hyperglycemia. *J Clin Endocrinol Metab* **89**:1200–6.

162. Mora S, Zamproni I, Beccio S, Bianchi R, Giacomet V, Vigano A. (2004). Longitudinal changes of bone mineral density and metabolism in antiretroviral-treated human immunodeficiency virus-infected children. *J Clin Endocrinol Meta* **89**:24–8.

163. Teichmann J, Stephan E, Lange U, *et al.* (2003). Osteopenia in HIV-infected women prior to highly active antiretroviral therapy. *J Infec* **46**:221–7.

164. Loiseau-Peres S, Delaunay C, Poupon S, *et al.* (2002). Osteopenia in patients infected by the human immunodeficiency virus. A case control study. *Joint Bone Spine* **69**:482–5.

165. Borderi M, Farneti B, Tampellini L, *et al.* (2002). HIV-1, HAART and bone metabolism. *New Microbiol* **25**:375–84.

166. Knobel H, Guelar A, Vallecillo G, Nogues X, Diez A. (2001). Osteopenia in HIV-infected patients: is it the disease or is it the treatment? *AIDS* **15**:807–8.

167. Johnson M, Grinsztejn B, Rodriguez C, *et al.* (2006). 96-week comparison of once-daily atazanavir/ritonavir and twice-daily lopinavir/ritonavir in patients with multiple virologic failures. *AIDS* **20**:711–8.

168. Noor MA, Flint OP, Maa JF, Parker RA. (2006). Effects of atazanavir/ritonavir and lopinavir/ritonavir on glucose uptake and insulin sensitivity: demonstrable differences in vitro and clinically. *AIDS* **20**:1813–21.

169. Yan Q, Hruz PW. (2005). Direct comparison of the acute in vivo effects of HIV protease inhibitors on peripheral glucose disposal. *J Acquir Immune Defic Syndr* **40**:398–403.

170. Zhang D, Chando TJ, Everett DW, Patten CJ, Dehal SS, Humphreys WG. (2005). In vitro inhibition of UDP glucuronosyltransferases by atazanavir and other HIV protease inhibitors and the relationship of this property to in vivo bilirubin glucuronidation. *Drug Metab Dispo* **33**:1729–39.

171. De Luca A, Cozzi-Lepri A, Antinori A, *et al.* (2006). Lopinavir/ritonavir or efavirenz plus two nucleoside analogues as first-line antiretroviral therapy: a non-randomized comparison. *Antivir The* **11**:609–18.

172. van Leth F, Phanuphak P, Stroes E, *et al.* (2004). Nevirapine and efavirenz elicit different changes in lipid profiles in antiretroviral-therapy-naive patients infected with HIV-1. *PLoS Med* 1(1):e19.

173. Clotet B, van der Valk M, Negredo E, Reiss P. (2003). Impact of nevirapine on lipid metabolism. *J Acquir Immune Defic Syndr* 34(Suppl 1):S79–84.

174. Tebas P, Yarasheski K, Henry K, *et al.* (2004). Evaluation of the virological and metabolic effects of switching protease inhibitor combination antiretroviral therapy to nevirapine-based therapy for the treatment of HIV infection. *AIDS Res Hum Retroviruses* 20:589–94.

175. Negredo E, Cruz L, Paredes R, *et al.* (2002). Virological, immunological, and clinical impact of switching from protease inhibitors to nevirapine or to efavirenz in patients with human immunodeficiency virus infection and long-lasting viral suppression. *Clin Infect Dis* 34:504–10.

176. Martinez E, Garcia-Viejo MA, Blanco JL, *et al.* (2000). Impact of switching from human immunodeficiency virus type 1 protease inhibitors to efavirenz in successfully treated adults with lipodystrophy. *Clin Infect Dis* 31:1266–73.

177. Estrada V, De Villar NG, Larrad MT, Lopez AG, Fernandez C, Serrano-Rios M. (2002). Long-term metabolic consequences of switching from protease inhibitors to efavirenz in therapy for human immunodeficiency virus-infected patients with lipoatrophy. *Clin Infect Dis* 35:69–76.

178. Ward DJ, Curtin JM. (2006). Switch from efavirenz to nevirapine associated with resolution of efavirenz-related neuropsychiatric adverse events and improvement in lipid profiles. *AIDS Patient Care STDS* 20:542–8.

179. Sax PE. (2006). Strategies for management and treatment of dyslipidemia in HIV/AIDS. *AIDS Care* 18:149–57.

180. Venter JC, Adams MD, Myers EW, *et al.* (2001). The sequence of the human genome. *Science* 291:1304–51.

181. Rotger M, Colombo S, Cavassini M, *et al.* (2006). Genetic Variability of CYP2B6 in Individuals with Extremely High Efavirenz Plasma Concentrations. 13th Conference on Retroviruses and Opportunistic Infections (CROI), 5–8 February 2006; Denver, CO, USA. [Abstract 572]

182. Friis-Moller N, Sabin CA, Weber R, *et al.* (2003). Combination antiretroviral therapy and the risk of myocardial infarction. *N Engl J Med* 349:1993–2003.

183. Saves M, Chene G, Ducimetiere P, *et al.* (2003). Risk factors for coronary heart disease in patients treated for human immunodeficiency virus infection compared with the general population. *Clin Infect Dis* 37:292–8.

184. Bergersen BM. (2006). Cardiovascular Risk in Patients with HIV Infection: Impact of Antiretroviral Therapy. *Drugs* 66:1971–87.

185. Friis-Moller N, Reiss P, El-Sadr WM, *et al.* (2006). Exposure to PI and NNRTI and risk of myocardial infarction: Results from the D:A:D study. 13th Conference on Retroviruses and Opportunistic Infections (CROI), 5–8 February 2006, Denver, CO, USA. [Abstract 144]

186. Castillo R, Pedalino RP, El-Sherif N, Turitto G. (2002). Efavirenz-associated QT prolongation and Torsade de Pointes arrhythmia. *Ann Pharmacother* 36:1006–8.

187. Ogedegbe AE, Thomas DL, Diehl AM. (2003). Hyperlactataemia syndromes associated with HIV therapy. *Lancet Infect Dis* 3:329–37.

188. Walker UA, Setzer B, Venhoff N. (2002). Increased long-term mitochondrial toxicity in combinations of nucleoside analogue reverse-transcriptase inhibitors. *AIDS* 16:2165–73.

189. Karras A, Lafaurie M, Furco A, *et al.* (2003). Tenofovir-related nephrotoxicity in human immunodeficiency virus-infected patients: three cases of renal failure, Fanconi syndrome, and nephrogenic diabetes insipidus. *Clin Infect Dis* 36:1070–3.

190. Izzedine H, Hulot JS, Vittecoq D, *et al.* (2005). Long-term renal safety of tenofovir disoproxil fumarate in antiretroviral-naive HIV-1-infected patients. Data from a double-blind randomized active-controlled multicentre study. *Nephrol Dial Transplant* 20:743–6.

191. Antoniou T, Raboud J, Chirhin S, *et al.* (2005). Incidence of and risk factors for tenofovir-induced nephrotoxicity: a retrospective cohort study. *HIV Med* 6:284–90.

192. Coca S, Perazella MA. (2002). Rapid communication: acute renal failure associated with tenofovir: evidence of drug-induced nephrotoxicity. *Am J Med Sci* **324**:342–4.

193. Creput C, Gonzalez-Canali G, Hill G, Piketty C, Kazatchkine M, Nochy D. (2003). Renal lesions in HIV-1-positive patient treated with tenofovir. *AIDS* **17**:935–7.

194. Gallant JE, Parish MA, Keruly JC, Moore RD. (2005). Changes in renal function associated with tenofovir disoproxil fumarate treatment, compared with nucleoside reverse-transcriptase inhibitor treatment. *Clin Infect Dis* **40**:1194–8.

195. Jones R, Stebbing J, Nelson M, *et al.* (2004). Renal dysfunction with tenofovir disoproxil fumarate-containing highly active antiretroviral therapy regimens is not observed more frequently: a cohort and case-control study. *J Acquir Immune Defic Syndr* **7**:1489–95.

196. Mauss S, Berger F, Schmutz G. (2005). Antiretroviral therapy with tenofovir is associated with mild renal dysfunction. *AIDS* **19**:93–5.

197. Peyriere H, Reynes J, Rouanet I, *et al.* (2004). Renal tubular dysfunction associated with tenofovir therapy: report of 7 cases. *J Acquir Immune Defic Synd* **35**:269–73.

198. Rollot F, Nazal EM, Chauvelot-Moachon L, *et al.* (2003). Tenofovir-related Fanconi syndrome with nephrogenic diabetes insipidus in a patient with acquired immunodeficiency syndrome: the role of lopinavir-ritonavir-didanosine. *Clin Infect Dis* **37**(12):e174–6.

199. Verhelst D, Monge M, Meynard JL, *et al.* (2002). Fanconi syndrome and renal failure induced by tenofovir: a first case report. *Am J Kidney Dis* **40**:1331–3.

200. Winston A, Amin J, Mallon P, *et al.* (2006). Minor changes in calculated creatinine clearance and anion-gap are associated with tenofovir disoproxil fumarate-containing highly active antiretroviral therapy. *HIV Med* **7**:105–11.

201. Gallant JE, Staszewski S, Pozniak AL, *et al.* (2004). Efficacy and safety of tenofovir DF vs stavudine in combination therapy in antiretroviral-naive patients: a 3-year randomized trial. *JAMA* **292**:191–201.

202. Izzedine H, Hulot JS, Villard E, *et al.* (2006). Association between ABCC2 Gene Haplotypes and Tenofovir-Induced Proximal Tubulopathy. *J Infect Dis* **194**:1481–91.

203. Nowak MA. (1992). Variability of HIV infections. *J Theor Biol* **155**:1–20.

204. Nowak MA, Bonhoeffer S, Shaw GM, May RM. (1997). Anti-viral drug treatment: dynamics of resistance in free virus and infected cell populations. *J Theor Biol* **184**:203–17.

205. Ho DDN, Avidan U, Perelson AS, Chen W, Leonard JM, Markowitz M. (1995). Rapid turnover of plasma virions and CD4 lymphocytes in HIV-1 infection. *Nature* **373**:123–6

206. Nei M, Jin L. (1989). Variances of the average numbers of nucleotide substitutions within and between populations. *Mol Biol Evol* **6**:290–300.

207. Ji J, Loeb LA. (1994). Fidelity of HIV-1 reverse transcriptase copying a hypervariable region of the HIV-1 env gene. *Virology* **199**:323–30.

208. Charpentier C, Nora T, Tenaillon O, Clavel F, Hance AJ. (2006). Extensive recombination among human immunodeficiency virus type 1 quasispecies makes an important contribution to viral diversity in individual patients. *J Virol* **80**:2472–82.

209. Kijak GH, McCutchan FE. (2005). HIV diversity, molecular epidemiology, and the role of recombination. *Curr Infect Dis Rep* **7**:480–8.

210. Rambaut A, Posada D, Crandall KA, Holmes EC. (2004). The causes and consequences of HIV evolution. *Nat Rev Genet* **5**:52–61.

211. Kalish ML, Robbins KE, Pieniazek D, *et al.* (2004). Recombinant viruses and early global HIV-1 epidemic. *Emerg Infect Dis* **10**:1227–34.

212. Robertson DL, Sharp PM, McCutchan FE, Hahn BH. (1995). Recombination in HIV-1. *Nature* **374**:124–6.

213. Robertson DL, Hahn BH, Sharp PM. (1995). Recombination in AIDS viruses. *J Mol Evol* **40**:249–59.

214. Marcello A. (2006). Latency: the hidden HIV-1 challenge. *Retrovirology* **3**:7.

215. Kulkosky J, Bray S. (2006). HAART-persistent HIV-1 latent reservoirs: their origin, mechanisms of stability and potential strategies for eradication. *Curr HIV Res* **4**:199–208.

216. Saksena NK, Potter SJ. (2003). Reservoirs of HIV-1 in vivo: implications for antiretroviral therapy. *AIDS Rev* **5**:3–18.

217. Pierson T, McArthur J, Siliciano RF. (2000). Reservoirs for HIV-1: mechanisms for viral persistence in the presence of antiviral immune responses and antiretroviral therapy. *Annu Rev Immuno* **18**:665–708.

218. Chun TW, Carruth L, Finzi D, *et al.* (1997). Quantification of latent tissue reservoirs and total body viral load in HIV-1 infection. *Nature* **387**:183–8.

219. Rouzine IM, Rodrigo A, Coffin JM. (2001). Transition between stochastic evolution and deterministic evolution in the presence of selection: general theory and application to virology. *Microbiol Mol Biol Rev* **65**:151–85.

220. Frost SD, Nijhuis M, Schuurman R, Boucher CA, Brown AJ. (2000). Evolution of lamivudine resistance in human immunodeficiency virus type 1-infected individuals: the relative roles of drift and selection. *J Virol* **74**:6262–8.

221. D'Amato RM, D'Aquila RT, Wein LM. (1998). Management of antiretroviral therapy for HIV infection: modelling when to change therapy. *Antivir Ther* **3**:147–58.

222. Calderon EJ, Torres Y, Medrano FJ, *et al.* (1995). Emergence and clinical relevance of mutations associated with zidovudine resistance in asymptomatic HIV-1 infected patients. *Eur J Clin Microbiol Infect Dis* **14**:512–9.

223. Larder BA. (1994). Interactions between drug resistance mutations in human immunodeficiency virus type 1 reverse transcriptase. *J Gen Virol* **75**(Pt 5):951–7.

224. Boucher CA, Cammack N, Schipper P, *et al.* (1993). High-level resistance to (-) enantiomeric 2'-deoxy-3'-thiacytidine in vitro is due to one amino acid substitution in the catalytic site of human immunodeficiency virus type 1 reverse transcriptase. *Antimicrob Agents Chemother* **37**:2231–4.

225. Boucher CA, O'Sullivan E, Mulder JW, *et al.* (1992). Ordered appearance of zidovudine resistance mutations during treatment of 18 human immunodeficiency virus-positive subjects. *J Infect Dis* **165**:105–10.

226. St Clair MH, Martin JL, Tudor-Williams G, *et al.* (1991). Resistance to ddI and sensitivity to AZT induced by a mutation in HIV-1 reverse transcriptase. *Science* **253**:1557–9.

227. Larder BA, Darby G, Richman DD. (1989). HIV with reduced sensitivity to zidovudine (AZT) isolated during prolonged therapy. *Science* **243**:1731–4.

228. Johnson VA, Brun-Vezinet F, Clotet B, *et al.* (2006). Update of the drug resistance mutations in HIV-1: Fall 2006. *Top HIV Med* **14**:125–30.

229. Vandamme AM, Sonnerborg A, Ait-Khaled M, *et al.* (2004). Updated European recommendations for the clinical use of HIV drug resistance testing. *Antivir Ther* **9**:829–48.

230. Hogg RS, Bangsberg DR, Lima VD, *et al.* (2006). Emergence of Drug Resistance Is Associated with an Increased Risk of Death among Patients First Starting HAART. *PLoS Med* **3**(9):356.

231. Quinones-Mateu ME, Arts EJ. (2002). Fitness of drug resistant HIV-1: methodology and clinical implications. *Drug Resist Updat* **5**:224–33.

232. Wainberg MA, Gu Z, Montaner JS, *et al.* (1995). Development of HIV-1 resistance to (-)2'-deoxy-3'-thiacytidine in patients with AIDS or advanced AIDS-related complex. *AIDS* **9**:351–7.

233. Gao Q, Gu Z, Parniak MA, *et al.* (1993). The same mutation that encodes low-level human immunodeficiency virus type 1 resistance to 2',3'-dideoxyinosine and 2',3'-dideoxycytidine confers high-level resistance to the (-) enantiomer of 2',3'-dideoxy-3'-thiacytidine. *Antimicrob Agents Chemother* **37**:1390–2.

234. Wakefield JK, Jablonski SA, Morrow CD. (1992). In vitro enzymatic activity of human immunodeficiency virus type 1 reverse transcriptase mutants in the highly conserved YMDD amino acid motif correlates with the infectious potential of the proviral genome. *J Virol* **66**:6806–12.

235. Wainberg MA. (2004). The impact of the M184V substitution on drug resistance and viral fitness. *Expert Rev Anti Infect Ther* **2**:147–51.

236. Deval J, White KL, Miller MD, *et al.* (2004). Mechanistic basis for reduced viral and enzymatic fitness of HIV-1 reverse transcriptase containing both K65R and M184V mutations. *J Biol Chem* **279**:509–16.

237. Perno CF, Cenci A, Piro C, *et al.* (2003). HIV fitness and resistance as covariates associated with the appearance of mutations under antiretroviral treatment. *Scand J Infect Dis Suppl* **35**(Suppl 106):37–40.

238. Van Rompay KK, Matthews TB, Higgins J, *et al.* (2002). Virulence and reduced fitness of simian immunodeficiency virus with the M184V mutation in reverse transcriptase. *J Virol* **76**:6083–92.

239. Devereux HL, Emery VC, Johnson MA, Loveday C. (2001). Replicative fitness in vivo of HIV-1 variants with multiple drug resistance-associated mutations. *J Med Virol* **65**:218–24.

240. Sharma PL, Crumpacker CS. (1999). Decreased processivity of human immunodeficiency virus type 1 reverse transcriptase (RT) containing didanosine-selected mutation Leu74Val: a comparative analysis of RT variants Leu74Val and lamivudine-selected Met184Val. *J Virol* **73**:8448–56.

241. Phillips AN, McLean AR, Loveday C, *et al.* (1999). In vivo HIV-1 replicative capacity in early and advanced infection. *AIDS* **13**:67–73.

242. Feng JY, Anderson KS. (1999). Mechanistic studies examining the efficiency and fidelity of DNA synthesis by the 3TC-resistant mutant (184V) of HIV-1 reverse transcriptase. *Biochemistr* **38**:9440–8.

243. Inouye P, Cherry E, Hsu M, Zolla-Pazner S, Wainberg MA. (1998). Neutralizing antibodies directed against the V3 loop select for different escape variants in a virus with mutated reverse transcriptase (M184V) than in wild-type human immunodeficiency virus type 1. *AIDS Res Hum Retroviruses* **14**:735–40.

244. Back NK, Nijhuis M, Keulen W, *et al.* (1996). Reduced replication of 3TC-resistant HIV-1 variants in primary cells due to a processivity defect of the reverse transcriptase enzyme. *Embo J* **15**:4040–9.

245. Quan Y, Gu Z, Li X, Li Z, Morrow CD, Wainberg MA. (1996). Endogenous reverse transcription assays reveal high-level resistance to the triphosphate of (-)2'-dideoxy-3'-thiacytidine by mutated M184V human immunodeficiency virus type 1. *J Virol* **70**:5642–5.

246. Wainberg MA, Drosopoulos WC, Salomon H, *et al.* (1996). Enhanced fidelity of 3TC-selected mutant HIV-1 reverse transcriptase. *Science* **271**:1282–5.

247. Margot NA, Waters JM, Miller MD. (2006). In Vitro HIV-1 Resistance Selections with Combinations of Tenofovir and Emtricitabine or Abacavir and Lamivudine. *Antimicrob Agents Chemother* **50**:4087–95.

248. Turner D, Brenner B, Wainberg MA. (2003). Multiple effects of the M184V resistance mutation in the reverse transcriptase of human immunodeficiency virus type 1. *Clin Diagn Lab Immuno* **10**:979–81.

249. Miller V, Phillips A, Rottmann C, *et al.* (1998). Dual resistance to zidovudine and lamivudine in patients treated with zidovudine-lamivudine combination therapy: association with therapy failure. *J Infect Dis* **177**:1521–32.

250. Balzarini J, Karlsson A, Perez-Perez MJ, *et al.* (1993). HIV-1-specific reverse transcriptase inhibitors show differential activity against HIV-1 mutant strains containing different amino acid substitutions in the reverse transcriptase. *Virolog* **192**:246–53.

251. Boucher CA, Lange JM, Miedema FF, *et al.* (1992). HIV-1 biological phenotype and the development of zidovudine resistance in relation to disease progression in asymptomatic individuals during treatment. *AIDS* **6**:1259–64.

252. Larder BA, Kellam P, Kemp SD. (1991). Zidovudine resistance predicted by direct detection of mutations in DNA from HIV-infected lymphocytes. *AIDS* **5**:137–44.

253. Tisdale M, Schulze T, Larder BA, Moelling K. (1991). Mutations within the RNase H domain of human immunodeficiency virus type 1 reverse transcriptase abolish virus infectivity. *J Gen Virol* **72**(Pt 1):59–66.

254. Larder BA, Kemp SD. (1989). Multiple mutations in HIV-1 reverse transcriptase confer high-level resistance to zidovudine (AZT). *Science* **246**:1155–8.

255. Gu Z, Salomon H, Cherrington JM, *et al.* (1995). K65R mutation of human immunodeficiency virus type 1 reverse transcriptase encodes cross-resistance to 9-(2-phosphonylmethoxyethyl)adenine. *Antimicrob Agents Chemother* **39**:1888–91.

256. Winston A, Stebbing J. (2004). The K65R mutation in HIV-1 reverse transcriptase. *J HIV Ther* **9**:25–7.

257. Nikolenko GN, Svarovskaia ES, Delviks KA, Pathak VK. (2004). Antiretroviral drug resistance mutations in human immunodeficiency virus type 1 reverse transcriptase increase template-switching frequency. *J Virol* **78**:8761–70.

258. Moyle GJ. (2004). The K65R mutation: selection, frequency, and possible consequences. *AIDS Read* **14**:595–7; 601–3.

259. Garcia-Lerma JG, MacInnes H, Bennett D, *et al.* (2003). A novel genetic pathway of human immunodeficiency virus type 1 resistance to stavudine mediated by the K65R mutation. *J Virol* **77**:5685–93.

260. Roge BT, Katzenstein TL, Obel N, *et al.* (2003). K65R with and without S68: a new resistance profile in vivo detected in most patients failing abacavir, didanosine and stavudine. *Antivir Ther* **8**:173–82.

261. Shah FS, Curr KA, Hamburgh ME, *et al.* (2000). Differential influence of nucleoside analog-resistance mutations K65R and L74V on the overall mutation rate and error specificity of human immunodeficiency virus type 1 reverse transcriptase. *J Biol Chem* **275**:27037–44.

262. Gu Z, Arts EJ, Parniak MA, Wainberg MA. (1995). Mutated K65R recombinant reverse transcriptase of human immunodeficiency virus type 1 shows diminished chain termination in the presence of 2',3'-dideoxycytidine 5'-triphosphate and other drugs. *Proc Natl Acad Sci USA* **28**:92(7):2760–4.

263. Gu Z, Fletcher RS, Arts EJ, Wainberg MA, Parniak MA. (1994). The K65R mutant reverse transcriptase of HIV-1 cross-resistant to 2', 3'-dideoxycytidine, 2',3'-dideoxy-3'-thiacytidine, and 2',3'-dideoxyinosine shows reduced sensitivity to specific dideoxynucleoside triphosphate inhibitors in vitro. *J Biol Chem* **269**:28118–22.

264. Miller V, Ait-Khaled M, Stone C, *et al.* (2000). HIV-1 reverse transcriptase (RT) genotype and susceptibility to RT inhibitors during abacavir monotherapy and combination therapy. *AIDS* **14**:163–71.

265. Ray AS, Basavapathruni A, Anderson KS. (2002). Mechanistic studies to understand the progressive development of resistance in human immunodeficiency virus type 1 reverse transcriptase to abacavir. *J Biol Chem* **277**:40479–90.

266. Sirivichayakul S, Ruxrungtham K, Ungsedhapand C, *et al.* (2003). Nucleoside analogue mutations and Q151M in HIV-1 subtype A/E infection treated with nucleoside reverse transcriptase inhibitors. *AIDS* **17**:1889–96.

267. Paredes R, Mocroft A, Kirk O, *et al.* (2000). Predictors of virological success and ensuing failure in HIV-positive patients starting highly active antiretroviral therapy in Europe: results from the EuroSIDA study. *Arch Intern Med* **160**:1123–32.

268. Gilliam BL, Chan-Tack KM, Qaqish RB, Rode RA, Fantry LE, Redfield RR. (2006). Successful Treatment with Atazanavir and Lopinavir/Ritonavir Combination Therapy in Protease Inhibitor-Susceptible and Protease Inhibitor-Resistant HIV-Infected Patients. *AIDS Patient Care STDS* **20**:745–59.

269. Hellinger J, Cohen C, Morris A, *et al.* (2005). Pilot study of saquinavir and lopinavir/ritonavir twice daily in protease inhibitor-naive HIV-positive patients. *HIV Clin Trials* **6**:107–17.

270. Deeks SG, Hoh R, Neilands TB, *et al.* (2005). Interruption of treatment with individual therapeutic drug classes in adults with multidrug-resistant HIV-1 infection. *J Infect Dis* **192**:1537–44.

271. Castagna A, Danise A, Menzo S, *et al.* (2006). Lamivudine monotherapy in HIV-1-infected patients harbouring a lamivudine-resistant virus: a randomized pilot study (E-184V study). *AIDS* **20**:795–803.

272. Turner D, Brenner BG, Routy JP, Petrella M, Wainberg MA. (2004). Rationale for maintenance of the M184v resistance mutation in human immunodeficiency virus type 1 reverse transcriptase in treatment experienced patients. *New Microbiol* **27**(Suppl 1):31–9.

273. Burgi A, Brodine S, Wegner S, *et al.* (2005). Incidence and risk factors for the occurrence of non-AIDS-defining cancers among human immunodeficiency virus-infected individuals. *Cancer* **104**:1505–11.

274. Herida M, Mary-Krause M, Kaphan R, *et al.* (2003). Incidence of non-AIDS-defining cancers before and during the highly active antiretroviral therapy era in a cohort of human immunodeficiency virus-infected patients. *J Clin Oncol* **21**:3447–53.

275. Engels EA, Pfeiffer RM, Goedert JJ, *et al.* (2006). Trends in cancer risk among people with AIDS in the United States 1980–2002. *AIDS* **20**:1645–54.

276. Bower M, Palmieri C, Dhillon T. (2006). AIDS-related malignancies: changing epidemiology and the impact of highly active antiretroviral therapy. *Curr Opin Infect Dis* **19**:14–9.

277. Boshoff C, Weiss R. (2002). AIDS-related malignancies. *Nat Rev Cancer* **2**:373–82.

278. Appleby P, Beral V, Newton R, Reeves G. (2000). Highly active antiretroviral therapy and incidence of cancer in human immunodeficiency virus-infected adults. *J Natl Cancer Inst* **92**:1823–30.

279. Monini P, Sgadari C, Toschi E, Barillari G, Ensoli B. (2004). Antitumour effects of antiretroviral therapy. *Nat Rev Cancer* **4**:861–75.

280. Stebbing J, Gazzard B, Mandalia S, *et al.* (2004). Antiretroviral treatment regimens and immune parameters in the prevention of systemic AIDS-related non-Hodgkin's lymphoma. *J Clin Oncol* **22**:2177–83.

281. Matthews GV, Bower M, Mandalia S, Powles T, Nelson MR, Gazzard BG. (2000). Changes in acquired immunodeficiency syndrome-related lymphoma since the introduction of highly active antiretroviral therapy. *Blood.* **96**:2730–4.

282. Rossi G, Donisi A, Casari S, Re A, Cadeo G, Carosi G. (1999). The International Prognostic Index can be used as a guide to treatment decisions regarding patients with human immunodeficiency virus-related systemic non-Hodgkin lymphoma. *Cancer* **86**:2391–7.

283. Sirera G, Videla S, Pinol M, *et al.* (2006). High prevalence of human papillomavirus infection in the anus, penis and mouth in HIV-positive men. *AIDS* **20**:1201–4.

284. Clifford GM, Polesel J, Rickenbach M, *et al.* (2005). Cancer risk in the Swiss HIV Cohort Study: associations with immunodeficiency, smoking, and highly active antiretroviral therapy. *J Natl Cancer Inst* **97**:425–32.

285. Palefsky JM, Holly EA, Ralston ML, *et al.* (2001). Effect of highly active antiretroviral therapy on the natural history of anal squamous intraepithelial lesions and anal human papillomavirus infection. *J Acquir Immune Defic Syndr* **28**:422–8.

286. Heard I, Schmitz V, Costagliola D, Orth G, Kazatchkine MD. (1998). Early regression of cervical lesions in HIV-seropositive women receiving highly active antiretroviral therapy. *AIDS* **12**:1459–64.

287. Minkoff H, Ahdieh L, Massad LS, *et al.* (2001). The effect of highly active antiretroviral therapy on cervical cytologic changes associated with oncogenic HPV among HIV-infected women. *AIDS* **15**:2157–64.

288. Lavole A, Wislez M, Antoine M, Mayaud C, Milleron B, Cadranel J. (2006). Lung cancer, a new challenge in the HIV-infected population. *Lung Cancer* **51**:1–11.

289. Hentrich M, Maretta L, Chow KU, *et al.* (2006). Highly active antiretroviral therapy (HAART) improves survival in HIV-associated Hodgkin's disease: results of a multicenter study. *Ann Oncol* **17**:914–9.

290. Hoffmann C, Chow KU, Wolf E, *et al.* (2004). Strong impact of highly active antiretroviral therapy on survival in patients with human immunodeficiency virus-associated Hodgkin's disease. *Br J Haematol* **125**:455–62.

291. Lopez-Caleya JF, Martin V, Martin L, Perez-Simon R, Carro JA, Alcoba M. (2006). [Prevalence of coinfection by human immunodeficiency virus and hepatitis C virus in the Leon Health Area: 1992–2000]. *Enferm Infecc Microbiol Clin* **24**:365–9.

292. Mohsen AH, Murad S, Easterbrook PJ. (2005). Prevalence of hepatitis C in an ethnically diverse HIV-1-infected cohort in south London. *HIV Med* **6**:206–15.

293. Saiz de la Hoya P, Bedia M, Murcia J, Cebria J, Sanchez-Paya J, Portilla J. (2005). Predictive markers of HIV and HCV infection and co-infection among inmates in a Spanish prison.. *Enferm Infecc Microbiol Clin* **23**:53–7.

294. Lewden C, Salmon D, Morlat P, *et al.* (2005). Causes of death among human immunodeficiency virus (HIV)-infected adults in the era of potent antiretroviral therapy: emerging role of hepatitis and cancers, persistent role of AIDS. *Int J Epidemiol* **34**:121–30.

295. Bica I, McGovern B, Dhar R, *et al.* (2001). Increasing mortality due to end-stage liver disease in patients with human immunodeficiency virus infection. *Clin Infect Dis* **32**:492–7.

296. Martin-Carbonero L, Soriano V, Valencia E, Garcia-Samaniego J, Lopez M, Gonzalez-Lahoz J. (2001). Increasing impact of chronic viral hepatitis on hospital admissions and mortality among HIV-infected patients. *AIDS Res Hum Retroviruses* **17**:1467–71.

297. Mocroft A, Brettle R, Kirk O, *et al.* (2002). Changes in the cause of death among HIV positive subjects across Europe: results from the EuroSIDA study. *AIDS* **16**:1663–71.

298. Rockstroh JK, Mocroft A, Soriano V, *et al.* (2005). Influence of hepatitis C virus infection on HIV-1 disease progression and response to highly active antiretroviral therapy. *J Infect Dis* **192**:992–1002.

299. Qurishi N, Kreuzberg C, Luchters G, *et al.* (2003). Effect of antiretroviral therapy on liver-related mortality in patients with HIV and hepatitis C virus coinfection. *Lancet* **362**:1708–13.

300. Stoff DM, Khalsa JH, Monjan A, Portegies P. (2004). Introduction: HIV/AIDS and Aging. *AIDS* **18**(Suppl 1):S1–2.

301. Smith G. (2005). *Statement of Senator Gordon H. Smith. Aging hearing: HIV over fifty, exploring the new threat.* Washington DC: United States Congress.

302. Farinpour R, Miller EN, Satz P, *et al.* (2003). Psychosocial risk factors of HIV morbidity and mortality: findings from the Multicenter AIDS Cohort Study (MACS). *J Clin Exp Neuropsychol* **25**:654–70.

303. Rempel HC, Pulliam L. (2005). HIV-1 Tat inhibits neprilysin and elevates amyloid beta. *AIDS* **19**:127–35.

304. Brew BJ. (2004). Evidence for a change in AIDS dementia complex in the era of highly active antiretroviral therapy and the possibility of new forms of AIDS dementia complex. *AIDS* **18**(Suppl 1):S75–8.

305. Esiri MM, Biddolph SC, Morris CS. (1998). Prevalence of Alzheimer plaques in AIDS. *J Neurol Neurosurg Psychiatry* **65**:29–33.

306. Kim YS, Joh TH. (2006). Microglia, major player in the brain inflammation: their roles in the pathogenesis of Parkinson's disease. *Exp Mol Med* **38**:333–47.

307. Wersinger C, Sidhu A. (2002). Inflammation and Parkinson's disease. *Curr Drug Targets Inflamm Allergy* **1**:221–42.

308. Koutsilieri E, Sopper S, Scheller C, ter Meulen V, Riederer P. (2002). Involvement of dopamine in the progression of AIDS Dementia Complex. *J Neural Transm* **109**:399–410.

309. Tanaka M, Endo K, Suzuki T, Kakita A, Takahashi H, Sata T. (2000). Parkinsonism in HIV encephalopathy. *Mov Disord* **15**:1032–3.

310. Mirsattari SM, Power C, Nath A. (1998). Parkinsonism with HIV infection. *Mov Disord* **13**:684–9.

311. Sui Z, Sniderhan LF, Fan S, *et al.* (2006). Human immunodeficiency virus-encoded Tat activates glycogen synthase kinase-3beta to antagonize nuclear factor-kappaB survival pathway in neurons. *Eur J Neurosci* **23**:2623–34.

312. Rumbaugh J, Turchan-Cholewo J, Galey D, *et al.* (2006). Interaction of HIV Tat and matrix metalloproteinase in HIV neuropathogenesis: a new host defense mechanism. *Faseb J* **20**:1736–8.

313. Daily A, Nath A, Hersh LB. (2006). Tat peptides inhibit neprilysin. *J Neurovirol* **12**:153–60.

314. Avraham HK, Jiang S, Lee TH, Prakash O, Avraham S. (2004). HIV-1 Tat-mediated effects on focal adhesion assembly and permeability in brain microvascular endothelial cells. *J Immuno* **173**:6228–33.

315. Amara S, Dezube BJ, Cooley TP, Pantanowitz L, Aboulafia DM. (2006). HIV-associated monoclonal gammopathy: a retrospective analysis of 25 patients. *Clin Infect Dis* **43**:1198–205.

316. Sachs J. (2005). *The End of Poverty*. New York: Penguin Press.

317. Kaiser Family Foundation. (2006). *ADAP Update, 2006*. Available at www.KFF.org accessed 9.11.07).

318. Egger M. (2007). Outcomes of ART in Resource-Limited and Industrialized Countries. 14th Conference on Retroviruses and Opportunistic Infections (CROI), 23–28 February 2007, Los Angeles, CA, USA. [Abstract #62]

319. UNAIDS. (2006). *Report on the Global AIDS Epidemic, 2006*. Geneva: UNAIDS.

320. Getahun R. (2007). Progress in the Global STOP-TB Program. International AIDS Society Conference, 23–25 July 2007, Sydney, Australia. [Abstract TuSy101]

321. Holguín A, Ramirez de Arellano E, Rivas P, Soriano V. (2006). Efficacy of antiretroviral therapy in individuals infected with HIV-1 non-B subtypes. *AIDS Rev* **8**:98–107.

322. Geretti AM. (2006). HIV-1 subtypes: epidemiology and significance for HIV management. *Curr Opin Infect Dis* **19**:1–7

Chapter 27

Maintaining and developing health systems to sustain HAART

Stephanie Nixon and Nina Veenstra*

Due to mounting political pressure and decreasing drug prices, the world is experiencing an unprecedented influx of support for the provision of highly active antiretroviral therapy (HAART) to people in need, with the goal of universal access shining in the distance. As a result, despite a decade of HAART in resource-rich countries, most lower- and middle-income countries are only now able to expand their armouries against HIV/AIDS to include treatment. This welcome development, however, has brought with it a range of challenges that are starting to come to light.

The most heavily affected countries in southern Africa started rolling out their HAART programmes in 2002, when Botswana established four central treatment sites [1]. Since then, progress has been rapid. South Africa claims to have the largest HAART programme in the world, with 175,000 people reportedly on treatment in the public sector in June 2006 [2]. Even less-developed countries like Malawi are overcoming significant barriers, such as human resource crises, to get significant numbers of people on treatment [3]. Part of this is testament to a new-found focus on health in Africa and the global resources that have been mobilized to assist in this regard.

This new reality has prompted a range of operational questions for governments, including:

◆ How well can our health workforce handle this demand?

◆ Will this focus on delivery of antiretroviral therapy (ART) compromise our ability to deliver other health programmes?

◆ How will we sustain funding for ART when international funding sources shift to a different priority?

◆ How well (or not) does this focus fit into our long-term vision for health?

While this chapter may not explicitly answer all these questions, it links them to a common theme, namely health systems. That is, they are all concerned with the impact that the greatly expanded scale-up of HAART could have on health systems, many of which are already stretched. Any analysis of HIV/AIDS must prioritize political, economic and social determinants of health. Nonetheless, attention to healthcare, and to the health systems through which services are delivered, is increasingly important. There is emerging evidence to demonstrate not only that health-care matters for population health in low-income countries [4], but also that the shift in regions highly affected by HIV from a 'prevention only' approach to one that embraces combined prevention, treatment and care strategies has represented a major change for health systems.

---

* Corresponding author.

This chapter focuses on countries where the impact of HAART on health systems is likely to be most significant; our analysis targets countries with fragile health systems, high HIV prevalence and generalized epidemics—the scenario in sub-Saharan Africa. The addition of HAART to HIV care in resource-rich countries in the 1990s was a significant development but did not threaten the stability of those health systems. In contrast, the greatly increased scale of the HIV epidemic in sub-Saharan Africa, married with the region's less resilient health systems, is likely to result in a very different scenario. Ongoing analysis of the impact of HAART delivery on health systems in the region is imperative for identifying and responding to challenges that have yet to be seen in the provision of HIV treatment. Furthermore, lessons learned from analysis of this region can offer warning signals for HAART provision in other parts of the world that may also not enjoy robust health systems.

This chapter contributes to this analysis by drawing on secondary data in the form of published studies. It considers assumptions about the potential impact of HAART on health systems in sub-Saharan Africa and contrasts them with lessons that are currently being learned through empirical research. To support this analysis, we first introduce the notion of health systems and the dominant approaches to health system strengthening over time. We then describe how the introduction of HAART can impede hard-won progress in terms of health system strengthening by shifting balances in undesired directions. Various long-term scenarios are presented that look at the future demand for healthcare as a result of the HIV epidemic, and issues affecting the supply of healthcare are highlighted. Finally, we conclude by arguing that the current exceptional and largely vertical approach to provision of HAART in sub-Saharan Africa is an appropriate response, provided it is accompanied by simultaneous efforts to ensure that the rise of HIV incidence is stemmed as quickly as possible.

Introduction to health systems

What constitutes a health system is not always clear. The World Health Organization (WHO) defines a health system as 'all the activities whose primary purpose is to promote, restore or maintain health' [5]. This definition includes not only formal health services, but also the activities of, for example, traditional healers, community health workers and home caregivers. Such activities remain integral to the continuum of care and should not be forgotten as HAART programmes draw our attention towards health facilities and the services they offer.

Even though health systems have developed around common understandings about medical science and disease, how they are structured and organized varies tremendously across countries [4]. In general, all health systems seek to improve the health of the population they serve. Less often considered are the responsibilities of health systems to respond to users' expectations and to protect them against the costs of ill health, these being the other two fundamental objectives of health systems [5].

To achieve their objectives, health systems perform a number of functions that offer a useful framework for examining the interaction between HAART and health systems. These functions were initially introduced in relation to health system reform [6], and later related to the health system objectives in the World Health Report 2000, whose theme was 'Health Systems: Improving Performance' [5]. They include:

- regulation/stewardship;
- financing; and
- the delivery of services.

For countries in sub-Saharan Africa, health systems are a work in progress, continuously being reshaped in an effort to improve these functions. Ideas about how best to strengthen health systems have shifted over time. However, the current expansion of access to HAART potentially involves an approach to health delivery that runs counter to many of the aims of health system strengthening in this region.

For the source of these aims, we must return to 1978 and the landmark Alma Ata Declaration on Health and its commitment to achieve 'Health for All by the Year 2000'. At the centre of this vision was the concept of primary healthcare (PHC), which encompassed a comprehensive approach to health addressing underlying social, economic and political determinants of wellness and illness [7]. Within this concept, the mandate of health systems is broader than simply the provision of primary healthcare services. We see the focus of health systems moving away from disease-specific technology and the culture of curative hospital care and towards a more integrated, holistic and proactive approach to wellness. A central goal of this approach is equity, and a human rights perspective is embraced to achieve such equity.

Although the PHC approach to health has received criticism over time for being idealistic [8], the philosophy holds important lessons. The healthcare 'reforms' that followed PHC in the mid-1980s emphasized a different set of principles, most notably the economic value of services. These reforms, associated with the neoliberal economic approach, aimed at increasing the role of market mechanisms in healthcare provision by expanding the role of the private sector, increasing 'cost-sharing', and focusing on efficiency [9]. The role of governments was minimized through fiscal limits on public healthcare spending and through decreased public regulation over health services as mandated by, for instance, World Trade Organization (WTO) agreements. Cost-recovery mechanisms such as user fees were particularly damaging because of their inequitable impact on healthcare utilization [e.g. 10]. The result was an approach to health that went against many of the principles espoused by PHC and lost sight of the goal of health for all.

The neoliberal economic policy approach remains visible today in both resource-rich and resource-poor countries. In sub-Saharan Africa, the approach was adopted by countries largely as a condition of World Bank/International Monetary Fund (IMF) loans or as a result of international pressure. However, as the damaging effects of policies on fragile health systems are becoming better documented, there is a renewed passion for many of the values articulated in the Alma Ata Declaration almost three decades ago [11,12]. Within this framework, we would see health systems strengthened through a shift in focus from curative to preventive care, and from understanding health within the medical model to an approach that concerns itself with the broader determinants of health. We would see health services shift from tertiary care delivered privately through centralized urban centres to an emphasis on primary care delivered publicly to all through a system that is decentralized and successfully covers rural environments. Community-driven perspectives would be given the kind of priority that top-down management currently enjoys. Long-term health system priorities would remain in focus while short-term crises were addressed. Finally, approaches to care would more often occur in an integrated way as opposed to vertical programming for disease-specific responses. It is within this context that we come to the question of how the greatly expanded roll-out of HAART could impact on health systems.

How HAART can shift the balance in health systems

It is imperative that people in need of ART receive the care and support services required to enable them to access and consistently use antiretroviral drugs. However, it is also crucial that these processes unfold in a way that, at worst, does not compromise already stretched health systems and, at best, serves to strengthen health systems in the process.

The goal of health systems strengthening through the delivery of HAART is a worthy target and can begin with acknowledgement of the ways in which the tensions described above could be exacerbated through delivery of antiretrovirals (ARVs). For instance, the spotlight on HIV treatment inevitably emphasizes a medical model focus instead of an approach that embraces the broader determinants of health as envisaged by PHC. It also seems to be leading to centralization of healthcare. For example, in South Africa, the response to HIV/AIDS has been shown to prioritize short-term delivery objectives decided by higher levels of government, which is at odds with the longer-term development objective of strengthening local government systems [13]. The impact of HAART on health systems is perhaps most clearly illustrated when considering the vertical versus horizontal programming debate.

Vertical versus horizontal approaches

The method of delivering HAART through specialized, 'vertical' programmes is not a new idea. Vertical programming, meaning separate health structures dedicated to the planning, management and implementation of selected disease-specific interventions, has been a public health approach used for decades [14]. The common rationale for verticalization (both then and now) is to provide greater capacity for a focused effort to reduce morbidity and mortality due to one specific disease [15]. Not surprisingly, the push to implement vertical programmes is stronger where epidemics, poverty and weakened health systems coincide, which is the case for HIV/AIDS in many countries, and especially in sub-Saharan Africa.

While this argument is compelling, there are related criticisms of this approach that are instructive for thinking about the scale-up of HAART. First, vertical programming often reflects a medical model response, which detracts from a more comprehensive approach to health that includes upstream determinants [16]. In the case of HAART, this is a call for developing treatment programming that includes attention to the social, political and economic forces that influence how well a person will be able to access, tolerate and adhere to ART. Moreover, it demands simultaneous investment in HIV prevention programming at individual, community, and structural levels in order to mount a comprehensive response to HIV/AIDS. This point cannot be overemphasized, since modelling has clearly demonstrated what might happen if treatment undermines prevention programmes; in such cases, treatment will most likely become unsustainable due to the high numbers of people requiring care [17].

Second, vertical approaches have historically assumed a top-down management approach as opposed to one that engages community participation. This is particularly salient in the context of HAART scale-up because the principle of GIPA, or the greater involvement of people with HIV/AIDS, is a fundamental component of effective and human rights-based responses and must remain at the centre of treatment programming.

Third, the quest to roll out and subsequently to scale up treatment as quickly as possible lends itself to preferentially targeting people who are easier to access, such as those with higher incomes and/or those who reside in urban areas. The result can be the widening of existing healthcare inequities, an issue that is currently receiving attention in South Africa [18]. Indeed, the rationing of limited supplies of antiretroviral drugs is a challenge in almost every setting; engagement of communities in determining how limited resources will be distributed builds community trust and respects the principles of a human rights-based approach [19].

A fourth concern involves the way in which vertical programming can result in multiple parallel disease-specific programmes operating separately. While these programmes may be effective in and of themselves, they have the potential to disrupt the efforts of local health systems to deliver comprehensive and integrated essential services [20]. A common harm involves the usurping of often limited supplies of health workers from existing systems to higher salary roles within vertical programmes being sponsored by international health non-governmental organizations

(NGOs) and donors [21]. Furthermore, this process may be seen as 'de-skilling' primary care workers as their expertise focuses to achieve narrow goals at the expense of their broader expertise on the health demands of communities [11].

The lesson for the scale-up of HAART is that all programmes need to be cognizant of health system targets. This can be done at a basic level through the inclusion of activities in vertical programme plans that are designed to counteract potential harms to broader health systems. A more proactive approach would be for all national HIV/AIDS programmes and global initiatives to be held accountable for not only minimizing harm to health systems, but also for health system strengthening through the inclusion of system indicators in their monitoring and evaluation frameworks [11,22]. Similarly, new initiatives can be expected to conduct systems impact assessments at the outset to identify potential damages before they begin. Some examples of the contributions that vertical programmes can make to strengthening health systems include fortifying elements of the general health service infrastructure that are required for the vertical delivery to be successful, such as laboratory facilities and drug supply chains [23].

Finally, while external funding for HAART programming is essential, it comes with the issue of who is setting health priorities. Responses to HIV/AIDS are designed and delivered at the country level. As such, the strategy created for scaling up delivery of HAART within and by countries should drive the allocation of external resources, not vice versa. In other words, financing should not only be predictable and sustainable, but also pliant enough to respect local priorities. The Commission on HIV/AIDS and Governance in Africa, convened by the United Nations in 2003 to clarify the data on the impact of HIV/AIDS on state structures and economic development and to assist governments in consolidating the design and implementation of policies and programmes that can help to govern their epidemics, advised that absorptive capacity will not be an issue if countries have more flexibility in financing their health systems [24]. Similarly, the potential for resources to be deflected towards HIV/AIDS could be minimized. Donor aid not only affects the nature of priorities, but also their time frames; the unpredictable nature of donor aid can compromise the sustainability of programmes and impair a country's ability to develop longer-term health strategies [25]. Sustainability of funding is an even more sensitive issue in the context of HAART, since treatment interruptions can have devastating effects on the development of viral resistance.

HAART and the HIV epidemic: four possible scenarios for health systems

The preceding discussion, while not in support of vertical programming, also rejects the idea that vertical programming should be abandoned altogether in favour of more horizontal approaches. We can appreciate that the current burden of disease and the political and economic milieu foster a tendency towards vertical programming for the mass delivery of HAART in sub-Saharan Africa. The rationale here is to reduce morbidity and mortality as a matter of urgency and later, ideally, incidence, through the potential preventive effects of decreasing viral load through treatment. This is a form of AIDS exceptionalism that is justified as an interim measure. However, this logic is based on the expectation that, in the medium term, HIV/AIDS will assume more manageable levels for the health system, at which time HAART programmes can become assimilated into general health services. HAART will then be delivered in a similar fashion to drugs for other chronic diseases, and the era of AIDS exceptionalism will be over.

The above justification of AIDS exceptionalism is based on one key question: will levels of HIV/AIDS become more manageable for health systems in the medium term? Unfortunately, this is a question that we are as yet unable to answer, given all the uncertainties about factors affecting the future demand for care. These uncertainties can be illustrated through a range of scenarios, outlined in Table 27.1, that hypothesize how HAART might affect HIV prevalence through:

• a change in the average survival time from infection to death ('AIDS deaths'); and

• a change in the rate of new infections.

The most hopeful scenario takes lessons from the demographic transition and has therefore been labelled the 'AIDS transition' [26].

These scenarios, unlike those recently developed for Africa or specific countries like South Africa [27,28], are narrow in their focus. In other words, they look quite explicitly at the management and impact of HAART and the resulting burden on health systems (keeping other factors constant). They therefore have to be put in context. In particular, matching the provision of HAART with aggressive prevention efforts has the potential to improve the outcome of all the scenarios. Similarly, if excessive attention is diverted away from prevention efforts, then even the outlook of the most optimistic scenario may appear quite bleak.

While scenarios might help us to understand how many people could potentially be HIV-infected and so require some form of care through the health system, they do not draw out the nuances of the potential burden. This is because HAART will not only affect health systems by increasing or decreasing the burden placed on them, but can also cause more subtle shifts within systems. These shifts are important for managers and policy makers, since they would ideally influence prioritization and resource allocation. The most obvious shift in the burden of HIV/AIDS care due to HAART would be from inpatient services to outpatient services. In Brazil, for example, the scale-up of the HAART programme (delivered through outpatient services) was accompanied by a gradual decline in hospital admissions among those on therapy [29]. In sub-Saharan Africa, such shifts have as yet not been reported because HAART programmes are still too new. However, we would hope to see a similar trend.

Table 27.1 Scenarios illustrating the potential demand for healthcare due to HIV/AIDS

Scenario	AIDS deaths	New infections	Resulting potential burden on health system
1. AIDS transition – the optimistic scenario	Decline as people access and adhere to treatment	Decline as treatment scales up (HAART has positive effect on prevention)	Initial increase in the number of people requiring care, with later stabilization to a much more manageable burden
2. Failed transition – AIDS deaths rebound	Decline initially as treatment scales up, but experience a rebound (due to problems with programme delivery – adherence, regimens)	Remain high (due to rebound in deaths – HAART has no effect on prevention)	Initial increase in the number of people requiring care, with some stabilization as deaths again increase (but burden remains greater than in scenario 1)
3. Failed transition – continued high rate of new infections	Decline as people go on treatment	Remain high (HAART has no effect on prevention)	Increase in the number of people requiring care, with this number remaining high
4. Failed transition – increase in the rate of new infections	Decline as people go on treatment	Increase (HAART has negative effect on prevention)	Massive increase in the number of people requiring care, with this number remaining high

Source: Adapted from [26]

The remainder of this section of the chapter reviews the current evidence on assumptions informing the various scenarios outlined in Table 27.1. Although limited, this evidence provides the best lessons for optimizing chances for AIDS transition to unfold.

The impact of HAART on AIDS deaths

The longer people living with HIV/AIDS (PLWHA) survive on HAART, the greater the number of patients that health systems will have to cope with, even if these people are, hopefully, less ill. Hence, a sustained reduction in AIDS deaths may be necessary for a successful AIDS transition, but will not in itself be able to achieve this. Established cohorts in Europe have witnessed sustained declines in the incidence of AIDS and death with HAART, despite the potential for long-term adverse effects [30]. In sub-Saharan Africa, the clinical success of HAART may be subjected to greater challenges. In particular, its success will depend on getting people on treatment early and maintaining adherence, both of which currently carry an uncertain prognosis for reasons highlighted below.

Early evaluations of HAART programmes in Africa demonstrated how their effectiveness is compromised when patients present late for treatment [31,32 for examples]. Survival probabilities have been found to decline incrementally, and a recent cost-effectiveness model constructed for southern Africa estimated that HAART plus antibiotics might prolong life for 6.7 discounted years if treatment is initiated 'late' (CD4 count of 200 cells/mm^3), or by 9.8 years if initiated 'early' (CD4 count of 350 cells/mm^3) [33]. Unfortunately, what most people fail to acknowledge is that decisions about if and when to seek therapy are dependant not only on government policy, but also on many other social, political and economic factors, which are discussed later.

Debates about adherence to HAART in Africa have, on the other hand, been ongoing. Most recently, concerns about suboptimal adherence in sub-Saharan Africa were allayed by a meta-analysis that concluded that there have been higher levels of adherence to antiretroviral regimens in this region than in North America [34]. This is despite the mixed successes with drug regimen compliance for other common diseases in sub-Saharan Africa, such as malaria and tuberculosis, and health infrastructure constraints that could potentially have contributed to 'antiretroviral anarchy' [35,36]. Therefore, we need to monitor adherence over the longer term to learn whether this early evidence remains relevant. The concern remains that many of the early HAART programmes, which have logically been the subject of adherence studies in sub-Saharan Africa until now, have captured a population and a set of circumstances that will not be the norm once treatment scales up.

Barriers to accessing HAART, and the potential for these to be broken down, are at the heart of concerns about late initiation of treatment and poor adherence. In sub-Saharan Africa, the most frequently cited barriers across a range of contexts have been stigma and cost [37–39]. When it comes to initiating treatment, perceptions of health facilities and the quality of their care also come into play. In general, there has been an assumption that HAART will assist to break down these barriers; however, this will not necessarily hold true. For example, although there has been some indication that HAART can reduce stigma in communities, this has not happened to the expected degree in workplace settings. People have continued to present late for treatment when it is offered by employers, thus limiting the potential benefits to patients and companies' returns for investments in workplace programmes [40].

If barriers to accessing HAART are not broken down, then patients could continue to access treatment late (or not at all) or default on treatment, thus compromising survival. At this stage, it is unclear how robust these barriers are, and what effect the HAART programme will have on them. Where daily survival is an issue, then HAART becomes pitched against many other challenges. This is perhaps most starkly illustrated in South Africa by the way that PLWHA have been found to compromise their health by transitioning on and off ART (without medical directive or supervision) simply to maintain a relatively low CD4 count, which qualifies them for a disability grant [41,42].

Therefore, although there is little doubt that we are already seeing improved survival for patients on HAART in sub-Saharan Africa, maintaining this effect may prove more challenging than in other contexts. If we do not succeed, then we will witness the failed AIDS transition associated with scenario 2 in Table 27.1. In the developed world, conditions under which HAART was introduced have remained relatively constant, while in this region, this is less likely to be the case. In particular, early programmes in the region have been well funded and supported, and often implemented without relying entirely on the functioning of local health systems. Challenges associated with the integration of HIV/AIDS treatment into fragile health systems, as well as the somewhat less stable social, political and economic context, all alert us to the need for vigilant monitoring and evaluation.

The impact of HAART on the rate of new infections

Central to the AIDS transition scenario described above is a reduction in HIV incidence. Indeed, assuming we witness a sustained decline in AIDS-related deaths in sub-Saharan Africa, scenarios 3 and 4 in Table 27.1 may still result in a failed AIDS transition. Furthermore, there are various ways in which the introduction of HAART could potentially result in declining HIV incidence, thus complicating any analysis of the situation in sub-Saharan Africa.

The most direct way that HAART can lead to a reduction in new infections, and hence in the number of people requiring treatment in the next decade, is by decreasing transmission rates through a reduction in HIV viral load. This effect has been demonstrated conclusively for both sexual transmission and vertical transmission [43–45 for examples]. However, it is still unclear what the impact of such an effect will be at a population level, because it depends on a number of other factors, including when people commence ART (i.e. their CD4 count) and the extent of discordant partnerships or sexual encounters. Such factors were investigated in a study in a township of South Africa, where the population impact of HAART on reducing sexual transmission was found to be relatively small [46].

A second question around incidence concerns the extent to which HAART may or may not influence behaviour change. Here, we are looking specifically at risky sexual behaviours, which were thought to have increased amongst men who have sex with men (MSM) after the introduction of HAART in North America [47]. However, it is important to note that such studies have not been able to conclusively prove a causal relationship between HAART and risky sexual behaviour, and that in the African context, failure to provide treatment could be even more damaging [48]. For instance, it has been suggested that some PLWHA, struggling with a lack of hope and a desire not to die alone, may spread HIV deliberately [49]. Clearly, this effect remains unknown.

Aside from the effect of HAART on risky sexual behaviours, there are other ways in which it can hinder or facilitate prevention programmes. It may be that the focus on treatment is deflecting attention and resources away from prevention. Conversely, the availability of treatment may reduce stigma and give hope, thereby encouraging the uptake of voluntary counselling and testing (VCT) leading to an improved awareness of status. Early evidence on the latter is encouraging, with a large study in Botswana demonstrating significant reductions in stigma. Although several factors were correlated, perceived access to ART was associated with decreased odds of holding at least one stigmatizing attitude [50].

The impact of HAART on the rate of new infections must also be viewed over a longer period of time to determine whether potential declines are sustained. Temporal trend analysis of HIV incidence rates in Brazil between 1996 and 2002 yielded a complex picture, with some level of decline and then rebound amongst men, but no clear evidence of this pattern amongst women. In two regions of Brazil, there was a marked difference between observed and expected incidence rates, but not in the other three regions [29]. Ultimately, it will be many years before we can start looking at such trends in the most heavily affected countries in sub-Saharan Africa. In other words, the second stage of the 'AIDS transition'—the reduction in HIV incidence—will still take many years to unfold in this region.

In sum, there are many features of the context in sub-Saharan Africa that might affect countries' ability to reduce HIV incidence. First, epidemics in the region are generalized, and this implies the need for a much broader and more extensive prevention strategy than might be employed in countries with concentrated epidemics. Where resources are limited, there is a greater chance that prevention efforts might falter as attention becomes focused on treatment. Second, PLWHA in conditions of poverty or political upheaval are unlikely to adapt their behaviour in the same way as those PLWHA in more developed societies once on treatment. The disability grant example documented above illustrated how the prioritization of health (whether one's own or that of another) may be valued differently under such circumstances.

The impact of HAART on the supply of health services

The future scenarios described in the previous section provide insight into potential demands on health services with the advent of HAART. However, it is also important to consider how HAART might affect the supply of healthcare, as this is a determining factor in deciding whether the HIV/AIDS burden will be manageable or not. In particular, the current human resource crisis is having a major impact on the capacity of health systems in sub-Saharan Africa. Since this issue is covered in another chapter of this book, it is only considered here in relation to two key questions:

- To what extent will health workers be prioritized or encouraged to begin treatment, hence reducing HIV-related absenteeism and attrition?
- To what extent will HAART improve the motivation and working conditions of healthcare workers, thereby discouraging migration from the public health system?

It is increasingly being acknowledged that healthcare workers are subject to the same stigma and discrimination as the communities they serve, making it difficult for them to seek care despite their knowledge of its benefits [51,52]. In some countries, such as Zambia, Malawi and Uganda, AIDS-related deaths have been shown to contribute significantly to health worker attrition [53–55]. In Zambia, it was estimated that deaths outnumbered resignations and that death rates alone could account for the nurse vacancy rate of 37% [56]. This suggests that any programmes helping health workers to obtain the necessary treatment might significantly improve the capacity of the health system to deliver.

Since nurses in particular have had to increasingly provide palliative care for those infected with HIV, levels of depression, stress and burnout have become a concern. These issues, among others, have been driving healthcare workers in sub-Saharan Africa into the private sector and abroad. HAART programmes were expected to change this trend. According to a September 2003 newspaper article published just prior to the implementation of South Africa's HAART programme: 'health workers' morale will be boosted as they will no longer be helpless when faced with destitute AIDS patients' [57]. However, current indications suggest that this shift in attitude has not materialized. Rather, the HAART programme has been seen as just another addition to the healthcare worker's already heavy workload [58]. It may be that too much emphasis has been placed on AIDS treatment as a means to improve health worker conditions.

Conclusion

This chapter has examined the ways in which the advent of HAART has impacted on health systems and their functions of stewardship, financing and service delivery. In terms of stewardship, HAART has generally steered fragile health systems away from the desired vision described in the Alma Ata Declaration. This shift is closely linked to financing trends, whereby countries have needed to accept donor aid to finance HAART programmes, even though much of this aid has come with controlling conditions and without any assurance of sustainability. As such, the immediate crisis of HIV/AIDS could be seen to have taken us some steps backward in our long-term development plans for health systems. But is this impact justifiable? To answer this question, we have to consider the issue of 'AIDS exceptionalism' and look at how we balance short-term delivery objectives with a more long-term developmental agenda in the health sector.

To date, AIDS exceptionalism has been supported in the health sector response as shown by the structuring of HAART programmes and other measures to address the burden of HIV/AIDS. It also makes sense given the exceptional nature of the burden; we would probably do the same for an outbreak of any communicable disease. However, we generally implement such measures knowing that the burden of illness will ultimately subside, thus allowing the health system to resume its commitment to longer-term development. In the case of HAART and the potential future demand for treatment, our most hopeful scenario suggests that pressures on the health system could stabilize to the point where HAART programmes can be integrated and managed in a similar manner to any other disease programme. However, this is not the only scenario facing fragile health systems, and evidence about the assumptions underlying the various scenarios is currently very limited. Furthermore, this optimistic scenario requires not only access and adherence to HAART, but a parallel injection of resources into prevention strategies to stem the tide of new infections.

This chapter argues that the current negative impact of HAART on health systems may be justified given our hopes that the AIDS transition will transpire. However, in the years to come, it will be essential that we accumulate evidence on the interactions between HAART and health systems in a way that allows us to revisit the scenarios outlined above. We need to move from a crisis-oriented response to one that is more strategic and, based on sound evidence, one that balances long- and short-term goals.

References

1. Government of Botswana. (2003). *Country report status of the 2002 national response to the UNGASS Declaration of Commitment on HIV/AIDS*. Gabarone: Government of Botswana.
2. South African Department of Health. (2006). *Press release: Response to an attack by Stephen Lewis on the Government of South Africa. 19 August 2006*. Available at http://www.doh.gov.za/mediaroom/index.html (Accessed 25 February 2007).
3. Palmer D. (2006). Tackling Malawi's human resource crisis. *Reproductive Health Matters* **14**: 27–39.
4. Beck E, Mays N. (2006). The HIV pandemic and health systems: an introduction. In: Beck EJ, Mays N, Whiteside A, Zuniga JM, eds. *The HIV pandemic: local and global implications*. Oxford: Oxford University Press. p3–20.
5. World Health Organization. (2000). *The World Health Report 2000. Health systems: improving performance*. Geneva:WHO.
6. Frenk J. (1994). Dimensions of health sector reform. *Health Policy* **27**:19–34.
7. World Health Organization. (1978). *Declaration of Alma Ata. International Conference on Primary Health Care, 6–12 September 1978, Alma-Ata, USSR*. Geneva: WHO.

8. Cueto M. (2004). The origins of primary health care and selective primary health care. *Am J Public Health* **94**:1864–74.

9. World Bank. (1993). *World Development Report 1993: Investing in health.* Washington, DC: World Bank.

10. Nabyonga J, Desmet M, Karamagi H, Kadama P, Omaswa F, Walker O. (2005). Abolition of cost-sharing is pro-poor: evidence from Uganda. *Health Policy Plan* **20**:100–8.

11. Global Health Watch. (2005). *Global Health Watch 2005–2006: An alternative world health report.* People's Health Movement, Medact and Global Equity Gauge Alliance. CapeTown: Global Health Watch.

12. People's Health Movement. (2000) *People's Charter for Health. First People's Health Assembly, 4–8 December 2000, Dhaka, Bangladesh.* Available at: http://www.phmovement.org/cms/en/contact

13. Blaauw D, Gilson L, Modiba P, Erasmus E, Khumalo G, Scheider H. (2004). *Governmental relationships and HIV/AIDS service delivery.* Johannesburg: Centre for Health Policy, University of Witwatersrand.

14. Mills A. (2005). Mass campaigns versus general health services: what have we learnt in 40 years about vertical versus horizontal approaches? *Bull World Health Organ* **83**:315–6.

15. Oliveira-Cruz V, Kurowski C, Mills A. (2003). Delivery of priority health services: searching for synergies within the vertical versus horizontal debate. *Journal of International Development* **15**:67–86.

16. Mills A. (1983). Vertical vs horizontal health programmes in Africa: idealism, pragmatism, resources and efficiency. *Soc Sci Med* **17**:1971–81.

17. Salomon J, Hogan D, Stover J, *et al.* (2005). Integrating HIV prevention and treatment: from slogans to impact. *PloS Medicine* **2**:50–6.

18. Stewart R, Padarath A, Milford C. (2006). Emerging threats to equitable implementation of ART in South Africa. *Acta Academica Supplementum* **1**:286–308.

19. Roseman M, Gruskin S. (2004). *HIV/AIDS & human rights in a nutshell.* Toronto: Harvard School of Public Health and International Council of AIDS Service Organisations (ICASO).

20. World Health Organization. (2006). *The African Regional Health Report: the health of the people.* Geneva: WHO.

21. Kober K, Van Damme W. (2004). Scaling up access to antiretroviral treatment in southern Africa: who will do the job? *Lancet* **364**:103–7.

22. Atun R, Lennox-chhugani F, Drobniewski F, Samyshkin Y, Coker R. (2004). A framework and toolkit for capturing the communicable disease programmes within health systems: tuberculosis control as an illustrative example. *European Journal of Public Health* **14**:267–73.

23. Travis P, Bennet S, Haines A, *et al.* (2004). Overcoming health-systems constraints to achieve the Millenium Development Goals. *Lancet* **364**:900–6.

24. Commission on HIV/AIDS Governance in Africa (CHGA). (2007). *"Securing Our Future." The Final Report of the United Nation's Commission on HIV/AIDS and Governance in Africa.* Addis Ababa: UN Economic Commission for Africa. Forthcoming.

25. Bulir A, Hamann J. (2003). *Aid volatility: an empirical assessment. IMF Staff Papers, Vol 50 No 1.* Washington, DC: International Monetary Fund.

26. Over M. (2004). Impact of the HIV/AIDS epidemic on the health sectors of developing countries. In: Haacker M, ed. *The Macroeconomics of HIV/AIDS.* Washington, DC: International Monetary Fund. p 311–344.

27. Metropolitan AIDS Solutions. (2006). *Live the Future. HIV and AIDS scenarios for South Africa: 2005–2025.* Cape Town: Metropolitan Holdings Limited.

28. Joint United Nations Programme on HIV/AIDS (UNAIDS). (2005). *AIDS in Africa: three scenarios to 2025.* Geneva: UNAIDS.

29. Dourado I, Amélia M, Barriera D, Maria A. (2006). AIDS epidemic trends after the introduction of antiretroviral therapy in Brazil. *Rev Saude Publica* **40**(Suppl):9–17.

30. Mocroft A, Ledergerber B, Katlama C, *et al.* (2003). Decline in the AIDS and death rate in the EuroSIDA study: an observational study. *Lancet* **362**:22–9.

31. Lawn S, Myer L, Orrell C, Bekker L, Wood R. (2005). Early mortality among adults accessing a community-based antiretroviral service in South Africa: implications for programme design. *AIDS* **19**:2141–8.

32. Weidle P, Malamba S, Mwebaze R, *et al*. (2002). Assessment of a pilot antiretroviral drug therapy programme in Uganda: patients' response, survival, and drug resistance. *Lancet* **360**:34–40.

33. Bachmann M. (2006). Effectiveness and cost effectiveness of early and late prevention of HIV/AIDS progression with antiretrovirals or antibiotics in Southern African adults. *AIDS Care* **18**:109–20.

34. Mills E, Nachega J, Buchan I, *et al*. (2006). Adherence to antiretroviral therapy in sub-Saharan Africa and North America. *Journal of the American Medical Association* **296**:679–90.

35. Harries A, Nyangulu D, Hargreaves N, Kaluwa O, Salaniponi F. (2001). Preventing antiretroviral anarchy in sub-Saharan Africa. *Lancet* **358**:410–4.

36. Stevens W, Kaye S, Gorrah T. (2004). Antiretroviral therapy in Africa. *Br Med J* **328**:280–2.

37. Mshana G, Wamoyi J, Busza J, *et al*. (2006). Barriers to accessing antiretroviral therapy in Kisesa, Tanzania: a qualitative study of early rural referrals to the national program. *AIDS Patient Care STDS* **20**:649–57.

38. Padarath A, Searle C, Sibiya Z, Williams E, Ntsike M. (2006) Understanding barriers and challenges to community participation in HIV and ARV services. 3rd Public Health Conference, "Making health systems work", 15–17 May 2006, Midrand, South Africa. [Poster Session P10]

39. Weiser S, Wolfe W, Bangsberg D, *et al*. (2003). Barriers to antiretroviral adherence for patients living with HIV infection and AIDS in Botswana. *J Acquir Immune Defic Syndr* **34**:281–8.

40. George G. (2006). Workplace ART programmes: why do companies invest in them and are they working? *African Journal of AIDS Research* **5**:179–88.

41. Leclerc-Madlala S. (2005). Juggling AIDS, grants and treatment in South Africa: predicaments of second phase HIV/AIDS. Anthropology Southern Africa Conference: "Continuity, Change and Transformation: Anthropology in the 21st Century", 22–24 September 2005, University of KwaZulu-Natal, Durban. [Abstract S-96]

42. Nattrass N. (2004). *Trading-off income and health: AIDS and the disability grant in South Africa. CSSR Working Paper No 82*. Cape Town: Centre for Social Science Research (CSSR).

43. Castilla J, Del Romero J, Hernando V, Marincovich B, Garcia S, Rodriguez C. (2005). Effectiveness of highly active antiretroviral therapy in reducing heterosexual transmission of HIV. *J Acquir Immune Defic Syndr* **40**:96–101.

44. Cooper E, Charurat M, Mofenson L, *et al*. (2002). Combination antiretroviral strategies for the treatment of pregnant HIV-1 infected women and prevention of perinatal HIV-1 transmission. *J Acquir Immune Defic Syndr* **29**:484–94.

45. Quinn T, Wawer M, Sewankambo N, *et al*. (2000). Viral load and heterosexual transmission of human immunodeficiency virus type 1. *N Engl J Med* **342**:921–9.

46. Auvert B, Males S, Puren A, Taljaard D, Caraël M, Williams B. (2004). Can highly active antiretroviral therapy reduce the spread of HIV?: A study in a township of South Africa. *J Acquir Immune Defic Syndr* **36**:613–21.

47. Katz M, Schwarcz S, Kellogg T, *et al*. (2002). Impact of highly active antiretroviral treatment on HIV seroincidence among men who have sex with men: San Francisco. *Am J Public Health* **92**:388–94.

48. Nattrass N. (2004). *The Moral Economy of AIDS in South Africa*. Cambridge: Cambridge University Press.

49. Leclerc-Madlala S. (2001). Infect one, infect all: Zulu youth response to the AIDS epidemic in South Africa. *Med Anthropol* **17**:363–80.

50. Wolfe W, Weiser S, Leiter K, *et al*. (2006). Impact of universal access to antiretroviral therapy on HIV stigma in Botswana. XVI International AIDS Conference, 13–18 August 2006, Toronto, Canada. [Abstract MOAXO301]

51. Kiragu K, Ngulube T, Nyumbu M, Njobvu P, Eerens P, Mwaba C. (2007). Sexual risk-taking and HIV testing among health workers in Zambia. *AIDS and Behaviour* **11**:131–136.

52. Zelnick J, O'Donnell M. (2005). The impact of the HIV/AIDS epidemic on hospital nurses in KwaZulu-Natal, South Africa: nurses' perspectives and implications for health policy. *J Public Health Policy* **26**:163–85.

53. Buve A, Foaster S, Mbwili C, Mungo E, Tollenare N, Zeko M. (1994). Mortality among female nurses in the face of the AIDS epidemic: a pilot study in Zambia. *AIDS* **8**:396.

54. Dambisya Y. (2004). The fate and career destinations of doctors who qualified at Uganda's Makerere Medical School in 1984: retrospective cohort study. *Br Med J* **329**:600–1.

55. Mukati M, Gonani A, Macheso A, Simwaka B, Kinoti S, Ndyanabangi B. (2004). *Challenges facing the Malawian health workforce in the era of HIV/AIDS*. Arusha, Tanzania: Commonwealth Regional Health Community Health Secretariat for East, Central and Southern Africa (CRHCS)/Washington, DC: United States Agency for International Development (USAID)/Support for Analysis and Research in Africa (SARA). Available at http://www.crhcs.or.tz (accessed 18 May 2008).

56. Feeley F. (2006). Fight AIDS as well as the brain drain. *The Lancet* **368**:435–6.

57. Cullinan K. (2003). Antiretroviral roll-out could be just the tonic – or a bitter pill. *Sunday Times*, September 28, 2003.

58. Chopra M, Kendall C, Hill Z, Schaay N, Nkonki L, Doherty T. (2006). Nothing new: responses to the introduction of antiretroviral drugs in South Africa. *AIDS* **20**:1975–7.

Chapter 28

Redefining HIV/AIDS care delivery in the face of human resource scarcity

Mario Roberto Dal Poz*, Norbert Dreesch and Dingie van Rensburg

Human resource challenges facing the globe
Nature and extent of shortages and deficits

In response to the burgeoning demands of and, needs for, HIV/AIDS care on existing human resources for health (HRH), the pressures on these resources have multiplied and steered many national health systems into ever deeper troubled waters as a result of dire and aggravating human resource shortages and deficits. This is especially the case in those countries hardest hit by the epidemic, and with the recent scale-up of antiretroviral therapy (ART).

The crux of the crisis is related to growing mismatches between demand and supply of human resources. For example, ART coverage in sub-Saharan Africa increased from 100,000 to 810,000 people between 2003 and 2006, and with the epidemic showing no signs of ebbing yet, coverage will certainly reach its maximum limit if a matching response in the supply of health workers in some form is not forthcoming.

In terms of human resources, on the other hand, the crisis manifests itself first of all in shortages in the numbers of healthcare workers, deficits in skills, gaps in skill mixes, and the appropriateness of the current workforce that must provide for the special care needs of people living with HIV/AIDS (PLWHA). Second, it is related to shortfalls in the number, capacities and competencies of managerial and supervisory personnel to optimally deploy, utilize and support the current health workers. Third, the crisis involves the preparation and fitness of the health workforce to meet prevailing demands and needs for care. This includes: the suitability of basic and pre-service training of new entrants to the core and allied or supplementary health professions; the need for retraining, in-service, and continuous training of existing personnel in the face of the rapidly changing supply and demand for healthcare; and, in particular, the need for refocusing the training of health workers to meet the special requirements of HIV/AIDS care.

The crisis exists in both developing and developed, poor and wealthy countries, though its nature varies greatly from one country to another, with stark regional, country, sector, area and class disparities contributing to and defining it. For example, the Americas (including Canada and the United States) harbour only 10% of the global burden of disease, yet almost 37% of the world's health workers live in this region and spend more than 50% of the world's financial resources for health there. In contrast, the African region suffers more than 24% of the global burden of disease but has access to only 3% of health workers and less than 1% of the world's

---

* Corresponding author.

financial resources [1]. Moreover, the scarcity of health workers in deprived rural areas, among lower socio-economic classes, and in the public health sectors of poor developing countries is a well-known distortion generally plaguing HRH deployment.

This multifaceted crisis in HRH is likely to worsen if strong political and financial commitments by governments and donors are not forthcoming to implement short- and long-term strategies to strengthen and expand HRH in general, and for HIV/AIDS care specifically. Nothing short of an international response is required, and one marked by solidarity [2]. However, the strategic uncertainty caused by the recent growth in philanthropic and other institutional leadership on the global health landscape is not conducive to producing such a response [3].

The *World Health Report 2006* considers that 'health workers are all people primarily engaged in actions with the primary intent of enhancing health' [1]. This is consistent with the World Health Organization's (WHO) definition of health systems as comprising all activities with the primary goal of improving health. The WHO estimates there to be a total of 59.2 million full-time paid health workers worldwide. These workers are in health enterprises whose primary role is to improve health, as well as additional workers in non-health organizations, such as nurses staffing a company or school clinic.

Health service providers constitute about two-thirds of the global health workforce. The WHO estimates a global shortage of 4.3 million health workers, with the situations in 57 countries (36 of them in sub-Saharan Africa) described as 'countries with critical shortage' where the estimated deficit is equivalent to 2.4 million doctors, nurses and midwives [1]. Such shortages mean sinking far below the WHO's threshold of workforce density necessary for interventions to meet the health-related Millennium Development Goals (MDGs), and where this threshold is not met, adequate coverage of essential interventions is very unlikely. Paradoxically, these workforce insufficiencies are often in countries with large numbers of unemployed health professionals, or where sufficient numbers of health workers are unequally distributed along private–public or rural–urban lines, resulting in significant secondary sector and area shortages. Poverty, imperfect private labour markets, lack of public funds, the push and pull of migration forces, bureaucratic red tape and political interference serve to exacerbate this paradox of shortages in the midst of underutilized talent.

Effects of human resource shortages on health personnel

The health workforce is heavily affected by the smouldering HRH crisis. Workers in health systems around the world are increasingly experiencing occupational stress, insecurity and burnout as they react to a complex array of forces, some old, some new. Demographic and epidemiological transitions drive changes in population-based health threats to which the workforce must respond. Financing policies, technological advances and consumer expectations can dramatically shift demands on the workforce in health systems. Workers seek opportunities and job security in dynamic health labour markets that are part of the global political economy. Expanding labour markets have accelerated international migration from poorer to wealthier and higher-bidding countries, intensified professional migration and concentration in urban areas, and stimulated large-scale flocking of health workers to the lucrative health sectors and industries at the cost of public health sectors and quality of care.

In many countries, several on the African continent, economic crises and health sector reform under structural adjustment have capped public sector employment and limited investment in health worker education and infrastructure. One consequence of these measures is that the supply of young graduates is drying up; another is the weakening of fragile public health systems, even to the point of crumbling and collapse. Although the scale-up of ART is also meant to strengthen health systems and relieve some of the pressure on personnel—and indeed has such outcomes—it nevertheless creates a series of pitfalls or dangers that hold unintended negative consequences for healthcare in general and for health human resources in particular [4,5]. Hence the call that ART scale-up should go hand in hand with comprehensive health systems development, upgrading of human resource capacity, and realistic targets.

Deficient skill mixes and distributional imbalances compound today's human resource problems. In many countries, the skills of limited yet expensive professionals are not well matched to the local profile of health needs. Amid a strong trend in recent decades towards specialization (even over-specialization) in most health professions—especially in more lucrative sub- and super-specialist areas—critical skills deficits and shortages have developed in the corps of generalist health professionals and specialists in public or community health, health policy and management, and health-related social sciences. At the same time, several now essential professions have lost their previous attraction and prestige as career paths due to shifting policies, compositions, values and disease profiles in the health sectors of countries, and within and among the health professions themselves. Among these, seemingly, are HIV clinicians—both doctors and nurses—in some resource-rich countries, where the field of HIV medicine is increasingly losing its erstwhile 'febrile allure of a hot, new topic' [6].

Many workers, especially in the public sectors of poorer developing countries and under-resourced rural areas, also face daunting working environments, including: poverty-level wages; lack of supervision and unsupportive management; insufficient social recognition; weak career prospects and development opportunities; lack of suitable infrastructure, equipment and medicines; and dilapidated facilities and amenities. Almost all countries suffer from a maldistribution of health workers characterized by urban concentrations and rural deficits, and access to care strongly determined by socio-economic class. These imbalances in provisioning, distribution and access are perhaps most disturbing from a regional perspective.

The exodus of skilled professionals in the midst of so much unmet health need places sub-Saharan Africa at the epicentre of the global health workforce crisis. This crisis packs a double punch since sub-Saharan Africa is also at the epicentre of the epidemic. Inasmuch as global funds are now being provided for antiretroviral treatment in African and other poor developing countries, these run the high risk of leaking away without the desired effects because decades of neglect have rendered public health systems and services and training institutions dangerously deficient, left health workers grossly unprepared and ill-equipped, and spurred many of the already meagre workforce to seek a better life elsewhere [3].

A deepening crisis requires reconsidering responses

The HRH crisis has the potential to deepen in the coming years if drastic measures of varying nature and intent are not implemented in a timely fashion. Demand for service providers will escalate markedly in all countries—rich and poor—as a result of changing profiles of disease and demands for care and support. Richer countries face a future of low fertility and large populations of elderly people that will increasingly shift towards chronic and degenerative diseases with accompanying high demands for high-tech and costly care. For the foreseeable future, growth in income, wealth and medical insurance coverage, technological advances, and more sophisticated health needs and care demands will require a more specialized workforce. At the same time, needs for basic care will increase because of families' declining capacity or willingness to care for their elderly and ill members. Without massively increasing the recruitment and training of health workers for the needs in wealthy countries, these growing gaps will exert even greater pressure on the outflow of health workers from poorer regions.

In poorer countries, large cohorts of young people will join increasingly aging populations, with both groups rapidly urbanizing, often amid growing poverty, constrained development and declining quality of health in deprived urban settings. Many of these countries are still struggling with unfinished agendas of infectious disease, the rise of new epidemics and the resurgence of old ones, and the rapid emergence of chronic illness complicated by the magnitude of the epidemic. The availability of effective vaccines and drugs to cope with these health threats imposes huge practical and moral imperatives to respond effectively. The chasm is widening between what can be done and what is happening on the ground. Success in bridging this gap will be determined in large measure by how well the health workforce is developed to secure effective health systems to render quality care.

In light of these changing trends and conditions in health and healthcare, redefining of care delivery, the composition of the workforce and the role of health personnel providing the care, as well as the training of health workers, has become imperative for appropriate responses to the challenges confronting nations. Such redefinition is even more pressing in the face of the extraordinary needs and demands generated by HIV, AIDS and ART. It therefore seems inevitable to purposefully explore alternative models and modes of care, as well as additional cadres of health carers, with a view to supplementing the current health systems and workforces in many countries. This should be accompanied by consistent attempts to reform, redirect and improve upon the current training of health workers to more closely align with, and adapt to, the prevailing and changing healthcare needs and demands of the day according to the country in question.

HIV/AIDS and the HRH crisis

HIV/AIDS, with its onslaught on national, regional and global health, poses unprecedented problems to the organization of healthcare. These problems manifest themselves most acutely in poor regions where the epidemic is most ravaging, especially in sub-Saharan Africa, and especially in the south-east African region [7]. The epidemic imposes particularly serious demands and problems on the human resources devoted to the attack on it at those very same levels affecting the national-, regional- and global-level organization of healthcare and its resources, including human resources. The epidemic's effects on HRH are diverse, pervasive and devastating. The complex disease conditions of HIV and AIDS, and the skills required to manage these, are often superimposed on already overstretched and dilapidated public health systems and facilities. This increases occupational stress and insecurity for the health workforce as the disease imposes huge work burdens, risks and threats on them. Dwindling morale, demotivation, compassion fatigue and burnout, declining productivity, increasing illness and absenteeism, and eventual attrition of staff through resignation, migration or death are increasingly recognized amid the loss of institutional memory.

The recent scale-up of ART in these countries has induced a further escalation of the pressure on existing health workforces. This scale-up was spurred by, among other things, the WHO/UNAIDS (Joint United Nations Programme on HIV/AIDS) '3 by 5' strategy, through which the WHO attempted to marshal global resources to place 3 million PLWHA in the developing world on ART by 2005, and was fuelled by the mobilization of massive amounts of funding and the advocacy of international and national pressure groups. In turn, this increasing pressure jeopardizes the very scale-up meant to counter the effects of the epidemic. The WHO, for one, faced severe neglect of human resources investment and planning from years of reductions in public sector spending. Thus, it was not possible to quickly and adequately supplement the plan for scale-up of treatment with matching strategies to develop and train personnel to meet the human resource demands it required. In fact, responding to the vast treatment needs as the driving force behind the scale-up efforts, it appeared that structural deficiencies greatly reduced national governments' capacity to implement the plan vigorously from the start, and had negative consequences for its subsequent course. At the same time, some governments embarked on the scale-up without being equipped to properly consider their real human resource capacity in the absence of human resource planning departments and staff; strategies to provide for both the human resource demands for scale-up and the effects of scale-up on existing human resources could not be developed simultaneously. In retrospect, suffice it to say that the abundance of funds and pharmaceutical agents did not, and still do not, compensate for lagging skills and severe backlogs in health worker capacity, leading to negative effects of ART scale-up on the workforce. One must therefore recognize that these developments have not left current health systems intact in the countries most affected by the disease. The expanding needs for care are leading to new, alternative models of care modes and a search for new, alternative pools of human resources to care for the infected and the ill. The call for 'care for the carers' has also grown louder and more intense.

In the above respects, HIV/AIDS is no different from other diseases that have attacked humanity before. Yet it differs in that, due to the very nature of the epidemic, addressing it requires changes in the conventional organization of prevention, treatment and care, as well as changes in the conventional composition of the health professions and workforce in those countries most affected. Health services in the orthodox mould alone cannot cope with the multidimensional demands and effects of this disease. A profound shift in attitudes to healthcare, the healthcare workforce and its training, planning and managing services, human resources and community participation must go hand in hand. Furthermore, as the disease decimates the workforce itself, it is necessary in both the public and private sectors to develop and implement strategies for rapid access to care and support for the staff affected by the disease, in order to reduce senseless losses from the corps of those who are needed to care for others.

The examples of smallpox, polio and, more recently, severe acute respiratory syndrome (SARS) and avian flu have demonstrated how a collective international response mobilizing the necessary financial and human resources can help to eradicate a life-threatening disease completely or contain an outbreak of global dimensions. Yet, other diseases such as tuberculosis (TB), multi-drug resistant tuberculosis (MDR-TB), malaria and HIV/AIDS have not been met with such a radical, collective response. In the case of HIV/AIDS, this may be because it develops over years and only emerges in its visibly life-threatening manifestations very late in its development. In terms of organizing a response at the global level with adequate human resources devoted to it, the world was slow to react; an initial WHO programme only took shape in the mid-1980s. But the dawning realization that this disease had numerous societal impacts and consequences that needed to be addressed on a broader scale led to the creation of an international human resource base in the joint UNAIDS programme to address national anti-AIDS development needs in a multidisciplinary manner.

Yet, despite early warnings in the 1980s about potential health and socio-economic consequences affecting entire nations, it took 20 years before a special session of the United Nations was devoted to HIV/AIDS in the year 2000. The MDGs including HIV/AIDS were developed, and a larger-scale funding mechanism, the Global Fund to Fight AIDS, Tuberculosis and Malaria (Global Fund), was set up to direct resources to the fight against all three diseases. However, the issue of human resources necessary to enhance access to HIV/AIDS prevention, treatment and care has emerged disconcertingly slowly. Investments in this essential component of HIV services delivery have been dwarfed by those devoted to the development of an adequate pharmaceutical, supplies and equipment response. In effect, one notices an almost inverse relationship between the global-level commitment to HIV as one of the specific priority diseases to be addressed by the MDGs, and the global development community's commitment to the production of the necessary human resources over the past 20 years of the epidemic. While the global disease burden has increased along with the earth's expanding population of more than 6 billion, only a tiny fraction (1%) of the global workforce is devoted to maintaining the health of all humans on the planet [1]. This is a somewhat disturbing figure given the relevance of the sector. It is therefore no surprise that the World Health Report of 2006 identified the need for an additional 4 million health workers—an almost unreachable goal given the previous global community response—to address the most burning health issues, including adequate attention to HIV/AIDS. The crisis in health services and human resource provisioning to deal with this specific disease has reached such levels that, in the meantime, all kinds of emergency adjustments and additions to the workforce, innovative skills transfer and other solutions are consistently sought.

The belated response, however, has prompted a strong call to action from many partners and governments. To cite one example, the Institute of Medicine (IOM) in the United States, under the aegis of its Committee on the Options for Overseas Placement of US Health Professionals, has proposed the creation of a global US Health Service to assist the US President's Emergency Program for AIDS Relief (PEPFAR) in offering a solution to the human resource crisis in many of the AIDS-afflicted countries targeted by the initiative [8]. In 2005, the Global Fund devoted its fifth round of calls for proposals to the strengthening of health systems and human resources, and has encouraged partners to include these elements in subsequent applications. In addition, the WHO announced a programme to focus on treatment, training, and retention of the health workforce for HIV/AIDS—known as 'Treat, Train, Retain'—with support from, among others, the recently created Global Health Workforce Alliance, established with funding from the Bill & Melinda Gates Foundation [9]. Therefore, momentum to address human resources and health system constraints in comprehensively implementing programmes for HIV/AIDS care has recently been mounting.

At the regional and national levels, responses were often lukewarm and delays even longer, for a variety of reasons. Moreover, responses to the epidemic in resource-poor countries were consistently crippled by financial deficits and shortages of human resources and managerial capacity. Today, Thailand, Uganda and a few other countries remain among the few shining examples of nations that confronted their epidemics head-on, both quickly and decisively. Strong political commitment allowed them to embark on concerted national action through comprehensive HIV/AIDS programmes steered by competent stewardship.

To complete the circle, the attitudes and behaviours of individuals and communities within their own sociocultural contexts have also contributed to slow—or outright lack of—action regarding the emerging epidemic. Denial, casting blame, and stigmatization have become part of the response (or non-response) to HIV/AIDS and ART, with crippling consequences for prevention, care delivery, and access and adherence to treatment.

HAART parameters defining human resource needs

Human resource needs depend on a multitude of factors. For HIV/AIDS interventions, they range from skills in consultation on preventive measures that need to be culture- and gender-sensitive and age-specific, to having the right neurological training to deal with psychiatric manifestations of AIDS. Thus, a considerable amount of specific clinical and psychological counselling skills, social support and knowledge of community organization may at any one time be needed to provide the required intervention. This will often need to go beyond the disease-stricken individual and address disrupted social institutions, relationships and functions as these are manifesting themselves in broken families, orphaned children and child-headed households.

At the same time, intervention technology may change. For example, when pharmaceutical treatment regimens were first offered, more than two dozen types of medication needed to be taken daily. Counselling and establishment of a treatment regimen, adherence information and many other nutrition- and regimen-related educational activities needed to be undertaken in line with these prescriptions. When pharmaceutical progress reduced intake to fewer pills per day, the corresponding counselling time, which translated into human resources needs, was reduced. With pressure to increase access to ART, potential time gains in individual attention were quickly offset by attending to an ever-increasing number of patients.

In the domain of laboratory testing, the same interplay between technology and human resource needs can be observed; when time-consuming HIV antibody tests started to emerge, the processing time needed more human attention and thus more full-time equivalent (FTE) staff time. With the arrival of quicker testing technology, human time and the type of health worker or volunteer undertaking the test changed both laboratory worker requirements and the distribution of tasks among team members. Again, now that ART has become more widely available, diagnostics for preparation of second-line pharmaceuticals may take up more time on the part of laboratory technicians, and there is likely to be an increased monitoring task to detect resistance in the treatment population. This will translate into additional laboratory technician time requirements, with back-up from researchers and national epidemiologists who need to be involved in strategy development.

Within this context, proxy calculation of staffing needs to reach the MDGs for HIV/AIDS can be performed. For example, once the prevailing HRH composition and the accompanying supplies, equipment and logistics chains have been properly analyzed, and the distribution of HIV prevention, treatment and care tasks among team members from the public and private sectors as well as from community-based organizations (CBOs) and faith-based organizations (FBOs) has been established, additional staffing needs can be assessed. This analysis very much depends on local circumstances in order to reach tangible levels of accuracy. For instance, if the provision of doctor-delivered services in the treatment cycle for ART throughout a given year requires an average of 30 minutes of patient contact, this translates into being able to see 16 patients per eight-hour day. Assuming a working year of 200 days (after deduction of leave, weekends, continuing education attendance, average illness absence, etc.), one staff member trained to the level of medical doctor could attend to between 250 and 300 patients per year if patients need to revisit once a month. This means that covering, say, 10,000 patients will take approximately 40 doctors.

A recent calculation estimates that ART caseload will remain at very high levels for years to come. Based on these estimates, 14 million patients will need to have access to highly active antiretroviral therapy (HAART) by 2015, and 18 million by 2025. This translates roughly into 57,000 and 73,000 (respectively) full-time, medically trained staff who would need to be available to meet those needs [10]. Given that these numbers will not be attained at current production capacity, and considering the uncertainty regarding political will to increase output, skills transfer and a change in organization of the HAART cycle need to be implemented based on analysis of the prevailing model of care in a particular country. An example of the amount of time that can be gained from an analysis of tasks and possible redistribution can be gleaned from initial results of a study of the impact of HIV/AIDS on the health workforce in Zambia (see Figure 28.1).

Establishing these simple relationships between a few variables can quickly provide guidance on the magnitude of scale-up needs in particular country contexts. It also allows quick assessment of systemic options on how to proceed to fill the gap. For example, if private practice is available and, say, private medical practitioners could be enticed and trained to be involved in HIV/AIDS care, public-private agreements could be established to purchase private practitioners' time. If, for instance, private practice could take care of 20% of treatment and follow-up needs,

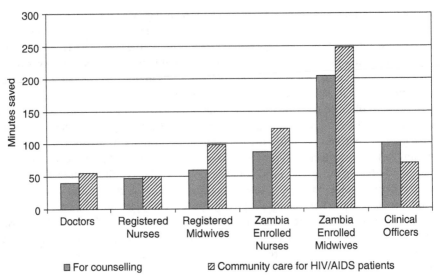

Fig. 28.1 Staff perceptions of time savings from increased community involvement in HIV/AIDS prevention, treatment and care, Zambia, 2005.

Source: [11].

this immediately translates into thousands fewer medical doctors needed. If company-based doctors and medical practitioners based at other state institutions, such as the military, could be enlisted to provide services at public clinics during off-hours, this would again reduce the demand. Most systems, while stretched for HRH in general, could still identify some efficiencies by enlisting human resources that are currently not fully utilized in innovative ways using an all-round analysis of total human resources availability throughout the health system.

Human resources for ART in less- and poorly-resourced contexts

The provision of ART, the models and modes of HIV/AIDS care, and the norms for staffing ART programmes in HRH-constrained regions, countries and areas cannot be similar, or applied to the same degree, as in better-resourced regions. This is partly the result of constrained budgets, but even more of absolute deficits in HRH and management capacity. The majority of developing countries, especially those hardest hit by the epidemic, cannot afford the luxury of expensive doctor-driven ART models; these are unfeasible in most countries and unsustainable in many others. As a result, other, less expensive models of ART, and those depending on more readily available professional and mid-level (auxiliary) workers, have to be explored because these offer the only options.

The roll-out of ART in South Africa provides useful lessons in this regard. It paints an HRH picture quite different from the situations prevailing, and the strategies opted for, in wealthy and well-resourced countries. In 2003, South Africa embarked on its ambitious ART programme, the biggest of its kind on the globe [12]. With more than 5 million South Africans living with HIV/AIDS, this public sector programme was designed to provide access to ART for more than a million people (a huge backlog built up over several years of denial and wavering response) during its first five years (i.e. by 2008). Of course, human resources would be key to the success of this endeavour. Staffing requirements were set as follows: the FTE professional staff required per 500 patients on ART would comprise one medical officer; two nurses; one pharmacist;

one dietician/nutritionist; and 0.5 social workers. Non-clinical FTE staff would include five lay counsellors or community health workers (CHWs) and two administrative clerks/data capturers.

Towards the end of the first two years (2003/4–2005/6), roughly 116,000 patients were on treatment in the public ART programme, meaning that a mere 30% of its original target of 381,177 patients were receiving ART. This initially slow roll-out, characterized by the missing of target dates and target numbers, had much to do with deficiencies in management capacity, but perhaps even more with the general unavailability of human resources, especially health professionals in certain essential categories (medical officers and pharmacists), in small towns and rural areas. Similarly, the absence of necessary capacity and mechanisms to train relatively large numbers of healthcare workers over a short period of time slowed down desired progress. Another result of the general scarcity of professionals in key categories to service the programme is that the focus has increasingly shifted towards the omnipresent professional nurse to assume more responsibilities in ART than the scope of his or her profession and practice would usually allow. This means that a primary healthcare (PHC)-oriented, nurse-driven and nurse-initiated ART model has emerged in public health service in HRH-deprived settings. It also means that professional nurses and nurse practitioners increasingly substitute for doctors and pharmacists, receiving additional training to take over the tasks and responsibilities traditionally rendered by these professionals. (This is indirect substitution; see substitution types listed later in this chapter.)

One has to bear in mind that among the countries in sub-Saharan Africa, South Africa is well equipped with HRH. The country's general ratio of 6.7 medical practitioners per 10,000 population (2004) far exceeds the average one per 10,000 in sub-Saharan Africa and compares favourably with those of its neighbours: Botswana's 2.65, Zimbabwe's 1.31, Lesotho's 0.56, Mozambique's 0.24, and Malawi's 0.18 per 10,000. However, South Africa's public sector doctors constitute a mere 2.9 per 10,000 compared with the 25.5 per 10,000 in its private sector, the latter approaching the average 28 per 10,000 of high-income countries [13,14]. Public sector ratios for health professionals are, however, worryingly carved away by high vacancy and turnover rates. Recently, the vacancy rate for all health professional posts in South Africa's public sector was 31% (52,597 unfilled posts). For medical practitioner posts, the vacancy rate was 27% (4222 unfilled posts) and for professional nursing posts, 25% (32,734 unfilled posts) [14–16]. The turnover rate of core medical staff was 27.8%, and for middle managers, 13.2% [17]. In recent years, the provisioning ratios of both doctors and professional nurses in South Africa's public sector have significantly deteriorated [18].

The pervasive shortfalls of health professionals in African countries bring the proper and appropriate staffing of ART programmes into serious question. The situation requires redefining the models of ART and HIV/AIDS care and, in particular, reconsideration of the nature and types of staffing for such care, as well as the appropriate models and methods of training for these health workers. It is from this position of absolute shortages of health professionals that the development of HIV/AIDS care delivery and ART in HR-constrained regions, countries and areas has taken a different course and forced profound mind-shifts by exploring unconventional strategies and introducing human resources for healthcare from outside the conventional health professional spheres/cadres. This is particularly the case in those areas most heavily stricken by HIV/AIDS.

Finding the right approach to increase access to human resources

The challenges of keeping and supplementing the conventional professional workforce at appropriate levels to service population health needs have been addressed in several overviews and discussion papers over the past few years [1,19,20]. The discussion has to be seen in the context of an ongoing, wider health systems debate, however, including the issue of how to organize a health system and its workforce most effectively to meet population health needs. The debate received a great deal of attention during the early years of the struggle to implement PHC programmes after the Alma Ata Declaration [21]. The search for optimum equilibrium between disease-driven and vertical organization of healthcare and its human resources, as opposed to a more integrated service delivery and multi-skill human resources concept, is as prominent today as it was then. This is particularly true as funds have been made available for specific disease target reductions/control in recent years, and in particular for HIV/AIDS. Suggestions that concentration and full investment of resources into HIV/AIDS will lead to a substantial strengthening of health systems have been proposed with a view to influencing government development policy for health in this way. But it is not immediately clear at which point a more horizontal approach to health systems strengthening will be needed to ascertain the service delivery system gains from focusing initially on specific disease programme support.

The debate over vertical versus horizontal health programme issues at stake has recently been summed up succinctly by Mills *et al*, [20]:

> A disease-specific focus leads to solutions for the specific program, whereas a health systems focus identifies a somewhat different set of reform priorities that relate to system-level changes and affect disease management across multiple diseases and conditions. The disease-focused responses can generally be implemented relatively quickly, whereas the systems-focused actions take longer. However, numerous, separate disease-specific responses can rapidly overwhelm frontline workers and managers.

> From early in the history of mass campaigns, the terminology used was of vertical and horizontal approaches ..., referring essentially to two key dimensions in program organization ...: the extent to which program management was integrated into general health systems management, especially at lower management levels, as opposed to kept strictly separate, and the extent to which health workers had one function as opposed to many functions.

> This debate is being given a new urgency by the introduction of treatment for HIV/AIDS. Immunization can be delivered using either a vertical or a horizontal approach. HIV/AIDS treatment, which requires continuing care, calls for strong health service backup. Nonetheless, such treatment services could be organized so that they isolate themselves from the broader health system—say, through separate clinics with their own workers and separate laboratories—or they could contribute to a greater degree of integration by sharing resources [20].

There are many examples of service organization between public and private providers in terms of sharing of premises, equipment and staff, but also of stubbornly maintaining the boundaries between the two sectors. The body of knowledge on what works well and what works less effectively and efficiently continues to grow. But the most important notion is that countries must each try to identify the most politically and culturally appropriate solution. For instance, Mills *et al.* [20] cite examples of government outsourcing of primary and HIV care functions to non-governmental organizations (NGOs), with the stewardship role essentially maintained by government, where a cooperative spirit has been fostered to facilitate this sharing of tasks and human resources. The success being achieved by the joint public-private venture in ART scale-up in Uganda is another model of good practice or rapid response that holds useful lessons—particularly with respect to developing and deploying human resources for ART—for strengthening and expanding the reach of the public health system in underserved rural areas in collaborative fashion [22].

There have been proposals to create efficiencies to reach the MDGs and their HIV/AIDS component by moving towards a more integrated workforce [23], but the complexities and organizational changes in a multi-stakeholder environment are daunting. An incremental approach to widening the spectrum of human resource skills utilization as coverage and experience with programme implementation increase is likely to be an easier and more pragmatic way forward.

The need and nature of paradigm shifts in redefining HIV/AIDS care and human resources

In the battle against HIV/AIDS, Marchal *et al.* [7] plead for true paradigm shifts in the areas of human resource management and policy making, education and international aid in order to deal effectively with the growing health workforce crisis. However, real paradigm shifts on human resources issues need to go beyond conventional strategies. For example:

- producing and training greater numbers of health professionals in the conventional mode, or redirecting the training;
- diverting or stopping the flow of health professionals to other countries, the private and NGO sectors, and better-resourced areas;
- introducing/producing new cadres of human resources to supplement and support health professionals;
- using the existing human resources pool more sparingly and enhancing performance by innovative management and incentives;
- introducing control measures to curb waste;
- establishing mutually beneficial public-private partnerships;
- realigning or revising the prevailing scopes of the professions and of practices.

As noted elsewhere, conventional health services alone cannot deal with the multidimensional demands and effects of HIV disease. The epidemic's impact is not limited to disease and death only; superimposed on it is also a 'social' epidemic. HIV/AIDS is also explicitly about the destruction and disruption of the very fibre of societies—of social institutions, relationships and essential social functions. Therefore, appropriate 'care' should reach beyond the best-known parameters of conventional and professional care. As well as forging a competent workforce to counter the epidemic and its disease complications, the strong dependency on the official and professional health workforce should also make way for additional forms and cadres of care not necessarily linked to a narrow 'disease-oriented' concept of health and conventional health professionals.

New cadres of human resources

Much headway has already been made in redefining the role of conventional health professionals and expanding the capacity of the conventional workforce in public settings lacking in health professionals. This is done by introducing new cadres of substitute and mid-level health workers, redefining the scopes and practices of the established health professions, and delegating tasks to lower-level health workers. More recently, under the pressure of healthcare needs generated by the epidemic and in the search for models of care that best fit the demands of the disease, this redefining of care delivery has been further boosted. It is no surprise that developing countries stand at the forefront of such a redefinition, because theirs is also a search for more affordable models of care commensurate with their scarce resources.

Dovlo's [24] concepts of 'substitution' or 'skill delegation to mid-level health workers' highlight the redefinition of the role of conventional health professionals that has already taken place in several African countries in an effort to come to terms with their drastic and growing HRH shortages and skills deficits. Such substitute health workers (SHWs) take on 'jobs, functions and roles that are normally the tasks of internationally recognized health professionals' [24]. Four types of substitution are identified:

- indirect substitution, or delegation of tasks to an existing but different profession (e.g. from doctors to nurses or pharmacists);
- direct substitution, or delegation of tasks from professionals to less-trained, mid-level health workers within the same professional sphere or scope of practice (e.g. using pharmacist, doctor, or nursing assistants in place of the scarcer pharmacists, doctors and professional nurses);
- delegation of non-technical tasks to lower-trained (even lay) cadres to relieve professionals of punishing workloads (e.g. using different kinds of CHWs, such as administrative clerks, lay counsellors, treatment/ directly observed therapy (DOT) supporters, or home-based carers, to support nurses); and
- intra-cadre skills delegation, or delegating tasks to less-trained cadres from the same profession (e.g. from medical specialist to general practitioner).

All these variations of substitution and task-shifting are increasingly being instituted in resource-poor developing countries in order to cope with shortages of expensive human resource and skills deficits. Needless to say, the demands of the epidemic and ART scale-up have stimulated and strengthened these developments in the HRH sphere of these countries. The scarcity of health professionals at the core of public sector ART programmes—doctors, professional nurses and pharmacists—renders direct substitution by mid-level workers increasingly inevitable as tasks and responsibilities such as physical examinations, simple diagnostics, initiating basic treatment, prescribing certain levels of medication, managing common conditions, and preparing and issuing of prescriptions are increasingly delegated to doctor, nursing and pharmacist assistants. Similarly, more and more CHWs in support of professional nurses are accepting responsibility for patient counselling, drug readiness training, home care for the chronically ill, adherence support, follow-up and tracing of defaulting patients. There is also a trend towards more comprehensive training and 'multi-skilling' of these CHWs.

The full spectrum and potential of substitute and mid-level health workers must be explored with a view to relieving the pressure on certain categories of health professionals by:

- fully employing the capabilities of lay and non-professional workers;
- searching beyond health departments for multidimensional solutions to the epidemic; and
- making optimal use of NGOs, CBOs, FBOs, etc. in order to muster a more comprehensive response to the epidemic.

Substitution with other professions and delegation of responsibilities and tasks to mid-level workers are complicated processes for the health professions concerned and are mostly met with resistance. These processes hold important consequences for both the scope of professions and scope of practice. The history and essence of the health professions show strong tendencies towards closing ranks, autonomy, collective self-monitoring, and thus considerable protectionism and dominance with respect to their domain [25]. This is certainly warranted for the purposes of upholding professional values and codes of conduct and in training new recruits, as well as ensuring high standards of healthcare practice, ample justification for maintaining professionalism and autonomy. However, we should realize that such protectionism also safeguards the non-professional interests of the profession and its members, especially where the professions are strong, and are not necessarily in synchronicity with population health needs and government priorities. In fact, clashes between competing interests and priorities are common, with negative consequences on all sides. Undermining the self-determination of the medical profession can severely degrade its prestige and, eventually, the quality of healthcare. In countries with weak professional statutory bodies and member associations, or where governments drive health reform agendas at any cost, there is a risk that the autonomy of the health professions and the standards of professional care and training will be compromised.

Against this backdrop, it cannot be assumed that the transformation of countries' current human resource distribution can be easily or quickly adapted to increase access to needed skills. The transfer of professional responsibilities and tasks, and changes in the scopes of professions and their practice, will not follow automatically. Purposeful and convincing programmes are necessary to facilitate such redirection. In addition, while the supposition remains that these new cadres of health workers will be supervised by the professions proper, the reality is that in many remote rural areas, impoverished urban settlements and poorly resourced health settings where supervisory capacity is meagre (either not readily available or even entirely absent), mid-level workers increasingly encroach upon the scope and practices of their mother professions and, in light of realities, have no option but to do so. A proper response to this reality must be found to ensure legitimacy and quality of care.

Exploring and using non-conventional human resource capacity

Note, however, that in most of the developments around human resources mentioned above, the trend is to expand, supplement and support the capacity of the conventional health professionals within the allopathic tradition. Redefining HIV/AIDS care delivery and the human resources needed to provide that care should go beyond that. Over and above conventional health professionals, HIV/AIDS-stricken and HRH-constrained countries require new, expanded and refocused cadres of HIV care and support workers in increased numbers to attend to the escalating social and socio-psychological needs that have sprung from the epidemic.

First among those outside the conventional circle is the proper but still elusive use of non-allopathic traditional health practitioners in AIDS care, not as a mere add-on to conventional HRH, but as a resource in its own right in the continuum of care. Their strength resides in their ability to mobilize communities towards implementing HIV/AIDS programmes, to raise HIV awareness, to draw clients into counselling and testing programmes, to promote adherence to treatment regimens, to monitor side effects, to share expertise in practitioner–patient communication skills, and to improve patient well-being and quality of life. Above all, the strength of traditional healers resides in their holistic approach, attending to the complete bio-psycho-social individual and taking care of and restoring relationships, families, communities and social functions damaged and disrupted by HIV and AIDS.

However, when moving outside the sphere of conventional healthcare, where such care represents the official health system, pleas for the incorporation and use of non-conventional or non-allopathic health practitioners will run even more against the grain of the conventional health professions and governments. Nevertheless, many nations and cultures use both traditional and alternative healing, and some practices are already well established, even professionalized, and are enjoying government recognition. Exploring these resources is neither new nor far-fetched. Since Alma Ata, the WHO has manifestly endorsed the importance of these sources of healthcare and has, specifically since the early 2000s, introduced mechanisms to promote traditional and alternative health resources. In many countries, much has been accomplished in terms of recognizing such health systems running in parallel with their official health systems. Progress in merging these healing traditions into one complementary national health system remains more modest and is limited to a few countries, with China and Zimbabwe often cited as examples of successful integration.

With respect to HIV/AIDS specifically, many African countries have made significant strides toward involving traditional health practitioners in AIDS-related programmes.

Lastly, another prerequisite is to promote and develop AIDS-competent communities, using the human resource reserves residing within communities to the fullest, and even introducing a community-centred approach to ART uptake rather than patient-by-patient ministration [26–28]. This would mean:

◆ promoting effective civil and community responses to HIV/AIDS;

◆ using local community dynamics and resources to shape the effectiveness of HIV/AIDS management efforts; and

◆ building health-enabling and health-supporting community environments and strategies for promoting these efforts, for accessing of health services and welfare grants, for organizing and supporting PLWHA and their carers, for countering denial, blame-casting and stigmatization, and for enhancing or repairing the damaged social fabric of communities.

In effect, it means community-led HIV/AIDS management.

Along with this goes the cultivation of HIV/AIDS-competent (or 'expert') patients, in other words, patients empowered and competent to pursue self-management and community involvement, in order to broaden the meaning of HIV/AIDS to include its social ramifications into modes of care, and to demedicalize parts of HIV care. Some of the care burden should be shed back onto households and communities in a self-care mode, while volunteering as a common good should be revived [1]. This implies a redefined relationship or 'contract' between providers and patients [5].

However, halfway through the time frame for achieving the MDGs, it is becoming increasingly clear that, as welcome as civil society contributions are, they need to be part and parcel of a multifaceted approach to service delivery, particularly when it comes to human resources planning and management. It is by now an oft-observed fact that at a time of global human resources crisis, and its particularly bad manifestation in countries most affected by HIV/AIDS and in need of HAART, there is bound to be an increase in workload arising from AIDS care and staff losses due to sickness and deaths from the disease itself. These problems need to be addressed in a concerted effort, and workloads consequently redistributed amongst all contributors in a fair manner.

Training of health workers, skills transfer, and creation of new cadres for an integrated workforce

The education and training of health workers are often used as powerful levers in the reform of national health systems. This implies the expansion of the education sector and the redirection of training health professionals with a view to addressing historical imbalances in access to education (e.g. to deprived groups), in the distribution of the workforce (e.g. to remote rural areas), and in the composition of the workforce (e.g. males/females, specialist categories), thus ensuring acceptable levels of equity in both the supply of, and demand for, healthcare. To this end, recruitment strategies and curriculum review and adjustment are commonly used to shift, for example, the emphasis to primary healthcare or to rural health. To prepare new recruits for the health workforce and to keep those in the loop primed for the challenges of changing healthcare environments, problem-based learning, community-based education and care, and continuing professional development have become common in the present-day health sphere.

One of the ways that countries have sought to expand access to primary healthcare and extend the corps of its providers is through skills transfer. This involves, first of all, a political will and acceptance by established professions and entrepreneurial interest groups to create new cadres or expand the remit of existing ones. Furthermore, organizational processes to generate consent from various stakeholders such as trade unions, professional and licensing authorities, public services commissions, and a number of other institutions, have to be assured. In addition, legislative procedures need to be in place to accompany a revised skills set, authority and responsibility distribution among the workforce. Personnel grading and assessment systems will ultimately have to be brought in line with new job profiles to reflect the revised spectrum of interventions and care of each staff category involved, as discussed by Buchan *et al.* [29]:

> Changing skill mix is not a panacea for all the ills of an organization. It has a role to play in improving organizational effectiveness and quality of care, but it must be recognized for what it is: a process for achieving change. An organization should not enter lightly in making changes in skill mix. It has to consider all four phases of the skill mix cycle:
>
> Evaluating the need for change;
>
> Identifying the opportunities and barriers for change;
>
> Planning for change;
>
> Making change happen [29].

Skills transfer is not a magic solution to human resource inadequacies and shortages in the workforce, whether for HIV/AIDS or any other services. It has been shown that when skills are transferred, the next-highest level is likely to experience an increased workload as a result of freed space, and thus savings in terms of HRH are unlikely to emerge. Caution is needed when engaging in skills transfer, and the organizational context within which it happens is of utmost importance [29].

These cautionary remarks should not mask the real possibilities for enhancing staff productivity and efficiency and increasing access to needed services. Evidence for successful skills transfer exists, much of it in the area of nursing [30]. There is ample proof that in human resource-poor countries and settings, the use of mid-level and substitute health workers is the only option to deal with human resource shortages and skills deficits. The arduous task for each health system and its human resources is, however, to analyze the existing distribution of tasks and skills and identify those that can be transferred without affecting norms and standards of quality of care. It is at this level that current institutional capacity deficiencies exist in many countries. Attempts to review and redefine parts of the workforce task distribution will also need to include a parameters analysis so that initial analysis, development of solutions, organization of all stakeholders, and support processes can be undertaken. As has been seen only too often, there is little point in having brilliant consultation and analyses come to no avail because no one at ministerial or health departmental level has either the capacity or the mandate to implement the recommendations or to provide monitoring and follow-up support to re-inform and adjust the implementation process.

Motivation, incentives and migration

An increasing body of knowledge has emerged on motivation and incentive needs of health workers [1]. Demotivating factors affecting the workforce have been identified as: insufficient salaries and incentives; inappropriate working conditions; lack of support and development opportunities; and the absence of supplies and equipment when needed. For HAART scale-up, one of the fundamental issues that need to be resolved in this respect lies in the question of how to convert increasingly available monetary volume into incentive schemes that are beneficial to all members of the workforce at facility sites. It is no secret that when incentives are introduced to one part of the workforce at a treatment site, those who do not benefit from them end up frustrated and demotivated because they happen to work on other aspects of the prevention, treatment and care spectrum of human illness. The 'poaching' phenomenon also needs to be addressed carefully when introducing incentive schemes so that benefits to some do not result in service dysfunction in other areas. A national consensus among partners and governments on how to introduce incentives throughout the system by all partners and across all programmes will help to address distortions and ensure equity and fairness in motivating the workforce.

Migration within countries between sectors, areas and health facilities, or emigration to other countries, deepens the crisis, and national planning and management of scarce human resources takes on new dimensions. Losses are observed at all levels; national planners and managers migrate to large-scale HIV/AIDS projects as managers, and clinical staff become part of specific treatment teams. The reasons for this are simple; projects recognize that salary levels are insufficient to provide a decent living standard and proper performance at work without having to resort to dual—or sometimes even triple—employment to feed one's family. Working conditions in projects tend to be better and lead to higher degrees of motivation as supplies and equipment are organized in a satisfactory manner. Partners do not operate under government fiscal constraints, and therefore they can more easily provide proper compensation.

However, there is a downside to this welcome injection of fresh capital for sustaining the workforce: those who do not benefit from access to better-equipped jobs view those migrating with envy, finding themselves left behind, demotivated and with higher workloads. In some instances, staff assigned to a facility may officially remain on the authorized list of positions at that facility but may have long ago moved on to work on a specific health priority programme. As a result, those left at the facility find themselves having to cope with an increased workload, while, at the same time, the post that has de facto been vacated cannot be filled because it is not officially vacant. At ministerial level, the situation is equally devastating when staff understandably leave for greener pastures in better-paying bilateral or NGO projects, including those for HIV/AIDS. Filling positions at lower government pay levels in a competitive labour market is not easy. It has been observed in some countries that, in effect, younger colleagues join the ministry ranks only for a few months to get trained and then turn towards better-paying jobs in the partner sector.

This situation will need to be addressed, and innovative government/partner situations will have to develop in order to provide the right stewardship, leadership and system management in countries to facilitate broad-based access to primary services, including HAART. Positions and capacity limits need to become part and parcel of a system design and management process that benefits population health development at large while attending to the most pressing HIV/AIDS prevention, treatment and care needs at the same time.

The overriding effects of inter-country migration of health professionals are that disparities and inequalities in health provisioning are created and aggravated between developed and developing countries; that the national health systems of developing countries are weakened to the point of collapse; and that the health of developing nations (as shown by health indicators) is destined to deteriorate. Similarly, intra-country migration of health professionals creates and aggravates health provisioning disparities and inequalities between sectors, areas, institutions and programmes. 'When a country has a fragile health system, the loss of its workforce can bring the whole system close to collapse and the consequences can be measured in lives lost' [1]. Of importance is that all forms of migration of health workers have similar distorting effects in common; they all generate inequities, imbalances, disparities and inequalities in HRH provisioning, which, in turn, create HRH shortages, scarcity of skills, and deficient skill mixes. These, in turn, all give rise to inequities in access, availability and coverage, compromising quality of care and, ultimately, affecting the outcomes of healthcare and people's health.

Conclusion

During the past two decades, HIV/AIDS has cast a dark cloud over the globe. In those countries most severely affected, the epidemic penetrates every corner of society and profoundly affects all dimensions of life and well-being. It is drawing deep contours around the nature of healthcare delivery and the HRH composition—at times creatively, but quite often causing depletion. In many ways, the prominence of the disease blurs our perspective and confuses our priorities through its dark prism, often with the unwanted and potentially dangerous effect of diverting attention and resources from other pressing concerns, and contributing to the neglect and crowding out of other essentials and priorities that are equally or even more important for health and survival [31].

As the countries hardest hit by the epidemic struggle to implement HIV/AIDS prevention, treatment and care programmes within the parameters of a generalized human resources crisis, the challenges to providing access to services and human resources in this area are formidable. In a way, every country is unique in its socio-economic, political and administrative environment within which solutions have to be found. Competition for human resources to service different MDGs is prevalent. Newly emerging diseases, and those needing rapid response such as SARS or avian flu, have to be attended to as well as the chronic care needs of ART. There is, unfortunately, no blueprint that can be applied across the board for countries with different ways of defining cadres, their education, knowledge and skills, their scope of authority to practice and the appropriateness of their educational sector for preparing the health workforce to serve population health needs. Countries also differ in their ways of financing healthcare and staff remuneration, of acting and interacting with the global donor and technical support community, and many other local factors. Health systems and services and human resources planners are thus confronted with the task of setting priorities and serving competing health targets with an appropriate organizational and human resources response, while at the same time sticking to tight budgets.

Should these efforts not succeed, Van Damme *et al.* [10] provide a sobering outlook on the sum total of human resources and HAART scale-up efforts:

> It is important to recognize the potential pitfalls related to the scaling up of ART, which could in itself further weaken the current prevention efforts. The focus, energy and resources, especially the already scarce human resources, could easily be absorbed by the formidable needs posed by the treatment programmes, resulting in an even greater reduction in the scale of prevention activities [10].

It is clear that all other health programmes will suffer equally if no integrated solution is found.

References

1. World Health Organization.(2006). *The world health report 2006. Working together for health.* Geneva: World Health Organization.
2. Smith MK, Henderson-Andrade N. (2006). Facing the health worker crisis in developing countries: a call for global solidarity. *Bull World Health Organ* **84**:426.
3. Garrett L. (2007). The challenge of global health. *Foreign Affairs* **86**:14–38.
4. McCoy D, Chopra M, Loewenson R, *et al.* (2005). Expanding access to antiretroviral therapy in sub-Saharan Africa: avoiding the pitfalls and dangers, capitalizing on the opportunities. *American Journal of Public Health* **95**:18–22.
5. Schneider H, Blaaw D, Gilson L, Chabikuli N, Goudge J. (2006). Health systems and access to antiretroviral drugs for HIV in Southern Africa: service delivery and human resource challenges. *Reproductive Health Matters* **14**:12–23.
6. Mascolini M. (2006). HAART, hubris, and humility. *IAPAC Monthly* **12**:424–435.

7. Marchal B, De Brouwere V, Kegels G. (2006). HIV/AIDS and the health workforce crisis: What are the next steps? *Tropical Medicine and International Health* **10**:300–304.

8. Committee on the Options for Overseas Placement of U.S Health Professionals, Fitzhugh M, Panosian C, Cuff P, eds. (2005). *Healers abroad: Americans responding to the human resource crisis in HIV/AIDS.* Washington D.C.: Institute of Medicine of the National Academies.

9. World Health Organization. (2006). *Press release. WHO launches new plan to confront HIV-related health worker shortages.* Geneva: WHO Press.

10. Van Damme W, Kober K, Laga M. (2006). The real challenges for scaling up ART in sub-Saharan Africa. *AIDS* **20**:653–656.

11. Ngulube TJ. (2006). *Perspectives from research and research synthesis of available data. Presentation at the Ministry of Health/WHO Meeting on HRH and HIV/AIDS.* Siavonga, Zambia: Ministry of Health of Zambia/WHO.

12. Department of Health of South Africa. (2003). *The Operational Plan for Comprehensive HIV and AIDS Care, Management and Treatment for South Africa.* Pretoria: South Africa: Department of Health.

13. Breier M, Wildschut A. (2006). *Doctors in a divided society: The profession and education of medical practitioners in South Africa.* Cape Town:HSRC Press.

14. South African Institute for Race Relations. (2006). *South Africa Survey 2004/2005.* Johannesburg: SAIRR.

15. Hall E, Erasmus J. (2003). Medical practitioners and nurses. In: A Kraak, Perold H, eds. *Human resources development review 2003: Education, employment and skills in South Africa.* Cape Town:HSRC Press. p522–553.

16. Padarath A, Chamberlain C, McCoy D, Ntul A, Rowson M, Loewenson R. (2003). *Health personnel in Southern Africa: Confronting maldistribution and brain drain. EQUINET Discussion Paper.* Harare, Zimbabwe: EQUINET.

17. Department of Health of South Africa. (2004). *Annual Report 2003/2004.* Pretoria, South Africa: Department of Health.

18. Day C, Gray A. (2005). Health and related indicators. In: Health Systems Trust, ed. *South African Health Review 2005.* Durban, South Africa: Health Systems Trust. p248–366.

19. Joint Learning Initiative. (2004). *Human Resources for Health. Overcoming the Crisis.* Boston: Global Equity Initiative, Harvard University.

20. Mills A, Rasheed F, Tollman S. (2006). Strengthening Health Systems. In: Jamison DT, Breman JG, Measham AR, *et al.*, eds. *Disease Control Priorities in the Developing World.* New York: Oxford University Press. p87–102.

21. World Health Organization. (1978). *Declaration of Alma Ata.* Geneva: World Health Organization.

22. Mugyengi PN, Kityo CM, Kibende S, *et al.* (2006). Scaling up antiretroviral therapy: experience of the Joint Clinical Research Centre (JCRC) access programme. *Acta Academica Supplementum* **1**:216–240.

23. Dreesch N, Dolea C, Dal Poz M, *et al.* (2005). An approach to estimating human resource requirements to achieve the Millennium Development Goals. *Health Policy and Planning* **20**:267–276.

24. Dovlo D. (2004). Using mid-level cadres as substitutes for internationally mobile health professionals in Africa. A desk review. *Human Resources for Health* **2**:1–12.

25. Fox RC. (1989). The professions of medicine and nursing. In: Fox RC, ed. *The sociology of medicine: a participant observer's view.* Englewood Cliffs, N.J: Prentice Hall. p38–71.

26. Mascolini M. (2006). HAART, hubris, and humility. *IAPAC Monthly* **12**:424–435.

27. Campbell C, Nair Y. (2006). Social capital and the fight against HIV/AIDS in Africa. Presentation at XVIth Congress of the International Sociological Association, 23–29 July 2006. Durban, South Africa.

28. Campbell C, Nair Y, Sibiya Z. (2005). Building 'AIDS competent' communities. *AIDS Bulletin* **14**:14–19.

29. Buchan J, O'May F. (2000). Determining skill mix: practical guidelines for managers and health professionals. *Human Resource for Health Development* **10**:111–118.

30. Buchan J, Dal Poz MR. (2002). Skill mix in the health care workforce: reviewing the evidence. *Bulletin of the World Health Organization* **80**:575–580.

31. Ssemakula JK. (2004). Through a glass darkly – the prism of AIDS. *Medilinkz* **7**. Available at http://medilinkz.org/Features/Articles/july2004/aidsdarkly.asp

Chapter 29

Closing the gap in the next decade of HAART: one world, one standard

Peter Piot, Julian Fleet* and Siddharth Dube

The global AIDS epidemic is no longer solely a public health problem. It has become one of the world's greatest social, economic and humanitarian crises. Since at least 2002, AIDS has been the world's leading cause of death among both men and women aged 15–59, causing one in every six deaths in this age group [1]. In highly affected countries, most of which have only begun to scale up HIV treatment services in the last few years, AIDS has caused life expectancies to plummet by 20 years [2]. With more that 25 million people dead, 40 million more currently infected with HIV, and 15 million children orphaned, AIDS has already caused the single greatest reversal in human development ever recorded [3] and presents a massive and sustained threat to the survival and well-being of individuals, and to the development, security, and even the viability of whole societies [4,5]. Without far stronger action to address it—not least in scaling up access to highly active antiretroviral treatment (HAART), the subject of this book—the impact of the pandemic upon human suffering and social upheaval in many countries will be even worse in the future.

One of the greatest advances in the recent history of the epidemic has been the development of HAART, and one of the greatest challenges has been providing sustainable access to the life-extending drugs that comprise HAART in some of the poorest and most underserved places in the world.

Overall, efforts to scale up access to HAART have proceeded relatively rapidly in recent years. As recently as June 2001, United Nations (UN) member states could not agree to include specific targets on antiretroviral therapy (ART) in the Declaration of Commitment adopted at the UN General Assembly Special Session on HIV/AIDS [6]. Yet, a growing recognition that AIDS is an exceptional crisis has increasingly led governments, industry and other powerful institutions to heed the calls of people living with HIV, civil society, the Joint United Nations Programme on HIV/AIDS (UNAIDS) and others for exceptional action to address the global epidemic. The Political Declaration on HIV and AIDS adopted at the 2006 UN High Level Meeting on HIV/AIDS committed governments around the world to revise national AIDS plans and targets in order to significantly scale up their response to AIDS and move to achieve universal access to HIV prevention, treatment, care and support by 2010. By the end of 2006, 90 countries had established targets to do so.

Earlier this decade, pharmaceutical companies began to decrease the prices of antiretroviral drugs in low-income countries, and generic versions of key AIDS drugs became increasingly available. At the same time, international donors and developing country governments alike

* Corresponding author.

mobilized substantial financial resources to expand access to HAART. In 2001, the member states of the World Trade Organization (WTO) agreed to significant clarifications and modifications in global trade rules that can be used to promote access to HIV-related medicines and other essential drugs [7,8].

This progress has helped change the way we look at drug access in developing countries, but it has not in itself been sufficient to address the ever-increasing need for therapies to tackle epidemics such as AIDS. In this concluding chapter, we argue that global efforts to ensure delivery of HIV treatment must progress much further if the AIDS epidemic and its impact are to be controlled [9].

Today, there is a looming gap between the need for treatment and its availability. The World Health Organization (WHO) estimates that only one in four people in need of ART was receiving it in June of 2006. Within this treatment shortfall lie several significant gaps that must be overcome. Chief among these is a financial gap. Despite the unprecedented mobilization of funding for the AIDS response in recent years, financing still falls far behind what is needed. A series of regional consultations and broad public debates in more than 100 low- and middle-income countries held in early 2006 revealed that lack of funds is one of the major obstacles to scaling up access to HIV prevention, treatment, care and support.

While ART prices have decreased significantly, many developing countries are still unable to afford the drugs, particularly the more expensive second- and third-line drugs to which clinicians and patients turn when initial regimens must be changed due to viral resistance or toxicity. Financing to implement exiting AIDS plans is also inadequate, and funding is often unpredictable and of insufficient duration.

At the same time, financial resource needs for AIDS are increasing. UNAIDS estimates that by 2010, the global AIDS response will require US$20–23 billion per year. In 2007, a record-breaking year from a funding perspective, US$9 billion was available, just half of what was needed. As more people become infected and treatment needs escalate, the need to remove obstacles related to pricing, tariffs and trade, regulatory policy, and research and development to speed access to affordable, quality HIV prevention commodities, medicines and diagnostics become ever more apparent.

Added to the funding gap is a growing prevention gap. Nearly 5 million people were newly infected with HIV in 2006. Vast numbers of people have little or no access to the information and commodities they need in order to protect themselves from the virus. Increasing infections continue to expand the ranks of those who will need HAART in future.

Finally, there is a technology gap, as shown by science's inability to date to develop an effective HIV vaccine (therapeutic or preventative), by the continuing struggle to develop effective female microbicides, and by the challenges posed by HIV drug resistance.

In the section below, we present a vision of the outcomes we must attempt to achieve in the next decade of HAART. We argue that the massive efforts and investments needed to achieve these outcomes are justified by the present and future threat posed by AIDS, and that these outcomes are feasible, as demonstrated by the equally unprecedented advances made in the first decade of HAART. Finally, we recommend strategies to help ensure that these vital outcomes are realized in the decade ahead.

A vision for the next decade of HAART

Action is required on many fronts to narrow the gap between the declared goal of moving toward universal access to HIV treatment and the realities that restrict access for poor people in many parts of the world. Priorities include: addressing barriers such as stigma and discrimination;

widening access to HIV testing and counselling; developing new medicines and diagnostic technologies; making new and existing medicines and technologies affordable; addressing the severe shortage of doctors, nurses, lab technicians, counsellors and other human resources; strengthening health and social system infrastructure, including pharmaceutical supply systems; and harmonizing national drug regulatory approaches.

These multiple priority areas for progress over the next decade can be summarized in three main goals, or 'pillars for action':

♦ Every country in the world must work to establish and meet ambitious, measurable targets for moving as close as possible toward universal access to effective HIV prevention and treatment, as well as treatment for opportunistic infections and palliative care for those in need. As a result of universal access: new HIV infections would be dramatically reduced; people living with HIV would lead longer, healthier, more productive lives; and deaths from advanced HIV infection would be significantly reduced.

♦ Governments, working in collaboration with academic institutions and the pharmaceutical and biotechnology industries, should research and develop: simpler, less toxic, better-tolerated antiretroviral drugs and other HIV treatments for all age groups; affordable and appropriate diagnostic tools; and preventive and therapeutic vaccines. These technologies should be affordable and otherwise suitable for use in developing countries.

♦ Agreements and systems should be firmly in place to ensure adequate, predictable and sustained financing for HIV treatment and prevention services.

In 2006, 13 new preventive AIDS vaccine clinical trials began in eight countries around the world. Three first-generation candidate microbicides are also currently being tested in large-scale efficacy trials in Africa, and if any of these prove successful, a microbicide could be ready for initial distribution within five years.

Why the effort is warranted

Achieving these goals in the next decade will entail an enormous commitment of political will, financial resources and human effort. We believe these efforts are justified on many grounds.

First, the reality is that all of the 40 million people currently living with HIV, and the millions more contracting HIV every year, will ultimately need sustained access to effective ART. In the countries worst affected by AIDS, such as those in southern Africa, the survival of the current generation—and the well-being of future generations—hinges on the immediate and massive scaling up of access to ART and related care. The need for access to life-saving treatment is a global humanitarian imperative.

Second, it is now well recognized that HIV prevention, treatment, care and support must be linked from planning through to delivery [10]. Simulations suggest that scaling up HIV treatment in tandem with HIV prevention is very likely to be the most cost-effective strategy [11]. All UN member states affirmed this approach in the Political Declaration adopted at the 2006 High Level Meeting on AIDS [9].

Third, wide, equitable and sustained access to HAART is key to keeping the AIDS response energized for the long run. In the past decade, it is treatment activism and breakthroughs in access that have replaced fatigue and despair with optimism and renewed energy in the AIDS response. The world would not be focused on scaling up toward universal access today were it not for the drive to provide widespread access to HAART through the activism of people living with HIV, campaigns such as the WHO/UNAIDS '3 by 5' initiative, and major programme support (e.g. provided by the Global Fund to Fight AIDS, Tuberculosis and Malaria, the US President's

Emergency Plan for AIDS Relief (PEPFAR), and UNITAID), and related efforts described in other chapters of this book. Treatment advocacy is critical to driving and sustaining the overall AIDS response, including HIV prevention.

Fourth, widespread access to ART, as well as to HIV prevention, care and support, remains not only a major global health issue, but also a matter of human rights. In 2001, the UN Commission on Human Rights adopted a resolution stating that the right to the highest attainable standard of health includes access to ART. Two years later, the Commission passed a resolution on access to medicines acknowledging that 'prevention and comprehensive care and support, including treatment and access to medication for those infected by pandemics such as HIV/AIDS, are inseparable elements of an effective response' [12].

Finally, the present-day scale and impact of the AIDS epidemic provide compelling reasons and precedents for undertaking far-reaching action on HIV treatment. High-income countries have prepared to take exceptional action when faced with even *potential* public health threats. For instance, in 2005, several industrialized countries prepared to stockpile Tamiflu® and to pre-order vaccine for their entire populations in the event of a possible outbreak of avian flu [13,14]. In virtually all low- and middle-income countries, AIDS is much more than a threat; in many countries, it is a real and present public health emergency [15] that national authorities, supported by their international community partners, must address.

People living with HIV in all developing countries should be able to benefit as fully as possible from the potential offered by HIV treatment, as is generally the case in high-income countries. An exceptional effort is justified by concerns for individual and social well-being, humanitarian and human rights imperatives, the effectiveness and dynamism of the AIDS response, and as a matter of government responsibility and accountability.

Can this vision be achieved?

We believe that the goals for the next decade of HAART delineated above are realistic and achievable. Realizing them will require extraordinary commitments of resources and political will, but these goals are no less feasible than the successes achieved in the first decade of HAART.

Consider, for example, the fact that in the early 1980s, there was doubt about the prospects for ever developing medicines that would lead to major gains in longevity and health for people infected by HIV. Today, about two dozen antiretroviral drugs are available in high-income countries, adding an average of more than 20 years to life expectancy after HIV diagnosis in those countries [16,17].

Even after antiretroviral drugs became widely available in wealthy countries, there was still widespread scepticism that these drugs could be used effectively across entire populations in low-income countries. Today, treatment rates, compliance and other indicators in a country such as Botswana are approaching those of high-income countries. Between 2003 and 2006, the number of people on HIV treatment in low- and middle-income countries rose more than fourfold to over 1.6 million [18].

Finally, prices of more than US$10,000 per patient-year for an antiretroviral regimen were considered an insurmountable barrier to providing HAART on a mass scale in developing countries. Today, the annual per-patient price for the least expensive WHO-recommended generic combinations is approximately US$150, and developing country governments and international donors have significantly increased their financial commitments to achieve large-scale access to HIV treatment.

Progress in each of these areas gives us good reason to hope and expect that large-scale access to HAART can be achieved in the years ahead.

A roadmap for action for the next decade of HAART

How should we move forward to quickly and effectively achieve the goals set out above? We discuss six key areas for action below, and refer readers seeking a fuller discussion of many of these points to the UNAIDS report, *Towards Universal Access: UNAIDS assessment on scaling up HIV prevention, treatment, care and support* [19], which was based on more than 100 inclusive consultations in low- and middle-income countries to develop solutions to the main obstacles to scaling up towards universal access.

Massive, urgent and simultaneous scaling up of HIV treatment and HIV prevention

The first priority must be to vastly speed up roll-out of the currently available first- and second-line antiretroviral drugs. Overall, HAART roll-out in developing countries today is slow and inadequate. According to WHO estimates, of the 38.6 million people living with HIV globally in mid-2006, there were approximately 6.9 million in low- and middle-income countries who required antiretroviral treatment. Yet, barely a quarter of those in need were receiving ART by the end of June 2006 [18].

Mechanisms to scale up treatment access in the five-year medium-term horizon have been closely analyzed in earlier chapters in this book. We draw particular attention to the need for: urgent improvements in treatment for opportunistic infections, particularly tuberculosis (TB); major reductions in prices for middle-income countries and for all second- and third-line drugs; increased political commitment to supporting low- and middle-income countries to use the flexibilities already provided in the WTO's Agreement on Trade-Related Aspects of Intellectual Property Rights (TRIPS Agreement); and steps to ensure sustainable supplies for scaling up, including a major expansion of capacity by pharmaceutical manufacturers.

Priority in each of these must go to the countries worst affected by AIDS, particularly those in the hyper-endemic southern African region. These countries require an exceptional and immediate effort in terms of scaling up HIV treatment and providing adequate monetary, educational and other support to survivors and affected households. This effort will require financial injections above the regular government budgets, as is accepted practice after natural disasters or armed conflict.

The future of HIV treatment will be determined not only by the quantity of treatment services, but also by their quality. This is particularly true for services that support patient adherence to their treatment regimens. Health workers require ongoing training and support in this area in order to avert the consequences of poor treatment adherence, including the possibility of an epidemic of multi-drug resistant HIV.

On the societal level, treatment cannot succeed separately from prevention. Because the success or failure of HIV prevention efforts will be a critical determinant of future treatment needs, universal access to effective HIV prevention must be a core element of the HAART agenda, meaning that HIV prevention and HIV treatment must be scaled up simultaneously and together. Greater access to ART reinforces prevention through increased HIV testing, which can contribute to a reduction in stigma and denial. Many countries that have made laudable progress in expanding treatment access continue to lag in their HIV prevention efforts, however, in large part because prevention requires dealing with 'taboo' subjects such as sex, homosexuality, sex work and illicit drugs. Far greater investment in HIV prevention programmes and commodities, informed by the internationally agreed-upon UNAIDS policy paper *Intensifying HIV prevention* [20], will be key to closing the gap on access to HAART.

Communication about HIV/AIDS plays a vital role in increasing knowledge about HIV prevention and treatment. Schools, media and community groups all have a part to play in supporting HIV/AIDS education, in particular by establishing and strengthening the link between HIV prevention and sexual and reproductive health.

Promoting knowledge of serostatus is vital to scaling up both HIV treatment and HIV prevention. With only a small fraction of the millions of people living with HIV aware that they are infected, far greater resources must be allocated to promoting and providing HIV counselling and testing. The Three C's—confidentiality, informed consent and counselling—must be at the core of HIV testing policies and services.

HIV prevention, like treatment, is underfunded at global and country levels. National governments need to increase domestic resources available for HIV prevention and recognize that investment in HIV prevention should be understood as a capital investment for the future.

Tackling social injustice, discrimination and AIDS-related stigma

Concerted efforts are also needed on a range of equity, social justice and human rights matters that will directly impact progress on both HAART availability and HIV prevention in the next decade.

We echo the calls of stakeholders and activists for far greater investment in efforts: to promote the human rights of people living with HIV and those most vulnerable to infection; to address the gender inequalities that fuel the epidemic; and to reduce HIV-related stigma and discrimination. Following through on this commitment will require greater support for combating homophobia, gender discrimination and the entrenched social norms that lead to the marginalization of sex workers, injection drug users, migrant populations and prisoners.

In particular, the epidemic is exacerbated in every regard by a widespread failure to tackle the social, cultural and economic factors that put women and girls at increased risk of HIV. The relatively low status of women and girls in many parts of the world and their frequent inequality in marriage and sexual relations limit their access to education and HIV information, and greatly reduce their capacity to protect themselves from infection. A far greater effort to address these core inequalities is essential to reducing HIV risk for millions of women and girls.

Fundamental principles of equity and human rights must guide ART roll-out, so that the most affected groups (e.g. sex workers) and underserved populations (e.g. the poor, women and children) have fair access to treatment. This requires not only the establishment of a fair process for setting priorities in the distribution of HIV treatment, but also consideration of special policies and outreach programmes to overcome barriers that marginalized or underserved communities face in obtaining services.

Extensive and meaningful involvement of people living with HIV and affected communities in HIV treatment programmes—and their empowerment, including through income support—is essential to overcoming the pervasive barrier of HIV related stigma.

Strengthening health and social sector human resources and delivery systems

Expanding the number of health and social sector workers and strengthening delivery systems are essential to scaling up HIV treatment in many low-income countries. Again, as more than two-thirds of the people needing treatment live in sub-Saharan Africa, this region should receive top priority in efforts to strengthen the health and social sectors.

The major steps needed to expand human resource capacity for delivering HIV services include:

- investments in training greater numbers of health and social services workers who can deliver HIV services;

- expansion of in-service training to empower and better equip service providers with the skills needed to care for patients living with HIV; and

- acceptance of 'task shifting' from more- to less-specialized health workers (e.g. from physicians to nurses, from nurses to community health workers and lay providers, including people living with HIV), including with regard to the delivery of HIV treatment services.

Concrete actions are also needed to retain the staff delivering HIV services. These include:

- instituting policy changes, codes of practice and ethical guidelines to minimize migration of health workers from lower-income to higher-income countries, and from public health systems to private sector HIV programmes;

- improving the workplace environment, including through ensuring infection control measures and commodities to prevent occupational transmission of HIV and other infectious diseases, as well as stress reduction and other occupational health safeguards;

- supporting staff and families living with HIV through access to HIV treatment, job security, protection against discrimination, social benefits and, where needed, adjustments in work demands; and

- financial and non-financial incentives for service in public health and social systems or in underserved areas, such as housing and education allowances, career development and training opportunities, and HIV treatment access for family members.

Countries with weak human resource capacity that are hard-hit by AIDS must consider emergency measures, such as those taken by Malawi to expand the capacity of its training institutions, top up wages for public health workers, and provide extra incentives for health workers in remote, rural areas [21]. Infusions of international staff who can deliver HIV services, while not an ideal long-term solution, may be the only way to urgently scale up HIV prevention and treatment services in some countries.

In the area of delivery system architecture, the development of clinical services for the delivery of HAART must also be used as an opportunity for the delivery of HIV prevention. Additionally, just as health settings provide increased opportunities for HIV counselling and testing, public health policy makers must recognize and fund non-health sectors and institutions, as well as communities, to deliver the HIV prevention services upon which the sustainability of treatment programmes ultimately depends.

Making pharmaceuticals and commodities affordable and available

Affordability of HAART remains critical to achieving treatment goals for the next decade. Despite the dramatic price decreases of the past decade, the high cost of medicines and diagnostic technologies continues to limit both the number of people who can be treated with available financial resources and the funds that can be allocated to other activities in the AIDS response, including HIV prevention. Many second-line and new generation antiretroviral drugs are priced far higher than first-line drugs. Even some first-line drugs are not available at the lowest possible prices in some low- and middle-income countries.

The pharmaceutical and diagnostic industry—that is, both innovator and generic companies—should offer existing and future essential HIV medicines and commodities at the lowest possible prices through rigorous differential pricing. While differential pricing means, by definition, that the prices of HIV medicines will remain higher in high-income markets, lower prices are needed for low-income countries, and fairer pricing, with structured and transparent price tiers, is needed for middle-income countries.

Innovator companies should expand their offers of voluntary licences for essential HIV medicines. Pharmaceutical companies—again, both innovator and generic—should ensure that their products are registered, quality-approved and differentially priced at the lowest possible levels in the countries concerned.

National authorities in low- and middle-income countries should employ the flexibilities now offered in the TRIPS Agreement as they deem appropriate. In tandem, high-income countries should take measures to ensure that their own trade authorities do not advocate bilaterally against such practices [22]. Also, because multiple sources of production and generic competition are crucial to sustaining affordability and the availability of adequate supplies, both government and the private sector should revisit their policies and practices to promote generic competition and the full engagement of both innovator and generic companies in meeting the increasing demand for antiretroviral drugs and other HIV medicines.

Even the most affordable drugs, however, cannot simply be dropped off at ports or in capital cities if they are to reach the people who need them. The importance of strengthening distribution systems for pharmaceuticals and other commodities has been raised earlier in this book. These improvements must be implemented on a priority basis in order to achieve significant, real and sustainable increases in access to HAART.

Finally, many antiretroviral drugs are not registered by the quality assurance authorities in the countries in which they are needed. We call for an overhaul of national drug regulatory systems to include harmonization of procedures and, wherever possible, national registration based on global references such as the WHO pre-qualification mechanism, or the linking of national registration to existing approvals by stringent drug regulatory authorities in high- or middle-income countries.

Securing adequate, predictable and sustained financing

Because there are millions of people already living with HIV, and because antiretroviral therapy is a lifelong treatment, more predictable, longer-term approaches to financing AIDS responses are required. UNAIDS estimates that by 2008, around US$22 billion will be needed annually to reach towards universal access to comprehensive HIV services, of which US$5.3 billion will be needed for HIV treatment.

These massive funding needs will require greater domestic and international spending, as well as efforts to ensure that countries have access to predictable and long-term financial resources to support national programmes. We recommend that major donors make 10-year commitments on financing the response to AIDS. At the same time, middle-income countries should substantially increase domestic budgetary financing of AIDS activities. A substantial proportion of low-income countries, especially those in which a relatively small proportion of the population is living with HIV, can afford to increase domestic financing for AIDS. Other low-income countries should also meet their commitments to increase spending on health and social services wherever possible [23]. We further recommend that governments seriously consider the potential for introducing universal health insurance that would cover HIV treatment, following the example of such diverse low- and middle-income nations as Kenya, Mexico, Rwanda and Thailand.

Financing HIV treatment involves more than raising resources, however. Financing is only meaningful when translated into affordable treatment for individuals. Many poor people cannot afford to purchase a condom, let alone antiretrovirals. Thus, we recommend that HIV treatment and prevention be provided free of charge at least to those who cannot pay, and to all in need whenever possible. We further recommend that donors and governments in the worst-affected countries undertake to meet related costs, such as for nutrition and transport to health services, as these factors often determine whether individuals can access and benefit from HIV treatment. Countries that have maximized treatment access or are moving to do so, including Botswana, Brazil, Ethiopia, Malawi, Senegal and South Africa, have all done so through universal access programmes that are free to consumers at the point of service delivery.

Accelerating innovation

The development of innovative new pharmaceutical products for HIV prevention and treatment remains crucial. While important scientific advances have been made in recent years in the development of new antiretroviral drugs, many of the newer products are not yet suitable for use in developing countries because of high prices [24] or complexity of administration [25,26].

While patents provide one type of incentive for innovation, particularly for the private sector, they also can be a barrier to affordable HIV medicines. For example, a key molecule of the most widely prescribed first-line antiretroviral regimen is protected by a related patent in over 20 sub-Saharan African countries, and offered by the innovator to least-developed countries at approximately four times the price of generic versions. As all WTO member states with major pharmaceutical production capacity now must comply with the minimum 20-year patent term and other obligations under the TRIPS Agreement, sources of supply for lower-cost generic medicines may be increasingly limited without steeper differential pricing by companies and greater recourse to the TRIPS Agreement's flexibilities.

Innovation must extend beyond the development of new medicines to include funding mechanisms for research and development of HIV pharmaceuticals and related technologies. A positive example of the latter type of innovation is the global network of 16 independent research organizations created by the Bill & Melinda Gates Foundation and known as the Global HIV Vaccine Enterprise.

Conclusion

More than 25 years into this epidemic, it is evident that AIDS can only be defeated through the kind of sustained, collaborative, global response that the world reserves for its greatest challenges. Because this epidemic spans generations, the true task facing us is not only to meet today's needs on an emergency footing, but also to take on extra responsibility for sustaining the response at increasingly high levels for another generation or more. A key part of this response must always be an exceptional effort for HAART, built on the principle of equity in HIV treatment and care for all of the world's peoples, to be central to a comprehensive response to AIDS.

Acknowledgements

The authors are grateful to Regina Castillo, Jantine Jacobi, Alasdair Reid, Susan Timberlake and Rania Al-Haddad for useful inputs.

References

1. World Health Organization. (2005). *Health and the Millennium Development Goals.* Geneva: World Health Organization. Available at http://www.who.int/mdg/publications/MDG_Report_revised.pdf

2. United Nations Population Division. (2004). *World Population Prospects: The 2004 Revision, database.* Available at http://esa.un.org/unpp/index.asp?panel=3

3. United Nations Development Programme. (2005). *Human Development Report 2005.* New York: United Nations Development Programme. Available at http://hdr.undp.org/reports/global/2005/pdf/ HDR05_complete.pdf

4. Batsy J. (2004). Mogae, Botswana's CEO and AIDS Crusader. *Agence France Presse,* Oct 31, 2004. Available at http://www.aegis.com/NEWS/AFP/2004/AF0410A7.html

5. McGregor L. (2002). Botswana Battles Against Extinction. *The Guardian,* July 8, 2002. Available at http://www.guardian.co.uk/international/story/0,3604,751071,00.html

6. United Nations General Assembly. (2001). *Declaration of Commitment on HIV/AIDS: "Global Crisis— Global Action".* New York: United Nations. Available at http://www.un.org/ga/aids/coverage/Final_ Declaration_HIVAIDS.html

7. World Trade Organization. (2001). *Declaration on TRIPS and Public Health. Doha, Qatar, November 2001.* Geneva: WTO. Available at http://www.wto.org/english/thewto_e/minist_e/min01_e/ mindecl_trips_e.htm

8. World Trade Organization. (2005). *Amendment of the TRIPS Agreement: Decision of 6 December 2005.* Geneva: WTO. Available at http://www.wto.org/english/tratop_e/trips_e/wt1641_e.htm

9. United Nations General Assembly. (2006). *High-level meeting on AIDS uniting the world against AIDS (Political Declaration, Para 20).* New York: United Nations. Available at http://data.unaids.org/pub/Report/2006/20060615_HLM_PoliticalDeclaration_ARES60262_en.pdf

10. UNAIDS. (2006). *Universal Access Assessment.* Geneva: UNAIDS. p3. Available at http://data.unaids.org/pub/InformationNote/2006/20060324_HLM_GA_A60737_en.pdf

11. Salomon JA, Hogan DR, Stover J, *et al.* (2005). Integrating HIV Prevention and Treatment: From Slogan to Impact. *PLos Medicine* **2**(1):e16.

12. Office of the High Commissioner for Human Rights. (2002). *Access to medication in the context of pandemics such as HIV/AIDS. Commission on Human Rights resolution 2002/32.* Available at http://ap.ohchr.org/documents/E/CHR/resolutions/E-CN 4-RES-2002–32

13. Watanabe C. (2006). Japan tamiflu stock below government goal. *Business Week,* November 30, 2006. Available at http://www.businessweek.com/ap/financialnews/

14. Left S. (2001). Row looming over anthrax drug patent. *Guardian Unlimited,* October 22, 2001. Available at http://www.guardian.co.uk/anthrax/story/0,1520,578769,00.html

15. Wook LJ, Piot P. (2003). Turning the Tide. *The Washington Post,* September 22, 2003.

16. Walensky RP, Paltiel AD, LosinaE, *et al.* (2006). The survival benefits of AIDS therapy in the United States. *J Infect Dis* **194**:11–19.

17. Schackman BR, Gebo KA, Walensky RP, *et al.* (2006). The Lifetime Cost of Current Human Immunodeficiency Virus Care in the United States. *Medical Care* **44**:990–997.

18. World Health Organization. (2006). *Progress in scaling up access to HIV treatment in low-and-middle income countries. Fact Sheet.* Geneva: WHO. Available at http://www.who.int/hiv/toronto2006/FS_Treatment_en.pdf

19. United Nations General Assembly. (2006). *Scaling up HIV prevention, treatment, care and support.* New York: United Nations. Available at http://data.unaids.org/pub/InformationNote/2006/20060324_HLM_GA_A60737_en.pdf

20. UNAIDS. (2005). *Intensifying HIV Prevention. UNAIDS policy position paper.* Geneva: UNAIDS. Available at http://data.unaids.org/publications/irc-pub06/jc1165-intensif_hiv-newstyle_en.pdf

21. IRIN (Integrated Regional Information Networks). (2006). Malawi: Health worker shortage a challenge to AIDS treatment. *IRIN News,* November 17, 2006. Available at http://www.irinnews.org/ Report.aspx?reportId=61598

22. Clinton WJ. (2000). *Executive Order 13155, Access to HIV/AIDS Pharmaceuticals and Medical Technologies, 10 May 2000*. Washington, DC: US Federal Register 65(93):30521–30523. Available at http://www.cptech.org/ip/health/africa/E013155.pdf

23. *The Abuja Declaration on HIV/AIDS, Tuberculosis and Other Related Infectious Diseases. Abuja, Nigeria, 26–27 April 2001*. Available at http://www.uneca.org/adf2000/Abuja%20Declaration.htm

24. Chequer P. (2005). Access to Treatment and Prevention: Brazil and Beyond. Rio de Janeiro, 2005. IAS Conference presentation, Rio de Janeiro, Brazil 2005.

25. Kumarasamy N. (2004). Generic antiretroviral drugs – will they be the answer to HIV in the developing world? *The Lancet* **364**:3–4.

26. World Health Organization. (2006). *Antiretroviral Therapy for HIV Infection in Adults and Adolescents in Resource-Limited Setting: Towards Universal Access. Recommendations for a public health approach. 2006 Revision*. Geneva: WHO. Available at http://www.who.int/hiv/pub/guidelines/WHO%20Adult%20ART%20Guidelines.pdf

Index